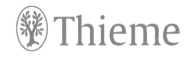

Speech-Language Pathology Casebook

Ryan C. Branski, PhD, CCC-SLP
Associate Professor
Department of Otolaryngology–Head and Neck Surgery and
  Communicative Sciences and Disorders
NYU School of Medicine
Associate Director, NYU Voice Center
New York, New York

Sonja M. Molfenter, PhD, CCC-SLP
Assistant Professor
Department of Communicative Sciences and Disorders
New York University
School of Culture, Education and Human Development
New York, New York

75 illustrations

Thieme
New York • Stuttgart • Delhi • Rio de Janeiro

Library of Congress Cataloging-in-Publication Data

Names: Branski, Ryan C., editor. | Molfenter, Sonja M., editor.
Title: Speech-language pathology casebook / [edited by]
  Ryan C. Branski, Sonja M. Molfenter.
Description: New York : Thieme, [2019] | Includes bibliographical
  references.
Identifiers: LCCN 2018059866| ISBN 9781626234871 (hardcover) |
  ISBN 9781626235342 (e-book)
Subjects: | MESH: Speech Therapy | Language Therapy | Case Reports
Classification: LCC RC423 | NLM WL 340.3 | DDC 616.85/506–dc23
  LC record available at https://lccn.loc.gov/2018059866

The views expressed in this book are those of the author and contributors, and do not reflect the official policy or position of the United States Government, the Department of Defense, Department of the Army or the Department of the Air Force.

Important note: Medicine is an ever-changing science undergoing continual development. Research and clinical experience are continually expanding our knowledge, in particular our knowledge of proper treatment and drug therapy. Insofar as this book mentions any dosage or application, readers may rest assured that the authors, editors, and publishers have made every effort to ensure that such references are in accordance with **the state of knowledge at the time of production of the book.**

Nevertheless, this does not involve, imply, or express any guarantee or responsibility on the part of the publishers in respect to any dosage instructions and forms of applications stated in the book. **Every user is requested to examine carefully** the manufacturers' leaflets accompanying each drug and to check, if necessary in consultation with a physician or specialist, whether the dosage schedules mentioned therein or the contraindications stated by the manufacturers differ from the statements made in the present book. Such examination is particularly important with drugs that are either rarely used or have been newly released on the market. Every dosage schedule or every form of application used is entirely at the user's own risk and responsibility. The authors and publishers request every user to report to the publishers any discrepancies or inaccuracies noticed. If errors in this work are found after publication, errata will be posted at www.thieme.com on the product description page.

Some of the product names, patents, and registered designs referred to in this book are in fact registered trademarks or proprietary names even though specific reference to this fact is not always made in the text. Therefore, the appearance of a name without designation as proprietary is not to be construed as a representation by the publisher that it is in the public domain.

© 2020 Thieme Medical Publishers, Inc.
Thieme Publishers New York
333 Seventh Avenue, New York, NY 10001 USA
+1 800 782 3488, customerservice@thieme.com

Thieme Publishers Stuttgart
Rüdigerstrasse 14, 70469 Stuttgart, Germany
+49 [0]711 8931 421, customerservice@thieme.de

Thieme Publishers Delhi
A-12, Second Floor, Sector-2, Noida-201301
Uttar Pradesh, India
+91 120 45 566 00, customerservice@thieme.in

Thieme Publishers Rio de Janeiro,
Thieme Publicações Ltda.
Edifício Rodolpho de Paoli, 25º andar
Av. Nilo Peçanha, 50 – Sala 2508
Rio de Janeiro 20020-906 Brasil
+55 21 3172 2297/ +55 21 3172-1896

Typesetting by DiTech Process Solution, India

Printed in The United States of America by   5 4 3 2 1
King Printing Co., Inc.

ISBN 978-1-62623-487-1
Also available as an e-book:
eISBN 978-1-62623-534-2

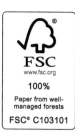

FSC
www.fsc.org
100%
Paper from well-
managed forests
FSC® C103101

I have been so blessed to have many mentors on my professional journey. I am particularly thankful for Dr. Thomas Murry who gave me my first job and has continued to be a critical advisor, colleague, and friend. I also owe a debt of gratitude to Sarah and TR for simply putting up with me. And finally, this book is for students. Enjoy the journey!

Ryan C. Branski, Ph.D., CCC-SLP

Speech-Language Pathology is a rewarding and exciting career that allows clinicians to work with individuals across the lifespan and in a variety of settings. I am grateful to have the opportunity to contribute to the future generation of clinicians through my teaching and my research and through this book. I would like to thank the faculty and staff of the Communicative Sciences and Disorders Department at New York University, and especially Dr. Christina Reuterskiöld, for her support and mentorship. Finally, I would like to recognize the contributors of cases that make up this casebook.

Sonja Molfenter, Ph.D., CCC-SLP

Contents

Foreword

A speaker at a recent convocation ceremony spoke eloquently about the importance of individual stories to get to know people, and for understanding the richness that diverse groups of people bring to our society. But he went further and argued that unless we hear and truly listen to these individual stories, we risk failing to appreciate that, regardless of the group these individual persons 'represent', they each have their own story and history and deserve to be treated as individuals, and not only as a member of the group. According to the speaker, paying attention to these individual stories will allow us to look beyond a label or stereotype and better understand the specific pathway that allowed this person to become who they are today.

The message in this convocation address made me think about the importance of individual stories for our understanding of individuals who experience communication disorders. Reflecting back on my own student days, I recollect how the content of a textbook or lecture really came alive when we were able to read or hear the personal story of someone who stuttered, had apraxia or aphasia, a hearing disorder, or experienced any other condition that affected communication or swallowing. All of a sudden, it became clear that most individuals showed some, but not necessarily all, characteristics of a condition, and that clinicians need to be very skilled at developing a treatment approach that is geared toward each individual client.

The two editors of this unique book are each immensely qualified researchers and clinicians. Dr. Branski is an Associate Professor at New York University and a speech-language pathologist with extensive clinical as well as research expertise who has published extensively especially in the area of voice disorders. Dr. Molfenter conducts research aimed at increasing the understanding of the physiology of both normal and disordered swallowing to inform and influence frontline clinical practice. In compiling the 80 case studies in this exceptional resource, the editors have gone beyond the disorder and brought individual stories to life. They did this by inviting expert clinicians to share case studies of clients they have worked with. Each story describes an individual client's history, how this story guided the clinician in their development of client-specific assessment and intervention approaches, and the outcome of this process. In doing so, the authors have not shied away from describing not only the successes, but also the challenges that they and their clients encountered. Readers are actively engaged through a series of questions and are provided with suggestions for further reading. Among the many case studies in this book, you will read the story of an adult who stuttered since he was 5 and how his willingness to give therapy yet another chance allowed him to become less stigmatized and more actively involved in self-help organizations. You will appreciate the complex story of a college student with Autism Spectrum Disorder who had difficulties with developing and maintaining friendships and how he was an active decision maker in treatment even if that involved a decision to terminate treatment. There is the story of a 90-year old man at the end of his life and his struggles with swallowing and quality of life. You will read about an 8-year old girl with dysphonia who was able to regain better voice quality through working creatively with her clinicians on improved voice skills. These and the many other case studies, or stories, will assist students as well as clinicians in recognizing the person behind the communication or swallowing disorder. Each case study, even in its brief format, will allow new as well as experienced clinicians to appreciate the importance of listening to each client's story, and how incorporating this story can help develop client-specific interventions and improve treatment outcomes. Indeed, reading these 80 stories will provide readers a rich glimpse of the fact that intervention for communication and swallowing disorders truly is 'a clinical art based on science.'

This book is one of a kind in compiling such a large collection of case studies, demonstrating how different communication and swallowing disorders manifest themselves in very individual ways in children and adults. It also demonstrates how clinicians can work with their clients in developing individualized assessment and treatment plans and how such a partnership will greatly enrich treatment. As such, instructors as well as clinicians will find this book to be a tremendously valuable teaching and clinical resource.

Luc De Nil, PhD
University of Toronto
Professor, Speech-Language Pathology
Acting Dean, School of Graduate Studies
Acting Vice-Provost, Graduate Research and Education
ASHA Fellow

Preface

Abraham Maslow stated, "I suppose it is tempting, if the only tool you have is a hammer, to treat everything as if it were a nail." Along this line of thought, every patient with a communication disorder requires unique problem solving and insight. And although didactic instruction is inherently valuable, true clinical skill involves implementation of theory to the human condition. This volume was constructed to encourage students and clinicians to seek out and employ their entire tool kit, not just a hammer, when managing complex communication disorders. More simply, we sought to provide clinical context to encourage the development of independent clinical decision-making skills.

The construction of a volume of cases has the potential to expose controversy. Surely, consensus regarding both the diagnoses and treatment employed is unlikely. Regardless, the intent is to encourage clinicians to be open to unfamiliar concepts and appreciate the diversity of approaches to challenging, and more routine, clinical conundrums. With that said, this volume, admittedly, suffers from an impressive lack of completeness reflective of the expansive breadth within the profession of speech language pathology. A wholly comprehensive casebook is an impossibility. Regardless, we hope you enjoy and learn from this compilation.

Contributors

Gemma Bailey, MHSc, S-LP, Reg. CASLPO
Speech-Language Pathologist
Hamilton Health Sciences
Regional Rehabilitation Centre
Hamilton, Ontario, Canada

Dana Battaglia, PhD, CCC-SLP
Assistant Professor and Department Chair
Department of Communication Sciences and Disorders
Adelphi University
Garden City, New York

Jenna Battipaglia, MS, CCC-SLP, TSSLD
Clinical Assistant Professor
Department of Communicative Sciences and Disorders
    Steinhardt School of Culture, Education, and Human
    Development
New York University

Risa Battino, MS, CCC-SLP
Speech-Language Pathologist
Montefiore Medical Center
Bronx, New York

Lisa M. Bedore, PhD
Professor and Chair
Department of Communication Sciences and Disorders, and
Director
Human Abilities in Bilingual Language Acquisition
    Laboratory (HABLA Lab)
Temple University
Philadelphia, Pennsylvania

Emily Berteau, BS (Hons)
Master's Student
School of Communication Science and Disorders
Florida State University
Tallahassee, Florida

Christie Block, MA, MS, CCC-SLP
Speech-Language Pathologist
New York Speech and Voice Lab
New York, New York

Annie Bradberry
Chair
International Stuttering Association

Nancy C. Brady
Associate Professor
Department of Speech Language Hearing Sciences
and Disorders
University of Kansas
Lawrence, Kansas

Susan Baker Brehm, PhD, CCC-SLP
Professor and Chair
Department of Speech Pathology and Audiology
College of Arts and Science
Miami University
Oxford, Ohio, and
Cincinnati Children's Hospital Medical Center
Cincinnati, Ohio

Alejandro E, Brice, PhD, CCC-SLP, ASHA Fellow
Professor
University of South Florida
St. Petersburg, Florida

Kelly A. Bridges, PhD, CCC-SLP
Clinical Assistant Professor
Director of Distance Education
Assistant Director of the M.S. Program
Department of Communicative Sciences and Disorders
Steinhardt School of Culture, Education, and Human
Development
New York University
New York, New York

Lisa D. Bunker, MS, CCC-SLP
Department of Communication Sciences and Disorders
University of Utah, and
Aphasia and Apraxia Research Program
VA Salt Lake City Health Care System
Salt Lake City, Utah

Paul W. Cascella
Associate Dean
San Jose State University
San Jose, CA

Jana Cason, DHS, OTR/L, FAOTA
Assistant Professor
Auerbach School of Occupational Therapy
Spaulding University
Louisville, Kentucky

Heather M. Clark, PhD
Associate Professor
Chair
Division of Speech Pathology
Department of Neurology
Mayo Clinic
Mayo Clinic College of Medicine
Rochester, Minnesota

Joanna Close, MS, CCC-SLP
Adjunct Clinical Supervisor
Pacific University
Forest Grove, Oregon

Ellen R. Cohn, CCC-SLP, ASHA Fellow
Professor
Department of Communication Science and Disorders
School of Health and Rehabilitation Sciences
University of Pittsburgh
Pittsburgh, Pennsylvania

Solaman J. Cooperson, PhD
University of Redlands
Redlands, California

Catherine J. Crowley, J.D., PhD
Professor of Practice
Teachers College
Columbia University
New York, New York

Barbara Culatta, PhD
Professor
Brigham Young University
Provo, Utah

James Curtis, MS, CCC-SLP, BCS-S
Laboratory for the Study of Upper Airway Dysfunction
Department of Biobehavioral Sciences
Teachers College
Columbia University
New York, New York

Sarah Diehl, MS, CF-SLP
Doctoral Student
Department of Hearing and Speech Sciences
Vanderbilt University Medical Center
Nashville, Tennessee

Amy L. Donaldson, PhD, CCC-SLP
Associate Professor
Department of Speech & Hearing Sciences
Portland State University
Portland, Oregon

Karen L. Drake, MA, CCC-SLP
Oregon Health Sciences University
Portland, Oregon

Megan Dunn Davison, PhD, CCC-SLP
Assistant Professor
Queens College
Flushing, New York

Kimberly A. Eichhorn, MS, CCC-SLP, ATP
Speech-Language Pathologist
Assistive Technology Professional
VA Pittsburgh Healthcare System
Pittsburgh, Pennsylvania

Erin Embry, MPA, MS/CCC-SLP
Associate Dean for Academic Operations
Clinical Assistant Professor
Department of Communicative Sciences and Disorders
Steinhardt School of Culture, Education, and Human
    Development
New York University
New York, New York

Kelly Farquharson, PhD, CCC-SLP
Associate Professor
Florida State University
Tallahassee, Florida

Christine Fiestas, PhD, CCC-SLP
Assistant Professor
Texas A&M University-Kingsville
Kingsville, Texas

Michael R Fraas, PhD, CCC-SLP
Associate Professor
Department of Communication Sciences and Disorders
Western Washington University
Bellingham, Washington

Jennifer C. Friberg, EdD, CCC-SLP, ASHA Fellow
Cross Endowed Chair in the Scholarship of Teaching and
    Learning
Associate Professor
Communication Sciences & Disorders
Illinois State University
Normal, Illinois

Dana Rissler Fritz, PhD, CCC-SLP
University of Missouri
Columbia, Missouri

Amy Fullerton, MA, CCC-SLP
Speech-Language Pathologist
Board Certified Specialist in Swallowing and
    Swallowing Disorders
UF Health Cancer Center
University of Florida
Gainseville, Florida

Jackie Gartner-Schmidt, PhD, CCC-SLP, ASHA Fellow
Professor
Department of Otolaryngology
University of Pittsburgh, and Director
Speech-Language Pathology-Voice Division
Co-Director
University of Pittsburgh Voice Center
University of Pittsburgh Medical Center
Pittsburgh, Pennsylvania

Shirley Gherson, MA, CCC-SLP
Clinical Voice Specialist
Department of Otolaryngology-Head and Neck Surgery
New York University Voice Center
New York, New York

Amanda I. Gillespie, PhD
Assistant Professor
Emory University School of Medicine
Director
Speech Pathology
Co-Director
Emory Voice Center
Atlanta, Georgia

Jessie L. Ginsburg, MS, CCC-SLP
Director of Clinical Services
Pediatric Therapy Playhouse
Los Angeles, California

Lynn Marty Grames, MA, CCC-SLP
Speech-Language Pathologist
Cleft Palate and Craniofacial Institute
St. Louis Children's Hospital
St. Louis, Missouri and
Adjunct Instructor
Department of Communication Sciences and Disorders,
    and Center for Advanced Dental Education
Saint Louis University
St. Louis, Missouri

Michelle Gutmann, PhD, CCC-SLP
Clinical Associate Professor
Speech, Language, and Hearing Sciences
Purdue University
West Lafayette, Indiana

Christine Hagie
Associate Professor
San Jose State University
San Jose, California

Anna Eva Hallin, PhD
Postdoctoral Researcher
Speech-Language Pathologist
Karolinska Institute
Department of Clinical Sciences
Intervention and Technology
Division of Speech Language Pathology
Stockholm, Sweden

Alease M. Holden MS, CF-SLP
Speech-Language Pathologist
Spencertown, New York

Emily M. Homer, MA, CCC-SLP
Speech-Language Pathologist
Students Eat Safely, LLC
www.emilymhomer.com

Jessica E. Huber, PhD
Professor
Speech, Language, and Hearing Sciences
College of Health and Human Sciences
Interim Associate Vice Provost for Faculty Affairs
Co-Director
Center for Research on Brain, Behavior, and
    Neuro-Rehabilitation (CEREBBRAL)
Purdue University
West Lafayette, Indiana

Myra J. Huffman, MS
Speech-Language Pathologist
Department of Psychological and Brain Sciences
University of Louisville
Louisville, Kentucky

Suzanne Hungerford, PhD, CCC-SLP
Professor
Graduate Coordinator
Communication Sciences and Disorders
SUNY Plattsburgh
Plattsburgh, New York

Lisa N. Kelchner, PhD, CCC-SLP, BCS-S, ASHA Fellow
Professor and Interim Chair
Department of Communication Sciences and Disorders
University of Cincinnati, and
Cincinnati Children's Hospital Medical Center
Cincinnati, Ohio

Debra L. Kerner, MS, CCC-SLP
Speech-Language Pathologist
McKinney, Texas

Shayne Kimble, MCD, CCC-SLP
Speech-Language Pathologist
Shriners Hospitals for Children
Houston, Texas

Kaitlin Lansford, PhD
Assistant Professor
School of Communication Science and Disorders
Florida State University
Tallahassee, Florida

Brooke Leiman MA, CCC-SLP, BCS-F
Board Certified Specialist in Fluency Disorders
Director of the Stuttering Clinic at National Therapy Center
Bethesda, Maryland

Kerry Lenius, PhD, CCC-SLP
Clinical Chief of Speech-Language Pathology
Clinical Assistant Professor
Department of Speech, Language and Hearing Sciences
College of Public Health and Health Professions
University of Florida
Gainesville, Florida

Nancy Lewis, MS, CCC-SLP; MPA
Speech-Language Pathologist
Centers for Disease Control and Prevention's Act
    Early Ambassador to New Mexico
University of New Mexico
Albuquerque, New Mexico

Savannah P. Little, MS
Illinois State University
Normal, Illinois

Kenneth J. Logan, PhD, CCC-SLP
Associate Professor
Director of Graduate Programs
Department of Speech, Language, and Hearing Sciences
University of Florida
Gainesville, Florida

Amy P. Lustig, PhD, MPH, CCC-SLP
Adjunct Professor
University of Pittsburgh
Pittsburgh, Pennsylvania, and
Clinical Educator, Speech-Language Pathology
Salus University
Elkins Park, Pennsylvania

Donald MacLennan, MA, CCC-SLP
Minneapolis VA Health Care System
Minneapolis, Minnesota

Toby Macrae, PhD, CCC-SLP
Associate Professor
School of Communication Science and Disorders
Florida State University
Tallahassee, Florida

Robert Maxwell, MA, CCC-SLP
Regional Clinical Director
Genesis Rehab Services
Eastern Territory/ Region 1 (Virginia)
Fredericksburg, Virginia

Lisa McQueen, MHSc, SLP (C) Reg. CASLPO
Speech-Language Pathologist
Status Only Lecturer
University of Toronto
Toronto, Ontario, Canada

Jyutika Mehta, PhD, CCC-SLP, FHEA
Associate Professor
Director
Neurophysiology Lab
Department of Communication Sciences and Disorders
Texas Woman's University
Denton, Texas

Carolyn B. Mervis, PhD
Distinguished University Scholar and Professor
Department of Psychological and Brain Sciences
University of Louisville
Louisville, Kentucky

Katie Micco, MS, CCC-SLP
Clinical Instructor
Department of Speech-Language Pathology
Duquesne University
Pittsburgh, PA

Jamila Minga, PhD, CCC-SLP
Assistant Professor
North Carolina Central University
Durham, North Carolina

Darlene Mariel Monda, MS, CCC-SLP
Clinical Assistant Professor
Department of Communicative Sciences and Disorders
New York University
New York, New York

Katie C. Miranda, MCD, CCC-SLP
St. Tammany Parish Schools
Covington, Louisiana

Alicia Morrison-Fagbemi, MA, CCC-SLP
Assistant Clinical Professor
Department of Communicative Sciences and Disorders
New York University
New York, New York

Kristen E. Muller, MA, CCC-SLP
Doctoral Candidate
Department of Speech Language Hearing Sciences
  and Disorders
University of Kansas
Lawrence, Kansas

Joseph Murray, PhD, CCC-SLP, BCS-S
Chief
Audiology/Speech Pathology Service
VA Ann Arbor Healthcare System
Ann Arbor, Michigan

Leslie Nitta, MS, CCC-SLP
Speech-Language Pathologist
Los Angeles, California

Billy T. Ogletree, PhD
Professor and Head
Department of Communication Sciences and Disorders
Western Carolina University
Cullowhee, North Carolina

José A. Ortiz, MA, CCC-SLP
Clinical Assistant Professor
LEAP Preschool Director
Department of Hearing and Speech Sciences
University of Maryland
College Park, Maryland

Mohamed (Mo) Oshalla, MHSc, SLP (C)
London-Elgin Speech & Language Services
St. Thomas, Ontario, Canada

Susan Ostrowski, MA, MS
Speech-Language Pathologist
Co-Founder, *Reading2Connect*
www.reading2connect.com

Megan S. Overby, PhD, CCC-SLP
Associate Professor
Department of Speech-Language Pathology
Duquesne University
Pittsburgh, PA

Elizabeth D. Peña, PhD, CCC-SLP
Professor
University of California, Irvine
Irvine, California

Maria Reséndiz, PhD, CCC-SLP
Assistant Professor
Texas State University
San Marcos, Texas

Michael de Riesthal, PhD, CCC-SLP
Associate Professor
Department of Hearing and Speech Sciences
Vanderbilt University Medical Center
Nashville, Tennessee

Luis F. Riquelme, PhD, CCC-SLP, BCS-S
Board Certified Specialist in Swallowing and
  Swallowing Disorders
Fellow, American Speech-Language-Hearing Association
Associate Professor, Speech-Language Pathology
Program Director, Certificate in Pediatric Dysphagia
New York Medical College
Valhalla, New York, and
Director, Center for Swallowing and Speech-Language
  Pathology
New York-Presbyterian Brooklyn Methodist Hospital
Brooklyn, New York

Abigail L. Rosenberg, MA, CCC-SLP
Speech-Language Pathologist
Children's Hospital of Philadelphia
Philadelphia, Pennsylvania

Ian Roth, MHSc, S-LP(C) Reg. CASLPO
Speech-Language Pathologist
University Health Network
Toronto, Ontario, Canada

Jennifer St. Clair, MS, CCC-SLP
Director of Clinical Education
Department of Communication Sciences and Disorders
Loma Linda University
Loma Linda, California

Jill E. Senner, PhD, CCC-SLP
Owner/Director
Technology and Language Center, Inc.
Oak Park, Illinois

Jordanna M. Sevitz, MS, CCC-SLP, TSSLD-BEA
Teachers College
Columbia University
New York, New York

Casey Sheren, MS
Speech-Language Pathology Clinical Fellow
Mount Sinai Hospital
Mount Sinai Health System
New York, New York

Lisa A. Simpson
Assistant Professor
San Jose State University
San Jose, California

Sarah Smits-Bandstra, PhD, SLP, Reg. CASLPO
Adjunct Professor
Department of Psychology
Social Science Centre, Room 7418
Western University
London, Ontario, Canada

Chelsea Sommer, MS
Speech-Language Fellow
Teachers College
Columbia University
New York, New York

Sarah Strathy-Alie, MHSc SLP (C)
Private Practice
Toronto, Ontario, Canada

Jamie Swartz, BS
University of South Florida
St. Petersburg, Florida

Casey Taliancich Klinger, PhD
Our Lady of the Lake University
San Antonio, Texas

Tina M. Tan, MS, CCC-SLP, BCS-S
Supervisor, Pediatric Speech and Swallowing Services
Department of Speech-Language Pathology
Rusk Rehabilitation
NYU Langone Health
Hassenfeld Children's Hospital
New York, New York

John A. Tetnowski, PhD, CCC-SLP, BCS-F, ASHA-F
Ben Blanco/BoRSF Endowed Professor in Communicative
    Disorders
Graduate Coordinator for Ph.D. Program in Applied
    Language and Speech Sciences
Board Certified Fluency Specialist and Mentor
Special Interest Group in Fluency and Fluency Disorders
    (SIG4) Coordinator
Fellow, American Speech-Language-Hearing Association
University of Louisiana at Lafayette
Lafayette, Louisiana

Amber Thiessen, PhD, CCC-SLP
Department of Communication Sciences and Disorders
University of Houston
Houston, Texa

Sara J. Toline, MA, CCC-SLP
Clinical Specialist
Cochlear Implant Center
Rusk Rehabilitation
NYU Langone Medical Center
New York, New York

Mitchell Trichon, PhD, CCC/SLP
Assistant Professor
Department of Communication Sciences and Disorders
La Salle University
Philadelphia, Pennsylvania

Michelle S. Troche, PhD, CCC-SLP
Associate Professor
Speech-Language Pathology Program, and Director
Laboratory for the Study of Upper Airway Dysfunction
Department of Biobehavioral Sciences
Teachers College
Columbia University
New York, New York

Shelley L. Velleman, PhD, CCC-SLP
Chair and Professor
Communication Sciences and Disorders
University of Vermont
Burlington, Vermont

Judy P. Walker, PhD, CCC-SLP
Associate Professor
Coordinator, Speech Therapy Telepractice Program
Department of Communication Sciences and Disorders
University of Maine
Orono, Maine

Julie L. Wambaugh, PhD, CCC-SLP
Professor
Department of Communication Sciences and Disorders
University of Utah, and
Research Career Scientist
VA Salt Lake City Healthcare System
Salt Lake City, Utah

Barbara D. Weinrich, PhD, CCC-SLP, ASHA Fellow
Professor Emerita and Research Associate
Department of Speech Pathology and Audiology
College of Arts & Science
Miami University
Oxford, Ohio, and
Cincinnati Children's Hospital Medical Center
Cincinnati, Ohio

Carol Westby, PhD
Consultant
Bilingual Multicultural Services
Albuquerque, New Mexico

Shane Wilmoth
Regional Adult Chapter Coordinator
National Stuttering Association

Erin Yeates
Speech-Language Pathologist
University Health Network
Toronto Rehabilitation Institute
Toronto, Ontario, Canada

Aaron Ziegler, PhD, CCC-SLP
Assistant Professor
NW Clinic for Voice & Swallowing
Department of Otolaryngology-Head & Neck Surgery
Oregon Health and Science University, and
Co-Founder, Co-President
PhoRTE LLC
Portland, Oregon

Jarrod B. Zinser, MS, CCC-SLP
School of Communication Science & Disorders
Florida State University
Tallahassee, Florida

1 Completely Normal Speech Is the Goal for a Child Born with Cleft Palate

Lynn Marty Grames

1.1 Introduction

An important concept, not often taught in our field, is that for the neurologically normal child born with a cleft, the goal is **normal speech**. Some children may present with maladaptive or compensatory articulations that require therapy, and these maladaptive/compensatory misarticulations are maladaptive motor patterns that require specific training at the phonetic level. A motor learning approach, in which the new motor pattern is practiced in increasingly complex motoric and linguistic functions, is an effective means of facilitating transfer to spontaneous speech.

1.2 Clinical History and Description

MC was a full-term male born with cleft of the secondary palate (posterior to the incisive foramen) and micrognathia (small, retrodisplaced mandible), consistent with a preliminary diagnosis of Pierre Robin sequence. In addition, he presented with mild shortening of limbs and digits, hip dysplasia, and macrocephaly associated with enlarged ventricles. His mother was also born with a cleft palate. Genetic evaluation yielded no specific diagnosis, asserting that MC's cleft was likely a unique presentation.

MC was admitted to the neonatal intensive care unit (NICU) at birth due to respiratory distress associated with his micrognathia, and feeding difficulties. The NICU followed an algorithm for conservative stabilization of his airway. When all conservative efforts failed, he underwent a 15-mm bilateral mandibular distraction at 4 weeks of age. This surgical procedure is designed to gradually lengthen the mandible, thereby increasing the space between the base of the tongue and posterior pharyngeal wall. The airway improved significantly with distraction, and MC was discharged home at 2 months of age with a combination of oral and nasogastric tube feeding. He was gradually weaned from tube feedings to become a fully oral feeder over the course of 1 month at home. He received early intervention services in the home.

At 4 months of age, he underwent bilateral myringotomies with ventilation tube placement to treat chronic middle ear effusion. Polysomnography (sleep study) at 12 months of age was normal. He underwent two-flap palatoplasty with repeat bilateral myringotomies and tubes at nearly 15 months of age.

1.3 Clinical Testing

Evaluation at 21 months of age yielded the following:
- Normal hearing acuity.
- Oral mechanism examination revealed intact palate with no evidence of fistula.
- Voice quality, pitch, and intensity were within normal limits.
- Resonance was difficult to assess due to limited phoneme inventory, but significant aberrant nasal emissions were observed.
- Articulation assessment via observation and imitation yielded a limited phoneme inventory. Consonants in the inventory included [m, h, ŋ], nasal stops, and both posterior and anterior nasal fricatives. Nasal stops and nasal fricatives are maladaptive articulations, believed to be compensatory, characterized by the supraglottal airstream being forced through the nose during speech and are frequently used as substitutions for oral pressure consonants. Vowel/diphthong repertoire was limited to [ɑ, æ, ʌ, ɛ, ɔ, ɑʊ]. Intelligibility of spontaneous speech was poor; MC's mother expressed concern regarding limited intelligibility.
- Language skills were assessed informally. MC used multisyllabic, but poorly intelligible utterances to request, negate, and comment. He exhibited age-appropriate social interactions and behaviors. The Bayley Scales of Infant Development-3rd Edition had been administered less than 2 months previously (chronological age 19 months) in his follow-up evaluation with the newborn medicine team (▸ Table 1.1).

1.4 Questions and Answers for the Reader

1. Does MC have a functional velopharynx?
   a) No.
   b) Yes.
   c) It is too early to tell.

Answer: c is correct. At present, his phonetic inventory consists of only vowels and consonants that do not require velopharyngeal closure. The addition of oral pressure consonants to his inventory will yield useful information about velopharyngeal function.

Table 1.1 MC's developmental testing prior to speech-language evaluation

The Bayley Scales of Infant Development, Third Edition (administered at chronological age of 19 months)	
Cognitive composite score = 100	
Cognitive scaled score = 10	Age equivalent = 19 mo
Language composite score = 109	
Receptive scaled score = 10	Age equivalent = 19 mo
Expressive scaled score = 13	Age equivalent = 24 mo
Motor composite score = 91	
Fine motor scaled score = 12	Age equivalent = 23 mo
Gross motor scaled score = 5	Age equivalent = 14 mo

a and b are incorrect. Until his phoneme inventory increases to include attempts at oral pressure consonants, velopharyngeal function is unknown. The velopharynx should remain open for [m, ŋ]. It does not close for nasal stops and nasal fricatives, since the air is forced through the nose for those consonants. Vowels and diphthongs can be produced without velopharyngeal closure at this early stage of development, without pressure consonants.

2. The treating clinician may consider teaching [p, b] first, so as to learn more about his velopharyngeal function. Will [p, b] increase his intelligibility if he has a limited vowel inventory?
   a) No.
   b) Yes.
   c) It is too early to tell.

Answer: a is likely correct. A limited vowel inventory will limit the number of words he can produce intelligibly once he has [p, b]. Given his current vowel/diphthong repertoire, the following functional words may still not be intelligible even if he uses [p, b]: bye, baby, boat, boot, bite, big, pee, poo, pig, piece.

c is possibly correct. The therapeutic process is likely to provide the answer to this complex issue.

b is incorrect. Just as a limited consonant inventory limits one's intelligibility, so too does a limited vowel inventory. With a full vowel repertoire, we can expand the number of intelligible words a child can produce once we begin adding consonants.

3. It is atypical for children with cleft-related articulation disorders to present with limited vowel inventory. Why might this child have a limited vowel inventory?
   a) He has apraxia.
   b) He has dysarthria.
   c) He maintains a posterior tongue carriage with pervasive nasal stop and fricative use.
   d) Any of the above.

Answer: d is correct. Only therapy progress will determine which of these options is correct. Given his history of enlarged ventricles and provisionally unique genetic diagnosis, one must be alert to the possibility of a neurologically based disorder, such as apraxia or dysarthria. Although he underwent mandibular distraction, which can result in stretching or severing of the inferior alveolar nerve, speech articulation deficits caused specifically by this are not reported. He also has a history of middle ear effusions, which may mean that he had conductive hearing loss during critical periods for speech and language learning.

1.5 Description of Disorder and Recommended Treatment

Given his normal hearing, cognition, and receptive-expressive language skills, treatment was initiated with the hypothesis that this was a disorder of speech motor learning, characterized by maladaptive nasal stops and fricatives that likely entered his inventory prior to palate repair and then became adapted for use in linguistically meaningful ways. However, given his hydrocephalus and history of bilateral mandibular distraction, the possibility of a motor speech component, either apraxia or

dysarthria, was also possible, which, if present, would become apparent as treatment progressed.

A motor learning approach to therapy was initiated. Vowels were the initial target to improve intelligibility once consonants were added to the inventory. Using this highly structured therapy approach, the child must learn to imitate the therapist in a structured way. In addition, and also critical to therapy success, is the need for the child to enjoy therapy. "Mr. Potato Head," or any construction toy or item with lots of pieces, is an effective tool for the structured imitation approach. For example, MC was given the body of the potato and was instructed to imitate the therapist raising her hand. When it did not happen, the therapist showed him, hand over hand, what was expected on command, and when he did so (with help), he got an item for the potato, such as the eyes, coupled with enthusiastic praise. This process was repeated until MC imitated independently. It took only minutes for him to adapt to the imitation–reward paradigm. The clinician quickly transitioned from gross motor to oral motor movements to mouth shaping, at which point instruction on vowel production was initiated. Tactile assist for mouth shaping was used as needed, and each phoneme's motor pattern, vowel or consonant, was given a new "name." For example, [i] was the "smile" sound, [o] was the "surprise" sound, [ɔ] was the "cute puppy sound," and [ɑʊ] was the "hit your thumb with a hammer" sound.

MC's vowel repertoire increased rapidly and it no longer seemed likely that a motor speech component was present. Therapy proceeded with a motor learning approach to consonant production. Oral pressure consonants are essential for yielding information about velopharyngeal function; [p, b] (we called them the "quiet and noisy lip sounds") were the first consonant targets. [p, b] are anterior, easy to see, and early developing. MC's limited consonant inventory included [m], and one bilabial consonant can be used to teach others. In MC's case, [b] was taught by plugging the nose as he produced repetitions of [ma]. Once the [b] was isolated, [p] was taught by whispering [b]. Multiple rapid productions of each isolated target were produced to establish the motor pattern. Once established, the motor pattern was practiced in increasingly complex patterns, so that it became habituated and could be easily called upon in rapid running speech. The progression of the therapy is shown in ▶ Fig. 1.1. However, some steps in the therapeutic process overlap, so that once a motor pattern becomes well established, the skill is addressed in multiple levels simultaneously, as shown in ▶ Fig. 1.2. Much early work was done in imitation, without pictures or objects, to establish the motor pattern. The addition of pictures or objects alters the task from imitation to word retrieval, and a child with normal language function may quickly revert to the undesirable motor pattern if the desirable motor pattern is not well established.

MC was weaned from the nose plugging after being consistently successful with all syllable imitation positions. Had he reverted to nasalization of [p, b] without nose plugging, it would have been clear that the distortion was obligatory in nature, due to velopharyngeal dysfunction, and he would have been referred for velopharyngeal imaging studies and management. However, MC was able to maintain good plosion on [p, b] without nasalization, nasal emission, turbulence, or grimacing. This observation strongly suggested that he was capable of nor-

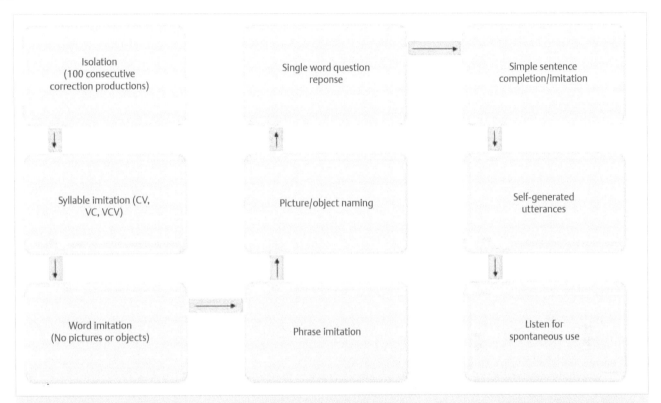

Fig. 1.1 Illustration of the motor learning process for a consonant, or allophonic pair, from the initial teaching of the motor pattern in isolation through increasingly complex motor and linguistic levels to transfer to spontaneous speech.

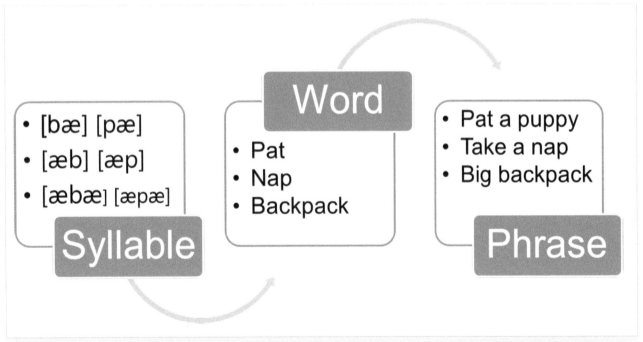

Fig. 1.2 Illustration of the process by which syllables, words, and phrases can be addressed in imitative sequences, pushing the target consonant to the next level of complexity. This is only of value if the target is produced correctly at the simplest level. There is no value in attempting a more complex level if the target motor pattern is not produced accurately at a simpler level.

mal velopharyngeal function, but had not yet learned to use his velopharynx appropriately. Just as a child may need to be taught how to use other articulators, such as tongue and lips in sound production, it is also possible for a child to need to be taught how to use the velopharynx.

Although a brief section of each therapy session was devoted to teaching a variety of consonants in isolation, therapy focused primarily on one place of articulation at a time. When [p, b] were well established in spontaneous speech, attention was turned to lingua-alveolar place, with [n] being taught first, then using it to teach [d] by nose plugging, followed by [t], which was stimulated by whispering [d]. These lingua-alveolar consonants were then advanced through syllable and word imitation, etc., using the same process as had been used for [p, b]. [s, z] were addressed next, then [f, v], followed by [ʃ, tʃ, dʒ]. Simple home practice activities that could be accomplished easily and quickly in a busy household were given each session, and follow-up was excellent. Weekly attendance was somewhat difficult due to multiple medical issues and family schedule conflicts.

1.6 Outcome

MC was discharged from therapy with excellent intelligibility at the chronological age of 5 years, 8 months, the week before he began kindergarten. He received a total of 56 individual therapy sessions, most of them 1 hour in length. Articulation testing using the Goldman-Fristoe Test of Articulation-2 in his last session yielded the following scores:
- Raw score: 2.
- Standard score: 109.
- Standard score projected range using the 95% confidence interval: 102 to 116.
- Percentile score: 67.

- Age equivalency: 6.3 years.

Spontaneous speech sampling revealed no concerns with regard to language skill. Voice quality, pitch, and intensity were within normal limits. Resonance was within normal limits. Following discharge, he performed well in an accelerated program at school. He participated in sports and functioned well socially. No further concerns with regard to speech production evolved and no further velopharyngeal management was indicated. He was scheduled for regular follow-up with his cleft palate team until facial growth is complete.

1.7 Key Points

- Normal speech is possible, and expected, for a neurologically normal child born with a cleft palate, with or without cleft lip or other oral structural anomaly.
- Nasal air escape during speech could be a function of articulation or of velopharyngeal dysfunction. This distinction must be made to provide appropriate treatment.
- If a child presents with abnormal or maladaptive motor articulation patterns, a motor learning approach can be an effective therapeutic program.

Suggested Readings

[1] Peterson-Falzone SJ, Trost-Cardamone J, Karnell MP, Hardin-Jones MA. The Clinician's Guide to Treating Cleft Palate Speech. 2nd ed. St. Louis, MO: Elsevier; 2016

[2] Zajac DJ, Vallino LD. Evaluation and Management of Cleft Lip and Palate: A Developmental Perspective. San Diego, CA: Plural Publishing; 2016

[3] Hardin-Jones MA, Chapman KL, Scherer NJ. Children with Cleft Lip and Palate: A Parent's Guide to Early Speech-Language Development and Treatment. Bethesda, MD: Woodbine House; 2015

2 Assessment and Treatment of Preschool Fluency

Sarah Smits-Bandstra

2.1 Introduction

J was a 4.1-year-old boy referred for fluency intervention by his parents after 17 months of therapy at another center where they considered his stuttering therapy to be unsuccessful. His parents were willing and able to participate in treatment.

2.2 Clinical History and Description

J's birth and medical history was notable for a loss of fetal heart tones prior to delivery and admission to the neonatal nursery for approximately 2 hours for postpartum monitoring. At 2.5 years of age, J experienced myoclonic episodes after pertussis vaccines. He had no family history of stuttering, speech, or language disorders. J met most developmental, speech, and language milestones on time with the exception of gross motor skills. He received physical therapy 1 hour per week for 6 weeks. He was discharged from therapy approximately 6 months ago. J was in good health and had no significant medical illnesses, injuries, or concerns. J passed a hearing screening within 1 month of referral.

J lived at home with his mother, father, and younger brother (8 months old) with whom he reportedly got along with well. English was the only language spoken in the home. J was described as a bright, imaginative, happy child. He began attending preschool 3 days per week 4 months ago. He also attended gymnastics, piano lessons, and swimming lessons on a weekly basis.

J began stuttering at around 18 months of age. He received clinician-directed stuttering therapy (parents were not trained in treatment) from the age of 2.5 to 4 years. Owing to insufficient improvements, his parents sought alternate treatment.

2.3 Clinical Testing

Assessment included a stuttering-specific case history, parent and preschool teacher interviews, videos from home, observation of parent–child interactions, and a clinic visit. The parents also recorded a written diary over a 1-week period describing the stutter, reactions to the stutter, and the contexts in which the stutter was more or less severe.

J's preschool teacher reported an increase in stuttering just prior to referral to the clinic. She noted that peers were kind and respectful and made no issue of the stuttering. She reported that his stuttering increased when asking a question, trying to get attention, or thinking of what to say. Informal assessment/screening of voice, articulation, receptive and expressive language, social skills, and resonance were unremarkable. Oral motor examination revealed mild limitations in range of motion for lip protrusion and retraction and occasional drooling.

A speech sample of 300 syllables was collected during unstructured play. During this sample, 5% of syllables were stuttered and 11% total disfluency (less than 10% is typical for preschool-aged children) was noted. Total disfluencies include typical disfluencies (revisions, interjections, one or two repetitions of whole words, phrase repetitions) and atypical disfluencies (also known as stutters). Atypical disfluencies can be defined as part-word repetitions (mo- mo- mo- mom), tense/rapid, and/or dysrhythmic whole- or part-word repetitions, prolongations, or blocks. In J's sample, 43% of total disfluencies were atypical. It is considered normal for preschool-aged children to demonstrate less than 50% of total disfluencies as atypical. J's disfluencies were most commonly slow, rhythmic part-word repetitions at the beginning of phrases (e.g., "Wha-wha-wha-what is that?"). Revisions and whole-word repetitions were also common (e.g., "I-I-I-you go up there."). Repetitions ranged in number from 2 to 10, with severe instances lasting 3 seconds in duration. No secondary behaviors (facial or body movements) were observed. J's father indicated J's speech during the sample was not representative and less severe than at home. J's father provided three videos from home that he felt were more representative.

Analysis of these videos yielded the following data:

- *Sample 1 (151 syllables)*: 8% syllables stuttered, 11% total disfluencies, 73% atypical.
- *Sample 2 (187 syllables)*: 13% syllables stuttered, 17% total disfluencies, 75% atypical.
- *Sample 3 (162 syllables)*: 12% syllables stuttered, 12% total disfluencies, 100% atypical.

Characteristics of atypical disfluencies included increases in pitch during a stutter, dysrhythmic repetitions, and repetitions ranging up to 16 units and 4 seconds in duration. J scored 6 on the KiddyCAT (Communication Attitude Test for Preschool and Kindergarten Children Who Stutter). This 12-item yes/no questionnaire for children younger than 6 years assesses a child's awareness of their stutter and their attitudes toward speaking (e.g., "Is talking hard for you?"). A typical score for a child who stutters of J's age is 4.89, indicating J was aware of his stutter and had developed some negative attitudes toward speaking.

2.4 Questions and Answers for the Reader

1. What information indicates that J is at risk for persistent stuttering?
   a) Stuttering for more than 12 months with no indication of improvement.
   b) Family history of stuttering.
   c) Indications of language delays.
   d) Unawareness and limited reaction to stuttering.

Answer: a is correct. Research shows that children who stutter for longer than 12 months without indications of recovery are more likely to continue stuttering.

b is incorrect. J's parents reported no family history of any type of speech or language disorders or stuttering. Instead, there are indications that stuttering may be congenital (loss of fetal heartbeat, fetal seizures).

c is incorrect. J showed no evidence on informal assessment or screening of language delays; instead, he showed evidence of motor delays (physical therapy, weak lips, drooling).

d is incorrect. Results of the KiddyCAT assessment indicated that J showed awareness of his stutter and some negative reactions to his stutter. Awareness and negative reactions to stuttering are risk factors for persistent stuttering.

2. What important assessment information was obtained outside of the initial clinic visit?
   a) Parent report/interview.
   b) Teacher report/interview.
   c) Parent–child interaction observation/video.
   d) KiddyCAT.

Answer: b is correct. Interviews with preschool teachers are usually done outside of the initial clinic visit due to difficulties with travel and scheduling.

a is incorrect. Although a case history can be completed at home or by telephone, a more detailed interview is typically done face -to -face (or through telepractice) with the clinician during a clinic visit.

c is incorrect. Although parent–child interaction observations or videos can/should be gathered from home, they are to supplement observations or videos taken during the initial clinic visit.

d is incorrect. Standardized stuttering assessments should be completed by a trained professional within a controlled setting to obtain valid and reliable results.

3. In addition to percent of syllables stuttered, what are the other important and necessary assessments to measure stuttering severity and the impact of stuttering on the child's life?
   a) Interviews with parents, teachers, and other significant caregivers.
   b) Child's awareness of stuttering and attitude toward speaking (e.g., KiddyCAT).
   c) Description of the types (repetitions vs. blocks) and categorizations (typical vs. atypical) of disfluencies, durations of the disfluencies, and secondary behaviors.
   d) All of the above.

Answer: d is correct. All of the aforementioned measures need to be incorporated to obtain a valid and comprehensive assessment of the impairments, activity limitations, and/or participation restriction associated with stuttering. Although it is important to speak directly to caregivers who spend time with the child, it is also important to administer assessment protocols directly with the child. It is also important to gather information from caregivers who spend time with the child and to directly assess/observe the child's stuttering behaviors. Finally, it is critical to directly assess/observe the child's stuttering behaviors as well as the child's awareness of the stutter and their reactions to and attitudes about stuttering and gather information from caregivers who spend time with the child.

4. J's previous therapy was not effective. What therapies for preschool children have the strongest evidence base?
   a) Treatment provided by a speech-language pathologist.
   b) Treatment provided by the parents, where the parents are trained by a speech-language pathologist.
   c) Wait and see—treatment is best provided after a child enters school.
   d) Treatment that focuses on having the preschool child self-monitor and self-correct stuttering using fluency-shaping techniques.

Answer: b is correct. Current meta-analyses of clinical trials research suggest that the Lidcombe program has the largest body of research support.[1] However, one study has shown Lidcombe and Demands Capacity treatments were equally effective.[2] Both of these treatments are parent-directed with clinicians training parents to deliver the treatment at home. Comprehensive treatment includes parent training to ensure generalization and transfer.[3]

a is incorrect. Treatments that include parental training and daily parent-directed practice at home are more successful than those that are administered solely by a speech-language pathologist.

c is incorrect. Preschool children are treated more effectively than school-age children. Early intervention is strongly recommended.[3]

d is incorrect. Preschool children do not generally have the metalinguistic or metacognitive skills to formulate language and simultaneously self-monitor fluency and use of fluency-shaping skills.[3]

2.5 Description of Disorder and Recommended Treatment

J presented as a child with beginning stuttering of moderate severity. Assessment information indicated several factors that put J at risk for persistent stuttering (congenital factors, stuttering for more than 12 months, and awareness/reactions to his stuttering). Therapy was recommended immediately. Therapy was provided by a student clinician with a clinical supervisor observing 75% to 100% of sessions. Therapy followed the Lidcombe Program, a stuttering treatment involving parent training in the clinic to provide the treatment to the child at home and other contexts. A detailed treatment guide can be freely downloaded from http://sydney.edu.au/health-sciences/asrc/docs/lp_treatment_guide_2016.pdf. The clinician also modeled other known facilitative communication strategies such as slow rate of speech. The clinician observed parent attempts at indirect strategies in interactions with the child. The parents reported these strategies to be very helpful in daily interactions at home and reported that the strategies positively influenced severity ratings for structured times. These "indirect" strategies were added to the Lidcombe program to individualize the treatment to meet client needs and parent wishes. They were employed as needed and gradually extinguished over time.

For approximately 23 weeks, in weekly sessions, the clinician trained the parents in Lidcombe techniques for stage 1, including demonstrations. The clinician consulted with J's parents weekly for updates on J's fluency patterns, progress, and areas of need outside of the clinic. Areas of need were discussed and problems were solved jointly between the clinician and parents.

Table 2.1 Stuttering severity: visits 1 to 12 (Lidcombe stage 1)

Visit no.	Visit date	Severity rating	Total disfluencies (%)	Syllables stuttered (%)	Atypical disfluencies (%)
1	January 28	7	23	15	67
2	February 2	4	12	1	9
3	February 9	3	19	5	26
4	February 16	7	10	3	27
5	February 23	5	10	5	45
6	March 2	5	5	2	35
7	March 23	4	8	2	22
8	March 30	4	6	1	16
9	April 6	5	9	1	15
10	April 13	5	8	2	21
11	April 20	4	4	1	25
12	April 27	4	3	1	15

Daily stuttering measures were taken by the parents to monitor fluency. Progress was measured through calculations of percentage syllables stuttered, ratings from the severity rating scale, reactions to stuttering, and parent report (see ▶ Table 2.1 and ▶ Table 2.2). The rating chart is freely available and can be downloaded from http://sydney.edu.au/health-sciences/asrc/docs/severity_rating_chart_2015.pdf.

2.6 Outcome

At the time of this report, J and his parents completed the first 13 weeks of stage 2 of the Lidcombe Program for childhood stuttering. J continued to show progress with fluent speech through stage 2. His most recent calculation of disfluencies in spontaneous speech was 0% syllables stuttered and 4.9% total disfluencies, 0% of which were atypical. He continued to respond positively to praise and showed no hesitations when asked to correct a disfluent utterance.

J's parents demonstrated exceptional understanding and use of Lidcombe and indirect home-programming techniques through implementation during structured and unstructured activities. They self-reported the use of strategies in the home and community settings and reported decreased severity ratings when they were implemented. J's stuttering decreased since his initial evaluation and his syllables were stuttered within normal limits for a 4-year-old across the last 13 consecutive weeks. J will continue to be monitored for the remainder of stage 2 (approximately 9 months).

Table 2.2 Stuttering severity: visits 13 to 23 (Lidcombe stage 1 continued)

Visit no.	Visit date	Severity rating	Disfluencies (%)	Syllables stuttered (%)	Atypical disfluencies (%)
13	May 6	4	5	1	5
14	May 13	3	4	0	1
15	May 27	2	5	1	10
16	June 10	2	4	0	0
17	June 17	3	4	0	0
18	June 24	4	4	1	25
19	July 1	2	3	0	0
20	July 8	1	4	0	0
21	July 15	1	4	0	9
22	July 22	1	4	0	10
23	July 29	1	5	0	0

2.7 Key Points

- Neither pre- nor posttreatment outcome measures are valid unless the representativeness of the clinic samples is determined and speech samples and reactions to stuttering are gathered across different contexts, speakers, and time.
- Parent-directed treatment is critical in fluency treatment for preschool children to ensure optimal effectiveness, generalization, and transfer.
- Treatment programs, such as the Lidcombe Program, can be modified to meet individual client and family needs (such as supplementation with indirect techniques) as long as effectiveness is monitored and maintained.
- It is unethical to continue with treatment programs without evidence of progress in a reasonable time period. Therapists without experience or training in current evidence-based practice in stuttering therapy are ethically obligated to consult with a specialist and/or refer the client to a specialist if outcome measures do not indicate improvement within 6 weeks of beginning treatment (for indirect treatment) or 2 to 3 months (for more general types of treatment).

References

[1] Nye C, Vanryckeghem M, Schwartz JB, Herder C, Turner HM, III, Howard C. Behavioral stuttering interventions for children and adolescents: a systematic review and meta-analysis. J Speech Lang Hear Res. 2013; 56(3):921–932

[2] Franken MC, Kielstra-Van der Schalk CJ, Boelens H. Experimental treatment of early stuttering: a preliminary study. J Fluency Disord. 2005; 30(3):189–199

[3] Guitar BG. Treatment of Stuttering: Established and Emerging Interventions. Baltimore, MD: Lippincott Williams & Wilkins; 2010

3 Working Collaboratively with a Young Child with Autism Spectrum Disorder

Ian Roth

3.1 Introduction

A 20-month-old boy is referred to a speech-language pathologist (SLP) because of red flags for autism spectrum disorder.

3.2 Clinical History and Description

WS was born following an unremarkable pregnancy and had what his parents—both of them pediatric medical professionals—described as a typical infancy involving a lot of babbling. At 16 months of age, they noticed a decrease in his babbling, which did not remit by the time he was seen for a speech and language assessment at 20 months. WS had a history of multiple ear infections, and had myringotomy tubes placed at 17 months of age. Audiological testing revealed no hearing loss at the time the tubes were placed.

3.3 Clinical Testing

A full case history was taken from both parents while WS played with toys in the room. This allowed him the opportunity to become familiar with the environment for 60 to 90 minutes and afforded the SLP and SLP student time to observe WS's play and spontaneous interaction skills. Two weeks later, the family returned for the more interactive components of the assessment. The Preschool Language Scales, 4th Edition (*PLS-4*) was attempted but was discontinued in favor of more informal assessment because WS did not follow instructions, with or without gestures. For this reason, it was difficult to determine accurate receptive language abilities for WS. It was concluded that social communication deficits likely prevented him from responding to instructions, as opposed to responding incorrectly, which would be more indicative of a receptive language impairment.

WS moved around the room for much of the assessment, occasionally stopping to touch a toy, but rarely played in functional or conventional ways. The clinicians found success interacting with WS by following his lead. WS did stop moving to watch a spinning toy that was deployed. While watching, WS tensed his entire body and flapped his hands. He made intentional requests by handing the toy to the SLP who was down at his level and silent, but with an open hand. WS made other requests by pulling an adult's hand toward objects he wanted/wanted help with. After the SLP initiated a dyadic activity (i.e., no materials) that involved moving WS's body side-to-side, when the SLP paused, WS moved his own body in a similar fashion to request the activity to continue.

WS was able to follow a point but he did not coordinate eye contact with gestures to request, and he did not initiate joint attention (i.e., a declarative gesture, such as pointing to show, while making eye contact). He was able to imitate some individual words but he did not use speech to communicate (i.e., to send a message to another person) during the assessment. Most of his spontaneous utterances were vowel sounds and did not appear to be communicative. His parents reported immediate echolalia, which was not observed during the assessment. WS drooled throughout the assessment. Eating and drinking were described as safe and efficient.

3.4 Questions and Answers for the Reader

1. Which of the following most closely approximates WS's communication profile?
   a) Receptive language delay, expressive language delay, social communication impairment.
   b) Apraxia of speech, expressive language impairment, social communication within normal functional limits.
   c) Autism spectrum disorder (ASD).
   d) Social communication impairment, expressive language impairment, receptive language unknown.

Answer: d is correct. Social communication is the primary impairment, given the low frequency of interactions, poor coordination of eye contact, and communication occurring primarily for the purpose of asking for help or other requests. WS's expressive language is also delayed, given his extremely limited expressive vocabulary. However, his social communication deficit may be largely to blame for his impaired expressive language as evidenced by his not using conventional, symbolic gestures or vocalizations to compensate for delayed speech. Receptive language may in fact be impaired, but without responding to most instructions, it is difficult to accurately assess WS's receptive language skills.

a is incorrect. Though he is at risk of a receptive language delay, there is not enough information to determine whether receptive language is in fact delayed because WS did not respond to most instructions, which in the absence of hearing loss may be indicative of a social communication impairment.

b is incorrect. Apraxia of speech cannot be positively identified based on the current assessment. Social communication is impaired, as evidenced by his not initiating joint attention, minimally coordinating eye contact with requests, using people's hands as tools, and not responding to his name or to simple instructions.

c is incorrect. ASD is not a communication profile. Children with ASD can present with a wide variety of communication profiles.

2. What referrals would you make to other health care/service providers?
   a) Developmental assessment.
   b) Dolphin-assisted therapy.
   c) Chelation therapy.
   d) General practitioner/pediatrician to halt all future vaccines.

Answer: a is correct. WS presented with impairments in social communication and language, and rarely engaged in conventional play. He displayed atypical repetitive movements. Given this profile, WS merits a referral to an interdisciplinary developmental team to determine whether he meets criteria for ASD or another developmental disability.

b is incorrect. Dolphin-assisted therapy and other interventions for which there is no scientific evidence are considered pseudoscience and should therefore not be recommended. Some are misled to believe that these activities are "worth trying" because they are harmless and might help. But recommending pseudoscientific interventions is considered unethical because they might provide a family with false hope and/or divert family resources away from interventions that are supported by evidence. In fact, children can be physically harmed by dolphins if not properly trained.

c is incorrect. Chelation therapy to remove mercury from the blood of a child with ASD or social communication impairment is considered extremely dangerous and scientifically unfounded in this population.

d is incorrect. Vaccines have been thoroughly studied and have been found safe and effective for the majority of children, including those at risk for ASD. There is no reason why a child suspected of or diagnosed with ASD should be denied the standard regimen of vaccines.

3. What immediate goals and strategies would you employ to begin speech and language intervention?
   a) Lip exercises to reduce drooling and to help WS speak.
   b) Verbal imitation to help WS repeat more words.
   c) Follow WS's lead to join him in his chosen activities. Then give WS opportunities to interact in positive ways.
   d) Wait until he starts saying words and then offer speech therapy.

Answer: c is correct. The assessment showed that allowing WS to lead play activities with adults resulted in more interactions. By creating situations where WS is interested in communicating with others, his primary social communication deficits are being addressed in ways that will allow him to see the value of interacting with people, which over time will prepare him for a greater variety of interactions, including specific, targeted speech and language interventions.

a is incorrect. WS's drooling was unlikely a significant factor in his communication impairment at that point. Nonspeech oral motor exercises have not been shown to improve speech skills in children. Even if his speech production improved, WS would still have social communication impairments and would likely still not communicate very often or for different reasons (e.g., to include others in his play).

b is incorrect. Verbal imitation would likely not have a significant impact on how effectively WS communicates at this point as it would not address his social communication impairments, which cause him to communicate so infrequently. In fact, placing WS in a position where he is expected to repeat what others say could detract from efforts to help him initiate intentional messages.

d is incorrect. WS's preverbal communication skills were delayed. Speech and language therapy should, therefore, target these skills, as it is essential to work within the child's zone of proximal development.

4. What role(s) might parents play in the intervention of their child with ASD?
   a) Clinician informant regarding the child's activities at home and in the community.
   b) Interventionist using similar strategies as the SLP and other clinicians.
   c) Child advocate for the implementation and ongoing coordination of services.

Answer: a is correct. Speech and language therapy is often carried out under ideal circumstances (e.g., quiet room; few distractions). However, for the intervention to be worthwhile, the targeted skills must improve the child's communicative effectiveness under typical circumstances in the child's natural environments. Parents' reports about how their children communicate at home, at school, and in the community must be considered strongly by the SLP to ensure the intervention is geared to that child's situation. Regular feedback from parents allows clinicians to better understand the impact that intervention is having on a day-to-day basis so that they can modulate it accordingly.

b is correct. Research has shown that children's communication skills improve when their parents use the same communication intervention strategies with them that their clinicians use. For this reason, parent education and parent training have been cited as important components of communication intervention for children, including those with ASD.

c is correct. In many communities, families with children who have special needs such as ASD do not have access to case managers to advocate for services or to coordinate current interventions to promote collaboration and generalization. In many cases, proper advocacy and service coordination does not occur, and so children do not receive the most prudent complement of services to maximize their progress. In some situations, parents assume this role. Parents often have the best knowledge of their children's needs, and are in a position where they can (on their own or in discussion with their service providers) determine when an intervention continues to be valuable and when it should be modified or discontinued. The SLP then must help parents to make these difficult decisions by educating them about the unique roles they play on their children's intervention teams and by deferring to parents around making educated decisions.

3.5 Description of Disorder and Recommended Treatment

Following the speech and language assessment, WS and his parents took part in an 8-week "block" of speech and language intervention to primarily address social communication and receptive language. Speech therapy followed a Naturalistic Developmental Behavioral paradigm, which involved coaching WS's parents to incorporate WS's interests into strategies they could use to promote social interaction at home and in the community. The SLP visited WS's childcare center to discuss how his teachers could use these same strategies in the classroom.

Immediately following his first treatment block, WS was diagnosed with ASD. WS's parents subsequently enrolled him in Applied Behavior Analysis (ABA) to address self-injurious behaviors and other behavioral concerns. The role of the speech pathologist changed over time as different areas of development became priorities for WS and his family. WS's parents arranged for cross-agency consultations between the ABA therapists and WS's SLP to ensure that the ABA therapists were using the same communication strategies employed in WS's speech therapy at home and in the childcare center. The SLP observed the ABA providers in person and on video, and then advised the rest of the team regarding modifications to WS's communication goals, strategies that could be added, and/or adjustments to how strategies were being used. At this time, the SLP only saw WS approximately monthly to monitor his progress and to update goals and strategies. Occupational therapy was also added to WS's intervention regimen. At one of the SLP monitoring sessions, it was decided that WS's speech production was emerging as a primary communication modality, and so intelligibility became a new priority that warranted a return to speech therapy.

3.6 Outcome

WS's communication skills improved steadily throughout his early intervention with the interprofessional team. Four years after his initial assessment, a speech and language reassessment using the Clinical Evaluation of Language Fundamentals, Preschool, 2nd Edition (CELF-P2) revealed average receptive language skills; a moderate impairment in expressive language skills; and speech was WS's primary mode of communication. His ABA program gradually ended as he entered a mainstream first grade class with one teacher and a special needs assistant. WS's parents made sure that he had regular, successful play dates with peers from the community.

A psychological evaluation in second grade reported a high average full-scale IQ with average-to-superior scores on all verbal and nonverbal subtests of the Wechsler Intelligence Scale for Children, 4th Edition (WISC-IV). Neuropsychological testing yielded scores that were above expected limits for affect recognition, average for memory for faces, but below expectations for theory of mind. His parents and teacher rated him on the Behavior Assessment System for Children, 2nd Edition (BASC-2). Their ratings demonstrated that WS was within normal limits for most behaviors, and that he was "at-risk" for problems at school, "atypicality," and study skills. None of their ratings were in the "clinically significant" range.

Today, WS is a happy 10-year-old boy who has been very successful in school and takes part in many extracurricular activities. His parents continue to arrange meaningful interactive activities across a variety of environments and with different peers to further his social communication skills. His is very much the model of a North American child.

Suggested Readings

[1] Morgan LJ, Rubin E, Coleman JJ, Frymark T, Wang BP, Cannon LJ. impact of social communication interventions on infants and toddlers with or at-risk for autism: A systematic review. Focus Autism Other Dev Disabil. 2014; 29(4): 246–256

[2] Prizant B. Uniquely Human: A Different Way of Seeing Autism. New York, NY: Simon & Schuster; 2015

[3] Schreibman L, Dawson G, Stahmer AC, et al. Naturalistic developmental behavioral interventions: empirically validated treatments for autism spectrum disorder. J Autism Dev Disord. 2015; 45(8):2411–2428

[4] Zwaigenbaum L, Bauman ML, Choueiri R, et al. Early identification and interventions for autism spectrum disorder: executive summary. Pediatrics. 2015; 136 Suppl 1:S1–S9

4 Clinical Decision Making for a Bilingual Child: Using Converging Information

Lisa M. Bedore, Casey Taliancich Klinger, and Solaman J. Cooperson

4.1 Introduction

Determining whether bilingual children have language learning disabilities is challenging as their language knowledge varies as a function of language experience. Using converging sources of information across assessment modalities likely yields the most reliable information as a foundation for treatment.

4.2 Clinical History and Description

BC was referred for language testing at age 5.2 years after failing a language screening administered in his prekindergarten class. BC spoke only Spanish before school entry and initiated regular exposure to English when he started prekindergarten. He employed both English and Spanish at home, but Spanish was used primarily. BC's parents indicated that his Spanish was stronger than his English, and that his vocabulary and speech intelligibility were good. They did note, however, that he did not consistently use grammatically correct Spanish utterances. BC's teacher also reported his Spanish was stronger than his English and indicated that grammatical accuracy and speech intelligibility were areas of concern. BC's vision and hearing acuity were within normal limits.

4.3 Clinical Testing

Standardized testing included the Bilingual English Spanish Assessment (BESA) semantics and morphosyntax subtests in English and Spanish.[1] The BESA is a standardized language assessment for Spanish–English bilinguals aged 4.0 to 6.11 years designed to identify Spanish–English bilinguals with language impairment. The semantics subtest evaluates semantic knowledge by having the child listen to short stories and answer questions about the stories. Example test item types include category generation, object function, and sentence completion. The morphosyntax subtest evaluates grammatical knowledge in English and Spanish with cloze task items and sentence repetition. Test items on the English and Spanish semantics and morphosyntax subtests are not translations of each other, but are specifically designed to evaluate semantic and morphosyntactic skills specific to English and Spanish.[1,2]

As a component of BC's assessment, language samples in the form of a narrative retell and tell were collected from wordless picture books in English and Spanish. The stories were recorded for transcription into the Systematic Analysis of Language Transcripts (SALT) software designed to assist clinicians and researchers in language sample analysis.[3] Standard measures were generated based on the narratives in each language, including mean length of utterance, number of different words, and total number of words. A summary of findings is provided in ▶ Table 4.1.

Table 4.1 Summary of clinical testing for BC

	Assess-ment tool	English score	Spanish score	Expected range of performance
BESA	Semantics	85[a]	80[b]	Expected mean = 100; SD = 15
	Morpho-syntax	70[b]	78[b]	Expected mean = 100; SD = 15
Language samples	MLU	4.07	3.54	ENG: 5.85–5.96 SPN: 5.63
	NDW	117	114	ENG: 69.75 SPN: 40.80
	NTW	489	269	ENG: 209.83 SPN:–[c]

Data from BC was reported for two analyzed narratives. Expected values obtained from published data available for a single narrative (Bedore et al.,[4] Muñoz et al.,[5] Simón-Cereijido and Gutiérrez-Clellen,[6] Uccelli and Páez[7]).

BESA, Bilingual English Spanish Assessment; ENG, English; MLU, mean length of utterance; NDW, number of different words; SD, standard deviation; SPN, Spanish; TNW, total number of words.

[a]1 SD below mean.

[b]More than 1 SD below mean.

[c]No published data available.

4.4 Questions and Answers for the Reader

1. PK is a 5-year-old girl who comes from a Spanish-speaking home. She was first exposed to English when she entered prekindergarten. She primarily receives school instruction in English. Her teacher expressed concern to the speech-language pathologist that although PK appears to follow simple directions that are given to her in English, most of PK's sentences in English are ungrammatical and her vocabulary skills in English are behind those of her peers. The bilingual clinician administered a language screening to PK in both English and Spanish, and PK passed a semantic and morphosyntax screening in Spanish and exhibited below-average scores in English for both of those domains. PK exhibited language-specific vocabulary (e.g., she generated more words about cooking/food in Spanish and when asked to name school supplies in English she named some of these in English but not in Spanish). Which of the following is likely true about PK's vocabulary skills?
   a) PK's vocabulary skills are distributed across her two languages and are reflective of her experiences with each language thus far and not necessarily an indicator of language delay.
   b) PK's vocabulary skills are delayed in both Spanish and English as there was little overlap in the words that she named for category-generation tasks.

c) PK's vocabulary skills are typical in Spanish and delayed in English as she is not exhibiting English vocabulary like her peers.

d) PK's vocabulary skills are low in both languages as she is regularly exposed to both languages.

Answer: a is correct. It is typical for a Spanish–English bilingual child to exhibit language-specific vocabulary skills based on their experiences in both languages. PK has had more experience with Spanish in the home and community setting, which is why she was likely able to name more foods, for example, in Spanish and less school supply items than in English.[8]

b is incorrect. Children learning two languages are likely to display language-specific vocabulary knowledge that is reflective of their experiences with those languages.[8]

c is incorrect. It appears that her Spanish vocabulary skills may be typical. Since she was recently exposed to English, the finding that her vocabulary is not yet like her peers is not indicative of a delay.[8]

d is incorrect. There is nothing to suggest that learning two languages caused her vocabulary skills in English to be lower than those of her peers. This answer is also incorrect as PK's vocabulary skills in Spanish are reflective of experiences she has had in Spanish.

2. TC is a 6-year-old bilingual girl exposed to Spanish from birth and exposed to English from the age of 1 year. She is currently in first grade in a school program in which instruction is entirely in English. Due to parent and teacher concerns, she was recently tested for a language disorder and she exhibited semantic and morphosyntactic deficits in both languages. A bilingual speech-language pathologist is planning to begin language intervention with her. The speech-language pathologist will treat and monitor progress in both languages and wants to know which intervention targets will benefit both languages. Which of these targets, if addressed in one language, is the most likely to have an effect on the other language?
   a) Verb tense markers.
   b) Gender agreement.
   c) Generating vocabulary items in different categories.
   d) Possessive 's (as in the girl's book).

Answer: c is correct. This goal, along with other goals that address knowledge of the semantic relationships among words, is likely to have effects in both languages.

a is incorrect. Because verb tense is expressed differently in English and Spanish (tense is expressed mainly with final consonants in English and with vowel and/or syllable alternations in Spanish), working on tense markers in one language is not likely to affect these structures in the other language.

b is incorrect. Spanish has gender agreement, but English does not. Working on this target in Spanish is unlikely to have any effect in English.

d is incorrect. English expresses the possessive in this way, but Spanish does not.

3. DC is a 6-year-old boy, bilingual speaker of Spanish and English. He speaks Spanish at home and first acquired English at 1 year of age. If DC is typically developing in terms of language, how is he most likely to differ from his monolingual English-speaking peers?

a) The accurate use of English tense markers.
b) Vocabulary size in English.
c) Correct use of English speech sounds.
d) The ability to use correct word order in English.

Answer: b is correct. Vocabulary knowledge may be distributed across languages, and thus a bilingual child may have a smaller vocabulary in a particular language compared to monolingual children.

a is incorrect. Typically, developing bilingual children are expected to exhibit similar performance to monolingual children in morphosyntax.

c is incorrect. For the most part, bilingual children develop the sound system of each language similarly to a monolingual child.

d is incorrect. We would expect typically developing bilingual children to show similar performance to monolingual children in morphosyntax.

4.5 Description of Disorder and Recommended Treatment

Language testing revealed deficits in both languages. A key indicator of language impairment was that BC's higher language score was below the mean for his age. Scores on both subtests of the BESA were at least 1 standard deviation below the mean in both languages. BC also produced many grammatical errors in his narrative language samples. One of the most prominent errors in English was the omission of verb tense markers. For example, BC said, "he try" instead of "he tried" and "he spill" instead of "he spilled." In Spanish, gender agreement errors were observed. These deficits in each language were consistent with a diagnosis of language impairment in bilingual children.[9,][10] He also tended to use nonspecific vocabulary such as "he" or "she" for all subjects and used only "happy" and "mad" as descriptors across the two stories. BC presented with errors typical of children with language impairment in both languages, and not only in his weaker language.

Language intervention for bilingual children should be delivered in both languages.[8,11] Therapy focused on skills that benefit both languages while recognizing particular deficits may be unique to one language. Because BC had difficulty generating specific vocabulary, intervention included organizing common vocabulary into categories and describing the functions of items. Working on these semantic skills may benefit both languages.[8] Vocabulary knowledge in each language is often dependent on the contexts in which a bilingual child uses each language. For example, knowledge of vocabulary related to household items may be greater in Spanish, and knowledge of academic vocabulary may be greater in English. In therapy, BC was asked to describe functions of different cooking utensils and various articles of clothing. This activity not only increased his knowledge of these particular vocabulary items, but also strengthened general knowledge of the semantic relationships between words. Because grammatical deficits were observed in each language, these structures were also targeted in therapy. Grammatical structures, such as tense markers, are almost entirely different in Spanish and English, so the benefits of instruction may be specific to each language.[12]

4.6 Outcome

BC received weekly language intervention that focused on building semantic and morphosyntactic skills in English and Spanish. Therapy addressed placing vocabulary items into categories (food, animals, clothing, etc.) and generating vocabulary items when given the names of these categories in both languages. For example, BC was presented with examples of clothing and school supplies to sort into categories. BC was also asked to describe the attributes that made the particular items members of these categories. Tense markers were targeted in English as well as the gender-appropriate use of articles in Spanish.

After 1 year of intervention, the BESA was readministered. His standard scores on the BESA semantics subtests were 90 in English and 85 in Spanish. His scores on the morphosyntax subtests were 85 in both English and Spanish. Although progress was noted, continued therapy was recommended.

4.7 Key Points

- A key difference between monolingual and bilingual language development is that language experiences are divided across two languages and contexts. As a result, bilingual children's skills in each language may be more variable than their typically developing monolingual peers, and their errors may resemble those of children with language impairment (e.g., tense marking and other grammatical errors as well as reduced vocabulary in each language).
- To make diagnostic decisions for bilingual children with risk for language impairment, it is important to consider performance in the stronger language. The stronger language may differ by domain (i.e., a child could have more developed vocabulary skills in English and more developed Spanish morphosyntax).
- A way to maximize communicative skill in bilingual children in intervention is to begin by selecting targets that support development in two languages.

Suggested Readings

[1] Kohnert K. Language Disorders in Bilingual Children and Adults. San Diego, CA: Plural Publishing; 2008
[2] Peña ED, Bedore LM, Lugo-Neris MJ. Language intervention for school-age bilingual children: Principles and application. In: McCauley RJ, Fey ME, Gillam RM, Eds. Treatment of Language Disorders in Children. 2nd ed. Baltimore, MD: Paul H. Brookes Publishing; 2017:245–274

References

[1] Peña ED, Gutiérrez-Clellen VF, Iglesias A, Goldstein B, Bedore LM. Bilingual English Spanish Assessment (BESA). San Rafael, CA: AR Clinical Publications; 2014
[2] Bohman TM, Bedore LM, Peña ED, Mendez-Perez A, Gillam RB. What you hear and what you say: language performance in Spanish–English bilinguals. Int J Biling Educ Biling. 2010; 13(3):325–344
[3] Miller J, Iglesias A. Systematic Analysis of Language Transcripts (SALT), Research Version 2016 [Computer Software]. Middleton, WI: SALT Software; 2016
[4] Bedore LM, Peña ED, Gillam RB, Ho TH. Language sample measures and language ability in Spanish-English bilingual kindergarteners. J Commun Disord. 2010; 43(6):498–510
[5] Muñoz ML, Gillam RB, Pena ED, Gulley-Faehnle A. Measures of language development in fictional narratives of Latino children. Lang Speech Hear Serv Sch. 2003; 34(4):332–342
[6] Simón-Cereijido G, Gutiérrez-Clellen VF. Spontaneous language markers of Spanish language impairment. Appl Psycholinguist. 2007; 28:317–339
[7] Uccelli P, Páez MM. Narrative and vocabulary development of bilingual children from kindergarten to first grade: developmental changes and associations among English and Spanish skills. Lang Speech Hear Serv Sch. 2007; 38 (3):225–236
[8] Peña ED, Kester ES, Sheng L. Semantic development in Spanish-English bilinguals: theory, assessment, and intervention. In: Goldstein BA, ed. Bilingual Language Development. 2nd Ed. Baltimore, MD: Paul H. Brookes Publishing; 2012:131–149
[9] Bedore LM, Leonard LB. Grammatical morphology deficits in Spanish-speaking children with specific language impairment. J Speech Lang Hear Res. 2001; 44(4):905–924
[10] Gutiérrez-Clellen VF, Simon-Cereijido G, Wagner C. Bilingual children with language impairment: a comparison with monolinguals and second language learners. Appl Psycholinguist. 2008; 29(1):3–19
[11] Thordardottir E. Towards evidence-based practice in language intervention for bilingual children. J Commun Disord. 2010; 43(6):523–537
[12] Bedore LM, Cooperson SJ, Boerger KM. Morphosyntactic development. In: Goldstein BA, ed. Bilingual Language Development and Disorders in Spanish-English Speakers. 2nd Ed. Baltimore, MD: Paul H. Brookes Publishing; 2012:175–192

5 Language Delay in a Bilingual Child

José A. Ortiz

5.1 Introduction

HN is a 5.6-year-old bilingual Spanish-English-speaking boy referred for speech-language evaluation at a university clinic due to concerns expressed by his mother regarding overall communication skills at home. She reported that HN exhibits difficulty with vocabulary and grammar, and that he is difficult to understand at times. In addition, she reported that he frequently exhibits difficulty following directions at home, requiring repetition.

5.2 Clinical History

HN's medical history was unremarkable. No history of ear infections was reported and a recent audiological evaluation indicated normal hearing acuity. HN reportedly achieved all developmental milestones within normal limits: he sat up at 7 months, walked independently at 9 months, began to feed himself at 2.5 years, dressed himself at 4 years, and he produced his first word at 8 months. No history of speech-language delays were reported in the family. HN was evaluated by a psychologist at age 3 and reportedly diagnosed with a mild, unspecified delay, but no follow-up services were provided. HN lived with his mother, father, and 2-year-old brother. In terms of language exposure, Spanish was reported to be the sole language spoken at home. At the time of referral, HN was enrolled in a monolingual English classroom, in a public school. According to his mother HN's classroom teacher reported no areas of concern regarding academic skills at the most recent parent–teacher conference. No concerns regarding literacy skills were reported.

5.3 Clinical Testing

HN was assessed by a bilingual speech-language pathologist. HN's language form-content skills were assessed via conversational language sample collected during the evaluation and the *Clinical Evaluation of Language Fundamentals, 4th Edition Spanish (CELF-4)*. A wordless picture book was used to elicit a narrative that was representative of HN's language use in connected speech. The CELF-4 was modified to appropriately assess dual-language use; code-switching was provided as needed and responses in either Spanish or English were accepted as correct. Standard scores, percentile ranks, and age-equivalencies were not calculated due to these modifications.

Overall, HN's language was characterized by age-appropriate utterance length but also by the use of simple rather than complex sentences, difficulty with age-appropriate vocabulary, subject–verb agreement errors, and frequent difficulty with age-appropriate morphosyntactic items. He was very talkative during the evaluation and did not hesitate to respond to any direct communication attempts. In general, he did not demonstrate difficulty communicating intent, but produced language that was not age-appropriate in terms of morphosyntactic and vocabulary use.

With regard to language comprehension, HN demonstrated significant difficulty following a variety of age-appropriate multistep commands. This deficit was noted in the administration of the Concepts and Following Directions subtest of the CELF-4 and during unstructured conversation. All oral directions were presented using a combination of both Spanish and English. HN demonstrated difficulty following many directions; he only successfully demonstrated comprehension of one- to two-step commands regardless of language. Significant difficulty was noted with auditory comprehension of sentences containing the following elements: multiple descriptives (e.g., the *big, white* ball), exclusion terms (e.g., all but, except, etc.), ordinal terms (e.g., first, next, last, before, after, etc.), spatial terms (e.g., right, left, next to, etc.), and temporal terms (e.g., before, after, while, etc.). When provided with cueing for attention and repetition of directions, performance improved but not significantly. Overall, a significant deficit in auditory comprehension was noted.

In terms of morphosyntactic usage, HN exhibited a pattern of errors not likely attributable to a language difference including: subject–verb agreement, gender agreement (Spanish only), and the absence of a variety of expected morphemes including plurals, possessives, and verb tense inflections. Subject–verb agreement errors were observed in a variety of contexts. For example, HN produced the sentence "He open the door," omitting the inflection for third person singular. This type of error was noted more frequently in English than Spanish, but it occurred across both languages. Gender agreement errors in Spanish were noted frequently. HN produced the sentence "La niño coger la bola (the boy get the ball)," using a feminine article with a masculine noun. The absence of specific morphemes was also noted on the Word Structure subtest of the CELF-4 and via analysis of the language sample. Production of English was marked by language transfer from Spanish, especially in the area of negation. For example, HN produced the sentence "I no want" which mirrors the Spanish "yo no quiero."

In the domain of vocabulary skills, HN demonstrated moderate difficulty with age-appropriate vocabulary. Although he frequently code-switched throughout the evaluation, when provided with the opportunity to label objects and actions, he produced labels much more consistently in Spanish than English. HN demonstrated significant difficulty identifying categories of objects and recognizing which items did not belong in a group (e.g., identifying the item that does not belong, because it is not part of a group of objects, such as food, clothes, etc.). In a fast-mapping task, he did not retain a novel vocabulary word that was presented to him. In addition, during connected speech, he was noted to employ inappropriate, unclear, or generic words. For example, he produced the utterance "Él quiere hacer la puerta (he wants to *do* the door)." This pattern of semantic usage was noted repeatedly throughout the evaluation.

In terms of pragmatic language ability, HN exhibited areas of concern with discourse level communication and narrative production including difficulty with age-appropriate eye contact and consistent responses to direct communication attempts.

HN frequently required multiple repetitions of directions prior to responding. In addition, he exhibited difficulty responding consistently to age-appropriate WH questions in Spanish and in English (i.e., where/donde, what/que, and when/cuando). This error pattern was improved by providing orienting cues (e.g., "are you listening?" or "look at me") before presenting an oral direction. His narrative production skills were limited; he produced only a heap narrative, consisting of a collection of seemingly unrelated ideas, with no distinguishable sequence, or expected story grammar elements. In addition, HN exhibited frequent use of self-talk during solitary play. Self-talk was not observed during interactive play with the examiner. HN also spoke at a reduced loudness level. Although he did not exhibit any delay in phonological production, his reduced loudness significantly affected overall intelligibility. However, HN was very responsive to requests for repetition in moments of reduced intelligibility (e.g., "No te escuché. ¿Puedes decirmelo otra vez, por favor?" or "I didn't hear you. Could you please say that again?").

5.4 Questions and Answers for the Reader

1. Based on the results reported, which specific area of language was much stronger in Spanish than in English?
   a) Phonology
   b) Literacy
   c) Vocabulary
   d) Syntax

Answer: c is correct. HN produced a significantly greater number of vocabulary words in Spanish than in English. Had the evaluation been conducted with only opportunities to produce vocabulary words in English during the labeling activity, HN would have appeared to exhibit substantially more difficulty.

a is incorrect. HN did not exhibit any difficulty with phonology.

b is incorrect. Literacy was not reported to be an area of concern.

d is incorrect. Although the client did exhibit somewhat stronger morphosyntactic skills in Spanish than in English (exemplified by language transfer in English), based on the information reported, a marked degree of difference between language in syntax as in vocabulary ability was not observed.

2. Why were standard scores, percentile ranks, and age equivalences not reported?
   a) The wrong test was selected.
   b) The test was modified to meet the language needs of the client.
   c) The client was not represented in the normative sample.
   d) The test was too long for the client given distractibility.

Answer: b is correct. The test was modified to meet HN's linguistic needs. Information was presented in both Spanish and English and responses were marked as correct in both languages. In addition, the normative sample does not include bilingual Spanish-English speakers.

a is incorrect. A limited number of norm-referenced bilingual assessment tools are available; the test was determined to be the most appropriate method of assessment with modifications to accommodate HN's needs.

c is incorrect. Bilingual individuals are represented in the normative sample of the CELF-4.

d is incorrect. Although HN's distractibility was a factor during assessment, it did not play into test selection.

3. What was an example of language transfer/influence from Spanish to English?
   a) The use of code-switching throughout the evaluation.
   b) Limited sustained attention.
   c) Difficulty with subject–verb agreement in English and Spanish.
   d) The production of negation in English that mirrored Spanish syntax.

Answer: d is correct. The production of negation in English as "I no want" is analogous to the Spanish "yo no quiero." This type of language transfer is common among sequential bilingual individuals (i.e., those individuals learning one language after another).

a is incorrect. Code-switching was a consistent characteristic of HN's language use, but this is not indicative of cross-linguistic transfer.

b is incorrect. HN's limited sustained attention did not affect language transfer.

c is incorrect. Subject–verb agreement was noted in both languages, albeit more frequently in English than in Spanish, which is indicative of emergence of the ability to produce subject–verb agreement, but it is unrelated to language transfer.

4. Given the results of the assessment, to support auditory comprehension what strategy would be most effective for the caregiver to utilize at home?
   a) Repeating information.
   b) Speaking louder to the client.
   c) Providing orienting cues to the client.
   d) Speaking at a slower rate.

Answer: c is correct. Orienting cues proved to be a very effective method of improving comprehension in moments of distractibility.

a is incorrect. Although repetition did support comprehension, providing orienting cues was noted to be very effective, reducing the need for repetition.

b is incorrect. Increased loudness level was not utilized as a strategy to support comprehension.

d is incorrect. Reduced rate of speech was not utilized as a strategy to support comprehension.

5.5 Description of Disorder and Recommended Treatment

HN's performance on the evaluation was indicative of a moderate delay in receptive and expressive language skills. His language use was characterized by frequent errors in subject–verb agreement, the absence of various expected form-content categories, frequent use of simple sentences, and limited vocabulary skills. In addition, HN exhibited significant difficulty with age-appropriate auditory comprehension in a variety of tasks. Narrative language production skills were characterized by the presence of frequent self-talk, lack of contingency in conversation, and the need for frequent redirection. Speech and language treatment once a week for 50 minutes was recommended to address difficulties in the areas of language form-content and pragmatic skills. In addition, ongoing parent education and training was recommended to maximize carry-over of treatment gains.

5.6 Outcome

HN received speech-language intervention once a week for 50 minutes starting approximately 1 month following the evaluation. Treatment was focused on the production and comprehension of specific aspects of morphosyntax, vocabulary skills, and narrative production. Given HN's tendency to frequently code-switch throughout the evaluation and at home, treatment was provided in a bilingual Spanish-English context. Language choice in treatment was directed by HN; the clinician allowed HN to select the most comfortable language for a given context. In addition, the clinician utilized both L1 and L2 as a means of reinforcing verbal directions; directions provided in one language were frequently repeated in the other, which substantially improved overall comprehension across treatment tasks. In addition, the provision of orienting cues proved to be effective to improve comprehension, resulting in a reduced repetition of oral directions.

Treatment was focused on morphosyntax and narrative production. Morphosyntactic targets included subject–verb agreement, gender pronouns, and gender agreement of articles, all of which were targeted in both Spanish and English, with the exception of gender agreement in articles, which is not a feature of English morphology. All treatment sessions were observed by HN's parents, who were also provided with fre-

quent home assignments to improve generalization of gains outside of the clinical environment. Over the course of two semesters of treatment, HN exhibited significant gains in appropriate subject–verb agreement in both English and Spanish. As HN's overall use of morphosyntax improved, focus was placed on narrative production skills. HN initially exhibited a great degree of difficulty producing a cohesive narrative without cueing. He initially produced a heap narrative and required frequent redirection to maintain attention to the task at hand. Limited sustained attention and a high level of distractibility proved to be persistent maintaining factors. However, over the course of 1 full year of treatment, HN's narrative production skills improved substantially. After this time, he produced a clearly defined chain narrative when given visual support and minimal redirection.

5.7 Key Points

- Early identification of speech and language issues is key.
- Identification of specific areas to be targeted in treatment within the context of bilingualism requires a knowledge of the specific linguistic characteristics in each language.
- Differential identification of specific linguistic skills in each language is fundamental to the identification of language delays/disorders in bilingual individuals.
- Appropriate treatment for bilingual clients requires the use of both languages in therapy sessions.

Suggested Reading

[1] Genesee F, Paradis J, Crago MB. Dual Language Development & Disorders: A Handbook on Bilingualism & Second Language Learning. Vol. 11. Baltimore, MD: Paul H Brookes Publishing; 2004

6 The Application of Dynamic Assessment of Narratives in an English Language Learner

Christine E. Fiestas, Elizabeth D. Peña, and Maria Resendiz

6.1 Introduction

It can be difficult to determine whether a child learning a second language has a language impairment (LI). Dynamic assessment (DA) is a three-phase evaluation process consisting of testing, teaching, and retesting. The teaching phase or mediated learning experience (MLE) is provided to support and teach a particular language skill. During this phase, the clinician has an opportunity to observe and measure the learning process and responsiveness to instruction while reducing bias linked to a student's lack of experience.

6.2 Clinical History and Description

HV, a first-grade bilingual boy aged 6.6 years, was referred for evaluation of LI. Information from both the teacher and the parents indicated that HV was exposed to both Spanish and English. His parents spoke Mexican Spanish and that was the main language used at home. His first exposure to English began in preschool; bilingual education was offered in his local school district. HV was enrolled in a first-grade bilingual class, where Spanish and English were both employed. An estimate of Spanish and English use throughout a typical week including weekdays and weekends across home and school was 76.8% Spanish and 23.2% English. He primarily employed Spanish at home, and both English and Spanish in school. Both parents and his teacher expressed concern regarding his communication skills across both languages. HV reportedly used short sentences and made grammatical errors in both languages.

6.3 Clinical Testing

HV's language evaluation included testing in both languages using the Dynamic Assessment of Narratives procedure.[1] The parallel stories, Two Friends and Bird and His Ring, wordless picture books, were used to elicit narratives in Spanish and English, respectively, at pretest and again (in the opposite language) at posttest following two MLEs of 30 minutes each. MLE sessions were conducted in English to target narrative story components (setting, character, temporal, and causal information) and episode structure (initiating event, internal response, attempt, resolution, and reaction). The scripts included components of mediated learning (intention to teach, meaning, transcendence, planning, and transfer).[2] During MLE, the scripts were adapted to respond to HV's strengths and needs. The goal of the MLE sessions was for HV to produce an organized and complete story.

At pretest, HV demonstrated weaknesses telling stories in both English and Spanish. He had particular difficulty including story components and story ideas. For example, he used general references for characters "un dinosaurio" (a dinosaur) and "a dog," and information about the story setting was not included. HV used temporal markers "y" (and), "luego" (then) in Spanish, and "and then" in English, but did not use words to indicate causality in either language. With respect to story ideas and language, he used concrete, literal language to describe events and used the mental state verb "pensar" (think) in Spanish. His stories were simple, consisting of multiple attempts and an ending in both languages, but no initiating event. His story in English included actions that were not goal oriented. Grammatically, HV consistently used the past tense in Spanish. He omitted the auxiliary form "___ pensando en una cosa" (___ thinking of something), and made both gender and number agreement errors with article/noun and subject/verb, such as "una serpienta" (a snake, feminine) for "un serpiente" (a snake, masculine), and "allí no encontraron" (they didn't find) for "allí no encontró" (he didn't find). In English, he omitted the copula (e.g., "they ___ friends") and predominately used third-person present tense in which he omitted the "s" morpheme ("then he wait_," "then he stop_"). He was more productive in Spanish as measured by the number of different words (NDW), mean length utterance (MLU), and total number of words (TNW): NDW = 45, MLU = 4.83, and TNW = 87. In English, his NDW = 22, MLU = 4.42, and TNW = 53.

Modifiability during the MLE sessions was scored according to the Mediated Learning Observation (MLO) Instrument,[3] a rating scale of clinician observations of applied narrative language learning skills during mediation sessions. Scores are based on four components of learning, namely, affect, arousal, elaboration, and behavior. Each of these four components includes three subscales totaling 12 items. Each item is scored on a Likert scale from 1 to 5 and lower scores indicate less clinician effort to support learning and higher modifiability; higher scores indicate more clinician effort and lower modifiability.

During the MLE session, HV demonstrated strengths, including a positive attitude, persistence, and cooperation during the tasks. However, across both mediation sessions, HV was sometimes unmotivated and displayed difficulty in task orientation (his understanding of the task). Lack of metacognitive skill (awareness of errors) and problem-solving skills was noted. Specifically, he had difficulty making plans for story telling even with support. During the intervention, HV verbalized only occasionally about a strategy and did not demonstrate flexibility in his use of strategies to remember what to include in stories. When HV did not know a word in English, he did not try to describe it or clarify his meaning despite prompting and reminders.

At posttest, which provides a clinician with the opportunity to observe modifiability and change, HV continued to demonstrate weaknesses in story production in both English and Spanish and he had persistent difficulty including story components. His character descriptions went from simple at pretest to omitted at posttest. For instance, he referred to characters in Spanish as "éste" (this) and in English as "this animal" instead of using specific terms "dog" or "cat." Setting information was not included at pre- or posttest; causality was also omitted. At posttest, he used the same temporal markers as pretest. HV's story ideas and language remained literal and concrete with the exception of more mental states in Spanish "querer" (want), "pensar" (think), and "está enojado" (mad). In both Spanish and English, HV included simple attempts and endings, but his episode structure did not improve in complexity. Grammatically, HV used "was + verb-ing" in English to express several events in the past compared to pretest where almost all events were expressed in the present. When he used present third person, he overgeneralized ("this animal who look 'ats' this," "he wanna 'gets' this"). His productivity slightly improved in English. As can be seen in ▶ Table 6.1, HV improved his posttest English NDW, TNW, TNU, and MLU. In Spanish, he produced NDW = 36, TNW = 62, TNU = 13, and MLU = 4.7. Although HV's stories improved slightly in English, his performance at posttest was greater than 1 SD below the norm on several measures compared to his first- and second-grade bilingual peers learning English who also received mediation in English.[4]

6.4 Questions and Answers for the Reader

1. YL is a 5-year-old girl in kindergarten referred for speech-language assessment because the teacher is concerned about her limited vocabulary use in the classroom. Intake history indicates that she speaks English as a second language and speaks Chinese at home. The parents report that this is her first year of school; she did not attend preschool. They report that she interacts appropriately with her siblings. DA focus on vocabulary learning indicates low scores on the Expressive One-Word Picture Vocabulary Test, 2000 Edition (EOWPVT-2000) in English—a standard score of 67. The MLE session indicates high levels of modifiability. Posttest scores show some modest change with use of descriptions and category names when she does not know a word. Her posttest score on the EOWPVT-2000 was an 85. Your next step is to:
   a) Make a diagnosis of a speech-language delay and recommend enrollment in speech-language therapy to increase vocabulary.
   b) Recommend monitoring language acquisition and retesting in 1 year after she knows enough English.
   c) Do not diagnose speech-language delay nor recommend intervention. You do provide the teacher with some ideas

of what can be done in the classroom to support vocabulary learning in English.

Answer: c is correct. Limited knowledge of English does not qualify as an impairment. Additionally, single-word vocabulary tests typically have poor diagnostic accuracy for LI. During DA, YL significantly improved on the test after a couple of intervention sessions resulting in improved scores at posttest. She was also highly responsive to MLE. Her high level of responsivity and her ability to make significant pretest to posttest changes even in her second language, which she has little experience with, suggest she does not have LI. If the classroom teacher is not familiar with typical second-language acquisition, it might be helpful for him or her to learn more about the normal progression. It may not be unusual for these children to show limited vocabulary in English. They may use descriptions and related words. Strategies to support comprehension for children who are in the process of learning English include demonstration, modeling, and visual supports during teaching.

a is incorrect. YL made significant pretest to posttest change and was highly responsive to the intervention. It seems that the patterns that she displayed are more like a typical child who is in the early stages of learning English.

b is incorrect. YL's performance is typical for a child who is in the early stages of learning English as a second language. Monitoring and testing is not warranted.

2. Why would DA be a valuable approach to language assessment for a student who is culturally and linguistically diverse (CLD)?
   a) DA allows you to obtain a standardized score on a language test.
   b) DA allows you to observe how children learn instead of what they already know.
   c) DA allows you to assess all children regardless of your proficiency in any of their languages.

Answer: b is correct. DA allows a clinician to observe the learning process and offer cognitive strategies to scaffoled learning during a language learning task and modify performance. Using a pretest, mediation, and posttest framework, lack of experience and unfamiliarity with an assessment task can be avoided by providing guided practice toward a particular skill. For many CLD children, unfamiliarity with testing procedures can hinder performance, which could lead to an inappropriate diagnosis of LI. The normative sample of most standardized language tests does not reflect the diverse language and demographic backgrounds of CLD children.

Table 6.1 Pretest and posttest narrative scores

		Total score	Story components	Story ideas and language	Story episode	NDW	TNW	TNU	MLU
Pretest	English	18	7	9	2	22[a]	53[a]	12[a]	4.4
	Spanish	20	6[a]	11	3	45	87	18	4.8[a]
Posttest	English	16[a]	7[a]	7[a]	2	34	71[a]	15	4.7[a]
	Spanish	19[a]	7[a]	10	2	36	62[a]	13	4.7[a]

MLU, mean length of utterances in words; NDW, number of different words; TNU, total number of utterances; TNW, total number of words.
[a]More than 1 SD below peers.

a is incorrect. The DA framework considers change from pretest to posttest, posttesting results, and observations of both modifiability and clinical judgment to make a diagnosis of LI, but not standardized test scores.

c is incorrect. If a child uses a language in which a clinician is not proficient, a translator may be necessary for assessment. Valuable information may still be obtained by conducting the mediation in English if a child is using English functionally and is well on their way to using English in the academic setting.

3. What is the best practice to assess HV's language abilities?
   a) Test in English since that is the language HV will eventually be using more of in school.
   b) Test in Spanish using an interpreter if necessary because HV uses Spanish more than English.
   c) Test in both languages using an interpreter as necessary to determine HV's overall language ability.

Answer: c is correct. The goal of assessing language skills is to gain information about communicative competence including the languages a child uses to function across different contexts. In HV's case, we are considering the languages needed at home and school. For a child who is learning English, we expect errors during the process of learning a second language or errors in a first language if not given sufficient exposure to develop these skills. Errors in either language can be mistaken for LI, and competency in both languages must be determined.

a is incorrect. Although important to determine HV's proficiency in English, this information alone does not provide a complete profile of HV's communication ability across the contexts in which he uses language.

b is incorrect. HV spends more time using Spanish than English. Although he is in the process of learning English, he receives significant input in English and it is necessary to determine how his skills are developing in both languages. If the clinician only speaks English, an interpreter may be needed to elicit a story as well as transcribe and review the language sample.

4. For a child learning English at school and using English functionally to communicate, but who speaks another language at home, what are the available options for conducting MLE?
   a) The mediation could be conducted in either language if both languages are used functionally.
   b) The mediation should only be conducted in the language that the child has more experience with.
   c) The mediation should never be conducted in the language that the child has less experience with.

Answer: a is correct. For children who are learning English and using the language functionally, mediation in English may be a possibility as well as mediation in the child's home language if the clinician is bilingual or an interpreter is available. There is a shortage of bilingual clinicians, and information gained from the mediation may be informative. For example, HV is using English more than 20% of the time during a typical week. He produced a simple story in English at pretest by generating sentences and drawing on his English lexicon. During mediation, the clinician would ensure that input was comprehensible, and make provisions for improving the child's abilities in English while providing individualized instruction. A bilingual child should be using English functionally in daily contexts for English mediation to be appropriate. Peña et al.[5]

reported that, by providing mediation in English to bilingual children in their less familiar language, they were still able to accurately classify children with and without LI. They did so by observing modifiability and substantial differences in learning behaviors during the MLE. Children in the process of learning English as a second language may demonstrate grammatical errors related to first language influence. However, these children should show good productivity in word production and be able to include most story elements even in the context of limited vocabulary.

b is incorrect. The clinician could still gain valuable information by conducting the mediation in the child's less proficient language.

c is incorrect and follows the same reasoning as the above choice.

6.5 Description of Disorder and Recommended Treatment

It is important to note that both HV's parents and teacher indicated concerns about his language abilities. HV's teacher likely compared HV to other bilingual first graders and noticed that he was not using either Spanish or English as competently as his peers. Likewise, HV's parents also noticed that he was not using Spanish in a manner that was consistent with their home and community expectations. For bilingual children, parents and teachers often provide reliable ratings of language performance.[6] Evidence from the story transcripts indicated that HV did not make much improvement from pretest to posttest in his inclusion of narrative components. Using only pretest measures may introduce bias into the assessment process for children from CLD backgrounds[2] especially when children are not familiar with an assessment task. Posttest measures following practice and mediation may better reflect language learning ability.[2] HV's performance at pretest was ≥ 1 SD below that of his bilingual first- and second-grade peers ($n = 24$) who also received mediation in English[4] on measures of productivity, including NDW, TNW, and TNU as compared to peer measures: NDW $M = 44.6 \pm SD = 19.6$; TNW $M = 124.3 \pm SD = 70.9$; TNU $M = 20.8 \pm SD = 9.1$. In Spanish, HV's inclusion of story components and his MLU were ≥ 1 SD below his peers on story components $M = 10.1 \pm SD = 0.9$ and MLU $M = 5.7 \pm SD = 0.9$. At posttest, HV's performance was below his peers (more than 1 SD below the norm) in both languages on narrative and productivity measures. Specifically, HV's total narrative score, story components, and measures of productivity, including TNW and MLU, were all below the performance of his bilingual peers: English total scores $M = 30 \pm SD = 7.9$; Spanish $M = 29.7 \pm SD = 7.6$; English story components $M = 11.2 \pm SD = 2.3$; Spanish $M = 11.4 \pm SD = 3.1$; English TNW $M = 139.4 \pm SD = 57.4$; Spanish $M = 132.3 \pm SD = 50.1$; English MLU $= M = 6.2 \pm SD = 1.2$; Spanish $M = 6.1 \pm SD = 1.3$. In English HV's story ideas and language were greater than 1 SD below his peers ($M = 14.5 \pm SD = 4.9$), although in Spanish, his inclusion of mental state verbs improved and thus his score on this measure was comparable to peers. HV did not appear to benefit from two sessions of mediation to improve narrative skills, while his typically developing peers improved. HV's performance at posttest was consistent with both parent and teacher concerns about his language.

With respect to modifiability, observations of HV's learning indicated difficulties predictive of LI (▶ Table 6.2). Difficulties with metacognition, flexibility, and task orientation are areas of modifiability that, with posttest measures, significantly increased correct classification of bilingual and CLD children with and without LI.[5] In terms of grammaticality, both pretest and posttest transcripts revealed high ungrammaticality in English and some ungrammatical utterances in Spanish. Grammatical errors in English included difficulty with third person, present tense, and copula and auxiliary omission "to be." In Spanish, HV's errors included gender and subject and verb number agreement, and omission of the auxiliary verb "estar."

The remediation plan for HV included bilingual intervention. Information gleaned from the MLE regarding HV's language learning should be employed to develop cognitive strategies for awareness and error recognition. In order to maximize progress in both languages, targets should be chosen to transfer across languages and improve language ability in both Spanish and English. Targets in both languages should include story grammar components of characters and setting with more description, the inclusion of initiating events, character plans to solve a problem, and attempts and outcomes to improve episode structure. To further improve story cohesion and sentence complexity, the use of words to mark the order of events and inclusion of causal information should be targeted. For example, targeting sentences that use "because" or "porque" to include causal information and relative clauses to give more detail about setting or character stimulate HV to use more complex utterances. Furthermore, HV did not use advanced or specific vocabulary. The inclusion of more detail when retelling stories should also help HV produce utterances with more specific vocabulary and more propositions. Grammatically, copula and auxiliary forms should be targets in both languages. HV was beginning to use past tense in Spanish and should be introduced to the past tense "ed" in English and contrasting that with the third person present form "s" morpheme.

6.6 Key Points

- Pretest and posttest in both languages can assess patterns in both languages.
- Observations during MLE should be incorporated into the treatment plan.
- Results from narrative assessment can guide intervention targeting grammar as well as vocabulary.

Table 6.2 Modifiability scores from MLE 1 and MLE 2

MLE components	Target	MLE 1		MLE 2	
		Score	Description	Score	Description
Internal social-emotional (affect)	Anxiety	1	Calm, little to no soothing required	1	Calm, little to no soothing required
	Motivation	3	Ambivalent, unsure about tasks	2	Curious, shows interest
	Tolerance to frustration	1	Persistent, wants to continue despite difficulty	1	Persistent, wants to continue despite difficulty
Cognitive arousal	Task orientation	2	Mostly understands tasks (75%)	3	Understands tasks some of the time (50%)
	Meta-cognition	2	Aware of most errors (75%)	3	Aware of some errors (50%)
	Nonverbal self-reward	1	Positive response to task regardless of difficulty	1	Positive response to task regardless of difficulty
Cognitive elaboration	Problem solving	2	Organized, but somewhat inefficient (<25% off task)	3	Sketchy plan, trial and error
	Verbal mediation	3	Talks occasionally	3	Talks occasionally
	Flexibility	3	Some evidence of more than one strategy and occasionally utilizes them	3	Some evidence of more than one strategy and occasionally utilizes them
External social-emotional (behavior)	Responsiveness to feedback	2	Positive but hesitant, requires some feedback	1	Very positive, maintains enthusiasm
	Attention	2	Focused, but distractible at times	2	Focused, but distractible at times
	Compliance	1	Cooperative	1	Cooperative

MLE, mediated learning experience.

Suggested Readings

[1] Miller J, Chapman RS. SALT for Windows-Research version 7.0. Madison, WI: Language Analysis Laboratory, Waisman Center, University of Wisconsin-Madison; 2002

[2] Miller J, Iglesias A. Systematic Analysis of English and Spanish Language Transcripts. Madison, WI: Language Analysis Laboratory, Waisman Center, University of Wisconsin-Madison; 2002–2004

[3] Squires KE, Lugo-Neris MJ, Peña ED, Bedore LM, Bohman TM, Gillam RB. Story retelling by bilingual children with language impairments and typically-developing controls. Int J Lang Commun Disord . 2014; 49:60–74

References

[1] Miller L, Gillam RB, Peña ED. Dynamic Assessment and Intervention: Improving Children's Narrative Skills. Austin, TX: Pro-Ed; 2001

[2] Peña ED, Gillam RB, Malek M, et al. Dynamic assessment of school-age children's narrative ability: an experimental investigation of classification accuracy. J Speech Lang Hear Res. 2006; 49(5):1037–1057

[3] Peña ED, Reséndiz M, Gillam RB. The role of clinical judgments of modifiability in the diagnosis of language impairment. Adv Speech Lang Pathol. 2007; 9:332–345

[4] Fiestas CE. The Dynamic Assessment of Narratives: A Bilingual Study. [doctoral dissertation]. 2008. Available at: http://www.lib.utexas.edu/etd/d/2008/fiestasc36454/fiestasc3645.pdf

[5] Peña ED, Gillam RB, Bedore LM. Dynamic assessment of narrative ability in English accurately identifies language impairment in English language learners. J Speech Lang Hear Res. 2014; 57(6):2208–2220

[6] Bedore LM, Pena ED, Joyner D, Macken C. Parent and teacher rating of bilingual language proficiency and language development concerns. Int J Biling Educ Biling. 2011; 14(5):489–511

7 Stuttering in Young Children

John A. Tetnowski

7.1 Introduction

The evaluation and management of stuttering is complex and several salient issues emerge. Primarily, parents frequently express uncertainty when a child begins to stutter and are unsure whether this speech pattern represents normal development or whether it warrants intervention. And upon the diagnosis of stuttering, parents are not sure whether they should intervene immediately, or wait to see whether the stuttering resolves over time. Finally, when parents wish to initiate treatment, they cannot find a "specialist" in their geographic area.

7.2 Clinical History and Description

GC was 2.5 years old and had been stuttering with "moderate-to-severe disfluencies" for 7 months according to his mother. She stated that he was advanced with "verbal expression," but she and her husband were quite concerned. Since there were no fluency specialists (FS) in her area, she reached out to an FS in another state and to a closed listserv associated with the Special Interest Group (SIG) on Fluency and Fluency Disorders in the American Speech-Language-Hearing Association. Through this outreach, GC's mother connected with the author for consultation via email and telephone. As an initial step, it was recommended that the mom record GC in several speaking conditions for review. Within 1 month, several short samples were made available to determine whether a complete assessment was indicated. In addition, GC's mother was also queried regarding his fluency. GC was an only child with an unremarkable birth and developmental history. He had one paternal uncle with a brief history of stuttering and recovery at a young age. In addition, GC's mother reported that GC is sometimes "stubborn" and has a "reactive temperament" (e.g., he is quick to get upset and slow to calm). In addition, GC's stuttering began just prior to his second birthday and although it varied since onset, GC's mother reported that his speech progressively worsened ("more bumpy" in his mother's words). GC had not received any previous therapy and was not particularly concerned by his stuttering. However, both parents expressed marked concern regarding his speech fluency.

7.3 Clinical Testing

As a result of the initial interactions, formal evaluation was recommended. GC and his mother drove approximately 3 hours for an evaluation of his speech and communication skills. GC cooperated completely. As suggested by his mother, his language was quite precocious for his age. GC interacted readily and completed all tasks. His articulation, voice, and language skills were subjectively judged to be within normal limits or even a bit advanced. As part of the assessment process, his speech was evaluated in several different settings and levels of linguistic demand. This information was elicited during a clinical assessment that included the use of several age-appropriate toys, pictures, and standardized tools. Tasks included naming and repetition tasks across various levels of length and linguistic complexity. The results of this assessment are presented in ▶ Table 7.1.

In addition to speech samples, a weighted stuttering-like disfluency (W-SLD) score, a formal stuttering assessment, specifically the Stuttering Severity Instrument-4 (SSI-4),[1] and an interview with GC's mother[2] were completed. GC obtained a W-SLD score of 35, an SSI-4 score of 24, which places him in the moderate severity range, and the interview revealed that both parents were greatly concerned about his stuttering and that they "wanted the 'best'" therapy for him. They also indicated that they did not know what to do when he stuttered and tried to not call it to his attention. Both parents were willing to "do whatever it takes" to get him through this period.

7.4 Questions and Answers for Reader

1. Based on the results of the clinical evaluation, this child's speech is:
   a) Normal for his age.
   b) Indicative of stuttering.
   c) Indicative of "normal" disfluencies.
   d) Unclear as to whether it is normal or abnormal.

Answer: a is incorrect. Stuttering frequencies in the range of 10% to 25% are abnormal. It is important to note that almost all of his nonfluencies are stuttering in nature. In some cases, a child may exhibit a large number of nonfluencies that are *not* stuttering. Almost all of GC's nonfluencies are stuttering. For example, the 25% level of stuttering at the one-syllable naming task is also the same as the overall level of nonfluency (also 25%). Thus, none of his nonfluencies were in the disfluency category.

b is correct. Stuttering is defined by the use of part-word repetitions, prolongations, blocks, and single-syllable word repetitions. High levels of stuttering across tasks (10%, 25%, etc.) are indicative of true stuttering. Distinction between stuttering and disfluency is critical.

c is incorrect. The clinician must differentiate between stuttering and disfluency. Disfluencies consist of multisyllabic word repetitions, phrase repetitions, interjections, revisions, incomplete phrases, and broken words.

d is incorrect. This child's speech is marked by true stuttering. The levels of stuttering are indeed outside of the normal range.

Table 7.1 Results of clinical testing for a 2.7-year-old child suspected of stuttering

Task	%SS	%nf	Dur	Type	
Single-syllable word naming	25	25	2 s	PWR	
Single-syllable word repetition	10	10	1 s	PWR	
Multisyllable word naming	10	12	2 s	PWR	PR
Multisyllable word repetition	5	5	2 s	PWR	
Dialogue with SLP	8.6	8.8	3 s	PWR	PR
Dialogue with parent	7.6	8.0	3 s	PWR	PR

Dur, duration of most typical stuttering; %nf, % of all nonfluencies (stuttered and nonstuttered types); %SS, % stuttered syllables; PR, phrase repetition; PWR, part-word repetition; SLP, speech-language pathologist; type, type of nonfluency.

2. Should therapy begin now or should the clinician offer an alternate choice?
   a) Begin direct treatment now.
   b) Begin indirect treatment now.
   c) Postpone treatment until age 3 years.
   d) Postpone treatment until he begins school.

Answer: a is correct. The child has been stuttering for over 6 months. Although it is possible that the child may spontaneously recover, the trend of "stuttering getting worse over time" indicates that persistent stuttering is a strong possibility.

b is incorrect. Although this answer is partially correct, in terms of beginning therapy now, early-intervention programs for young children like the Lidcombe Program, family-focused therapy, and parent–child interaction therapy are effective and efficacious. All of these programs use direct intervention strategies rather than simply modifying the environment as the primary means of treatment.

c is incorrect. This child has been stuttering for over 6 months and his stuttering is getting worse; these findings justify initiating treatment.

d is incorrect. This child has been stuttering for over 6 months and his stuttering is getting worse; these findings justify initiating treatment.

3. Which of the following are risk factors for "persistent" stuttering?
   a) He is an only child.
   b) He is male.
   c) He has an uncle who also stuttered.
   d) He has not been in previous therapy.

Answer: b is correct. Males are between 2 and 12 times more likely to stutter than females.

c is correct. A genetic history of stuttering is a risk factor for stuttering; this link does not have to be a sibling, but can be a parent, grandparent, or other relative.

a is incorrect. No evidence suggests that an "only child" is more likely to stutter than children with siblings.

d is incorrect. There is no evidence that being in previous therapy (or not) puts a child at a higher (or lower) risk for persistent stuttering.

4. If therapy is recommended, what is the best and most efficient type of intervention and in what format should it be administered?
   a) Indirect treatment from a local speech-language pathologist who is not an FS.
   b) Direct treatment from a local speech-language pathologist who is not an FS.
   c) Direct treatment from a distant speech-language pathologist who is an FS that the parent can drive the child to for therapy.
   d) Direct treatment from a distant speech-language pathologist who is an FS and is willing to provide distance therapy through video/teleconferencing.

Answer: d is correct. Recent research, specifically on the Lidcombe Program, suggests that distance intervention (e.g., webcam delivery) can be as effective and efficient as face-to-face therapy for young children who stutter.

a is incorrect. Indirect therapy has not been shown to be as effective as direct therapy for young children with persistent stuttering.

b is incorrect. The mother was not comfortable with the local options since none of them were board-certified specialists in fluency disorders.

c is incorrect. This is not the best answer. For this parent, the nearest board-certified FS was 3 hours of driving time away.

7.5 Description of Disorder and Recommended Treatment

GC presented with stuttering. Furthermore, positive "risk factors" for persistent stuttering included (1) significant stuttering across settings greater than 3%, (2) a high W-SLD score of 35, (3) male, (4) stuttering progressively worse for more than 6 months, (5) a reactive temperament, (6) a relative who stuttered, and (7) parental concern.

Since GC lived almost 3 hours away from an FS, it was recommended that the Lidcombe Program for Early Stuttering[3] be implemented via webcam. The Lidcombe Program for Early Stuttering is a behaviorally based intervention program that targets the elimination of stuttered speech through appropriate reinforcement for fluent speech. Much of this program is carried out by a parent trained by a speech-language pathologist. This program has been shown to be highly efficacious through multiple randomized control trials. The treating speech-language pathologist was trained through the Lidcombe Training Consortium. Recent evidence suggests that the Lidcombe Program has sufficient efficacy when implemented in this manner (i.e., through a webcam).[4] Treatment was scheduled for weekly sessions with daily practice at home to be mediated by GC's mother. Daily text messages were employed to track progress as well as address any problems or questions. Daily severity ratings (SRs) were also texted based on the level of complexity and demand of the assigned task(s). An SR was assigned to each task on a 10-point scale, with a score of 1 indicating *no stuttering* and a score of 10 indicating *very significant stuttering*. GC's parents were trained on this method to ensure agreement between the therapist and mother. As therapy continued, GC's love for books emerged and many therapeutic activities revolved around books and other enjoyable activities. One of the primary concepts underlying the Lidcombe Program is that therapy must be enjoyable and, after a short time, it was apparent that GC greatly enjoyed the individual time with his mother that often involved shared reading and interaction experiences.

Table 7.2 Results during "free conversation" task

Date	SR(Mom)	SR(SLP)	%SS
6/21/2016			9.8
6/28/2016	5	5	5.8
7/12/2016	6	5	4.9
7/19/2016	4	4	4.2
7/26/2016	6	6	6.8
8/2/2016	5	4	4.5
8/10/2016	3	2	2.2
8/23/2016	2	2	2.3
8/30/2016	2	2	2.3
9/6/2016	2	2	2.6
9/13/2016	2	3	2.4
9/20/2016	2	2	2.1
9/27/2016	1	1	1
10/4/2016	1	1	1
10/11/2016	1	1	0.9
10/18/2016	1	1	1
11/3/2016	1	1	1.15
11/8/2016	2	2	1.7
11/22/2016	1	1	0.17

%SS, % stuttered syllables; SR(Mom), severity rating by mom; SR(SLP), severity rating by speech-language pathologist.

7.6 Outcome

Over 18 sessions across 5 months, GC's stuttering decreased from 8.6% in dialogue to under 0.2%. The 18 sessions were approximately 1 week apart until success was apparent, and visits were then scheduled at biweekly intervals and eventually reduced to monthly. Therapeutic tasks were based on the level at which GC could interact and receive significant verbal rewards for "unambiguously stutter-free speech." These tasks and proper reinforcement were demonstrated for GC's mom to implement daily at home. The initial activity was a one-sentence, carrier-sentence completion task (e.g., This is a _____). As shown ▶ Fig. 7.1, GC maintained SR levels of 2 or less within a short time and maintained this level over extended periods.

GC progressed through two- and three-sentence tasks in a similar fashion and more online activities were eventually implemented. These activities included games, but as noted earlier, often revolved around shared-reading activities. These tasks included asking questions about a book after it was read to him and eventually progressed to GC telling a story about a book independently. Of note, books were never read verbatim to GC, but were paraphrased as he followed the pictures. In that regard, his storytelling was never memorization, but rather his interpretation of the story. He initially obtained an SR score of 3 and eventually progressed until he had 22 consecutive days with an SR of 1. In addition to SR scores, the percentage of stuttered syllables (%SS) was calculated during free conversation at the beginning of each session. The results are shown in ▶ Table 7.2, along with the SR score provided by both the treating speech-language pathologist and GC's mom.

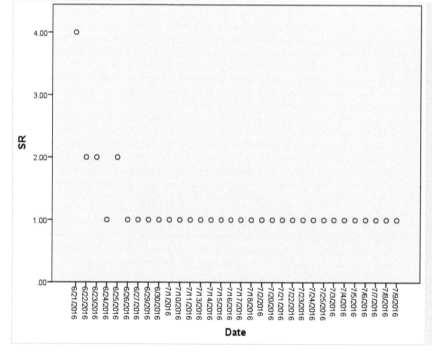

Fig. 7.1 Daily Severity Ratings (SR) over the course of treatment. SR of 1 indicates no stuttering and a score of 10 indicates very significant stuttering.

7.7 Key Points

- The risk for persistent stuttering is based on published risk factors.
- The awareness of the parents and their willingness to participate in treatment are critical to therapeutic success.
- A distance model of intervention may be effective when in-person sessions are infeasible.

Suggested Readings

[1] Bernstein Ratner N, Guitar B. Treatment of very early stuttering and parent-administered therapy: the state of the art. In: Bernstein Ratner N, Tetnowski JA, Eds. Current Issues in Stuttering Research and Treatment. Mahwah, NJ: Lawrence Erlbaum Associates; 2006:99–124

[2] Goodhue R, Onslow M, Quine S, O'Brian S, Hearne A. The Lidcombe Program of early stuttering intervention: mothers' experiences. J Fluency Disord. 2010; 35(1):70–84

[3] Ambrose NG, Yairi E. Normative disfluency data for early childhood stuttering. J Speech Lang Hear Res. 1999; 42(4):895–909

References

[1] Riley GD. Stuttering Severity Instrument 4th ed. Austin, TX: Pro-Ed; 2009.

[2] Westby CE. Ethnographic interviewing: asking the right questions to the right people in the right ways. J Child Com Dis. 1990; 13:101–112

[3] Packman A, Onslow M, Webber M, et al. The Lidcombe Program treatment guide. 2014 Available at: https://sydney.edu.au/health-sciences/asrc/docs/lp_treatment_guide_0314.pdf.

[4] Bridgman K, Onslow M, O'Brian S, Jones M, Block S. Lidcombe Program webcam treatment for early stuttering: a randomized controlled trial. J Speech Lang Hear Res. 2016; 59(5):932–939

8 Evaluation and Intervention for a Young Child with Severe Intellectual Disability

Billy T. Ogletree

8.1 Introduction

This case describes a communication evaluation and intervention sequence for BT, a 3-year-old boy with severe intellectual disabilities. BT's communication disorder is consistent with significant delay associated with severe intellectual impairment. Critical features of communication-based services are featured. Children with severe intellectual disabilities benefit from early intervention with a broad therapeutic focus on partners and environments.

8.2 Clinical History and Description

BT was delivered via cesarean section at 27-week gestation and presented as "small for date" with a familial history significant for intellectual disabilities. BT participated in a developmental follow-up clinic after an 8-week neonatal intensive care stay. He was initially identified as "low" tone and moderately hearing impaired. In addition, BT's extremely slow emergence of developmental milestones resulted in a team (including a speech-language pathologist [SLP]) diagnosis of severe intellectual disability at 8 months. Impaired vision was also suspected at that time.

BT received home-based early intervention conducted by an early interventionist working in conjunction with his parents. Efforts emphasized general development throughout much of BT's second year. The SLP involved in BT's initial diagnosis consulted with the early intervention specialist throughout this treatment. At 18 months, BT was rolling over, sitting, and reaching for objects with both hands. He was also wearing bilateral hearing aids and corrective glasses. BT looked at the faces of others and at objects of interest. By 24 months, he was reaching for objects with persistence and repairing failed communication attempts by adding vocalizations without consonants (primarily vowelized squeals). By 36 months, BT was standing and communicating to request and protest with reaches, vocalizations, and some aberrant behaviors. He received direct speech and language intervention services for 12 months and was referred for testing to create his Individualized Education Plan.

8.3 Clinical Testing

BT's assessment was tri-focused.[1] This framework pursued assessment targets relating to the child, his communicative partners, and relevant environments. BT's early care was coordinated by the early intervention provider network (IDEA Part C). On his third birthday, BT participated in a complete developmental/educational team evaluation conducted through his local school district. The team considered all areas of development including emergent communication. SLP evaluation was initiated by a review of BT's general records and consulting with team partners with respect to BT's sensory impairments. A pre-evaluation staffing with BT and his parents was then initiated. Specifically, BT's parents were questioned regarding communication goals. BT was also informally observed, and his parents agreed to attend and participate in communication testing by assisting with sampling and through some limited test administration. His parents also requested that information be shared as testing progressed. A questionnaire regarding BT's emergent language and general health and development was administered. BT's parents were also provided with the words and gesture form from the MacArthur Communicative Development Inventories (CDI)[2] with the instruction to complete the form prior to BT's formal evaluation.

BT's evaluation occurred in his home with his parents present. BT's hearing aids were confirmed to be in working order, and BT wore his glasses throughout the duration of the evaluation. BT's parents were instructed to initiate play in a typical manner. BT's parents brought favorite toys from BT's room and introduced them in a variety of games and routines. During these activities, BT and his parents were observed and data specific to expression of communicative intent, coordinated attention, affect, and play were recorded. Partner targets such as parent responsiveness to his emergent communication were also observed. After approximately 10 minutes, the SLP joined play and gradually introduced communicative temptations and play probes from the Communication and Symbolic Behavior Scales (CSBS).[3] BT's mother periodically assisted with temptation tasks, and data regarding learner and partner assessment targets were collected. The Communication Matrix[4] and the Communication Complexity Scale (CCI)[5] were completed. As materials were gathered and put away, the SLP shared observations from the assessment session and sought parental confirmation or clarification about their perceptions of BT's abilities as well as routine environments and parental perceptions of communication opportunities as a function of these settings.

BT's CSBS assessment (learner findings) revealed that he was an intentional nonsymbolic communicator who requested and protested with gestural forms (e.g., reaches) accompanied by vocalizations without consonants. He occasionally used behavior (e.g., pushes) to protest. His CCI scores ranged from 7 to 9, indicating the presence of triadic gaze and the use of communicative vocalizations and object reaching and offering. BT's Communication Matrix administration revealed level IV behaviors characterized by requests for objects with conventional communicative forms consistent with CSBS and CCI results.

Assessment of BT's partners revealed that some did not respond to his nonsymbolic communication attempts. BT's environmental assessment identified potential environmental modifications to increase communication opportunities.

8.4 Questions to the Reader

1. A tri-focused framework was implemented in this case. One clear benefit of this framework is that:
   a) It is immediately more cost-efficient.
   b) It addresses assessment from a broad-based inclusive perspective.
   c) It only provides objective data points for intervention planning.
   d) It only provides subjective data points for intervention planning.

Answer: b is correct. A tri-focused framework broadens the SLP's view of BT's communication by providing objective and subjective data on BT's learning abilities, the competence of his partners, and the communicative-friendliness of his environments. Data in each of these domains allow for a comprehensive intervention that is likely to result in intervention gains.

a is incorrect. Tri-focused assessment is likely to result in long-term savings but will be more immediately labor-intensive for BT's SLP.

c and d are incorrect. Tri-focused assessment generates both objective and subjective data.

2. Implementing a preassessment staffing provided:
   a) The opportunity to discuss parental involvement in the assessment process while making some early observations of BT.
   b) Time for the initiation of standardized testing.
   c) Specific information regarding BT's sensory status.
   d) Team members the opportunity to meet BT and his family.

Answer: a is correct. Preassessment staffing allowed for the determination of the aspirational expectations of the assessment process. It also provided a platform for the discussion of assessment roles for the parents and an opportunity to observe BT.

b is incorrect. No testing is conducted during preassessment staffing, rather it is a time for assessment planning and some initial observations.

c is incorrect. Although informal observations may assist with a better understanding of BT's sensory status, specific information would require testing or record review.

d is incorrect. The SLP conducted the preassessment staffing by herself with BT and his parents.

3. The MacArthur Communicative Development Inventories (CDI)[2] is
   a) An informant tool for parents to complete form specific to emergent communicative abilities.
   b) A structured communication sampling sequence for use by the SLP.
   c) An instrument for assessing emerging grammar.
   d) An instrument for a comparing play stages to emergent communication abilities.

Answer: a is correct. The CDI is an assessment instrument that allows parents to record emergent gestures, words, and early phrases.

b is incorrect. The CDI does not include a specific sampling sequence but instead allows parents to observe and record early communicative forms.

c is incorrect. Although the CDI allows for recording of emergent phrases, it does not target more advanced grammar.

d is incorrect. The CDI does not address emergent play.

4. Both the Communication and Symbolic Behavior Scales (CSBS)[3] and the Communication Matrix[4] were administered. These two measure are similar in that:
   a) They were specifically designed for children presenting with severe intellectual deficits.
   b) They involve clinician-directed communication sampling.
   c) They were designed for children communicating at the presymbolic to emergent symbolic levels.
   d) They assess play.

Answer: c is correct. Both measures were designed to assess presymbolic to emergent symbolic communication.

a is incorrect. The Communication Matrix was designed to assess the specific communication abilities of persons with severe disabilities.

b is incorrect. The Communication and Symbolic Behavior Scales includes clinician-directed communication sampling.

d is incorrect. The Communication and Symbolic Behavior Scales specifically assesses emergent play.

8.5 Description of Disorder and Recommended Treatment

Initially, BT presented as a child with a significant developmental delay possibly attributed to his shortened gestation and small presentation at birth (i.e., Intrauterine Growth Restriction).[6] BT's diagnosis became more clear with the familial presence of intellectual impairment and as the gap in his developmental status and chronological age widened. His dual sensory impairment also provided diagnostic clarity. In sum, the most appropriate diagnosis for BT was severe intellectual disability. This diagnosis occurs under neurodevelopmental disorders in DSM-5 and is used when significant measured intellectual and adaptive deficits are present within the developmental period.[7]

Prelinguistic Milieu Teaching (PMT) with parent responsivity training[8] was determined to be an appropriate therapeutic strategy. PMT utilizes turn-taking within typical routines. As expectancy is established, routine interruptions are interjected to create communicative opportunities, and prompt sequences are employed to solicit intentional communicative acts. Given BT's use of requests and protests, initial treatment efforts focused on expansion of communicative behaviors to include comments and/or greetings. BT's occasional use of behaviors communicatively could also be addressed through PMT. That is, conventional communicative means such as gestures or vocal behaviors could be targeted as replacements for any aberrant forms.

PMT is a preferred treatment choice for children emerging into nonsymbolic intentional communication.[9] It has empirical support for children with intellectual disabilities, and its effectiveness can be enhanced with parental involvement.[10] In BT's case, parental training included a focus on routine creation and milieu instructional strategies as well as emphasis on recognizing and responding to nonsymbolic communication. Parental involvement within everyday environments makes PMT a tri-focused friendly intervention option.

8.6 Outcome

After 6 months of intervention, BT had expanded his intentional communication to include nonsymbolic commenting and greeting expressed through distal gestures (e.g., points and waves). This broadened his communicative repertoire and provided increased social opportunities. BT also had replaced existing aberrant behaviors previously used to communicate (pushes) with a more appropriate head nod paired with vocalizations. BT's treatment would now shift to expanding his requesting behavior vertically through the introduction of symbol forms such as objects and photographs. Objects and photographs will also now be used in schedules to assist with daily transitions.

Finally, in this same time frame, BT's parents and other stakeholders participated in the creation of gesture dictionaries to assist with the recognition of nonsymbolic forms. Communication opportunities had also been infused into most of his daily life environments creating practice for nonsymbolic communicative behavior.

8.7 Key Points

- Evidence supports positive outcomes for young children with disability who receive early intervention services.[11]–[13] Of course, these services are most effective when utilizing evidenced-based practices.
- The larger focus on partners and environments provided a broad platform for intervention likely to promote meaningful change.
- The ability to communicate for more purposes will make BT a more successful communicator and will contribute a more positive perception of his communicative competence.

Suggested Readings

[1] Brady NC, Bruce S, Goldman A, et al. Communication services and supports for individuals with severe disabilities: Guidance for assessment and intervention. Am J Intellect Dev Disabil. 2016; 121(2):121–138

[2] Snell ME, Brady N, McLean L, et al. Twenty years of communication intervention research with individuals who have severe intellectual and developmental disabilities. Am J Intellect Dev Disabil. 2010; 115(5):364–380

[3] Hebbeler K, Spiker D, Bailey D, et al. Early intervention for infants & toddlers with disabilities and their families: participants, services, and outcomes. Final report of the National Early Intervention Longitudinal Study (NEILS). 2007. Available at: http://www.sri.com/neils/pdfs/NEILS_Report_02_07.pdf

[4] Warren SF, Fey ME, Finestack LH, Brady NC, Bredin-Oja SL, Fleming KK. A randomized trial of longitudinal effects of low-intensity responsivity education/prelinguistic milieu teaching. J Speech Lang Hear Res. 2008; 51(2): 451–470

References

[1] Siegel-Causey E, Bashinski S. Enhancing initial communication and responsiveness of learners: a tri-focus framework for partners. Focus Autism Other Dev Dis. 1997; 12(2):105–120

[2] Fenson L, Marchman VA, Thal DJ, Dale PS, Reznick JS, Bates E. MacArthur-Bates Communicative Development Inventories: User's Guide and Technical Manual. 2nd ed. Baltimore, MD: Brookes; 2007

[3] Wetherby AM, Prizant B. Communication and Symbolic Behavior Scales. Baltimore, MD: Paul H. Brookes; 2001

[4] Rowland C. Communication Matrix. 2009. Available at: www.communicationmatrix.org

[5] Brady NC, Fleming K, Thiemann-Bourque K, et al. Development of the communication complexity scale. Am J Speech Lang Pathol. 2012; 21(1):16–28

[6] Resnik R. High-risk pregnancy series: an expert's view. Obstet Gynecol. 2002; 9(3):490–496

[7] American Psychiatric Association. Diagnostic and Statistical Manual of Mental Disorders: DSM-5. Washington, DC: American Psychiatric Association; 2013

[8] Yoder PJ, Warren SF. Effects of prelinguistic milieu teaching and parent responsivity education on dyads involving children with intellectual disabilities. J Speech Lang Hear Res. 2002; 45(6):1158–1174

[9] Warren SF, Yoder PJ. Facilitating the transition from preintentional to intentional communication. In: Wetherby A, Warren SF, Reichle J, Eds. Transitions in Prelinguistic Communication. Baltimore, MD: Paul H. Brookes; 1998:365–384

[10] Fey ME, Warren SF, Brady NC, et al. Early effects of responsivity education/prelinguistic milieu teaching for children with developmental delays and their parents. J Speech Lang Hear Res. 2006; 49:526–547

[11] Bailey DB, Jr, Hebbeler K, Spiker D, Scarborough A, Mallik S, Nelson L. Thirty-six-month outcomes for families of children who have disabilities and participated in early intervention. Pediatrics. 2005; 116(6):1346–1352

[12] Hebbeler K. First five years fund briefing. Presentation given at a Congressional briefing on June 11, 2009, to discuss Education that works: The impact of early childhood intervention on reducing the need for special education services. Available at: http://www.sri.com/neils/pd fs/FFYF_Briefing_Hebbeler_-June 2009_test.pdf

[13] Hebbeler K, Spiker D, Bailey D, et al. Early intervention for infants & toddlers with disabilities and their families: participants, services, and outcomes. Final report of the National Early Intervention Longitudinal Study (NEILS). 2007. Available at: http://www.sri.com/neils/pdfs/NEILS_Report_02_07_Final2.pdf

9 Assessment and Treatment of a School-Aged Speech Sound Disorder

Kelly Farquharson

9.1 Introduction

This case reviews the complex issues associated with persistent speech sound disorders in a child. In particular, this case highlights the importance of considering decoding and spelling skills while assessing and treating school-aged children with speech sound disorders.

9.2 Clinical History and Description

B is a 9-year-old boy who just began fourth grade. He has received school-based speech-language therapy services since kindergarten for remediation of a speech sound disorder. In kindergarten, many speech sounds were problematic, but he is now only targeting the /r/ sound. Recently, B's fourth grade teacher reported that he has very poor spelling and will not read aloud in class. She initially thought B was shy, but now reports that he clearly has difficulty decoding words. Although B's current speech therapy sessions focus only on /r/ sound production, this report from his teacher suggested that additional testing was indicated to determine whether his speech sound disorder impacted his literacy skills.

9.3 Clinical Testing

Clinical testing must go beyond traditional articulation testing. B's assessment battery examined speech production (Goldman–Fristoe Test of Articulation, 3rd Edition [GFTA-3][1] and speech sample), receptive and expressive language (Clinical Evaluation of Language Fundamentals, 5th Edition [CELF-5][2]), word decoding (Woodcock Reading Mastery Test, 3rd Edition [WRMT-3][3]), and spelling abilities (Test of Written Spelling, 5th Edition [TWS-5][4]). All measures have a mean standard score of 100 with an average range of 85 to 115. Results of the standardized assessments are presented in ► Table 9.1.

B's receptive and expressive language abilities were within normal limits. Interestingly, his GFTA-3 score was only slightly below normal limits as is often the case with older children with one speech sound error. B's speech sample also revealed distortions and substitutions with the /r/ phoneme in all word positions. His /r/ error was quite obvious and, although intelligibility was not greatly impacted, it is clear that he is aware of, and embarrassed by, this aspect of his speech.

Two subtests from the WRMT-3 were administered: word identification and word attack. The word identification subtest requires reading of decontextualized real words that increase in complexity as the test advances. The word attack subtest requires phonemic decoding of nonwords. The

stimuli words follow the rules of English, but do not carry meaning. As such, this subtest examines the ability to apply knowledge of letter–sound correspondence. The results of the two subtests are combined to create an overall composite, which was below the average range in B's case. B's score on the word identification subtest indicated that he had some sight word skills, but he experienced difficulty decoding more complex word structures. This finding was substantiated by the word attack subtest, which revealed moderate impairment in the use of letter–sound correspondence for decoding. This deficit is particularly relevant as B is in fourth grade and interacts with novel and advanced vocabulary in most academic subjects.

Finally, the TWS-5 was administered to quantify B's spelling abilities. His score was below normal limits. In his written narrative, he produced multiple spelling errors as well as missing and incorrect punctuation and capitalization. His spelling errors comprised 38% of his writing sample. Importantly, his errors were reflective of letter substitutions that mapped onto his current speech production errors (e.g., "w" written in place of "r," or "r" omitted in vocalic contexts). Additional errors reflected an immature knowledge of letter–sound correspondence (e.g., "wach" instead of "watch"), many phonetic spellings (e.g., "educashun" instead of "education"), and homophone confusion (e.g., "two" vs. "to"). Collaboration with the teacher further corroborated that these types of errors are pervasive in B's spelling on classroom-based measures.

Table 9.1 Results of Brandon's speech, language, and literacy assessments

Construct	Assessment (subtest)	Standard or scaled score
Speech sound production	GFTA-3	83
Receptive and expressive language	CELF-5	103
	Sentence comprehension	10
	Word structure	11
	Recalling sentences	10
	Formulating sentences	9
Word reading	WRMT-3	80
	Word identification	87
	Word attack	76
Spelling	TWS-5	77

CELF-5, Clinical Evaluation of Language Fundamentals, 5th Edition; GFTA-3, Goldman–Fristoe Test of Articulation, 3rd Edition; TWS-5, Test of Written Spelling, 5th Edition; WRMT-3, Woodcock Reading Mastery Test, 3rd Edition.

9.4 Questions and Answers for the Reader

1. Should services be provided to a fourth grade student who has difficulty with only the /r/ sound?
   a) No, because this deficit does not adversely affect educational performance.
   b) Yes, but only if the parent requests services.
   c) No, because if he cannot produce the sound by fourth grade, he will likely never produce it.
   d) Yes, because it may be impacting educational performance and that will vary for each case.

Answer: d is correct. The American Speech Language Hearing Association (ASHA) and the U.S. Department of Education have clearly indicated that an adverse impact on educational performance should be determined on a case-by-case basis. Blanket policies that suggest that a single speech sound error does not create educational impact are not appropriate. As evidenced by this case, a connection between a speech sound disorder and literacy is common.

a is incorrect. The evidence in the case supports that B is experiencing difficulties within the classroom. Although his speech sound disorder may be considered "mild," it has evolved into a disorder that is impacting his reading and spelling abilities.

b is incorrect. According to the Individuals with Disabilities Education Act (IDEA) as well as the ASHA Scope of Practice documents, children with communication impairments are entitled to services that can assist them in accessing the classroom curriculum.

c is incorrect. Children are able to make progress in speech sound production past the fourth grade. Certainly, for older children, it is more challenging for the child and the clinician to make a change in speech production. However, like any child, B deserves the opportunity to make this change and to acquire the necessary skills for classroom success.

2. Why might B be experiencing difficulties with spelling in fourth grade?
   a) He has weak alphabet knowledge.
   b) He has not developed the appropriate phonological and orthographic representations.
   c) He was never taught letter–sound correspondence.
   d) He has an underlying language impairment.

Answer: b is correct. It is very likely that B experienced limitations in the development of phonological representations, which leads to difficulty mapping sounds to letters. This deficit could be a result of a persistent speech sound disorder. However, causal directionality of this relation is unclear.

a is incorrect. As a fourth grader, B is able to identify letters of the alphabet, but is unable to complete the orthographic mapping necessary for accurate word decoding.

c is incorrect. we cannot assume that B was or was not taught any specific skill. We can only make clinical judgments based on his current performance on tasks.

d is incorrect. B's language scores were normal.

3. Why is it important to test B's receptive and expressive language if there does not appear to be a weakness in those areas?
   a) It is possible that, after years of a speech sound disorder, language can become weak over time.
   b) A language impairment would ensure he gets the services that he needs.
   c) It is not important to test receptive and expressive language.
   d) It is a common practice to test receptive and expressive language.

Answer: a is correct. For some children with speech sound disorders, language is normal early in elementary school. However, over time, expansion of language skills in children with severe or persistent speech sound disorders may be reduced, particularly if literacy skills are impacted. This deficit is primarily related to an impaired phonological system; thus, the connection between phonemes and graphemes is a challenging concept. As that system progresses, problems with word reading and spelling are likely to evolve. The less a child reads or practices spelling, the likelihood of issues with semantics and morphosyntax skills is increased.

b is incorrect. Children should receive the services that they need, regardless of the area of communication that is impacted.

c is incorrect. Language can become weakened over time in the presence of a speech sound disorder. Furthermore, as classroom demands increase, language requirements become more complex. As such, it is crucial to ensure that language abilities are age appropriate.

d is incorrect. There are theoretical and clinical reasons why testing language is important. Although it is a common aspect of a communication evaluation, the choice to test language should be clinically and empirically driven.

4. What is the recommendation for a speech-language pathologist (SLP) who does not have access to standardized tests of reading and spelling?
   a) Use clinical judgment to guess a child's reading and spelling skills.
   b) Collaborate with a classroom teacher, reading specialist, or school psychologist.
   c) Examine the child's classroom tests and assignments for patterns of strength and weakness.
   d) Both b and c.

Answer: d is correct. It is often the case that the appropriate test(s) are not available. Collaboration with relevant service providers is encouraged. It is also clinically meaningful to examine what the child has produced in the classroom. An analysis of decoding and spelling patterns can be determined using classroom materials and can also lend insight into how the student is functioning in the classroom.

a is incorrect. Although newer clinicians are being training in reading and spelling assessments and interventions, it is never appropriate to guess. Collecting data from the child, the teacher, the parent(s), and the environment are the best ways to make informed clinical decisions.

b alone is incorrect. Collaboration can be difficult due to time constraints or the fluctuation of an itinerant clinician's schedule. Although collaboration is strongly encouraged, the SLP should be able to supplement that information with his/her own assessment of the child's classroom performance.

c alone is incorrect. Although this approach is an appropriate method to examine how a child is functioning within the classroom, it is best that the SLP is able to pair this information with other data from the classroom teacher or related service professionals.

9.5 Description of Disorder and Recommended Treatment

B's diagnosis was persistent speech sound disorder, as evidenced by continued difficulty achieving appropriate articulation. In particular, B continued to exhibit difficulty with the production of the /r/ phoneme. Although B's speech sound disorder was limited to one phoneme, the disorder impacted his literacy skills in the areas of decoding and spelling. Thus, he experienced difficulty accessing fourth grade curriculum as (1) his speech production was unclear and, although not unintelligible, certainly noticeable and distracting to his peers and teachers, (2) he was unwilling to read aloud in class due to social embarrassment related to a persistent speech sound disorder, (3) he was experiencing difficulty decoding words due to poor phonological and orthographic representations, and (4) he was experiencing difficulties in spelling because his letter–sound correspondence was affected by the persistent speech sound disorder.

Treatment was altered to target both expressive (i.e., speech sound) and receptive (i.e., decoding and spelling) phonological skills. Specifically, sessions focused on not just phoneme production but also his knowledge of the linguistic use of those phonemes. Therapy materials included curriculum-based vocabulary and spelling words ranging in complexity from second to fourth grade levels. Where appropriate, B highlighted the /r/ phoneme within a word so that he could practice correct speech production skills on highly relevant words that he was likely to see in the classroom. Therapy activities included phonological awareness (e.g., rhyming, blending, and phoneme deletion), phonics (e.g., letter manipulation, orthographic knowledge), and morphological awareness (e.g., explicit instruction of prefixes and suffixes). Tasks related to these three areas, employing vocabulary and spelling words from his curriculum, provided repeated practice identifying sounds and letter similarities and differences. Importantly, therapy activities were contextualized (e.g., no flashcards) in hopes of generalizing speech production and letter–sound skills to decoding and spelling opportunities in other settings.

9.6 Key Points

- In this case, the speech sound disorder appears to be more complex than difficulty with speech sound production.
- Continued difficulty with speech sound production throughout a child's academic experience is likely to lead to difficulties with literacy skills (e.g., decoding and spelling).
- The connection between phonology and literacy is an intimate one; children with weak phonological representations often experience difficulty with mapping phonemes onto graphemes.
- For all children with speech sound disorders, early phonological awareness and reading skills should be monitored to avoid persistent reading and spelling issues later in elementary and middle school.

Suggested Readings

[1] Foy JG, Mann VA. Speech production deficits in early readers: predictors of risk. Read Writ. 2012; 25(4):799–830

[2] Lewis BA, Avrich AA, Freebairn LA, et al. Literacy outcomes of children with early childhood speech sound disorders: impact of endophenotypes. J Speech Lang Hear Res. 2011; 54(6):1628–1643

[3] Lewis BA, Freebairn LA, Taylor HG. Correlates of spelling abilities in children with early speech sound disorders. Read Writ. 2002; 15(3–4):389–407

[4] Raitano NA, Pennington BF, Tunick RA, Boada R, Shriberg LD. Pre-literacy skills of subgroups of children with speech sound disorders. J Child Psychol Psychiatry. 2004; 45(4):821–835

References

[1] Goldman R, Fristoe M. Goldman–Fristoe Test of Articulation. 3rd ed. Circle Pines, MN: Pearson; 2009

[2] Semel E, Wiig EH, Secord WA. Clinical Evaluation of Language Fundamentals. 5th ed. Circle Pines, MN: Pearson; 2013

[3] Woodcock R. Woodcock Reading Mastery Test. 3rd ed. Circle Pines, MN: Pearson; 2011

[4] Larsen SC, Hammill D, Moats L. Test of Written Spelling. 5th ed. Austin, TX: Pro-Ed; 2013

10 Assessment and Treatment of Pediatric Dysphonia with a Complex Medical History

Abigail L. Rosenberg

10.1 Introduction

Dysphonia refers to "abnormal pitch, loudness, and/or vocal quality resulting from disordered laryngeal, respiratory, and/or vocal tract functioning".[1] The prevalence of dysphonia in the pediatric population ranges from 1.4% to 6.0%.[2]

10.2 Clinical History and Description

EB was an 8-year-old girl who presented with a breathy voice, low volume, and difficulty being heard at home and school. Vocal quality had been consistent since she began speaking. EB described feeling "winded" while speaking and needed to breathe every few words. She was adequately hydrated and rarely engaged in concerning vocal behaviors. EB's medical history included extreme prematurity, prolonged intubation as an infant, chronic lung disease, repaired patent ductus arteriosus (PDA), and paralyzed right diaphragm status post plication.

10.3 Clinical Testing

Clinical testing was completed in conjunction with an otolaryngologist to assess laryngeal function and voice quality. Flexible laryngoscopy revealed false vocal fold compression with phonation and mild arytenoid tilt. The true vocal folds were smooth and straight with no obvious immobility; however, due to false vocal fold squeeze, complete glottic closure could not be fully visualized. Microlaryngoscopy, bronchoscopy, and laryngeal electromyography (EMG) were then completed, revealing acquired grade I posterior subglottic stenosis and normal vocal fold innervation with full closure (▶ Fig. 10.1).

Acoustic analyses included fundamental frequency for sustained vowels and connected speech, pitch range, and maximum phonation time. Frequency measures were within the normal range for EB's age/sex. Pitch range was restricted at the upper register (262.26–601.44 Hz), and maximum phonation time was significantly lower than anticipated (5.91 vs. 14–17 seconds).

Perceptual measures of voice quality were completed using the Consensus Auditory Perceptual Evaluation of Voice (CAPE-V), which judges the voice on overall severity, roughness, breathiness, strain, pitch, and loudness (▶ Fig. 10.2). EB presented with a moderate rating for overall severity and breathiness and mild ratings for the remaining parameters. EB also participated in stimulability trials to test therapy techniques targeting enhanced vocal quality, reduced laryngeal tension, and improved breath support.

10.4 Questions and Answers for the Reader

1. Based on EB's presentation, there was concern for vocal fold immobility, prompting completion of a laryngeal EMG. Which of the following cranial nerve branches would negatively impact vocal fold mobility if damaged, and what in EB's medical history would cause concern for damage of this nerve?
   a) Trigeminal nerve.
   b) Hypoglossal nerve.
   c) Recurrent laryngeal nerve (branch of vagus nerve).
   d) Pharyngeal branch of vagus nerve.

Answer: c is correct. The recurrent laryngeal nerve innervates all intrinsic laryngeal muscles except the cricothyroid. Damage to this nerve would weaken or paralyze the affected side, resulting in breathiness, hoarseness, or weak vocal quality. EB's medical history is significant for PDA repair, which is a cardiac surgery. The left recurrent laryngeal nerve loops under the aorta, making it vulnerable to injury during heart surgery.

a is incorrect. The trigeminal nerve innervates muscles related to jaw movement. Damage may impact articulation and chewing.

b is incorrect. The hypoglossal nerve innervates the majority of muscles in the tongue. Damage may cause tongue deviation and muscle wasting.

d is incorrect. The pharyngeal branch of the vagus nerve innervates many muscles of the pharynx and soft palate. Damage to this branch may negatively impact resonance and/or swallowing.

2. Voice disorders can negatively impact a child's education. What is one reason why this may be?
   a) Children with voice disorders typically have co-occurring learning impairments.
   b) Children with voice disorders may have limited participation in classroom activities.
   c) Children with voice disorders have frequent illnesses and often miss school.
   d) Children with voice disorders typically have co-occurring hearing loss and so cannot hear classroom instructions.

Answer: b is correct. Spoken communication is critical to classroom learning. Children may self-limit class participation to hide their voice disorder, which may reduce the amount of practice or feedback they receive.

a is incorrect. While children with learning disabilities may also have voice disorders, the two are not directly correlated.

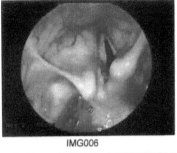

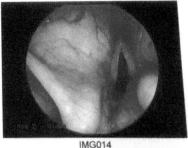

IMG006

IMG014

IMG015

IMG019

Fig. 10.1 Microlaryngoscopy and bronchoscopy images (with permission of Karen B. Zur).

c is incorrect. While some voice disorders may have underlying medical influences, children with voice disorders are not more likely to miss school due to illness.

d is incorrect. It is possible that children with conductive hearing loss due to middle ear fluid may speak loudly, which could result in vocal fold damage. Generally, there is not a high co-occurrence of hearing loss and voice disorders.

3. Based on EB's clinical presentation, which of the following would be an appropriate treatment recommendation?
   a) Resonant voice therapy.
   b) Surgical intervention (for vocal folds).
   c) Pushing/pulling adduction exercises.
   d) Indirect intervention only, such as vocal hygiene.

Answer: a is correct. Resonant voice therapy aims to unload tension from the vocal folds, with emphasis on easy vibrations further up in the vocal tract such as the mouth and nose. Resonant voicing is often produced with "vocal folds that are barely touching or barely separated," resulting in a stronger, clearer voice with minimal vocal fold impact stress. It also requires "the least amount of lung pressure to vibrate the vocal folds." This is appropriate for EB, as it can help achieve an improved vocal quality while reducing strain and without requiring high lung volume.

b is incorrect. Microlaryngoscopy and laryngeal EMG revealed normal vocal fold innervation and normal laryngeal function and motion; therefore, surgical intervention for the vocal folds would be inappropriate.

c is incorrect. These exercises can be beneficial for individuals with weak vocal fold closure and quiet, breathy voice. However, they can also result in increased strain and tension. As EB presented with strain and false vocal fold squeeze with phonation, this would not be recommended.

d is incorrect. Vocal hygiene is an important component of voice intervention, as it helps create healthy voice habits and serves as a foundation for direct therapy. While it can be beneficial on its own, its effectiveness is reduced compared to voice hygiene plus direct voice therapy. As EB successfully achieved an improved vocal quality using trial techniques during the assessment and demonstrated few negative vocal behaviors, her treatment should not be limited to vocal hygiene alone.

10.5 Description of Disorder and Recommended Treatment

EB presented with moderate dysphonia characterized by breathiness, perceptual component of strain, reduced breath support, and low volume. She frequently spoke on inhalation, which negatively impacted her ability to be heard. Vocal quality was not appropriate for her age/sex. Voice therapy was recommended to address breath support, identification and use of appropriately timed breathing breaks within longer sentences or songs, and use of forward focus and resonant voicing to reduce strain. In addition to voice therapy, physical therapy was recommended to help increase trunk strength in relation to breath support.

Specific therapy techniques to target improved voice quality and strain reduction emphasized the use of forward focus voicing. EB used kazoos, noise makers, straw phonation, and humming to unload tension from her vocal folds and establish forward focus. These activities were motivating and brought attention to feelings of vibration around her nose and lips. They also provided immediate auditory and sometimes visual feedback as to whether successful voicing was achieved. For example, forward focus voicing created a fuller kazoo sound and increased airflow through the straw, which was used to move a tissue across the table. As EB became successful with these techniques, external materials were faded and she practiced producing words, phrases, and then sentences while still maintaining the targeted voice placement. Breath support and timing were addressed by establishing a consistent breathing pattern and pairing breathing exercises with motivating voice tasks including tongue twisters, jokes, and popular song lyrics.

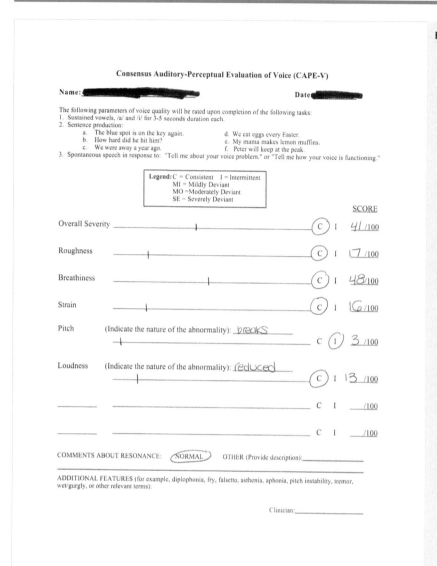

Fig. 10.2 Initial assessment CAPE-V results.

10.6 Outcome

EB participated in weekly voice therapy across several months and progressed toward achievement of all goals. Her breath support improved with phrases and eventual carry-over to structured conversation. She also established appropriate breaks to reduce inhaled phonation. She initially benefitted from reading passages and marking of appropriate breathing breaks; at completion of therapy, she appropriately timed breaks without cuing during structured tasks in 80% of opportunities, with improvement noted during semi-structured tasks and conversation. EB participated in resonant voice therapy and use of forward focus. Gains were notable within structured tasks, with some carry-over to conversation given clinician cuing. She successfully maintained forward focus to produce sustained nasal syllables, to chant nasal syllables with changing intonation, to produce nasal phrases, and to read short passages. She also completed weekly home exercises regarding breath support and vocal quality.

Reevaluation was completed following therapy. EB presented with significantly improved, though persistent, mild-moderate dysphonia. Pitch range was within expectations and CAPE-V measurements were improved for all parameters. EB demonstrated greatly improved breath support, including identification of more appropriate breathing breaks to reduce instances of inhaled phonation. EB's parents and teachers reported that she was more easily heard. Some variability in volume and vocal quality persisted, particularly during extended conversations. She demonstrated the knowledge and skills required to achieve efficient voicing with adequate loudness and breath support.

10.7 Key Points

- Pediatric voice disorders are common and can negatively impact a child's ability to be heard and understood.
- Collaboration with an otolaryngologist is necessary to identify any underlying physical dysfunction related to a voice disorder, and to make appropriate recommendations.
- Children can participate in direct voice therapy and should not be limited to indirect intervention, such as vocal hygiene, based on age alone.

- Treatment for voice disorders often includes a combination of techniques to address various symptoms and/or causes.

Suggested Readings

[1] National Center for Voice and Speech 1998. Available at: https://www.ncvs.org/freebooks/vocologyguide.pdf

[2] Hooper CR. Treatment of voice disorders in children. Lang Speech Hear Serv Sch. 2004; 35(4):320–326

11 Augmentative and Alternative Communication in a Child with Congenital Porencephaly

Jill E. Senner

11.1 Introduction

Pediatric neurodevelopmental disorders can result in multiple impairments affecting cognition, motor skills, hearing, and vision. In some cases, children may not be able to communicate using natural speech. Augmentative and alternative communication (AAC) can support these children with complex communication needs.

11.2 Clinical History and Description

JF was a 30-month-old boy referred for AAC evaluation to identify strategies and assistive technology to improve his ability to communicate. He had been receiving early intervention services, but his expressive communication remained limited to two sign approximations (more and eat) and making choices between objects presented in a field of three by reaching with his left hand.

Brain abnormalities were detected on a 20-week ultrasound and labor was induced at 37 weeks of gestation due to concerns about JF's lack of growth. Labor was complicated by fetal heart rate decelerations and nuchal cord. At birth, JF was diagnosed with congenital porencephaly, which resulted in quadriplegic cerebral palsy (CP) and cortical visual impairment (CVI).

JF lived at home with his mother and father, although his paternal grandparents frequently assisted with his care. English was the only language spoken in the home. JF was not yet sitting alone or crawling. He was reportedly dependent on a care-giver for all activities of daily living. He had a Zippie IRIS manual wheelchair for mobility but was dependent on a care-giver to push it. Occupational therapy and physical therapy reports obtained noted that JF demonstrated decreased muscle strength and poor head control. He was reported to consistently attempt to use his left hand to play and assist in functional activities.

JF underwent surgery at 24 months to correct strabismus in both eyes; however, his left eye still turned inward. He had diagnoses of CVI, nystagmus in both eyes, and strabismic amblyopia in the left eye at the time of the assessment, and glasses were prescribed. JF's hearing was within normal limits.

The report from his primary speech-language pathologist indicated that JF babbled using open-mouth vowel sounds, bilabials /m/ and /w/, and sometimes /g/. He demonstrated the ability to vary his intonation and pitch. He cried to protest or when upset.

11.3 Clinical Testing

Assessment occurred over two visits and included an AAC Intake Questionnaire, caregiver interview, observation, testing, and device trials. During the evaluation sessions, JF was smiling and engaged. Upon arrival, he responded to a greeting by waving his left hand. When asked to follow commands within his motor capabilities (e.g., "look up"), he did so upon request. An open mouth posture with intermittent drooling was noted at rest. During the sessions, JF produced an approximation of the sign for "eat" (he put his fist near his mouth) to request a snack and smiled while moving his head slightly upward (paired with a vocalization) to indicate acceptance of the food item offered. His mother presented him with pureed and mechanical soft foods. She reported that he was unable to masticate crunchy or chewy foods. Some anterior loss of material was noted due to poor lip closure. JF reached toward toys presented with his left hand.

The Prelanguage Inventory from Evaluating Acquired Skills in Communication, Third Edition (EASIC-3, an inventory designed for children with developmental disabilities), was administered using a combination of testing, observation, review of records, and informant interview. JF's mother and paternal grandfather served as informants. JF's receptive skills were as follows: he turned his head to attempt to locate environmental sounds, turned his head and smiled in response to voice, consistently inhibited when told "no" in a normal voice, demonstrated comprehension of several common objects (e.g., cup, crayon and paper, toothbrush, toy car, tissue), responded to 4/4 commands (to show/give me) with gestures involving an object, responded to verbal commands with gestures, and demonstrated the ability to match 4/4 identical objects. Receptive skills were consistent with the 24-month developmental level. In addition, JF demonstrated appropriate symbolic play (e.g., he pretended to cook with toy pots and pans, tried to feed a baby doll) and he manipulated objects to achieve a desired outcome (e.g., he operated a variety of large-button and switch-adapted toys). Expressive communication was limited. JF produced a sign approximation (eat) to gain adult attention to obtain a desired food item out of reach, used eye gaze to get assistance (e.g., he stopped trying to open a container and looked at the evaluator for several seconds), produced a sign approximation of "more" (putting his hands together) to indicate recurrence, rejected items by shaking his head "no," accepted items by smiling and looking upward, initiated a greeting by waving to his grandfather upon entry to the room, and reached for desired items. JF demonstrated difficulty indicating basic needs (e.g., he had no way to request "drink" so he refused food until a caregiver presented him with a drink, he cried to indicate physical discomfort) and was unable to request actions or objects out of his immediate reach. ▶ Table 11.1 provides a summary of JF's nonverbal communication.

The Visual Identification section of the AAC Evaluation Genie iPad app was used to evaluate JF's ability to visually track and identify a single icon from 5″ to 1″ in size. AAC Evaluation Genie is an informal diagnostic tool that is intended to assist with identifying skill areas that relate to the language representation

Table 11.1 EASIC-3 functions of nonverbal communication

Score	Function of communication	Items	Comments or examples
+	Requests for objects	24, 25	Reached toward desired toys
+	Requests of action	25, 26	Signed "more"
+/E	Calling/attention	13, 14	Signed "eat," gazed at evaluator for assistance
+	Rejection/negation	19, 20	Shook head "no," refused food (turned head away)
+	Affirmation	19	Smiled and looked upward (occasionally included a vocalization)
+	Recurrence	26	Signed "more"
+	Greeting	21	Smiled, waved

+, present in spontaneous nonverbal communication; +/E, spontaneous in elicited nonverbal communication.

methods commonly found on augmentative communication systems. On this informal probe, JF used the three middle fingers on his left hand to access the iPad. He was 50% accurate in selecting 5" buttons from a field of two using direct selection. His accuracy dropped to 25% in a field of four. Due to chance accuracy using direct selection with his left hand, alternate access methods were trialed using high-interest, low-cognitive demand activities (e.g., switch-accessible iPad and computer games). Eye gaze was attempted on an available SGD (speech-generating device), but was not effective likely due to his nystagmus. Similarly, optical head pointing was not accurate due to poor head control. Two-switch step-scanning was then attempted. In this access method, two switches were placed vertically, one to the right and one to the left of JF's left hand. The green switch on the left was used to "move" between items presented and the red switch to the right of his hand was used to make selections on an iPad app. Following modeling, JF demonstrated emerging understanding of the functions of both switches; however, his accuracy was 50% from a field of 15.

Partner-assisted auditory and visual scanning was done on pages printed out from an SGD. During partner-assisted scanning, a communication partner points to (or holds up) each symbol while saying each word or phrase, "scanning" through the child's choices. JF appropriately smiled to affirm and occasionally shook his head "no" to reject items presented. During a play-based activity (bubbles), JF independently selected "go" several times as well as "more" and "want" at appropriate times during the activity.

11.4 Questions and Answers for the Reader

1. What conclusion can you draw about the appropriateness of AAC interventions for this child based on the description provided?

a) JF is unable to communicate using his natural speech alone, therefore AAC is appropriate.

b) JF is too cognitively impaired to use an AAC system.

c) JF cannot point accurately and alternate access methods are not mastered at this time, therefore JF is not an appropriate candidate for AAC.

d) JF cannot use an AAC system due to his visual impairments.

Answer: a is correct. According to the National Joint Committee for the Communication Needs of Persons with Severe Disabilities (NJC), all individuals with severe expressive communication impairments that interfere with the development of oral language should have access to AAC systems or devices to promote effective communication.

b, c, and d are incorrect. According to the NJC, "the currently accepted evidence in the literature suggests that no specific skills are prerequisite for successful use of AAC in the broadest sense."

2. What therapeutic intervention strategies would be most appropriate for JF at this time?

a) Use of partner-assisted scanning with a light tech paper-based system.

b) Motor training to improve two-switch step-scanning skills.

c) Use of a light tech paper-based communication system for immediate communication needs plus motor training to more complex skills required for adaptive access.

d) AAC is not appropriate for this child.

Answer: c is correct. "A longitudinal program designed to meet the person's immediate communication needs with a number of readily accessible approaches, which also 'invests in the future' through a systematic motor or speech therapy program to train more complex skills, may be fruitful and ultimately, more balanced".[1] This is referred to as a "balanced approach to intervention or parallel training."

a is incorrect. Although JF needs a system to meet his immediate communication needs, abandoning motorically complex options completely would not prepare JF for use of an SGD in the future.

b is incorrect. Although JF needs practice to improve his access, waiting to provide a means of communication until this is mastered would delay access to language opportunities.

d is incorrect. According to the NJC, all individuals with severe expressive communication impairments that interfere with the development of oral language should have access to AAC systems or devices to promote effective communication.

3. What features would need to be present in an SGD for JF?

a) Auditory cues or previews.

b) Indirect access methods.

c) Core vocabulary.

d) All of the above.

Answer: d is correct. JF required a system with a large amount of vocabulary to meet his current and developing language needs, as well as auditory cues due to his poor vision and alternate access (i.e., scanning) options due to his limited fine motor skills.

4. What type of training (if any) should JF's caregivers receive?
   a) Caregivers do not require any special training.
   b) Caregivers should only be trained in operating the device (e.g., turning it on/off, programming messages).
   c) Caregivers should be trained in operating the device and in modeling use of the device.
   d) Caregivers should join an online group so they can ask other parents of children using SGDs for advice when needed.

Answer: c is correct. Parents must have sufficient skills in operating the communication system, the language of the device, and strategies for reinforcing communication (e.g., modeling and responding to children's communication) to support children learning to use an AAC system.

a is incorrect. Recent analyses of communication partner training programs suggest that there is consistent evidence that communication partner instruction not only improves the skills of communication partners but also has a positive impact on the communication of people who use AAC.[2] Parents are the primary communication partners for their young children and they need training in operating the device as well as ways to integrate use of the device into naturally occurring activities.

b is incorrect. Parents do need to know how to operate the device; however, they also need to know how to support communication with the device.

d is incorrect. Parent and family support has been identified as a contributor to positive outcomes for individuals who use AAC; however, information from online groups may not be always accurate or relevant.

11.5 Description of Disorder and Recommended Treatment

JF's CP affected his oral motor skills for both feeding and communication. His phonemic repertoire was severely limited and he was unable to produce oral speech, characteristic of severe dysarthria. JF had receptive language skills at approximately the 24-month level, but his nonverbal expressive skills were limited. At 24 months, children typically have 200- to 300-word expressive vocabularies and are using short, incomplete sentences. In this case, a clear discrepancy evolved between what JF understood and what he could communicate.

A feature-matching process was completed in which JF's skills were matched to features of available SGDs. JF required a system with dynamic display and a large amount of vocabulary to meet his current and developing language needs, as well as auditory cues due to his poor vision and alternate access (i.e., scanning) options due to his limited fine motor skills. Three devices with these features were trialed during the assessment sessions, and the most appropriate synthetic speech, dynamic display SGD was obtained through the state lending library for a 6-week trial period. A core vocabulary that included some phrase-based branches was selected that allowed for a balance of novel sentence construction and quick messages. Concurrently, a printout of the device screens provided JF an immediate means of communication when accessed via partner-assisted scanning and nonverbal yes and no responses. In addition, weekly diagnostic speech therapy commenced to (1) teach the language of the communication system, (2) improve JF's two-switch step scan-

ning skills in a variety of high-interest, lower-cognitive demand iPad and computer games, and (3) instruct communication partners how to operate JF's technology and to support his communication in the home environment. Communication progress was monitored via language sampling.

In therapy, JF participated in a number of play-based activities designed to improve language skills using his book and SGD. During the trial period, JF smiled and vocalized excitedly when provided with opportunities to communicate using his book and device. Objective measures indicated that JF used his communication book to generate a number of action + object phrases to request objects and actions (e.g., "play music," "eat yogurt," "drink milk," "go outside,"), used two-word combinations to greet communication partners (e.g., "good morning + mom"), terminated activities (e.g., "all done," "stop"), and expressed feelings (e.g., "hungry," "tired").

Two-switch step-scanning training was provided throughout the trial period using a combination of high-interest, low-cognitive demand games as well as opportunities for operation of the SGD during play-based activities. JF's accuracy increased to 60% in a field of 15 during the trial period. On the communication device, JF generated similar messages on occasion; however, they were often interspersed with unintended messages due to decreased accuracy.

The success of an interaction between a child using AAC and a communication partner depends heavily on the skills of the partner. Being an effective communication partner of a child using AAC often requires parents to change long-established ways of communicating. Because JF spent most of his waking hours with his mother and grandfather, both caregivers were trained in operating the book and device and they also received instruction in partner-augmented input (PAI), a modeling strategy whereby communication partners use the child's AAC system themselves by pointing to the symbols on the child's communication board or device while simultaneously talking.

11.6 Outcome

Based on data collected during the 6-week trial period, the SGD was recommended for purchase. JF continued to benefit from weekly therapy to improve his language and use of two-switch step-scanning. An occupational therapist provided consultation regarding optimal switch placement to improve JF's access, and JF's grandfather fabricated a switch mount based on her recommendations (see ▶ Fig. 11.1).

Six months after the assessment, JF began a blended preschool program with both students with disabilities and neurotypical peers. School staff were trained to provide PAI throughout JF's day using an eight-step training model.[3] JF continued to be a multimodal communicator, using a combination of signs, vocalizations, a light tech book, and a synthetic speech, dynamic display SGD. He was a very social and engaging child who continued to eagerly expand his communication skills.

11.7 Key Points

- There are no specific prerequisites for AAC use.
- Intervention that balances a child's immediate communication needs with systematic therapy to teach more complex skills is appropriate for young children with CP.

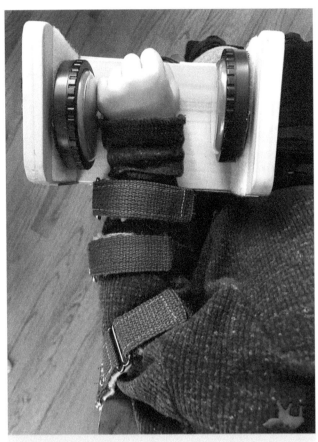

Fig. 11.1 Switch mount.

- Feature matching is a systematic process by which a child's strengths, abilities, and needs are matched to available tools and strategies and can aid in the selection of an appropriate SGD.
- Parent instruction should be viewed as an essential part of AAC assessment and intervention and should be routinely provided upon receipt of an SGD.

Suggested Readings

[1] National Joint Committee for the Communication Needs of Persons with Severe Disabilities (NJC). Augmentative and alternative communication. Available at: http://www.asha.org/NJC/AAC

References

[1] Beukelman D, Mirenda P. Augmentative and Alternative Communication: Supporting Children and Adults with Complex Communication Needs. 4th ed. Baltimore, MD: Paul H. Brookes; 2013

[2] Kent-Walsh J, Murza KA, Malani MD, Binger C. Effects of communication partner instruction on the communication of individuals using AAC: A meta-analysis. Augment Altern Commun. 2015; 31(4):271–284

[3] Senner JE, Baud MR. The use of an eight-step instructional model to train school staff in partner-augmented input. Commun Disord Q. 2017; 38 (2):89–95

12 The Importance of Reassessment following a School-Based Individualized Education Plan (IEP) Referral: A Case of Cluttering

Jenna Battipaglia

12.1 Introduction

In the public school setting, speech-language pathologists (SLPs) are faced with large caseloads of students who have often been evaluated by other professionals. The optimal approach when treating a new student is to conduct a thorough assessment to ensure accuracy and consistency of previous diagnoses and goals prior to the initiation of treatment.

12.2 Clinical History and Description

MA was an 11.4-year-old monolingual English-speaking girl with exposure to Arabic. She just entered sixth grade and was in a general education classroom setting with an individualized education plan (IEP) for Special Education Teacher Support Services (SETSS), as well as speech-language therapy twice a week in a group of three students. According to the IEP, MA had received speech and language services since Kindergarten. MA's IEP classification was "learning disability" and, according to her teacher, she was reading at a second grade level and was frequently getting in trouble for "calling out, disrupting class, and talking back to the teacher." It was also noted that MA's handwriting was "messy" and that she spoke at an increased rate, causing her to be unintelligible to both familiar and unfamiliar listeners 80% of the time. MA's speech and language goals primarily focused on organizing thoughts and ideas to increase verbal and written expression, increasing spelling/grammar/punctuation skills, and answering WH questions with supporting details to increase reading comprehension.

12.3 Clinical Testing

During MA's initial speech and language therapy session, an informal assessment was performed, including reading grade-level text, answering WH questions, writing a paragraph following a prompt, and playing a "getting to know you" game with other students in the group and the clinician. Throughout the session, MA called out, interrupted the other group members, and required redirection to task. MA had noticeable difficulty reading aloud and answered two out of five WH (What and Who) questions correctly. MA's written paragraph included phonemic transpositions, omitted words and letters, little to no punctuation, spelling errors, and an overall disorganized structure and hard-to-read handwriting. During the "getting to know you game," MA had difficulty taking turns with communication partners, maintaining topics, sustaining attention, and controlling impulses. She consistently displayed tachylalic (fast rate) speech, which included phonemic transpositions as well as articulation errors, repetition of multisyllabic words and

phrases, telescoping (over-coarticulating), monotone prosody, and maze behaviors (revisions or repetitions). MA appeared to lack awareness of these features.

Following the initial session, data were reviewed and analyzed. Although the receptive and expressive language goals included in MA's IEP, as well as attention concerns, were consistent with the clinician's findings, parameters of fluency, voice, and pragmatic language were not considered in her current treatment plan. The clinician also contacted MA's mother who reported that MA has "always been like this" and "no one ever mentioned that her fast rate of speech was something we should address."

The Predictive Cluttering Inventory or PCI[1] was then administered. The PCI is an informal checklist addressing the following domains of communication: Pragmatics, Speech-Motor, Language Cognition, and Motor Coordination–Writing Problems. Items within each parameter are rated on a scale of 0 (*never*) to 6 (*always*). Scores from each section are then added together to obtain the total score. The PCI was completed by the SLP as well as the SETSS and classroom teachers. PCI scores of 120+ are indicative of cluttering, scores between 80 and 120 are indicative of coexisting stuttering and cluttering, and scores below 80 suggest no fluency disorder.

12.4 Questions and Answers for the Reader

1. What is cluttering?
    a) Speech presenting as difficult to understand.
    b) Speech is characterized by incorrect productions and disorganization.
    c) Speech produced at an extremely fast rate.
    d) Speech with the inclusion of words that are unnecessary or meaningless without the speaker's awareness.
    e) All of the above.

Answer: e is correct. Cluttering is dysfluent speech characterized by an extremely fast rate, which is often difficult to understand. Cluttering also contains incorrect productions and disorganization, with the inclusion of words that are unnecessary or meaningless without the speaker's awareness.

a is incorrect. Speech presenting as difficult to understand is only one characteristic of cluttering. Alone, this could be attributed to other speech or language disorders and would require further assessment and referral to specialists.

b is incorrect. Speech characterized by incorrect productions and disorganization is only one characteristic of cluttering. Alone, this could be attributed to other speech or language disorders and would require further assessment and referral to specialists.

c is incorrect. Speech produced at an extremely fast rate is only one characteristic of cluttering. Alone, this could be attributed to other speech or language disorders and would require further assessment and referral to specialists.

d is incorrect. Speech containing the inclusion of words that are unnecessary or meaningless without the speaker's awareness is only one characteristic of cluttering. Alone, this could be attributed to other speech or language disorders and would require further assessment and referral to specialists.

2. Which speech characteristics did the clinician attribute to cluttering?
    a) Phonemic transpositions, exposure to Arabic, unintelligibility, impulsivity.
    b) Poor reading comprehension, disorganized writing, impulsivity, grammatical errors.
    c) Impulsivity, unintelligibility, tachylalia, lack of awareness.
    d) Impulsivity, poor topic maintenance, difficulty with turn-taking, difficulty sustaining attention.

Answer: c is correct. Impulsivity, unintelligibility, tachylalia, and lack of awareness are the most salient features of cluttering listed earlier. The clinician took these characteristics into account when deciding to administer the PCI.

a is incorrect. A client's exposure to or speaking of another language has no correlation with the presence of cluttering.

b is incorrect. Although concomitant features, these characteristics alone are not indicative of cluttering.

d is incorrect. Although concomitant features of cluttering, impulsivity, poor topic maintenance, difficulty with turn-taking, and difficulty sustaining attention are all indicative of pragmatic language and attention issues when presented alone, people who clutter exhibit one or more features within the following areas: language, pragmatics, cognition, speech, and motor.

3. What do you predict MA's PCI scores will be?
    a) Below 80; no fluency disorder present based on the case history and presenting features.
    b) Between 80 and 120; coexisting stuttering and cluttering based on the case history and presenting features.
    c) 120+; classic cluttering based on the case history and presenting features.
    d) This test is not necessary to administer based on the case history and presenting features.

Answer: c is correct. 120+; this is a classic case of cluttering based on the case history and presenting features.

a is incorrect. There is a clear presence of fluency disorder based on tachylalia, unintelligibility, and repetition of multisyllabic words and phrases.

b is incorrect. While there may be features consistent with stuttering, it is not clear from the case history and assessment information that this is truly the case.

d is incorrect. The PCI is necessary to administer based on the case history and presenting features. It is better to administer a test or checklist than subjectively rule out a possible disorder.

4. How will MA's treatment plan be affected if the diagnosis of cluttering is confirmed?
    a) MA's treatment plan will not be affected if diagnosis of cluttering is confirmed.
    b) MA's treatment plan will be adjusted to add a cluttering goal to her current group speech therapy sessions.
    c) MA's treatment plan will be adjusted to add visual cues for slowed speech rate and overarticulation within the classroom setting.
    d) MA's treatment plan will include an additional speech-language therapy session mandate, additional IEP goals targeting self-awareness, decreased rate, and varying prosody, as well as collaboration with and education for the team and reinforcements in the classroom as well as in the home.

Answer: d is correct. MA's treatment plan will include an additional speech-language therapy session mandate, additional IEP goals targeting self-awareness, decreased rate, and varying prosody, as well as collaboration with and education for the team and reinforcements in the classroom as well as in the home. If diagnosis of cluttering is confirmed, not only will the clinician add an individual speech therapy session as well as cluttering-specific goals but also include collaboration with and education for the entire team. This increased collaboration will include both the special education and classroom teachers, as well as MA's mother. This collaboration will include reinforcement in the classroom as well as at home as an aid in the achievement and generalization of MA's treatment goals.

a is incorrect. MA's treatment plan will be affected if diagnosis of cluttering is confirmed.

b is incorrect. It will be necessary for MA to have an additional individual speech session to address her new cluttering goals.

c is incorrect. While it will be necessary to add cluttering reinforcement within the classroom setting, this will not be the only addition to her treatment plan.

12.5 Description of Disorder and Recommended Treatment

MA's PCI scores were 161, 162, and 176 on the Pragmatics, Speech–Motor, Language Cognition, and Motor Coordination–Writing Problems domains, respectively, confirming that MA presented with cluttering as well as symptoms consistent with attention deficit hyperactivity disorder (ADHD). MA's checklists contained several "*always*" scores of 6. These features contributed to her learning, speech, and reading/writing delays, as well as difficulties in the classroom. A referral was also made to a pediatric neurologist to further evaluate impulse control and high levels of distractibility. Prognosis for improvement of cluttering features was good, pending increased awareness and support of therapy techniques in the classroom and home.

The clinician added goals to the IEP to address these issues, including reduced rate of speech, increased cluttering awareness, and varying prosody. An individual speech and language treatment session, in addition to MA's current speech and language group session, was implemented within the IEP to specifically address cluttering. MA's updated treatment plan included auditory biofeedback and discrimination tasks as well as verbal and visual cueing techniques.

MA's treatment plan involved cooperation from the entire team to support and generalize speech and language goals within the classroom. The SLP provided education regarding cluttering to the SETTS and classroom teachers, as well as MA's mother. In addition, strategies, such as slowed speech rate, overarticulation, and increased prosody, and cues, such as visual (e.g., a picture of a turtle to cue slower speech rate) and verbal (e.g., "Remember your 'turtle talk'!") were proposed in all contexts, such as the speech room, classroom, and at home. It was also suggested that MA increase reading at home while listening to an audiobook at half speed using her finger or tracking implement to increase awareness of tachylalic rate and reading comprehension skills.

12.6 Outcome

Since implementing MA's new treatment plan, success was noted in several areas. Auditory biofeedback and discrimination of her own productions significantly increased her awareness within the first month of treatment. Her speech rate during reading and conversational speech improved, and she was understood by unfamiliar listeners 60% of the time. MA's SETSS and classroom teachers reinforced strategies in the classroom, which increased MA's awareness in all contexts within the school setting.

MA's mother facilitated a pediatric neurology assessment and MA was diagnosed with ADHD. Methylphenidate-based sustained release (10 mg) was initiated, which resulted in decreased impulsivity and disruptions within the classroom and speech group setting. This increase in focus was associated with improved reading comprehension and organization of verbal and written expression. Although MA was previously unaware of cluttering features interfering with daily communication, as her awareness increased, so did her confidence. She was no longer complacent in receiving lower marks on assignments and sought to do better in her schoolwork.

MA's mother reported changes at home, including implementing a structured 30-minute "reading time" every evening, which she and her daughter enjoyed together, as well as MA's increased awareness during all conversations with family members of her speech rate. MA also demonstrated more willingness to "sit down and do homework after school," which had been a daily struggle for the family.

12.7 Key Points

- Often small components of speech or language difficulty are symptoms or characteristics of a larger issue.
- Conduct an initial informal assessment when treating a new client, even if an existing treatment plan is already in place.
- Seek collaboration with team members and family to reinforce therapeutic goals across contexts.
- Parent/caregiver and team education is an important and necessary role of the speech-language therapist.

Suggested Readings

[1] St. Louis K, Hinzman A. Studies of cluttering: perceptions of cluttering by speech-language pathologists and educators. J Fluency Disord. 1986; 11:131–149

[2] Manning WH. Clinical Decision Making in the Diagnosis and Treatment of Disorders. Albany, NY: Delmar Publishers; 1996

References

[1] Daly DA. Predictive Cluttering Inventory (Measurement Instrument). 2006. Available at: http://associations.missouristate.edu/ica/Translations/PCI/daly-cluttering2006.pdf. Last accessed March 31, 2016

13 Prioritizing Communication Supports for an Adolescent with Intellectual Disability

Paul W. Cascella, Lisa A. Simpson, and Christine Hagie

13.1 Introduction

Families and educational teams (e.g., special and general educators, speech-language pathologists, and school psychologists) often find it difficult to prioritize speech therapy goals and communication services for school-age young adults with moderate-to-severe intellectual disabilities. Multiple options exist and may include a particular focus on (1) next-step developmental milestones, (2) ensuring communication opportunities and environmental supports, (3) actualizing functional communication across daily routines, and (4) practicing communication skills associated with adult employment and living.

13.2 Clinical History and Description

LH was a 16-year-old adolescent diagnosed with severe intellectual disability requiring extensive support and assistance to participate in home and school routines. His hearing was within normal limits. He had mild myopia, corrected with glasses. His birth, medical, and health histories were unremarkable. At the time of assessment, LH was enrolled in general education academic classes and one elective (drama), and participated in community-based instruction one afternoon per week. He could work for approximately 25 minutes on familiar tasks and enjoyed collecting car magazines, bowling, eating lunch, and watching others play basketball and handball. His individualized education plan (IEP) included goals related to socialization, community awareness, speech-language skills, and assistive technology (via occupational therapy).

13.3 Clinical Testing

LH's communication was evaluated for several consecutive hours during homeroom, academic classes, lunch, and an occupational therapy session via interview, observation, and direct interactions. His mother was also interviewed via telephone in addition to his special education teacher, math teacher, and occupational therapist. Direct interaction included incidental treatment strategies to determine their utility for enhancing communication (i.e., dynamic assessment tasks). No standardized speech-language tests were administered, in part, because none include students like LH in the normative sample. Instead, a communication profile was constructed to identify receptive skills, expressive forms and functions, and the partner strategies that enhanced communication. Rating scales were referenced, including the Functional Communication Profile-R,[1] the Communication Matrix,[2] and the Augmentative and Alternative Communication Profile.[3]

13.3.1 Receptive Skills

LH identified the names of familiar people, objects, and activities. He also acted on one-step, context-specific verbal directions. LH responded to his own name and the meaning conveyed in a speaker's tone of voice. He associated objects with specific routines (i.e., his backpack represented school) and he identified pictures of familiar people and objects. His mother and teachers commented that he understood the steps associated with daily routines, but did not always comply with adult directions. In addition, LH's attention span and comprehension varied based on his interest in an activity.

13.3.2 Expressive Communication

LH utilized a variety of communication functions. He labeled familiar objects, commented (i.e., "wait," "your turn"), greeted, and conveyed farewell. He requested attention, people, action, discontinuation, help, and reoccurrence. He asked questions ("you stay lunch?"), directed people ("don't touch"), and expressed physical state ("hungry," "pain"). LH protested, made choices, and communicated emotional state (i.e., happy, angry). LH sometimes initiated communication and attempted to repair communication breakdowns by repeating the same message and actions. With regard to communication forms, LH vocalized, produced one to three-word sentences ("let's go," "right there," "no"), and had a core spoken vocabulary of about 100 words, including people's names, object labels (i.e., "puppy," "ice cream," "TV," "juice," "movies"), and context-specific social words (i.e., "hi," "yeah," "oh shit," "wow"). LH occasionally imitated single-word models. He used body orientation, whole body actions, and head nods/shakes. His gestures included reaching, showing, pointing, a high-five, waving, and pushing toward/away. LH used 15 modified sign language words and although he previously used a low-tech voice output communication aid, it was not observed. LH sometimes used physically aggressive behaviors and social withdrawal to communicate his unwillingness to participate in daily routines.

13.3.3 Communication Supports

Several communication supports enhanced LH's communication. He imitated words ("LH, say…"), and he responded to verbal prompts (i.e., "tell me what you want") and verbal encouragement (i.e., "I like that you told me…"). LH was more verbal when others used an upbeat tone of voice and verbal enticements (i.e., talking up an activity so that it sounded extra special). LH responded to some phonetic cues (i.e., modeling the first sound of a word) and a cloze (fill-in-the-blank) procedure. For example, when a teacher said "it's time for snack, let's get the _____," LH could fill in the word "juice." He benefited from transition comments that told him about upcoming activities and he used a daily routine photograph schedule. His peers and teachers were observed to readily interpret LH's idiosyncratic actions by stating these interpretations. LH benefitted from extra time to answer questions and comply with requests. He responded to verbal choices and imitated some sign language models paired with key spoken words.

13.4 Questions and Answers for the Reader

1. At age 15, an IEP was revised to eliminate objectives that focused on concept identification (i.e., colors, shapes, and size), mean length of utterance, and speaking with plural markers (i.e., book vs. books) and adjectives. This shift meant that the new IEP had less emphasis on:
   a) Communication forms and functions.
   b) Situational employment objectives.
   c) Partner's behaviors.
   d) Content-form-use objectives.
   e) Developmental objectives.

Answer: e is correct. These skills are milestones expected during childhood communication development.

a is incorrect. Forms are modes of expression (i.e., words, gestures, and body orientation) and functions are reasons for communication (i.e., to protest, request, and direct others).

b is incorrect. Situational employment objectives are task-specific skills.

c is incorrect. Partner's behaviors state how others support LH's communication.

d is incorrect. While there are content and form objectives, there are no pragmatic skills in LH's original IEP.

2. Which of the following assessment activities is the most relevant for a 16-year-old with Down syndrome and severe intellectual disability?
   a) An oral motor exam and diadochokinetic rates to estimate functional intelligibility skills.
   b) An observation of the student during recess activities to estimate social communication skills.
   c) Administration of the verbal subtest of the Wechsler Adult Intelligence Scale to estimate expressive language.
   d) Standardized testing with the Test of Pragmatic Language to measure social communication skills.
   e) Standardized testing with the Goldman–Fristoe Test of Articulation to measure functional intelligibility skills.

Answer: b is correct. A recess observation enables the clinician to gather information about social communication among peers; the clinician can identify initiation skills, overt communication actions, responses to others' communication, and naturally occurring communication successes and breakdowns.

a is incorrect. Neither an oral motor exam nor diadochokinetic rates estimate functional intelligibility skills.

c is incorrect. Given this student's degree of intellectual disability, an updated result from the Wechsler will only confirm already known information.

d is incorrect. The Test of Pragmatic Language requires more verbal comprehension skills than typically evidenced by persons with severe intellectual disability.

e is incorrect. The Goldman-Fristoe Test of Articulation measures baseline articulation skills but not functional intelligibility skills.

3. You receive a referral for a 19-year-old student who says about 20 single words. She is very social and well-liked by her peers. A prior assessment report noted that her vocabulary, morphology, and syntax are at the 18-month level, consistent with her diagnosis of severe-to-profound intellectual disability. Her educational team recommends a low-tech voice output device to enhance expressive communication. Which of the following actions is a likely first step before introducing the student to the device?
   a) The student could practice identifying, via discrete picture-identification tasks, the vocabulary words that will be programmed on the device.
   b) The student could practice shaping her right index finger into a pointing motion while looking at herself in a mirror.
   c) The student's teachers could show her how to sequence two picture cards.
   d) The student's teachers could create a list of messages that she might want to communicate.
   e) The student could practice clear pronunciation of the words that will be programmed on the device.

Answer: d is correct. It is important to consider the student's perspective prior to programming her communication device.

a is incorrect. The student is less likely to learn vocabulary words when they are practiced in a decontextualized setting without naturally occurring reinforcement.

b is incorrect. The student is less likely to learn a pointing gesture when it is practiced in a decontextualized setting without naturally occurring reinforcement.

c is incorrect. Picture sequencing is a developmental task that implies the student will follow a typical developmental trajectory, something less likely given her age and degree of intellectual disability.

e is incorrect. Pronunciation practice is not related to using a voice output communication device.

13.5 Description of Disorder and Recommended Treatment

Young adults with severe intellectual disability require a variety of communication supports to participate in educational, home, and community activities. For LH, a communication supports framework identified his abilities and how he could be encouraged to actualize these skills through the actions of his communication partners. For some families and educational teams, this model is confusing, as it states that someone like LH has communication skills, albeit atypical. Less emphasis is placed on describing LH as disordered or speech-language impaired. The model shifts intervention responsibility from the speech-language pathologist to family members, teachers, and peers. In doing so, the model emphasizes the quantity and quality of others' actions while they assist him to actualize his skills. Finally, the communication supports model pays less attention to LH's developmental communication age (27 months) and the development of next-step sequential objectives (i.e., skills expected at 28–34 months). Instead, it identifies how LH communicates in specific situations and what others can do to provide him with support, especially during communication breakdowns.

13.6 Outcome

LH's team held a series of meetings to decide how (1) his communication partners could be trained in a communication supports model, and (2) his IEP could be modified to focus on practical communication skills at school and in future community work and living. For the former, the team reviewed LH's communication profile and discussed how they could incidentally embed strategies into his routine. For the latter, the team used the Brigance Transition Skills Inventory and increased LH's exposure to community situations during school hours.[4] In the community, team members also attempted to identify (1) the communication demands of specific settings, and (2) whether LH's current skills were sufficient or needed support. LH's communication was relatively unchanged since the team shifted to the current plan. In contrast, his mother and team reported that they changed how they think and act about his communication. For example, LH practiced remaining quiet while riding public transportation, a skill that team members did not previously consider. He continued to use his photograph orientation schedule, but with photos that represented community activities. In addition, his teacher provided him with fewer verbal directions to encourage problem solving within communication breakdowns.

13.7 Key Points

- A communication supports model advocates identifying current skills and how others can support these skills during daily routines.
- Direct speech-language intervention is a lower priority for older students with severe intellectual disability. Communication programs and supports are not the sole responsibility of a speech-language pathologist.
- Families and team members have a vested interest in communication skills and should be encouraged to provide incidental supports during daily routines.

Suggested Readings

[1] Downing JE. Teaching Communication Skills to Students with Severe Disabilities. 2nd ed. Baltimore, MD: Paul H. Brookes; 2005
[2] National Joint Committee for the Communication Needs of Persons with Severe Disabilities. 2016. Available at: http://www.asha.org/NJC/. Last accessed May 7, 2016

References

[1] Kleinman LI. Functional Communication Profile. Austin, TX: LinguiSystems; 2003
[2] Rowland C. The Communication Matrix. 2016. Available at: http://www.communicationmatrix.org/. Last accessed May 7, 2016
[3] Kovach TM. Augmentative and Alternative Communication Profile. Austin, TX: LinguiSystems; 2009
[4] Brigance AH. Brigance Transition Skills Inventory. North Billerica, MA: Curriculum Associates; 2010

14 Language Impairment in a Child with Suspected Fetal Alcohol Spectrum Disorder

Mohamed (Mo) Oshalla

14.1 Introduction

Fetal alcohol spectrum disorder (FASD) is a neurological disorder caused by in utero alcohol exposure. It is commonly perceived as an acquired brain injury. Various physical and neuropsychological sequelae of the disorder manifest themselves as a result of exposure to alcohol at any time during pregnancy, with different windows during fetal development being affected in different ways. As a spectrum disorder, severities vary, and some persons with FASD do not show the physical characteristics typically associated with more severe presentations, such as a thin upper lip or flat philtrum, among other facial features. However, common features of many individuals with FASD are deficits of varying degrees in the development of language, verbal reasoning, and executive functioning.

14.2 Clinical History and Description

AJ was referred by her stepmother for evaluation due to concerns regarding the clarity of her speech and overall language abilities. AJ's father and stepmother were also concerned that AJ's exposure to alcohol in utero may underlie her school and behavioral difficulties.

At the time of referral, AJ lived with her father, stepmother, and two younger siblings. She attended fourth grade in a public school. She was born in Wales and, according to her father, was exposed to alcohol and illicit drugs in utero. She moved to Canada with her father when she was approximately 4 years old. She reportedly uttered her first words at around 10 months, and her father recalls no developmental concerns during infancy or toddlerhood. AJ took her first steps at around 13 months and progressed through feeding stages with no concerns. In infancy, she was identified with "tongue-tie" and underwent frenectomy. AJ's father and stepmother also expressed concern that she may have witnessed traumatic events associated with illicit drug use when she visited her biological mother prior to moving to Canada with her father, who has sole custody of AJ. Although AJ was reportedly toilet trained early, she began to wet the bed again at 4.5 years old. AJ was recently diagnosed with attention deficit hyperactivity disorder (ADHD) and received medication to manage her symptoms. This has helped to reduce behavioral outbursts at home and at school.

AJ frequently had verbally aggressive outbursts during what would be considered typical family interactions. Specifically, she frequently screamed and name-called without apparent provocation. This behavior was preceded by verbal instruction/direction by her parents or by "typical" sibling social interactions. Similar outbursts occurred at school, especially during unstructured social time with peers.

At school, AJ was a B student and enjoyed writing. Reading was challenging for her, but she reportedly put in extra effort at literacy tasks. She was reportedly seen twice by a speech-language pathologist (SLP) during third grade to assess language expression or comprehension as possible contributor(s) to signs of inattentiveness and/or verbally aggressive outbursts. The results of this evaluation were not shared, but AJ's stepmother reported that AJ was identified with "problems" in putting sentences together and in paying attention to oral instructions when there were numerous distractions in the classroom. According to her stepmother, and in keeping with the mandate of the local school board, the attending SLP provided consultation to her teachers following this evaluation and no direct intervention.

14.3 Clinical Testing

This evaluation took place over three visits ranging from 45 minutes to 1 hour each visit. Assessment took place in a clinic setting with adequate lighting and no ambient noise. AJ's stepmother was present during all test sessions but was seated behind AJ to avoid influencing her responses.

Expressive language: An expressive language sample was elicited and recorded with AJ's consent. Her mother provided a recording of a conversation they had recently had.

AJ generally kept her contributions brief (a single statement or utterance without elaboration), regardless of the manner with which her utterances were elicited (i.e., questions, cloze statements, indirect requests, or gestural cues). Many of her responses were vague, she only partially answered the question, and/or she appeared to misinterpret the question entirely. However, a recording of a conversation in the car with her mother revealed a more fluid exchange with spontaneous and more elaborate utterances.

The following are examples of question-and-answer exchanges in clinic:

Q: Let me get to know you. Don't look at her [jokingly, as AJ looks to her mother], you know yourself, you're old enough.
A: I'm 9.

Q: What do you like to do when you're not at school?
A: Crafts?

Q: Crafts. What kind of crafts do you enjoy the most?
A: Making stuff.

Q: What do you make?
A: Play-Doh.

In addition to informal interview, the Formulating Sentences subtest of the Clinical Evaluation of Language Fundamentals, 5th Edition was recorded for analysis. Most of AJ's sentences included the definite article (the) or were stated in the first or third person. When the first person was used, it was in reference to the self or spoken as a quote of what a character in the illustration may have said. Errors in sentence formulation primarily occurred when the words given to AJ were abstract, such as adverbs, adjectives, or conjunctions. The following is a list of AJ's errors on this task where she earned 0 points out of 3, with the target word underlined:

Quickly hurry up [unintelligible] soccer.
Best work?
If he fall he [unintelligible] back up.
Instead can I get this book instead of robots.
It's closed until the afternoon.
Although I like your bike.
Unless I get my homework done I can play with you guys.

In responses to other subtests, AJ made errors in irregular past tense verb conjugation.

Receptive language: AJ demonstrated an understanding of single-step oral instructions for therapy tasks. Receptive language was better assessed formally (see standardized testing results). Where permitted, she was provided with repetition of instructions or test items. She asked for repetition of the trial items for the Word Classes and Formulated Sentences subtests. During the trial items for Structured Writing, she required several prompts and repetition of instructions to complete the trial.

AJ demonstrated some difficulty in answering interview questions. In the above dialogue sample, she answered an indirect request by responding to one phrase of the statement as if that phrase was a question. Both "what" questions were also answered incorrectly.

Narrative retell: Every session consisted of an open invitation for AJ to provide a narrative of her choosing to share. She required prompting to contribute to her narrative following the completion of every statement. Articulation difficulties limited the clarity of her speech. The following is a transcription of an attempt to elicit a narrative:

Q: Where did you have Christmas dinner?
A: I [unintelligible] and I opened up the presents. And we ate dinner at church.

Q. Tell me about the presents you got.
A: [unintelligible]. [unintelligible] stuff.

Q: Spy stuff? Oh, I didn't know you were into that! Tell me a bit more about spy stuff. [Long pause]. Imagine I don't know what spy stuff is….
A: Spying on people?

Q: OK, so you said spy stuff. Does that mean more than one thing?
A: [shrug].

Q: I'm asking you, you got the present! Did you get one present that was a spy present or more than one present that was a spy present?
A: One thing.

Q: Ok. Tell me about the one thing that you got.
A: You can change the volume in it and speak into it. [unintelligible] you can change voices when you're talking into it.

Speech (articulation and phonology): Articulation was examined using the Linguisystems Articulation Test (LAT). The following speech-sound errors were found:
- [θ] becomes [f] in all word positions.
- [z] becomes [ð] in word-medial position.
- [s] becomes [θ] in word-medial position.
- Deletion of the final consonants [n], [r], [z], [θ], [t], [d] in most words.
- Initial consonant cluster reduction, especially with the clusters [gl], [st], [sk], and [sp].
- Glide deletion in the middle of a word (e.g., crayon becomes (/kran/)).

AJ's overall intelligibility was affected by these speech-sound errors. The SLP required AJ to repeat many of her utterances in the clinic. The clinician conducted a PROMPT (Prompts for Restructuring Oral Motor Phonetic Targets) speech analysis observation (SAO) to determine the levels of the motor speech hierarchy to be targeted during therapy. It was determined through the SAO that PROMPT levels 4 (labiofacial) and 5 (lingual) were the most appropriate targets for AJ.

A phonological awareness screening was conducted using the Phonological Awareness subtest of the Clinical Evaluation of Language Fundamentals—Preschool, 2nd Edition. AJ received a score of 19 and did not meet the minimum criterion number of 20 for a child 6 years, 11 months. Her errors occurred in syllable blending, syllable segmentation, and rhyme production.

Fluency: AJ's speech was fluent. No stuttering-like behaviors were noted.

Attention: AJ demonstrated adequate attention for the informal and formal tasks necessary for this assessment.

Social communication: AJ responded to greetings with smiles, eye contact, and a wave of the hand. She maintained a friendly demeanor and was generally interested in participating in testing and therapy tasks. It was suspected that turn-taking in conversations was limited due to expressive language difficulties and not social communication difficulties. Throughout all sessions, AJ was pleasant and cooperative. No remarkable adverse behavior was noted, and she demonstrated adequate attention during the course of this evaluation.

Literacy: Reading and writing was screened using the CELF-5 Reading and Writing Supplement. Results are detailed below. Spelling, grammar, mechanics, and complexity are considered in the scoring of these subtests.

The following spelling errors occurred:
- *Nedid* (needed).
- *Raincote* (raincoat).
- *Warter* (water).
- *No* (know).
- *Wat* (what).

The following grammatical errors occurred:
- Incorrect pronoun use (*their* instead of *her*).
- Incorrect verb conjugation (*ask* instead of *asked*).

Table 14.1 Percentile rank and clinical interpretation of performance for each subtest of the Clinical Evaluation of Language Fundamentals, 5th Edition (CELF-5)

Subtest	Percentile rank	Interpretation of performance
Word classes	37	Average
Following directions	37	Average
Formulated sentences	2	Below average—moderate impairment
Recalling sentences	25	Low average
Understanding spoken paragraphs	16	Borderline
Word definitions	16	Borderline
Sentence assembly	5	Below average—mild impairment
Semantic relationships	2	Below average—moderate impairment
Reading comprehension	2	Below average—moderate impairment
Structured writing	0.1	Below average—severe impairment

Table 14.2 Percentile rank and clinical interpretation of performance for each composite category of the *Clinical Evaluation of Language Fundamentals, 5th Edition* (*CELF-5*)

Composite categories	Percentile rank	Interpretation of performance
Core language index	8	Below average—mild impairment
Receptive language index	18	Low average/borderline
Expressive language index	5	Below average—moderate impairment
Language content index	16	Borderline
Language memory index	12	Below average—mild impairment

The Test of Problem Solving-3-Elementary (TOPS-3) was used as a formal means of assessing abstract reasoning, interpretation, and critical thinking skills. It was administered in one session. Results are summarized in ▶ Table 14.3.

Sentence complexity: AJ's sentences used the conjunctions *so* and *but*, but her answers for this task were circular. That is, she repeated the content of the lead sentence she was expected to complete and did not contribute further to the paragraph, as instructed. Unfortunately, due to this error, AJ did not earn points; to earn points, she was required to add two more sentences.

▶ Table 14.1 and ▶ Table 14.2 summarize AJ's subtest and composite performances, respectively, on the Clinical Evaluation of Language Fundamentals-5 (*CELF-5*). This test battery was administered over two sessions, each of which occurred in the late afternoon.

14.4 Questions and Answers for the Reader

1. Why was AJ's articulation test not scored? If you think it should have been scored, explain your rationale for the clinical utility in doing so.
   a) The test should have been scored, as the results could have been used for progress monitoring should her parents choose to receive therapy for speech-sound production.
   b) Given her age, any standardized test results would have yielded below-average performance. Therefore, given what is known about speech-sound developmental expectations, a spontaneous sample with an error analysis would yield more clinical utility than standardized test results.
   c) Using the test to gather information about stimulability suffices to augment the results of the analysis of the spontaneous speech sample and to help with goal setting should her parents choose to address speech-sound errors in therapy.
   d) b and c.
   e) None of the above.

Answer: d is correct. Many standardized tests of articulation will concur with clinical impressions regarding the severity of a child's articulation errors, especially for children AJ's age, where it is universally expected that all children would acquire accuracy of all phonetic targets and possess 100% intelligibility. Therefore, using the test's format to guide stimulability testing is more clinically useful than scoring the test and relying on its scores to guide clinical impressions or goal setting. A carefully analyzed spontaneous speech sample from a natural conversation (if that is possible) is a more robust baseline measure of performance.

a is incorrect. While standard scores or percentile ranks may be useful measures of progress in other domains (e.g., expressive language), criterion references are better suited for progress monitoring in articulation, given the lack of sensitivity of articulation tests in acknowledging minimal improvements in performance, especially at AJ's age.

2. Why did the clinician choose to use these tests to examine this student? Consider only the available background information.
   a) Behavioral outbursts may be indicative of challenges in AJ's oral receptive language ability, as she may be unable to comprehend increasingly complex oral communication, especially under emotional duress.
   b) Verbally or physically aggressive behavior may be a result of AJ's reduced ability to express herself in a manner clearly understood by others.
   c) AJ's behavior may be a result of a reduced capacity for social reasoning, regardless of her core oral language skills.
   d) Any difficulty in others' ability to understand AJ's speech, especially when she is in a heightened emotional state, may further influence AJ's level of verbal or physical aggression.
   e) This battery of tests simply has to be done to get the most comprehensive clinical impression of AJ.
   f) None of the above.
   g) a through e.
   h) a through d.

Table 14.3 Percentile rank and clinical interpretation of performance for each reasoning subskill of the Test of Problem-Solving, 3rd Edition (TOPS-3)

Subskill	Percentile rank	Interpretation of performance
Making inferences	12	Below average—mild impairment
Sequencing	35	Average
Negative questions	38	Average
Problem solving	32	Average
Predicting	14	Below average—mild impairment
Determining causes	2	Below average—moderate impairment
Total test	16	Borderline

Answer: h is correct. Difficulty in oral language comprehension may lead AJ to feel "lost" or confused when she either does not understand or cannot remember complex oral instructions. While students around her may be executing the tasks required of them in the classroom, AJ will not. This may give rise to a number of emotions that—if exacerbated by accumulating classroom demands—may manifest themselves in unwanted or aggressive behaviors. If AJ attempted to express her frustrations verbally, she may encounter difficulty in expressing her complex thoughts and feelings in a manner that can be understood by her teacher or students around her. If others indicate they do not understand her due to her impaired speech clarity, this may further exacerbate AJ's emotional state and lead to further undesired behavior.

e is incorrect. There are numerous other standardized tests available to assess student skills and to corroborate and/or support clinical impressions.

3. If the laws in your state or province allowed for SLPs to make diagnoses, would you diagnose this child with a language disorder? If not, why not? What information do you think is missing?
   a) Yes, because test results indicate below-average global language abilities. I do not need additional information to make this diagnosis.
   b) Yes, because test results indicate below-average expressive language abilities. I do not need additional information to make this diagnosis.
   c) No, because AJ's verbal reasoning skills—higher-level abilities required to navigate social situations—are borderline.
   d) No, because a diagnosis of a language disorder requires differentiating AJ's language skills from her skills in other developmental domains. I need additional information from a comprehensive psychometric evaluation.
   e) None of the above.

Answer: d is correct. For a language disorder to be diagnosed, language skills must fall at least 2 standard deviations below the mean of other domains of development as measured by intelligence or neuropsychological tests. That is, language skills alone must be significantly impaired compared to other domains of development. Otherwise, the language impairments

identified may be a part of a more global delay. If a language impairment is identified by an SLP, a differential diagnosis of language disorder must be ruled out by broader psychometric testing. Impairments in reasoning identified by an SLP must also be isolated to verbal reasoning (vs. visuospatial reasoning, for example) and further supported by both language-specific and global developmental testing to rule in language disorder.

4. Could AJ be diagnosed with FASD? Why or why not? Use the following website as your starting point: http://www.nofas.org.
   a) Yes, she has FASD. No more information is needed to make a definitive diagnosis.
   b) Yes, she could have FASD, but more information is needed from other domains of development to make a definitive diagnosis.
   c) She is unlikely to have FASD given her history and clinical profile.
   d) No, she cannot have FASD given that she is already diagnosed with ADHD.

Answer: b is correct. Given the broad spectrum of FASD presentations and current best practice in the diagnosis of this disorder, language and verbal reasoning impairments are a piece of the puzzle. Other professions that need to be involved in the diagnosis can shed light on other domains of development that are not the purview of the SLP, such as developmental pediatrics, occupation therapy, and psychology. These professionals can, in turn, provide information regarding physical development and facial features, sensory and fine motor development, and intelligence, respectively.

a is incorrect. This answer assumes that only information documented by the SLP is sufficient to make this diagnosis. It is not.

c is incorrect. Many of the behaviors reported are present in children without FASD. However, these behaviors are also seen in children with FASD. Her behaviors and history alone cannot rule in or out FASD.

d is incorrect. It is a definitive statement that does not take into consideration that FASD and ADHD can be comorbid disorders.

14.5 Description of Disorder and Recommended Treatment

AJ's areas of concern were primarily in expressive language at the word and sentence level. She also showed some difficulties in narrative retell, although this skill was not examined formally. Her Core Language Index placed her in the 8th percentile rank with a statistically significant discrepancy between her receptive and expressive language skills (18th and 5th percentiles, respectively). AJ's literacy skills were moderately-to-severely impaired relative to children her age, and this was at least in part due to demonstrated difficulties with phonological awareness. Furthermore, AJ demonstrated difficulties in making inferences, predicting, and determining causes of events when given visual and verbal stimuli concurrently. Finally, her intelligibility was affected by several articulation and phonological processing errors that made her difficult to understand in a quiet setting.

The following recommendations were made following the evaluation.

- Professional supports:
  - Speech-language therapy to focus on articulation and language skills. It was advised that the treating clinician target PROMPT motor speech hierarchy stages 4 and 5 (labiofacial and lingual movement), specifically.
  - Learning support in school: one-on-one pull-out support for specific impairments in addition to participation in classroom group learning activities.
  - Further psychometric evaluation to rule in/out a language or other learning disorder/disability and to assist with FASD diagnostic formulation.
  - Sharing of assessment results with AJ's primary care physician to facilitate further supports, as needed.
- Classroom environment:
  - Provide AJ with preferential seating close to her instructors.
  - Ensure AJ is facing the teacher during instructions.
- Academic instruction and programming:
  - Reduce the use of rhetorical language.
  - Incorporate language instruction within the context of AJ's preferred activities.
  - Provide opportunities for AJ to engage in oral sentence formulation activities.
  - Provide AJ with a "buddy" with whom she can exercise her narrative skills as they develop.
  - Use barrier games to encourage expressive language and theory of mind development.
  - Use picture cards or photographs to help elicit stories from AJ. Explicitly teach AJ the components of a story and have her practice story retelling either with picture cues or from memory.
- Home environment:
  - When giving AJ instructions orally, ensure that AJ is facing the person giving the instruction, give instructions slowly, ensure comprehension of oral instructions by having her repeat them, and avoid the use of figurative or rhetorical language.

14.6 Outcomes

AJ presented with many strengths. She was a social girl who participated readily in the evaluation. In spontaneous speech recorded by her mother offsite, AJ engaged in conversational turn-taking and provided spontaneous contributions and elab-orations typical of a child her age in a casual setting. Furthermore, she displayed strengths in her ability to use visual and verbal information to sequence events, answer negative questions, and solve problems in a manner broadly similar to children her age. AJ presented with strengths in her ability to draw similarities among single spoken words, follow multiple-step, complex directions, and remember verbatim short statements spoken to her.

AJ's family attended several speech-language therapy sessions targeting speech-sound production. During her attendance, she demonstrated perceptible success in the production of /s/ and /z/ in one- and two-syllable words in all word positions using the PROMPT method for tactile cueing and immediate auditory feedback of her utterances. However, this was not observed to generalize to the sentence level or made spontaneously. Unfortunately, therapy stopped after four sessions due to lack of resources and AJ was discharged to the care of her parents and school.

14.6.1 Key Points

- FASD can manifest in several domains of development, including language, making it necessary to implement a multidisciplinary approach to its differential diagnosis.
- Language and speech-sound impairments can more broadly impact children's successful interactions with people in their environments. The effects of these impairments can be observed in children's behavior, which can vary from harmless indifference to verbal and/or physical aggression.
- While an important part of a thorough evaluation, the clinical utility of standardized tests does not necessarily lie in the scores derived from them.
- Although ideally all individuals with speech, language, or other impairments should receive the services they need, the unfortunate reality is that not all will receive them due to lack of resources.

Suggested Readings

[1] Astley SJ. Diagnostic Guide for Fetal Alcohol Spectrum Disorders: The 4-Digit Diagnostic Code. Seattle, WA: University of Washington; 1994

[2] American Psychiatric Association. Diagnostic and Statistical Manual of Mental Disorders. 5th ed. Arlington, VA: American Psychiatric Publishing; 2013

[3] Paul R. Language Disorders from Infancy through Adolescence: Listening, Speaking, Reading, Writing, and Communicating. St. Louis, MO: Elsevier; 2012

[4] Reid N, Dawe S, Shelton D, et al. Systematic review of fetal alcohol spectrum disorder interventions across the life span. Alcohol Clin Exp Res. 2015; 39 (12):2283–2295

15 Speech Rehabilitation following Cleft Palate Repair

Catherine Crowley and Chelsea Sommer

15.1 Introduction

Cleft palate can yield significant limitations to speech intelligibility. In addition, compensatory misarticulation can persist following surgical correction of the cleft. This case outlines the differentiation between cleft palate speech and compensatory misarticulation, as well as appropriate therapy approaches for this challenging population.

15.2 Clinical History and Description

MR, a 6-year-old English-dominant Spanish bilingual girl born with cleft of the hard and soft palate, underwent primary palate repair when she was 12 months old. From 12 months to 6 years of age, she produced typical cleft palate speech errors. At the age of 6, MR underwent secondary palate surgery to extend the velum to improve velopharyngeal closure. Concurrently, MR had myringotomy tubes placed due to recurrent middle ear infections. Conductive hearing loss is common in children with cleft palates, as the tensor veli palatini, the primary muscle responsible for eustachian tube opening, inserts into the soft palate. With a cleft, the tensor veli palatini cannot regulate air pressure and opening between the mouth and middle ear, making children with cleft palates more vulnerable to middle ear infections.[1] MR was referred by the head surgeon of the local cleft palate team who performed her surgery.

15.3 Clinical Testing

In the evaluation of cleft palate patients, a clinician's perceptual skills are the "gold standard" for assessment.[2] Assessment included an oral examination; assessment of resonance; and assessment of all sounds in isolation, syllables, single words, and sentences. Oral mechanism examination revealed no fistulae and grossly adequate movement of the velum and articulators. Resonance was normal. With regard to speech, poor articulatory placement for all high-pressure sounds was observed. These "high-pressure," or oral sounds, are sounds that require complete closure of the velopharyngeal mechanism so that the nasal passageway is occluded and all sound exits through the mouth. High-pressure sounds in English include /p, b, t, d, k, g, s, z/. Patients with cleft palate can produce nasal sounds, such as /m/, /n/, and /ŋ/ and low-pressure sounds, such as /w/, /l/, and /r/, which do not require full closure of the velopharyngeal port. In MR's case, however, high-pressure, low-pressure, and even nasal sounds were replaced by typical errors in cleft palate speech, including pharyngeal fricatives, glottal stops, and nasal emissions. MR's only consistently accurate placement was the bilabial, voiced nasal phoneme /m/ and all vowels.

During the initial assessment, MR produced the /p/ sound in isolation at three different times. This moment was captured on video and can be seen in ▸ Video 15.1. All other sounds except for /m/ were produced with incorrect placement (such as producing an /n/ by closing the lips) and often in an incorrect manner (such as producing a stop /t/ instead of a continuant /s/) and/or voicing (such as producing a /p/ as a /b/). MR also demonstrated the ability to imitate bilabial placement of the /p/ and /b/ after a few attempts using a multisensory approach with visual, tactile, kinesthetic, and auditory cueing.

15.4 Questions and Answers for the Reader

1. Why was MR able to produce a /p/ sound only three times during the evaluation?
   a) To be able to consistently produce the /p/ sound, MR would need a third surgery.
   b) MR was stimulable for the high-pressure /p/ sound, but she needed more therapy to produce consistent productions.
   c) MR had the adequate structure following the surgery; however, MR did not have adequate physiology for the /p/ sound.
   d) MR had lip weakness and needed to work on lip strengthening before she could produce the /p/ consistently.

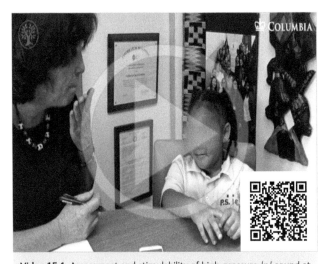

Video 15.1 Assessment and stimulability of high-pressure /p/ sound at initial consult. This is the first time the authors worked with this client. They assessed her speech sounds and probed for stimulability. MR was stimulable for the /p/ sound, as demonstrated in this clip.

e) MR's surgery had not fully healed and would improve even without speech therapy after a few more weeks of healing.

Answer: b is correct. By producing the /p/ sound correctly, MR demonstrated that the secondary palate surgery was a success and she could create adequate velopharyngeal closure. MR was only able to produce the /p/ sound three times in response to a multisensory approach to stimulate the sound. The elimination of compensatory errors, or "cleft palate speech," involves motor learning and requires much practice and repetition to eliminate compensatory cleft palate speech errors.

a is incorrect. MR did not need another surgery following her secondary palate repair. MR needed more speech therapy. By producing the high-pressure /p/ sound only once during the initial evaluation demonstrates that she had adequate structure and function, and is not in need of another surgery, only speech therapy.

c is incorrect. MR had adequate structure and function after her secondary surgery as demonstrated by her production of the high-pressure /p/ sound, which indicated appropriate palatal function.

d is incorrect. Lip strengthening and other nonspeech oral motor exercises, such as horn blowing and straw sucking, are not evidenced based and will have no positive effect on MR's speech.

e is incorrect. Once the surgeon confirms that the patient is ready for speech therapy, there is little healing left. More importantly, because MR did not have correct articulatory placement, that is, a bilabial placement, MR's /p/ sound production is very unlikely to improve without therapy where she can learn correct placement.

2. Why did MR present with incorrect articulatory placement for so many speech sounds, including all high-pressure sounds and also most low-pressure and nasal sounds?
   a) The levator veli palatini, the most important muscle in velopharyngeal closure, could not function correctly for the low-pressure and nasal sounds.
   b) In addition to the cleft palate speech errors with the high-pressure sounds, MR's speech had many phonological processes unrelated to velopharyngeal insufficiency.
   c) MR had many speech errors that were consistent with apraxia of speech.
   d) Due to a conductive hearing loss, MR could not hear the sounds correctly, and produced the sounds the way she heard them.
   e) For MR's case, the compensatory misarticulations affected virtually her entire sound system.

Answer: e is correct. Although a child with an unrepaired cleft palate can generally produce the nasal sounds and the low-pressure sounds, in MR's case all but the /m/ and vowels were produced with inconsistent placement and mostly with incorrect manner and voicing. In MR's case, the compensatory misarticulations affected virtually her entire sound system, meaning that she had to relearn almost all sounds needed for speech with the exception of the /m/ and the vowels.

a is incorrect. Although the levator veli palatini is the most important muscle in velopharyngeal closure, this muscle has minimal involvement in the production of low-pressure and none with nasal sounds.

b is incorrect. MR did not demonstrate any phonological processes. Phonological processes are separate from cleft palate speech errors.

c is incorrect. Often children with cleft palate speech are misdiagnosed with apraxia, as they must relearn correct placement for sounds, resulting in inconsistent errors and groping as they work to relearn correct production for the mislearned sounds post–cleft palate repair. In this case, MR did not have apraxia of speech as vowel production was consistent and any inconsistent productions could be attributed to relearning correct production of sounds.

d is incorrect. While MR might hear sounds with distortions with a conductive loss, this is unlikely to cause classic cleft palate speech errors such as glottal stops and pharyngeal fricatives, and also unlikely to cause such poor placement of articulation for virtually all sounds.

3. Why did MR need another cleft palate surgery to address her speech issues if she had her cleft palate repaired at an excellent hospital with an American Cleft Palate-Craniofacial Association ACPA–certified cleft palate team?
   a) Even the best surgeons have patients who need a secondary repair for speech, even if the initial repair is flawless.
   b) The hospital had a change in personnel and the surgeon who did MR's surgery was inexperienced.
   c) MR received speech therapy from a speech-language pathologist who did not have any understanding of how to address cleft palate speech.
   d) MR's mother failed to follow postoperative procedures after the first cleft palate surgery, causing the velopharyngeal insufficiency.
   e) MR did not have any health insurance to cover speech therapy postsurgery.

Answer: a is correct. MR required another cleft palate surgery because after her primary palate repair she continued to display velopharyngeal insufficiency. Even the best cleft palate surgeons have patients who need a secondary palate surgery. The role of the speech-language pathologist is to work with the patient after the initial cleft palate surgery to determine whether the speech errors are simply compensatory errors needing more speech therapy or consistent with velopharyngeal insufficiency, indicating the need for a secondary cleft palate surgery.

b is incorrect. While it is possible to have inexperienced or even less-than-competent surgeons on cleft palate teams, even the best cleft palate surgeon will have patients who need a secondary speech surgery, even when the first surgery was flawless. In MR's case, she had an excellent and experienced surgeon do her first cleft palate repair.

c is incorrect. It is important that the speech-language pathologist has a full understanding of how to address cleft palate speech; however, without a secondary surgical intervention, MR's velopharyngeal mechanism would not have functioned adequately. MR needed that surgery to have the anatomical and physiological ability to close the velopharyngeal mechanism and produce high-pressure speech sounds.

d is incorrect. MR's mother went to all necessary meetings for MR following her palate repair. MR's velopharyngeal insufficiency was caused by her lack of tissue and muscle needed for velopharyngeal closure.

e is incorrect. Whether MR received speech therapy postsurgery has no impact on the fact that she needed a secondary speech surgery.

4. Would speech therapy have benefited MR even before she had her secondary speech surgery at the age of 6 years?

   a) No. Without velopharyngeal closure, MR would never have been able to produce any of the high-pressure sounds.

   b) Yes. With high-quality multisensory speech therapy, using nasopharyngoscopy feedback, MR could have had excellent production of the /p/ and /b/ phonemes.

   c) Yes. Speech therapy could have focused on lip and tongue strengthening so that after she had her surgery, she would require very little speech therapy.

   d) Yes. Speech therapy could have focused on reducing her hypernasality making her speech more intelligible.

   e) Yes. Speech therapy could have focused on correct articulatory placement so she would require less speech therapy after the surgery.

Answer: e is correct. It is generally beneficial to receive speech therapy before surgery to improve speech outcomes after surgery. If MR had been receiving speech therapy before surgery, she would not be able to make the high-pressure sounds but would have good placement and manner. Therapy postsurgery could have focused on having the air and sound come through the mouth, something MR could not do without the speech surgery. Additionally, with good placement and manner of articulation, MR's intelligibility would have been significantly better presurgery.

a is incorrect. Without velopharyngeal closure, MR would never have been able to produce any of the high-pressure sounds. Yet, speech therapy presurgery could have benefited MR by improving placement of articulation and intelligibility.

b is incorrect. High-quality multisensory speech therapy is helpful when providing feedback; however, without the secondary speech surgery, using only this method would not generate excellent production of the /p/ and /b/ sounds.

c is incorrect. Lip and tongue strengthening exercises would have had no impact on MR's speech before or after surgery.

d is incorrect. Resonance is a function of the size and shape of the resonance cavity. Speech therapy cannot reduce hypernasality, where there is no change in the size or shape of the cavity. Only surgery can change the size and shape of the cavity.

15.5 Description of Disorder and Recommended Treatment

MR had compensatory misarticulation secondary to velopharyngeal insufficiency. Prior to the secondary surgery, MR did not have the requisite anatomy and physiology for production of high-pressure sounds. The compensatory misarticulations formed as MR attempted to replicate the sounds she heard but that she could not make correctly because she had velopharyngeal insufficiency. Treatment involved moving sound by sound through the traditional hierarchy for cleft palate speech therapy discrimination, production of single sounds, the sound

in syllables, single words with no other high-pressure sounds followed by similarly constructed sentences, and, finally, conversation. Because cleft palate speech therapy requires drills and many repetitions, the therapy itself must be varied and fun to keep the child, and the family, focused and engaged.

In this case, each hierarchical step had different, including multisensory, single-sound games, practicing the target sound in syllables, single-word cleft palate speech therapy games, and cleft palate speech storybooks that target voiced and voiceless cognates. ▶ Video 15.2 demonstrates how the cleft palate speech therapy hierarchy was implemented with MR. To optimize therapy outcomes, MR's mother became a critical member of the therapy team acquiring the pertinent cleft palate speech therapy strategies MR was working on. Throughout the week, the mother worked with MR on repetition and drills to enhance motor relearning.

Therapy initially focused on appropriate placement of nasal sounds, as they are critical for the eventual placement of high-pressure sounds. Once correct placement of the nasal sounds /m/, /n/, and /ŋ/ was achieved, /p/ was introduced as it is a bilabial, voiceless sound and thus less likely to engage the vocal folds to yield a glottal stop. MR could employ the bilabial /m/ to model appropriate placement for the /p/. With practice, the /p/ was relatively easy for MR.

In the cleft palate speech therapy hierarchy, clinicians should begin with discrimination of the compensatory error and the correct production so that the patient can perceive and understand the difference between the incorrect production and the correct target production. The next step is to work on the target sound in isolation. This means that the sound is targeted without a vowel after it (e.g., say "p" not "pa" as the prompt). Next, the clinician can combine the target sound with vowels in the "Acevedo Spoke." In this approach (▶ Video 15.2), the target sound is in a circle in the middle of the page with spokes from the target sound to vowels around the outside of the page. The first combinations on the Acevedo Spoke involve the target sound in the initial position "pa, pe, pi, po, pu" followed by in

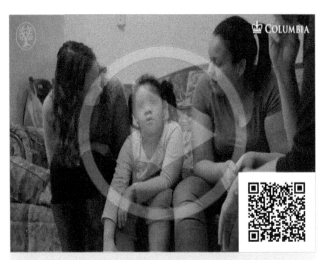

Video 15.2 Hierarchy for cleft palate speech therapy. This demonstrates the speech therapy hierarchy to follow when working with a child who has had cleft palate speech.

the final position "ap" "ep" "ip" "op" "up" and then placing the target sound in the medial position surrounded by a combination of vowels "apa" "epe" "ipi" "opo" "upu." Next, the clinician will move on to placing the target sound in words (in the initial, medial, and final positions). Following successful use at the word level, the clinician can use cleft palate speech therapy books, which can be found for free at leadersproject.org. Finally, the target sound should be practiced in spontaneous speech during conversation.

15.6 Outcome

Beginning 2 weeks after surgery, and with the approval of her surgeon, speech therapy was initiated approximately three times per week for 8 months. She also received school-based therapy twice per week. Over 8 months of therapy, MR improved from minimal intelligibility (20% for trained listeners and family members and 10% for others) to mostly intelligible speech even without known context (90% for trained listeners and family members and 75% for others). MR's mother actively participated in the therapeutic process and continued to provide home practice and support. MR's school-based speech-language pathologist collaborated with the university speech-language pathologist clinic team to ensure therapy speech goals were consistent and synergistic.

MR continues to have difficulty with the /k/ and /g/ sounds. MR can produce /k/ in seemingly more difficult clusters such as "school" and the /ŋ/ placement is helpful as a placement transition for words such as "pink" and "ringing." The rationale underlying this success is likely related to the nasal /ŋ/ which is also a velar sound and the tongue is in the same place for production of /k/ and /g/. The final sounds to address will be /ʧ/, /ʃ/, and /ʤ/. Based on her progress to date, her prognosis for developing these sounds is good.

15.7 Key Points

- Collaboration among all members of the interdisciplinary team ensures optimal outcomes.

- When a child can produce one high-pressure sound, the child has adequate velopharyngeal closure.
- Screen for hearing; children with cleft palate often have a conductive hearing loss due to the improper insertion of the tensor veli palatini muscle.
- Parental involvement in intervention is essential for success.
- Eliminating compensatory cleft palate speech is a motor learning skill and needs to be practiced frequently throughout each day.

Suggested Readings

[1] Crowley C. Cleft palate practice books. Leadersproject.org. 2014. Available at: http://www.leadersproject.org/cleft-palate-directory/cleft-palate-practice-books/. Last accessed June 2016

[2] Crowley C. Cleft palate therapy word games. Leadersproject.org. 2016. Available at: http://www.leadersproject.org/english-cleft-palate-directory/cleft-palate-therapy-word-games/. Last accessed June 2016

[3] Crowley C, Baigorri M, Sommer C. Speech sound assessment and stimulability. Leadersproject.org. 2016. Available at: http://www.leadersproject.org/2016/06/06/speech-sound-assessment/. Last accessed June 7, 2016

[4] Crowley C, Baigorri M, Sommer C, Acevedo D. What to do before the cleft palate is repaired to improve speech outcomes after surgery. Leadersproject.org. 2016. Available at: http://www.leadersproject.org/2016/05/30/strategies-before-the-cleft-palate-is-repaired/. Last accessed June 5, 2016

[5] Sommer C, Crowley C, Baigorri M, Acevedo D. Cleft palate speech therapy hierarchy. Leadersproject.org. 2016. Available at: http://www.leadersproject.org/2016/05/30/cleft-palate-speech-therapy-hierarchy/. Last accessed May 29, 2016

References

[1] Peterson-Falzone SJ, Hardin-Jones MA, Karnell MP. Cleft Palate Speech. 4th ed. St. Louis, MO: Mosby Elsevier; 2010

[2] Baylis A, Chapman K, Whitehill TL, The Americleft Speech Group.. Validity and reliability of visual analog scaling for assessment of hypernasality and audible nasal emission in children with repaired cleft palate. Cleft Palate Craniofac J. 2015; 52(6):660–670

16 Disorder, Difference, or Gap? A School-Age Disability Evaluation

Catherine Crowley and Casey Sheren

16.1 Introduction

This case describes a teenager previously diagnosed as "severely language impaired" based on a private, score-based evaluation. The emphasis is on the assessment of language and dialect acquisitional history and prior academic experiences to determine whether to characterize the deficits as a true language disorder or related to dialectal and/or academic issues.

16.2 Clinical History and Description

SD was a 13-year-old girl from a multilingual and multidialectal, low socioeconomic background. When SD was 7 years old, she and her younger siblings were removed from their biological mother and spent the next 4 years living in foster care. By fifth grade, SD had attended five different schools and was exposed to Puerto Rican Spanish, African-American English, Spanish-influenced English, and code-switching, but had minimal exposure to Standard American English. At the age of 11, SD was adopted by two university professors. Standard American English was spoken at home and at school.

Shortly after adopting SD, her mother expressed concerns regarding her processing skills, as well as her expressive and receptive language. Specifically, she worried about SD's vocabulary development and verb conjugations. She reported that SD demonstrated difficulty in school with text comprehension. Her performance on state tests was in the very lowest range.

Approximately 1 year following her adoption (age 12), SD underwent a score-based speech and language evaluation employing standardized assessment tools. Her performance on the Recalling Sentences subtest, a test of knowledge of syntax of Standard American English, suggested "significantly disordered language."

This evaluation employed test scores in isolation without considering language and dialect, educational history, or instability of her home environment. The parents referred SD to a university-based clinic to address these deficits. After reviewing the initial report, reevaluation was indicated to consider SD's sociolinguistic background and prior life experiences as well as linguistic and academic progress since initial evaluation.

16.3 Clinical Assessment and Evaluation

In addition to an in-depth parent interview, SD's primary seventh-grade teacher was interviewed (▶ Video 16.1). In addition, SD was observed in the classroom and samplings of recent schoolwork were obtained and reviewed. SD's teacher previously worked in the inner city where SD grew up, making her a particularly reliable source of information. She explained that SD's greatest weaknesses were vocabulary and comprehension

of academic content. She noted that when SD first arrived at her new school as a sixth grader, she was hesitant to speak up when she did not understand something. Since then, though, SD's teacher described "so much progress" and "great strides in writing."

To examine SD's acquisition of syntax, the Crowley and Baigorri School-age Language Assessment Measures (SLAM) subway assessment was administered (▶ Video 16.2).[1] SD was presented with a picture of a man whose shoe was caught in the subway door and posed with questions to elicit complex sentence structures and personal narrative. SD demonstrated age-appropriate ability to follow a line of questions, integrate and

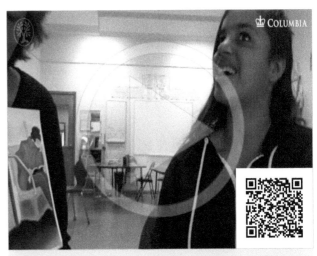

Video 16.1 The teacher interview. SD's seventh-grade teacher shares her perspective on the academic progress SD made since arriving at her new school.

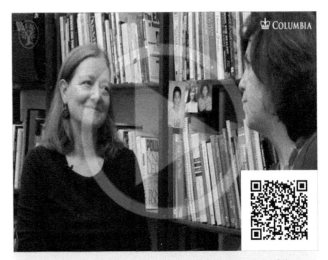

Video 16.2 Clinical interactions with the student. Two clips of the student responding to assessment questions during the author's administration of her language evaluation.

organize her thoughts, and express these ideas employing appropriate Standard American English grammatical structure. For example,

Evaluator: What happened?

SD: There was probably a big crowd and he didn't get out, so then his foot got stuck.

Evaluator: Did this ever happen to you?

SD: Almost. When we were going back to the apartment, it happened to my mom because she was swiping it the wrong way.

Evaluator: What would you do if this happened to you?

SD: I would probably start yelling. I know it would hurt.

As noted in the sample, SD had acquired many features of Standard American English. She used modal and conditional tenses ("I would probably" and "It would hurt"), Standard American English noun–verb agreement ("we were"), copula and auxiliary "be" forms ("there was" and "she was swiping"), and complex sentences including causation and temporal elements ("when," "so then," "because," and "I know [that]").

Review of the prior score-based evaluation revealed that SD fully acquired all aspects of Standard American English dialect over the past 18 months and considerable expansion of vocabulary. This information provided longitudinal information regarding language acquisition. For example, she described "treaty" as "A treaty is like a contract"; a "souvenir" as "something to remember where you were, something precious to someone who got it"; a "committee" as "a whole group of people in deciding what to do"; a "negotiation" as "trying to work something out"; a "decade" as "a very long time"; and "award" as "you achieved in something, a reward, you get an award to show your effort." Her mother indicated that the family worked together building vocabulary with SD and her sister at breakfast and there is considerable focus in school as well.

Additionally, SD demonstrated metalinguistic understanding of language and an ability to use language to solve problems, make inferences, and compare and contrast. Further evidence of her linguistic skills included her quick understanding of humor and her ability to follow complex plots and character development in ongoing television shows (▶ Video 16.3).

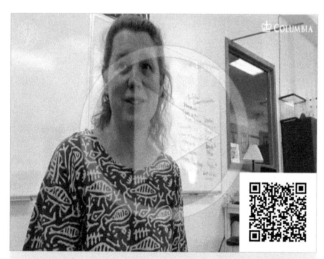

Video 16.3 The parent interview. SD's mother shares with the evaluator that SD is able to follow complex plots and character development in ongoing television shows.

16.4 Questions and Answers for the Reader

1. Why was the teacher interview particularly salient in the differential diagnosis?
   a) SD's teacher is a close friend of SD's adoptive family and has had the opportunity to witness SD's behavior and interactions both in school and in informal, familial settings.
   b) SD's teacher herself is from the same linguistic background as SD and, therefore, can provide insight into whether SD's communication represents a language difference or a true disorder.
   c) SD's teacher had done extensive linguistic research, looking at dialectal differences between Spanish-influenced English, African-American English, and Standard American English and brings an important knowledge base to SD's case.
   d) SD's teacher previously taught in the inner city where SD grew up and, therefore, could provide information about how SD compared to other children of her same cultural and linguistic background.

Answer: d is correct. Because SD's teacher had taught in the same community where SD grew up, she had an understanding of SD's academic and linguistic experiences leading to more valid and reliable responses to the author's questions.

a is incorrect. Because the teacher knew SD from school over the past 2 years, the teacher knew the family, but did not have a relationship with the family outside of school.

b is incorrect. SD's teacher is a monolingual speaker of Standard American English. While she has insight into whether SD has a language difference or a language disorder, she is not from the same linguistic background.

c is incorrect. SD's teacher did not do academic research on different dialects of American English. However, as a result of her prior experience teaching in the diverse inner city where SD grew up, she was able to identify basic characteristics of Spanish-influenced English and African-American English.

1. Why did SD's understanding of long-running television shows with complex plots and characters influence the author's conclusions?
   a) SD's watching television takes away from time when she should be working to fill academic gaps through reading comprehension practice.
   b) These skills demonstrate strong cognitive skills and strong cohesive syntactical skills, as she used noun phrases and complex sentences to describe the stories.
   c) SD is able to hear the television from a far distance, suggesting that her hearing is within normal limits.
   d) The characters in the television shows that SD watches have diverse dialects of American English, which may be slowing the rate of her acquisition of Standard American English.
   e) SD's ability to follow complex plots in television shows but not in novels suggests that her deficits are a result of a true language disorder.

Answer: b is correct. An understanding of complex plots and character development requires the ability to analyze, compare, synthesize, problem solve, make inferences, make meaningful predictions, and other academic language skills. SD's ability to express these concepts syntactically indicated high-level academic language skills.

a is incorrect. SD's ability to describe plots and character development in complex, ongoing television shows provided another piece of evidence that her language skills were age appropriate and that her issues were related to academic gaps only.

c is incorrect. The information learned about SD's language skills that related to her television watching did not relate to her hearing.

d is incorrect. There is no evidence that hearing different dialects on a television show would slow the rate of her acquisition of Standard American English.

e is incorrect. Information from the parent about SD's understanding of the television shows was especially valuable because it isolated SD's language skills from her academic gaps. While weak language skills can affect reading comprehension, in this case, SD demonstrated strong academic language skills, thereby offering further evidence distinguishing a language disorder from pure academic gaps.

1. What conclusion can we draw from SD's rapid acquisition of Standard American English in the 18 months she was in her new school prior to speech-language evaluation?
   a) SD had previous exposure to Standard American English in previous academic settings and home environments.
   b) SD has a strong facility to acquire language and understand metalinguistics.
   c) SD's new school has enabled her to be able to correct the grammatical mistakes of her previous speech and language.
   d) SD did a great deal of preparation for her subsequent evaluation, engaging in rigorous study sessions both at school and at home, to memorize the features of Standard American English.
   e) SD actually did not acquire Standard American English, supporting that she does have a true language disorder, in addition to language differences and academic gaps.

Answer: b is correct. SD's ability to use modal and conditional tenses, Standard American English noun–verb agreement, copula and auxiliary "be" forms, and complex sentences including causation and temporal elements indicates that she rapidly acquired Standard American English in the 18 months she was in her new school. A student with severe language impairment, or even mild language impairment, would not demonstrate this level of linguistic and metalinguistic competence, especially after only such a short period of exposure to the new dialect.

a is incorrect. Prior to being adopted by her current parents, SD was exposed to Puerto Rican Spanish, African-American English, Spanish-influenced English, and code-switching, but had minimal exposure to Standard American English. Therefore, her acquisition of Standard American English cannot be attributed to prior exposure to the dialect.

c is incorrect. During SD's initial speech and language evaluation, she did not exhibit "grammatical mistakes," but rather language and dialect differences that represent characteristics of rule-governed systematic dialects of American English. SD's new school and home environments provided her with the exposure to Standard American English that she needed to acquire features of the dialect; it was not a matter of "correcting grammatical mistakes."

d is incorrect. SD did not "prepare" or "study" for her second speech-language evaluation. Rather, she spontaneously acquired the features of Standard American English with adequate exposure to the dialect, which supports that she has the facility to learn language. The outcome of SD's initial evaluation reflects that SD previously lacked exposure to Standard American English, the sole dialect that was taken into account during that initial evaluation.

e is incorrect. SD's performance revealed that she fully acquired Standard American English in the 18 months that she was exposed to it across all parameters of language, including syntax, morphology, semantics, and pragmatics.

1. What is one reason the private clinician who performed SD's first speech-language evaluation incorrectly diagnosed SD as having severe language impairment?
   a) The clinician violated IDEA 2004, the Federal law on special education, by relying on standard scores in a test that was significantly biased against SD.
   b) SD did not cooperate fully with the evaluation.
   c) The clinician did not use a more appropriate standardized test to diagnose SD.
   d) As a clinician in a private practice, the speech-language pathologist did not have much experience with speakers of dialects other than Standard American English and should not be expected to know about other dialects.
   e) The clinician administered the test in Standard American English but took into account SD's language and dialect acquisitional history.

Answer: a is correct. IDEA 2004 specifically states that evaluation materials cannot be racially or culturally biased. By failing to consider SD's background, the evaluator came up with a diagnosis that was wrong, derived from seriously biased test materials. Evaluation materials that do not take into account a student's cultural or linguistic background violate IDEA 2004, the Federal law on special education, as well as sound assessment procedures.

b is incorrect. Nothing in the evaluation indicated that SD failed to cooperate.

c is incorrect. It is true that the clinician did not use an appropriate standardized test. But it is also unlikely that any standardized test exists that can take into account the impact of SD's prior experiences, including the multiple changes in homes and schools, and the shifts in exposure between Spanish and English including several different dialects of English.

d is incorrect. Although the clinician who did the private speech-language evaluation probably mostly sees speakers of Standard American English, a professional must be able to provide culturally and linguistically appropriate evaluations for all.

e is incorrect. Nothing in the initial score-based evaluation indicated that the evaluator took into account SD's language and dialect acquisitional history. Failure to do so resulted in a seriously flawed diagnosis.

16.5 Differential Diagnosis

Upon review of both prior and current assessment, it was determined that SD presented with academic deficits as well as language differences, but certainly not a disorder or disability. SD demonstrated age-appropriate syntactic structures in Standard American English acquired, indicating a high level of language skills. She also demonstrated age-appropriate semantic knowledge through precise definitions of grade-level vocabulary words. Moreover, SD acquired metalinguistic skills and grade-level academic language skills in her ability to make inferences, compare and contrast, analyze and synthesize complex ideas, and solve problems.

16.6 Recommended Treatment and Outcome

SD's current school and teacher provided a stimulating environment, which was likely contributory to SD's progress toward academic success. To supplement the exposure to high-level vocabulary at school, SD's parents were encouraged to introduce new words into structured discussions meaningful to SD. To allow SD to maintain and express her diverse cultural identity, her parents were advised not to limit SD to speaking only Standard American English at home with her siblings. This diversity of language was thought to allay her concerns that she would "become white" when she "speaks white," and support an additive model for continued acquisition of the new dialect.

16.7 Key Points

- Differential diagnosis in speech and language requires more than measuring and reporting scores. Evaluators should consider influences of the student's language and dialect acquisitional history in the analysis of linguistic abilities and have knowledge of the variability and influences of morphology and syntax across those dialects and languages.
- Parent and teacher interviews offer valuable information about the student's abilities across contexts.
- Informed clinical opinion and direct observations are critical to gather evidence and gain a more holistic understanding of the student's strengths and weaknesses.
- Remain up-to-date on the research and best practices for culturally and linguistically appropriate evaluations.

Suggested Readings

[1] American Speech-Language-Hearing Association (ASHA). Knowledge and skills needed by speech-language pathologists and audiologists to provide culturally and linguistically appropriate services. American Speech-Language-Hearing Association. 2004. Available at: http://www.asha.org/policy/KS2004–00215.htm. Last accessed June 10, 2016

[2] Burns FA, de Villiers PA, Pearson BZ, Champion TB. Dialect-neutral indices of narrative cohesion and evaluation. Lang Speech Hear Serv Sch. 2012; 43(2): 132–152

[3] Crowley C. Understanding assessment: The critical questions. Leadersproject.org. 2015. Available at: http://www.leadersproject.org/2015/03/18/the-critical-questions/. Last accessed June 10, 2016

[4] Crowley C, Grossman C. Grammar fundamentals for a pluralistic society. Leadersproject.org. 2014. Available at: http://www.leadersproject.org/ceu-courses/-grammar-fundamentals-for-a-pluralistic-society/. Last accessed June 10, 2016

Reference

[1] Crowley C, Baigorri M. School-age language assessment measures. Leadersproject.org. 2015. Available at: http://www.leadersproject.org/disability-evaluation/school-age-language-assessment-measures-slam/. Last accessed June 10, 2016

17 Social Communication Intervention for a Child with Autism Spectrum Disorder

Amy L. Donaldson

17.1 Introduction

Social communication challenges are a core feature of autism spectrum disorder (ASD).[1] Effective interventions targeting such skills have the potential to significantly impact the quality of life for children with ASD and their families.

17.2 Clinical History and Description

GM was a 4-year, 4-month-old girl with autism. GM attended a developmental preschool program 3 days per week for 4 hours. GM was referred for assessment and intervention by her parents based on concerns regarding her social communication skills and engagement with others. GM was first diagnosed on the spectrum at 3 years, 5 months and received speech-language and early intervention preschool services since diagnosis. Her medical history was otherwise unremarkable with no previous diagnosis of known genetic syndromes, reports of serious medical or neurological conditions (e.g., encephalitis, concussion, seizure disorder, diabetes, congenital heart disease), sensory impairments such as vision or hearing loss, and/or serious motor impairment.

17.3 Clinical Testing

The Autism Diagnostic Observation Schedule–2 (ADOS-2)[2] was administered to confirm diagnosis and gain information regarding GM's social communication and interaction skills. Throughout administration of the ADOS-2, GM demonstrated limited initiation of communication bids, limited responsiveness to her name, delayed and immediate echolalia, and lack of coordination of nonverbal and verbal communication. In addition, GM repeatedly regarded herself in the mirror throughout the assessment, particularly when manipulating a play object.

In addition, a sample of GM's expressive language use was analyzed using the Systematic Analysis of Language Transcripts (SALT).[3] Results of this analysis yielded information about the complexity of her expressive language. She demonstrated a mean length of utterance (MLU) of 2.93. MLU is a measure of the number of words per utterance, as well as the number of morphemes used in that utterance. Children of GM's age typically demonstrate an MLU in words of 4.08. Her spontaneous language comprised primarily requests for action/object and an occasional comment. Her language sample was notable for periods of "self-talk" (delayed echolalia of TV scripts), which did not appear to be directed toward the clinician or related to the play context. Finally, the Auditory Comprehension subscale of the Preschool Language Scale–5 (*PLS-5*)[4] was administered to assess GM's receptive language skills. She achieved a standard score of 67 (mean = 50; standard deviation = 15).

17.4 Questions and Answers for the Reader

1. Would further assessment be valuable to examine GM's social communication and interaction skills? If so, what kind?
   a) No further assessment is needed. The ADOS-2 provides adequate information regarding social communication skills.
   b) No further assessment is needed. Speech-language pathologists (SLPs) are best suited to target language and speech production skills. Social communication and interaction is the domain of school psychologists.
   c) Yes, further assessment is needed. Communication occurs within social interaction; therefore, it is important to have multiple examples of communication within meaningful social contexts.
   d) Yes, further assessment is needed. However, not for social communication. Examine GM's expressive language (syntax, semantics, and morphology) through a norm-referenced standardized measure to compare her performance to same-age peers.

Answer: c is correct. Given the decontextualized nature of most norm-referenced standardized measures, particularly those focusing on core language skills,[5] further assessment of GM's social communication within meaningful social contexts is warranted. Although the ADOS-2 allows for observation of social communication and interaction skills within a semistructured environment, the primary communication partner within the assessment is an examiner unknown to the child. As such, observing a child's performance within a familiar social context and/or with a known communication partner provides the examiner with the opportunity to observe a range of performance.

As such, in addition to the assessment described above, we observed GM and her neurotypical sibling HM (age 5 years, 5 months) within a 10-minute sibling interaction. They were provided with novel play materials (e.g., floor puzzle, play-dough) that were appropriate to their age and developmental level and that their parents had reported were objects/activities of high interest on a Play Interest Survey.[6] The clinician provided no support or instructions. We observed that GM rarely initiated social communication with HM and that when she did so, HM did not consistently respond. GM also demonstrated limited engagement in the play activity (block design toy), but rather manipulated a piece in her hands while engaging in "self-talk." HM appeared to "guard" the materials, often blocking GM's access to the activity with her body. One main difference noted between the ADOS-2 administration and this observation was GM's overall decrease in initiations toward her communication partner. We hypothesized that GM's reduction may be due, in part, to the lack of responsiveness by her sister, HM, whereas, during the individual assessment, the clinician was prompt in responding to all GM's communication bids.

a is incorrect. Although the ADOS-2 can provide information regarding a child's social communication skills, including initiation and response to communication bids and various types of communicative functions, the semistructured format may not provide adequate opportunities to assess particular behaviors of interest. An ADOS-2 contributes valuable information to a comprehensive evaluation of an individual for diagnostic purposes.

b is incorrect. Social communication might be best conceptualized as use of communication within social contexts and for interacting with others. As such, there is rarely a time when one does not employ their social communication skills. While speech-language therapy with children often focuses on the "appropriateness" of communication (i.e., correct use of morphology, phonology, syntax, and/or semantics), one cannot do so to the exclusion of the "effectiveness" of communication (i.e., successful use of communication skills for interaction). As such, assessment and intervention for social communication skills is well within the realm of an SLP's scope of practice[7] and should be a regular part of any assessment protocol.

d is incorrect. As indicated above, the ADOS-2 in isolation is insufficient to fully assess GM's social communication skills. Her performance on the receptive language portion of the PLS-5 was within normal limits for her age. Given her MLU during the language sample, further testing of her expressive language skills using a norm-referenced standardized measure may have been warranted. However, social communication skills were the primary area of concern for the family and reason for referral.

2. What type(s) of intervention might support GM's social communication growth and facilitate interaction with others?
   a) A combination of evidence-based social communication interventions that include a peer or sibling in targeted interactions.
   b) Clinician-directed intervention that focuses on increasing GM's vocabulary skills.
   c) Extinguishing GM's "self-talk"/delayed echolalia.
   d) Naturalistic intervention focusing on increasing speech intelligibility.

Answer: a is correct. Based on the expanded assessment results demonstrating HM's influence on both GM's frequency and diversity of social communication bids and HM's own patterns of decreased interaction and shielding of toys, the team (clinician and parents) discussed how to best approach increasing and improving the social engagement and social interactions of the siblings. The team agreed that both children could benefit from learning strategies to facilitate and improve their social interactions with each other. This approach considers both communication partners equally responsible for communicative and social success and creates an environment where both communication partners learn strategies to grow their skills.[8] Two evidence-based practices for targeting social communication skills were specifically selected for this sibling dyad: video modeling (VM) for supporting the skills of the child with ASD; and peer mediation (sibling mediation) for teaching social communication strategies to the neurotypical sibling.[9] The intervention was implemented following a strengths-based model that capitalized on the children's motivation as the context for

learning and maximized strengths to support areas of challenge.[10] (VM and peer mediation is described in more detail below.)

b is incorrect. Increasing GM's vocabulary was not the focus of her parents' referral for services; improving her social communication as a core feature of ASD was their primary focus. To date, there has been no evidence of a clinician-driven vocabulary-specific intervention resulting in collateral benefits to social communication skills and/or social engagement for children with ASD.

c is incorrect. Although self-talk can disrupt social interactions and engagement with others, following principles of naturalistic developmental behavioral intervention, the team decided to address GM's self-talk within the sibling dyad social communication intervention in the following manner: (1) incorporate use of highly preferred objects and activities as the teaching context to increase interactions and language related to context[11]; and (2) coach LH in responding to all of GM's communicative bids, even if they were self-talk, in an effort to engage in ongoing interaction. We call this the "as if" principle —the communication partner responds "as if" the child was directing the communication to them and is context-appropriate. By responding, the communication partner opens up the opportunity for further interaction and ongoing communication.

d is incorrect. Speech intelligibility was not an area of concern for GM.

3. Why should clinicians consider including siblings or peers when targeting the social communication skills of children with ASD?
   a) Because siblings and peers can be good teachers for children with ASD—they can show them how to communicate.
   b) Because effective communication requires everyone's participation; therefore, both the child with ASD and peer/sibling can learn strategies to facilitate success and develop meaningful relationships.
   c) Because families want peers and siblings to feel sorry for children with ASD and help them at school.
   d) Because children with ASD do not want friends; therefore, it is the SLP's job to establish friendships for them.

Answer: b is correct. Social communication skills are integral to developing and sustaining peer relationships.[12] In addition, social and communicative competence is considered key to school success.[13] And, as children progress through school, communicative and social expectations become increasingly complex.[14] Although social communication skills are often the target of intervention, many children with ASD demonstrate difficulty with generalization of social communication skills to natural contexts, particularly within peer relationships.[15,16] As such, inclusion of peers and/or siblings in intervention is warranted, not only to support generalization of skills, but also to facilitate development of meaningful relationships.[8] Further, it takes two people to effectively communicate; as such, supporting the communication of both individuals promotes success and creates equity in relationships.

a is incorrect. While peers and siblings can certainly serve as models for each other and for children with ASD, a strengths-based approach to intervention encourages equity in peer and sibling relationships.[10] To build lasting relationships between children with disabilities and neurotypical children, it is important to maintain balance with regard to power and responsibility.[8] As such, in peer-inclusive or sibling-inclusive interventions, the author and her colleagues assist children in developing *their own* skills, rather than teaching others (except what would occur within a natural interaction).

c is incorrect. As indicated above, authentic relationships occur when children are provided natural and equitable opportunities for interaction. Recent research indicates that friendship may be an important context for development of communication, particularly production of different types of communicative functions or speech acts. Bauminger-Zviely and colleagues[17] found that preschool-age children with ASD demonstrated greater frequency and variety of speech acts during conversation with friends as compared to nonfriend peers. In addition, they found these children demonstrated increased frequency and variety when engaged in conversation with neurotypical friends. They stated, "friendship may enable children to converse in a more socially complex and co-regulated way."

d is incorrect. Children with ASD seek interaction and friendship, but may do so in a manner that differs from neurotypical children. Although previous research has indicated that children with ASD may report fewer friendships and challenges maintaining friendships,[18] other research has indicated that children with ASD report levels of friendship satisfaction similar to neurotypical peers.[19]

17.5 Description of Disorder and Recommended Treatment

With an understanding of the range of GM's social communication skills and how her communication partner's responsiveness potentially impacts her performance, we employed a two-element intervention that involved both GM and her sibling. For 10 weeks (two times per week for 50 minutes), the family participated in "Socialsibs," a social communication intervention that combines two methods: VM and peer mediation (in this case, sibling mediation).

VM is an intervention method that provides direct intervention to the child with ASD and has been identified as effective for targeting social communication skills.[9,15,16,20] In VM, the child with ASD watches a video of a peer and/or adult demonstrating a discrete skill/target behavior and then practices the skill.

Peer mediation (or in our case, sibling mediation) refers to direct coaching of a peer to elicit and facilitate the child with autism's social communication skills[21] and/or direct training of a peer to increase their own initiations and responsiveness to the child with ASD.[22,23] Peers have been successfully taught to initiate interactions, maintain interactions, and prompt a variety of play, motor, and communicative behaviors in children with autism.[9,24]

Using VM, GM targeted the following social communication behaviors with HM: (1) responding to communication bids; (2) requesting objects; and (3) turn taking. The procedure for VM included: (1) video recording of the target behavior as demonstrated by HM during an interaction with the clinician; (2) playback of video for GM, with discussion of target behavior; (3) clinician-supported practice of the target behavior using the same play materials from the video; and (4) fading support of the VM, as well as clinician prompts, as GM demonstrated increased accuracy in spontaneous production of the behavior.[25]

We found it important to explain in age-appropriate, literal language the function of the behavior and why it is important, particularly when first introducing a target behavior. By pausing after the behavior was demonstrated within the VM and discussing these points, the child associated the model of the behavior with the intent. For example, when targeting responding to communication bids, the VM included at least three to five clear exemplars of the target behavior (with the sibling as the model). When the skill was first taught, after each demonstration of the behavior the video was paused and the clinician described the behavior (e.g., "I asked HM about her picture and she told me what she colored") and identified its importance (e.g., "I didn't know what she drew. I liked learning about her picture").

The sibling-mediated intervention followed the model of Pierce and Schreibman[26,27] by teaching HM to use strategies based on Pivotal Response Training[28] to change her *own* social communication behaviors when interacting with GM. Based on family priorities, the age of the participants, and the length of the intervention (10 weeks), three strategies were selected for sibling mediation; they included (1) gaining attention; (2) responding to all communication bids; and (3) providing GM with a choice between two objects/activities.

To teach each strategy, the clinician brought HM into an individual treatment room (separate from GM) and explained the skill in developmentally appropriate and literal language. For example, when teaching the strategy of gaining attention, the clinician said, "Have you ever noticed that when you talk with GM it seems like she might not hear you? I have some ideas to help make sure that she is listening when you tell her something." The clinician would then explain each component of the strategy in turn (often using age-appropriate visual supports), and role-play use of the skill with HM. This initial training of the strategy lasted approximately 10 minutes. HM then practiced using the strategy directly with GM, with facilitation and feedback from the clinician. The clinician provided graduated prompts from most to least support as needed to facilitate use of the strategy within play activities. Also, the clinician provided verbal praise (e.g., "You did it!") to reinforce HM's performance of a target behavior. It can be tempting for the clinician to direct attention to the child with ASD in an effort to facilitate interaction; however, this strategy can leave the sibling without a clear understanding of his/her performance. As such, we directly reinforced the sibling's attempts at using the strategy, regardless of their success in eliciting the desired behavior from the child with ASD.

17.6 Outcome

Overall, GM increased all targeted social communication behaviors (i.e., responding to HM's communication bids; requesting objects from HM; turn-taking) and maintained generalization of the first two skills at a 1-month follow-up. Although engagement was not a specifically targeted behavior, we also measured GM's engagement with HM within sibling interactions over the course of intervention to see whether targeting specific social communication behaviors might have a more global impact on GM's social engagement. She increased joint engagement (siblings are involved in activity or object together and GM coordinates attention between object and activity) and decreased object engagement (GM is involved solely in playing with object, not attending to HM) over the course of intervention. HM increased the use of attention-getting strategies and responded to GM's communication bids more frequently than prior to intervention. However, she did not demonstrate an increase in offering GM choices within play interactions.

Following intervention, the girls' parents reported an increase in responsiveness and initiations by GM. In addition, they reported an increase in the frequency of social interactions between the siblings and noted a difference in the quality of the interactions, as characterized by increased spontaneous verbal interactions, imitation during play, and reciprocity since the start of intervention. The parents also reported that HM independently and spontaneously taught the children's cousins the gaining attention strategy, which increased GM's participation in play during extended family visits in their home.

17.7 Key Points

- Traditional norm-referenced standardized measures, even those intended to identify social communication and interaction challenges, may not provide adequate information for intervention planning. Assessment of skills within multiple social contexts and/or across communication partners will provide clinicians with a range of performance, as well as a starting place for intervention planning.
- Siblings and peers are integral to social communication intervention for children with ASD and other social communication challenges. Successful social interaction requires two people and too often adult communication partners scaffold performance. Although this strategy may assist in acquiring new skills, it can be a detriment to generalization of skills and relationship building. As such, inclusion of peers and/or siblings in intervention promotes communication success and relationship equity.

Suggested Readings

[1] Sam A; AFIRM Team. Modeling. Chapel Hill, NC: National Professional Development Center on Autism Spectrum Disorder, FPG Child Development Center, University of North Carolina. 2016. Available at: http://afirm.fpg.unc.edu/modeling

[2] Sam A; AFIRM Team. Peer-Mediated Instruction and Intervention. Chapel Hill, NC: National Professional Development Center on Autism Spectrum Disorder, FPG Child Development Center, University of North Carolina. 2015. Available at: http://afirm.fpg.unc.edu/peer-mediated-instruction-and-intervention

References

[1] American Psychiatric Association. Diagnostic and Statistical Manual of Mental Disorders. 5th ed. Washington, DC: American Psychiatric Association; 2013

[2] Lord C, Rutter M, DiLavore PC, Risi S, Gotham K, Bishop S. Autism Diagnostic Observation Schedule. 2nd ed. Los Angeles, CA: Western Psychological Services; 2012

[3] Miller JF, Chapman RS. Systematic Analysis of Language Transcripts (Version 6.1)#[Computer software]. Madison, WI: University of Wisconsin—Madison, Waisman Center, Language Analysis Laboratory; 2000

[4] Zimmerman IL, Steiner VG, Pond RE. Preschool Language Scales–5th ed. (PLS-5). San Antonio, TX: The Psychological Corporation; 2011

[5] Donaldson AL, Olswang LB. Investigating requests for information in children with autism spectrum disorders: Static versus dynamic assessment. Int J Speech Lang Pathol. 2007; 9(4):297–311

[6] Quill K. Do-Watch-Listen-Say. Baltimore, MD: Paul H. Brookes Publishing Co.; 2000

[7] Landa RJ. Assessment of social communication skills in preschoolers. Ment Retard Dev Disabil Res Rev. 2005; 11(3):247–252

[8] Donaldson AL. Siblings of children with ASD: promoting social communication. Perspect Lang Learn Educ. 2015; 22(1):31–38

[9] National Autism Center. Findings and Conclusions: National Standards Project, Phase 2. Randolph, MA: National Autism Center; 2015

[10] Donaldson AL, Krejcha K, McMillin A. A strengths-based approach to autism: neurodiversity and partnering with the autism community. Perspectives of the ASHA Special Interest Groups. 2017; 2:56. doi:10.1044/persp2.SIG1.56

[11] Baker MJ, Koegel RL, Koegel LK. Increasing the social behavior of young children with autism using their obsessive behaviors. Res Pract Persons Severe Disabil. 1998; 23(4):300–308

[12] Rotheram-Fuller E, Kasari C. Peer relationships: challenges and interventions. In: Hollander E, Kolevzon A, Koyle JT, Eds. Textbook of Autism Spectrum Disorders. Arlington, VA: American Psychiatric Publishing; 2011:555–564

[13] Zigler E, Gilliam WS, Jones SM. A Vision for Universal Preschool Education. New York, NY: Cambridge University Press; 2006

[14] Brinton B, Fujiki M. Social development in children with specific language impairment and profound hearing loss. In: Smith P, Craig H, Eds. Blackwell Handbook of Childhood Social Development. Malden, MA: Blackwell Publishing; 2002:588–603

[15] Ferraioli SJ, Harris SL. Treatments to increase social awareness and social skills. In: Reichow B, Doehring P, Cicchetti DV, Volkmar FR, Eds. Evidence-Based Practices and Treatments for Children with Autism. New York, NY: Springer; 2011:171–196

[16] Schreiber C. Social skills interventions for children with high-functioning autism spectrum disorders. J Posit Behav Interv. 2011; 13(1):49–62

[17] Bauminger-Zviely N, Golan-Itshaky A, Tubul-Lav G. Speech acts during friends' and non-friends' spontaneous conversations in preschool dyads with high-functioning autism spectrum disorder versus typical development. J Autism Dev Disord. 2017; 47(5):1380–1390

[18] Kasari C, Locke J, Gulsrud A, Rotheram-Fuller E. Social networks and friendships at school: comparing children with and without ASD. J Autism Dev Disord. 2011; 41(5):533–544

[19] Petrina N, Carter M, Stephenson J, Sweller N. Perceived friendship quality of children with autism spectrum disorder as compared to their peers in mixed and non-mixed dyads. J Autism Dev Disord. 2016; 46(4):1334–1343

[20] Wang S, Chui Y, Parrila R. Examining the effectiveness of peer-mediated and video-modeling social skills interventions for children with autism spectrum disorders: a meta-analysis in single-case research using HLM. Res Autism Spectr Disord. 2011; 5(1):562–569

[21] Kuhn LR, Bodkin AE, Devlin SD, Doggett RA. Using pivotal response training with peers in special education to facilitate play in two children with autism. Educ Train Dev Disabil. 2008; 43(1):37–45

[22] Goldstein H, Kaczmarek L, Pennington R, Shafer K. Peer-mediated intervention: attending to, commenting on, and acknowledging the behavior of preschoolers with autism. J Appl Behav Anal. 1992; 25(2):289–305

[23] Strain PS, Odom SL. Peer social initiations: effective intervention for social skills development of exceptional children. Except Child. 1986; 52(6):543–551

[24] Zhang J, Wheeler JJ. A meta-analysis of peer-mediated interventions for young children with autism spectrum disorders. Educ Train Autism Dev Disabil. 2011; 46(1):62–77

[25] Shukla-Mehta S, Miller T, Callahan K. Evaluating the effectiveness of video instruction on social and communication skills training for children with autism spectrum disorders: A review of the literature. Focus Autism Other Dev Disabil. 2010; 25(1):23–26

[26] Pierce K, Schreibman L. Increasing complex social behaviors in children with autism: effects of peer-implemented pivotal response training. J Appl Behav Anal. 1995; 28(3):285–295

[27] Pierce K, Schreibman L. Using peer trainers to promote social behavior in autism: Are they effective at enhancing multiple social modalities? Focus Autism Other Dev Disabil. 1997; 12(4):207–218

[28] Koegel RL, Schreibman L, Good A, Cerniglia L, Murphy C, Koegel L. How to Teach Pivotal Behaviors to Children with Autism: A Training Manual. Santa Barbara, CA: University of California; 1989

18 Reading Comprehension Difficulties in a School-Age Student

Anna Eva Hallin

18.1 Introduction

This case report describes comprehensive language and literacy assessment in a 10-year-old who scored poorly on the English Language Arts summative reading comprehension test at the end of fourth grade.

18.2 Clinical History and Description

SH was a healthy monolingual, English speaker with good hearing and vision. She reportedly started talking late, around age 2, and saw a speech-language pathologist (SLP) weekly between the ages of 3 and 4 years. She was then discharged as she was performing at age-expected levels. SH was described as quiet and kind. She functioned well socially and focused satisfactorily in the classroom, but rarely participated in class discussions. She had no difficulties with early reading and writing skills, and at the time of assessment, read fourth-grade texts fluently and accurately. However, her performance on reading comprehension tasks varied greatly depending on text, topic, and task. She particularly struggled with understanding social studies and science texts. Her writing was described as simple with occasional grammatical errors, but she used appropriate writing conventions and her spelling was within normal limits. SH met most standards in mathematics, but she often required support with word problems.

18.3 Clinical Testing

18.3.1 Standardized Testing

Conventional and comprehensive standardized tests of both oral and written language were administered. See ▶ Table 18.1 for a summary of results. SH did not have difficulties with the technical aspects of reading (e.g., word recognition/decoding, fluency, and accuracy). She had average oral expression scores but below average receptive skills, and below average comprehension when oral or written information was presented in paragraphs.

18.3.2 Curriculum-Based/Informal Tasks and Portfolio

In addition to standardized testing, materials from the classroom were employed to gain additional insight into SH's difficulties with reading comprehension. Two "think-aloud" tasks using fourth grade science/social studies texts were employed; SH had difficulty understanding central content words and her performance was not enhanced with morphological or context clues; she did not understand complex syntax, and struggled when asked to find the main idea of a paragraph, draw infer-

ences, and summarize content. When asked what she usually does when she does not understand text, SH replied that she "sometimes re-reads." When SH was asked to retell a short narrative, she was fluent with all main elements of the story, indicating that narrative language was one of her strengths. SH used simple and repetitive sentence structure as well as limited and/or nonspecific vocabulary in written samples obtained from her classroom teachers. Her narrative texts were longer and more elaborate than expository texts, which were brief and contained more grammatical errors.

18.4 Questions and Answers for the Reader

1. One well-established model of reading comprehension is the Simple View of Reading, which states that to comprehend a text you need both good decoding/word recognition skills to be able to read fluently and accurately, and good language skills to understand the decoded text. In other words, reading comprehension can be expressed as the product between decoding and linguistic comprehension. Even though linguistic comprehension in this model is a complex construct, this model is a meaningful starting point when assessing reading comprehension difficulties. The following statements about the Simple View of Reading are true except one:
   a) A student may have reading comprehension difficulties weak decoding skills, due to weak linguistic comprehension skills, or both.
   b) A student with reading comprehension difficulties due to weak decoding skills only will typically understand the text if it is read to him/her.
   c) A student with reading comprehension difficulties will typically struggle with understanding all types of texts.
   d) A student with weak oral language skills will most likely also have weak reading comprehension skills.
   e) When assessing reading comprehension difficulties, both decoding abilities and oral language abilities should be carefully mapped out.

Answer: a is true. A student with weak decoding skills but good linguistic comprehension skills has a specific reading disability ("dyslexia"), a student with good decoding skills but weak linguistic comprehension skills may have language impairment without phonological processing difficulties (or, if linguistic difficulties are subclinical, they might be called "poor comprehenders"), and a student with weaknesses in both areas may have a language impairment with phonological processing difficulties.

b is true. For students with isolated decoding difficulties, listening to texts is a way to compensate for their decoding difficulties when learning about a topic.

d is true. Oral language skills are the foundation of written language skills.

Table 18.1 Summary of a selection of SH's oral and written standardized test results

	Test	Subtests/scales	Percentile rank
Written language	Test of Written Spelling: TWS-5	Spelling of single words	23
	Test of Word Reading Efficiency: TOWRE-2	Sight word efficiency	50
		Phonetic decoding efficiency	63
	Gray Oral Reading Test: GORT-4	Rate	71
		Accuracy	37
		Reading comprehension (oral)	15
Oral language	Clinical Evaluation of Language Fundamentals: CELF-5	Reading comprehension (silent)	9
		Core language score	13
		Expressive language index	39
		Receptive language index	10
		Understanding spoken paragraphs	11
	Peabody Picture Vocabulary Test: PPTV-4	Receptive vocabulary	9

e is true. The intervention and accommodations for a student with reading comprehension difficulties due to weak decoding compared to a student with weak (oral) linguistic comprehension are very different. Always assess both areas.

c is false. Texts vary significantly in their demands on both decoding and linguistic comprehension skills.

2. SH's case is an illustration of the common phenomenon typically referred to as "illusory recovery"—when children with developmental language disorders seem to catch up with their peers in later preschool years, but exhibit language processing difficulties at a later stage again. What is the most likely explanation of this phenomenon?
   a) Language processing demands increase throughout the school years.
   b) Language processing difficulties in children often worsen over time.
   c) Language processing difficulties often spontaneously reappear following puberty.
   d) Preschool language assessments typically fail to capture language ability.
   e) School-age language assessments are more sensitive than preschool assessments.

Answer: a is correct. The introduction of reading and writing and the increasing academic and social demands in the school-age years can lead to reemerging language difficulties when language processing demand exceeds a child's language processing ability.

b and c are incorrect. The effects of a developmental language disorder change over time, but internal processing does not typically worsen and, furthermore, is not associated with puberty.

d and e are incorrect. Although it is important to ensure that standardized tests are reliable and valid, no universal differences exist in tests for different ages.

3. All of the following statements highlight the importance of including curriculum- or classroom-based tasks in addition to standardized language assessment tools as a component of comprehensive language assessment in school-aged children except:
   a) Curriculum-based tasks are essential when setting appropriate language goals.
   b) Curriculum-based tasks will quantify a student's language skills compared to peers.
   c) Curriculum-based tasks may capture subtle language processing difficulties.
   d) Curriculum-based tasks may guide language intervention procedures.
   e) Curriculum-based tasks reflect the language demands in the student's everyday life.

Answer: a is true. School-based SLPs must write language goals that are aligned with the curriculum and should focus on functional language and communication.

c is true. Curriculum-based tasks and texts might reveal both language processing difficulties and strengths that standardized tests might not capture due to the specific language demands of the academic curriculum.

d is true. A dynamic informal task may show what type of support and intervention strategies are most beneficial for the student.

e is true. Students spend most of their time in school, and it is important that the language assessment reflects the demands that the student must meet.

b is false. Although curriculum- and classroom-based tasks might give an indication of how a student is performing relative to grade or age benchmarks, standardized tests of language and literacy with an appropriate normative sample would be the appropriate quantitative comparison.

4. The complexity of text depends on many interacting factors, such as word difficulty, syntactic complexity, text structure, discourse style, genre features, background knowledge of the reader, and level of reasoning and inferencing required, as well as text format, length, and layout. Given this information, which of the following statements is accurate:
   a) Additional factors, such as ability to focus and areas of interest are not important to take into account when assessing reading comprehension.
   b) It is important to assess reading comprehension with a wide range of texts and comprehension tasks.
   c) Texts that are difficult for one reader will most likely be difficult for another reader of the same age.
   d) The format of a reading comprehension task or a reading test does not influence performance.

e) Only a limited number of factors can be targeted in language intervention to improve reading comprehension.

Answer: b is correct. Research has shown that different reading comprehension tasks do not identify the same students as having reading comprehension difficulties. Several different texts and tasks have to be used in assessment.

a is incorrect. Because of the complex process of comprehension, both text factors and reader factors are important to take into account in assessment and intervention.

c and d are incorrect. See explanation b above.

e is incorrect. Reading comprehension can be improved through targeting both micro and macro aspects of language as well as working with comprehension strategies and improving background knowledge of the reader.

18.5 Description of Disorder and Recommended Treatment

Assessment results with the knowledge that SH had a previous diagnosis of language impairment suggest that SH's language processing difficulties persist, but now primarily impact her ability to comprehend complex and academic texts. Students like SH, who have language impairments or subclinical linguistic difficulties without major deficits in oral and/or written phonological processing such as non-word repetition and decoding, are often referred to as poor comprehenders. These students often perform poorly in the classroom and run the risk of not being detected as readily as those students with expressive difficulties or decoding difficulties.

In this case, it was recommended that SH receive individual and small-group language treatment and support, both inside and outside the classroom. The main goal of treatment was to improve reading comprehension in social studies and science. These goals were written to align with the Common Core Standards (http://www.corestandards.org/). A secondary goal was to strengthen expository written language skills. Based on SH's test profile, treatment initially focused on comprehension monitoring and strategies including note taking and activating background knowledge, strengthening of vocabulary skills with a subfocus on morphology, and structured work with complex syntax and embedded phrases. The starting point was materials from social studies, science, and math. Later targets included identifying and contrasting different expository text structures.

18.6 Outcome

Midway through fifth grade and following SLP intervention for one semester, follow-up assessment was performed using a "think-aloud" protocol with curriculum-based texts. In addition, the specific reading comprehension strategies employed by SH spontaneously in the classroom setting was assessed. SH identified the main idea in short paragraphs on four out of five occasions and demonstrated improved comprehension monitoring. SH stopped and commented on words she did not know and demonstrated the ability to use the context and her own background knowledge or morphology to infer the meaning of unfamiliar words. Her performance in the comprehension of complex sentence structures improved. In the classroom, she more readily asked for help and accepted more assistance from her peers when she had difficulty understanding a task or instructions. The teacher reported that SH performed better on homework assignments involving reading comprehension, but that her difficulties with writing expository texts were even increasingly prevalent given the academic demands in fifth grade. SH reported that she enjoyed reading her social studies textbook more than before and her parents reported that SH was more willing to do homework assignments than in previous years.

SH will likely require continued support in oral and written language throughout her school years. Ideally, however, the intensity of support will decrease over time as SH gains independence with the targeted comprehension strategies and with language knowledge gained through intervention.

18.7 Key Points

- Speech and/or language impairment identified in the preschool years may appear to resolve, but as linguistic demands increase, significant language processing difficulties may reemerge. Students with good reading accuracy and fluency, but with significant difficulties with reading and listening comprehension, may go undetected.
- Language difficulties categorized as mild to moderate based on standardized test scores may still have severe consequences for academic achievement, in addition to students' well-being.
- Reading comprehension is complex and challenging to quantify. Multiple complementary approaches must be employed including both well-constructed standardized tests of oral and written language as well as curriculum- and standard-appropriate informal tasks to ensure language intervention goals are curriculum-based and functional for the student.

Suggested Readings

[1] Hogan TP, Adlof SM, Alonzo CN. On the importance of listening comprehension. Int J Speech-Language Pathol. 2014; 16(3):199–207

[2] Keenan JM, Meenan CE. Test differences in diagnosing reading comprehension deficits. J Learn Disabil. 2014; 47(2):125–135

[3] Wallach GP. Improving clinical practice: a school-age and school-based perspective. Lang Speech Hear Serv Sch. 2014; 45(2):127–136

19 Childhood Apraxia of Speech

Megan S. Overby and Katie Micco

19.1 Introduction

This case study discusses the differential diagnosis and treatment of a preschooler who presents with expressive language delay and suspected childhood apraxia of speech (CAS).

19.2 Clinical History and Description

KJ was a 3.5–year-old, nonverbal boy with reported "strong" receptive language skills and no significant family history of speech-language difficulties. Perinatal history included induction at 36 weeks due to maternal preeclampsia and a birth weight of 5.6 lb. According to parent report, KJ did not latch successfully during breastfeeding and presented with limited babbling and sound play in infancy, although developmental motor milestones were met. During his first 2 years, KJ produced occasional vowel-like productions with few attempts at consonant-vowel combinations; first words ("da" and "muh") emerged at approximately 25 months of age but were "lost" shortly thereafter. He was reported to drool excessively until age 3. KJ demonstrated strong communicative intent and primarily communicated through leading/guiding, vocalizing, and gesturing, although he occasionally hit and bit others when frustrated. Socially, he was often withdrawn, especially with peers in preschool or with unfamiliar communication partners.

19.3 Clinical Testing

Pure-tone hearing screening indicated KJ responded to 500, 1,000, 2,000, and 4,000 Hz at 25 dB. Examination of oral mechanism structures and function revealed lips were symmetrical both at rest and when retracted. The hard and soft palates appeared normal in shape and color and the soft palate was observed to rise upon production of "ah." Adequate voicing and breath support were demonstrated across three trials of sustained vowel phonation (mean length = 10 seconds), though nasal resonance was noted during one trial. On the Preschool Language Scale-5 ,[1] KJ's subscale performance was as follows: auditory comprehension = 97 (percentile rank = 42) and expressive language = 64 (percentile rank = 1). Because KJ presented with a highly limited sound repertoire and lack of functional speech, standardized assessment of speech-sound production skills was not attempted.

Diadochokinetic (DDK) rates for alternating and sequencing oral movements were assessed. Given a clinician model, KJ demonstrated difficulty imitating single consonant (C)–vowel (V) productions of "puh," "tuh," and "kuh;" although placement of "puh" and "tuh" was obtainable, productions were inconsistent and contained voicing errors. Despite multiple attempts, KJ was unable to produce "kuh," sound repetitions, or alternating phoneme sequences (i.e., "puhtuhkuh").

Informal motor speech examination assessed KJ's accuracy, timing, and smoothness when producing increasingly complex syllable shapes. Given maximum cues (clinician verbal model, visual cues, gestural support, and verbal placement cues), he produced CV, VC, and C_1VC_1V syllables. In some VC combinations, KJ failed to mark the final consonant or segmented the production (e.g., /u-m/). He often simplified C_1VC_1V to CV or segmented it to C_1V–C_1V with equal lexical stress. KJ simplified C_1VC_1 and C_1VC_2 shapes to CV even when maximal cues were provided. His phonetic inventory across all syllable shapes was /m/, /b/, /d/, /n/, an approximation of /w/, and schwa vowel. He was not stimulable for any voiceless phonemes or other vowels, though vowel approximations were possible with manual cues.

19.4 Questions and Answers for the Reader

1. A 4.5-year-old girl's performance on the Diagnostic Evaluation of Articulation and Phonology[2] was 57% inconsistency score, articulation SS = 72 and phonology SS = 88. Speech-sound errors included "fife," "ive," and "vie" for "five"; "shish" and "fi" for "five"; and "wain" and "yai" for "rain." However, stimulability testing revealed she was able to correct many of her articulatory errors at the phoneme level when provided a slowed auditory model. Her DDK for "patty-cake" was within 1 standard deviation of her age mean. Paternal history was significant for speech delay because of errors on the /s/ sound. Based on these results, the most likely diagnosis is:
   a) Dysarthria.
   b) Childhood apraxia of speech.
   c) Phonological disorder.
   d) Articulation disorder.
   e) Typical speech-sound development.

Answer: c is correct. Errors are primarily unsuppressed developmental phonological process errors (assimilation, gliding, and final consonant deletion) in the absence of neurological or motor speech movement/planning impairment.

a is incorrect. dysarthric speech-sound errors are typically predictable, regardless of speaking task, and are most commonly distortions and omissions, with distortions being the most prevalent.

b is incorrect. Although inconsistency and significant family history may occur in children with CAS, speech-sound errors are typically omissions and distortions with evidence of motor speech movement/planning deficits. Deficits may appear in the accuracy, timing, and smoothness of sound sequences and/or transitions between sounds, as well as disruptions in prosody at various linguistic levels. In this example, normal DDK rates imply normal motor speech movement gestures, though careful observation of such gestures is required. Additionally, in this case, most speech-sound errors are substitutions.

d is incorrect. Articulation errors are due to errors in the placement of the articulators, not motor movement/planning. Although a case could be made that this client demonstrates an articulation disorder as well as a phonological disorder, her stimulability for phonemes suggests that any articulation disorder is mild and possibly resolving. Hence, phonological impairment is the better answer (although clinicians may wish to monitor the client's articulatory status).

e is incorrect. By age 3, consonant assimilation and final consonant deletion typically disappear, although gliding may still be present. Initial consonant deletion is atypical at any age.

2. A 6-year-old boy diagnosed with CAS has the following phonetic inventory: /b/, /d/, /m/, /n/, /s/, /schwa/, and "ah." His syllable shape inventory includes CV, VC, C_1VC_1V in direct imitation and C_1VC_1 in simultaneous production with the clinician. His mother says he adores cars and trucks and also asks that her son learn to say the name of the family dog, "Snowflake." What would you recommend as initial therapy goals?
   a) "on, mom, done, beep, see, nah, tuhtah!, Snowflake."
   b) "no, yes, apple, baa-baa, mama, uh-oh."
   c) /p/, /t/, /k/, /g/, /f/ in isolation, then in words, then in sentences.
   d) "all done, go, no, yes, me, mine, you, is, are, I, mommy, daddy, home, eat, milk."
   e) "bun" vs. "fun;" "not" vs. "rot;" "sun" vs. "one."

Answer: a is correct. For children with limited repertoires, create four to seven meaningful target words representing different parts of speech (e.g., nouns, verbs, exclamations, adjectives) using primarily syllable shapes and phones within the child's inventory. "Tuhtah!" introduces a voiceless phoneme, but the syllable shape and vowels are familiar; new vowel /i/ is a visible high front vowel in contrast to the central-low vowels produced. Prosody can be addressed with multisyllabic targets or monosyllables using rising and falling pitch contours to ask a question, demand attention, or "whine!" "Snowflake," an important parent/child goal, introduces a new syllable shape, possibly achievable through forward chaining of /s/ and /n/ already in the inventory (e.g., "sn," "sno," snof," "snofay," and/or "snoflay," and then possibly "snowflake").

b is incorrect. These targets do not include sounds primarily in the child's repertoire. "Baa-baa" is not particularly meaningful for this 6-year-old boy.

c is incorrect. A developmental "traditional" approach does not support the acquisition of gestures for motor speech movement/planning.

d is incorrect. Although these meaningful targets can build syntax, they are not composed of sounds within the child's phonetic inventory and include challenging new gestures for motor speech movement/planning.

e is incorrect. These maximal opposition pairs contrast the target to a sound within the inventory across several possible feature contrasts (e.g., place, nasality, manner, voicing). Such pairs may assist in overall system-wide phonological change in children with a phonologically based speech-sound disorder, but do not address deficits in motor speech movement/planning.

3. In treating a client with CAS, the clinician first identified the level of cueing support (e.g., simultaneous production—direct imitation—delayed imitation) as well as the number and type of multisensory cues (clinician verbal model, visual cues, gestural support, and verbal placement cues) needed for accurate, smooth, and appropriately timed movements/productions. For each target, the clinician shaped the client's independence for targeted speech-sound production by fading the number and type of multisensory cues. What therapy strategy was used?
   a) Melodic intonation therapy.
   b) Cycles phonological approach.
   c) Vertical therapy.
   d) Core vocabulary approach.
   e) Dynamic temporal and tactile cueing (DTTC).

Answer: e is correct. DTTC is a type of integral stimulation (i.e., imitation tasks combined with motor learning principles)[3] in which the clinician shapes the child's productions with multisensory cues to achieve accurate, well-timed, and smooth movement gestures in speech.

a is incorrect. In this therapy, the client intones simple two-to-three-syllable phrases containing high-frequency words or social phrases, tapping out each syllable as it is produced, while the clinician provides auditory models and visual cues.

b is incorrect. This linguistic approach addresses the gradual suppression of phonological processes through listening to correct speech-sound models and learning the kinesthetic and auditory feedback associated with correct target production.

c is incorrect. A vertical approach is an intense (often massed) practice on one or two targets until a specific level of mastery (typically conversational level) is attained, after which new targets are practiced.

d is incorrect. Although the child's motor speech movement/planning may be considered, this approach's focus is consistent production of functional words selected with parent, child, and/or teacher input, and not necessarily incorporating the child's phonetic repertoire.

19.5 Description of Disorder and Recommended Treatment

Although no standardized diagnostic markers for CAS exist, KJ's characteristics were most consistent with a diagnosis of CAS. He demonstrated difficulty with consistent production of consonant and vowels combinations (e.g., VC, CV_1CV_1), accurate timing and production when transitioning between sounds, simplification of more complex syllable shapes, and disturbances in lexical prosody. Additional indicators of motor speech movement/planning deficits included a profoundly limited sound repertoire for consonants and vowels, vowel neutralization, and speech-sound production improvement with multisensory cues and imitative models. KJ's difficulties in breastfeeding and excessive drooling imply some early deficits with oral motor control/planning, a separate but sometimes comorbid condition with verbal motor control/planning difficulties. It is important to note that a diagnosis of CAS does not depend on any single deficit, but on a combination of difficulties suggesting motor speech movement/planning problems.

A DTTC approach was recommended. KJ's family assisted in the development of the treatment plan so that goals were functional and meaningful. Treatment was scheduled for three times a week for 30 minutes.

Table 19.1 Cumulative percent correct for target "mama" across 30 treatment sessions.

	Treatment session										
	1	2	3	4	5	6	7	8	...	30
Daily data (no. of correct/total targets) [a]	5/10	1/11	4/20	5/22	6/26	8/25	13/26	15/26		25/25
Daily percent correct	50	9	20	23	23	32	50	58		100
Cumulative data(no. of correct/total targets) [b]	5/10	6/21	10/41	15/63	21/89	29/114	42/140	57/166		624/780
Cumulative percent correct	50	29	24	24	24	25	30	34		80

[a] Calculate by dividing the number of targets correct each session by the total number of targets produced each session.
[b] Calculate by dividing the total number of targets correct for all sessions by the total number of targets produced for all sessions.

19.6 Outcome

KJ's initial therapy goals included the use of his current sound repertoire to produce functional words or approximations, expanding C and V repertoires, and improving prosody. Seven functional targets across various language functions were "dada," "mama," "whoa," "beep," "me," "no," and "do." Three to four repetitions of targets ("mini-blocks") were practiced in a distributed, variable manner. Initially, KJ required simultaneous productions, but transitioned to direct imitation given verbal placement, visual placement, and gestural cues. Clinician cues were faded with repetitive practice and KJ began to self-cue with gestural prompts. After 15 sessions, he was still unable to produce /p/ in the final position, but during a moment of frustration, spontaneously produced "off." Because it could be elicited with verbal and visual placement cues in subsequent sessions, "off" was added as a target as were VC combinations "on" and "odd."

Production of /i/ and /o/ was prompted with manual gestures using arm movements mimicking each vowel's distinctive oral motor movement and mouth shape. Approximations of target words in isolation were obtained with limited carryover in simple syllable shapes. Prosody using rising and falling intonation activities was achieved for "whoa." Because cumulative percent correct is more useful in accounting for performance variability than daily percent correct, it was used to monitor progress for all targets. KJ achieved 80% cumulative percent correct (▸ Table 19.1) for accuracy (including appropriate lexical stress) for "mama" after 30 sessions.

19.7 Key Points

- CAS presents as a complex symptom and cannot be identified by the presence or absence of any single deficit.
- The family of the client should be actively involved in the development of the treatment plan.
- Speech motor movement/planning gestures should be included using multisensory cues, fading cues as soon as possible.

Suggested Reading

[1] Maas E, Gildersleeve-Neumann C, Jakielski KJ, Stoeckel R. Motor-based intervention protocols in treatment of childhood apraxia of speech (CAS). Curr Dev Disord Rep. 2014; 1(3):197–206

References

[1] Zimmerman I, Steiner Pond R. Preschool Language Scales-5 (5th ed.). Bloomington, MN: Pearson; 2011.
[2] Dodd B, Hua S, Crosbie S, Holm A, Ozanne A. Diagnostic evaluation of articulation and phonology (DEAP). San Antonio, TX: Pearson; 2006.
[3] Maas E, Robin DA, Austermann Hula SN, et al. Principles of motor learning in treatment of motor speech disorders. Am J Speech Lang Pathol. 2008; 17(3): 277–298

20 Severe Speech-Sound Disorder with Motor Involvement

Sarah Strathy-Alie

20.1 Introduction

AB was a 5.1-year-old girl referred for speech assessment and possible treatment by her parents after being discharged from preschool speech and language services.

20.2 Clinical History and Description

AB's parents were aware of delays in her speech development from the age of 18 months (i.e., no spoken words); however, AB did not undergo formal assessment due to limited access in the rural region where they resided. The family moved to a more urban center when AB was 3.6 years of age. At that time, AB's family doctor suspected a global developmental delay and referred her for further assessment. Audiological assessment revealed normal hearing acuity and examination by an ear, nose, and throat (ENT) specialist was unremarkable. Occupational therapy (OT) assessment revealed average fine and gross motor skills. Assessment by a speech-language pathologist (SLP) indicated that AB could follow most simple one- and two-step directions and understood a variety of vocabulary, but had difficulty following longer, more complex instructions at an age-appropriate level. Her expressive language consisted of mostly unintelligible single words and her speech was limited to almost exclusively vowel sounds. Through publicly funded preschool speech-language services, AB received two blocks of weekly speech therapy, eight sessions each, focused on the production of bilabial speech sounds (/p/, /b/, /m/). Psychological assessment at age 4.11 years indicated AB had average nonverbal reasoning skills.

20.3 Clinical Testing

The assessment included a parent interview, oral-motor examination, and administration of the Goldman–Fristoe 2 Test of Articulation, four subtests of the Clinical Evaluation of Language Fundamentals Preschool-2 (CELF-P2), the Bus Story Test, and a spontaneous language sample. Informal literacy testing was conducted and AB named approximately half of the alphabet letters, but not the corresponding sounds, and could not yet read simple words (e.g., cat, mom). The Goldman–Fristoe 2, Bus Story, and language sample were video-recorded for later transcription and more in-depth review.

AB was born following a typical pregnancy and delivery. No family history of speech or language disorders was reported. English was the language spoken at home.

The CELF-P2 indicated moderate delays in receptive language and severe delays in expressive language. The Bus Story transcription consisted of single word attempts, approximately 10% of which could be interpreted (e.g., /d^m/ for *jump*, /d^k/ for *stuck*), paired with frequent gestures (e.g., wagging finger for

bad, arm motion for *jumping over*). AB's spontaneous language also yielded a combination of single word attempts and gestures. AB scored below the first percentile on the Goldman–Fristoe 2 and produced a very limited number of consonant and vowel sounds. AB's speech movements were analyzed based on the Motor Speech Treatment Hierarchy[1] to determine the types of speech movements that were impaired. Difficulty with movement and coordination of the jaw, lips, tongue, and sequencing of speech sounds were observed.

20.4 Questions and Answers for the Reader

1. What information can the SLP obtain from a spontaneous language sample?
   a) A judgment of overall intelligibility in a more natural speaking context.
   b) The child's ability to produce specific speech sounds and motor movements in connected speech.
   c) The child's mean length of utterance (MLU).
   d) All of the above.

Answer: d is correct. A spontaneous language sample is useful for judging the production of both specific speech sounds and movements as well as overall intelligibility in more natural, connected speech. Measures of expressive language skills, including MLU, may also be available from the sample.

a is incorrect. The SLP can judge overall intelligibility from the sample, but also evaluate production of discrete speech sounds and movements in connected speech and calculate MLU.

b is incorrect. The SLP can assess production of discrete speech sounds and movements in connected speech, but also judge overall intelligibility and calculate MLU.

c is incorrect. The SLP can calculate MLU, but also assess production of discrete speech sounds and movements in connected speech and judge overall intelligibility.

2. How would AB's speech–sound disorder (SSD) impact her scores on language testing?
   a) Difficulty producing morphological markers for expressive grammar testing.
   b) Difficulty labeling pictures with intelligible words.
   c) Difficulty pointing to pictures in response to verbal directions.
   d) a and b.
   e) b and c.

Answer: d is correct. Scores on both subtests of expressive language would be impacted by AB's very limited speech–sound inventory and difficulty sequencing speech sounds in words.

a is incorrect. Difficulty with coordinating and sequencing body movements is separate from difficulties with movement of the speech articulators. AB's OT assessment results would support the ability to point to discrete pictures.

b is incorrect. Although AB had difficulty producing the sounds required for morphological markers (e.g., /s/ and /z/ for plural and possessive forms), she also had difficulty producing and sequencing sounds and syllables to label pictures.

c is incorrect. Although AB had difficulty producing and sequencing sounds to label pictures in a way that could be interpreted clearly by the tester (e.g., "dass" for *trophy*), she also had difficulty producing the sounds required for morphological markers.

e is incorrect. Because c is incorrect this is not the correct response.

3. What would the SLP likely note during AB's oral-motor examination?
   a) A short, thick lingual frenulum (ankyloglossia or tongue-tie).
   b) Difficulty with sequential and alternating movement repetitions (e.g., "puh-puh-puh," "puh-tuh-kuh").
   c) A bifid uvula.
   d) Enlarged tonsils.

Answer: b is correct. A child who has an impairment in controlling and sequencing speech movements would have difficulty performing sequential and alternating movement repetitions.

a is incorrect. A short frenulum rarely impairs speech production. Additionally, AB was seen by an ENT who did not report any concerns.

c is incorrect. A bifid uvula may be related to a submucous cleft palate or velopharyngeal insufficiency, but would not impact speech movement and control. Additionally, AB was seen by an ENT who did not report any concerns.

d is incorrect. Enlarged tonsils could result in hyponasal speech and/or mouth-breathing, but would not directly impact speech movement and control. Additionally, AB was seen by an ENT who did not report any concerns.

4. What should the SLP consider when choosing target vocabulary and phrases for therapy?
   a) Information from parents regarding AB's communication needs at home.
   b) AB's current speech abilities and the abilities she needs to develop.
   c) Information from teachers regarding AB's communication needs at school.
   d) All of the above.

Answer: d is correct. It is important to combine movements/sounds AB is already producing with those she has difficulty with for her to be successful. Demands of her communicative environments must also be considered so that words and phrases are functional.

a is incorrect. The home is only one of AB's communicative environments, and if targets are not considered with regard to speech difficulty, AB may experience limited success.

b is incorrect. If targets are chosen exclusively based on AB's acquisition of speech sounds and patterns, they may be limited in functionality for daily activities.

c is incorrect. School is only one of AB's communicative environments, and if targets are not considered with regard to speech difficulty, success may be limited.

20.5 Description of Disorder and Recommended Treatment

AB was determined to have a severe-to-profound SSD with motor involvement, as well as moderate receptive language delay and severe expressive language delay. Motor speech involvement is a term used to describe a subgroup of children with SSD who present with speech characteristics suggesting subtle motor involvement.[2] AB had difficulty sequencing sounds and syllables in longer words and had a limited vowel repertoire, but she did not display groping behaviors or inconsistent errors as in childhood apraxia of speech and no muscle impairment was noted, as in dysarthria.

AB's parents initially agreed to weekly speech therapy, 45 minutes per session. After significant gains following the first 10 weekly treatment sessions, treatment was increased to twice weekly sessions, 30 minutes per session. The initial goals included, but were not limited to, improved jaw control and movement for vowel sounds /ɑ/ and /æ/; improved lip contact for /m/, /b/, and /p/; increased lip rounding for /u/, /o/, and /w/; and expanded repertoire of syllable shapes and functional vocabulary. AB's parents were involved in goal-setting and provided a list of words and phrases that that would be useful to AB in daily activities. Sessions followed a consistent pattern structured to support motor learning[3] and included the following: (1) a shared book-reading activity to introduce a functional target word or phrase; (2) one or two turn-taking activities that consisted of short, quick turns using the target to establish the movement/sound (massed practice); (3) one or two activities with greater time between turns, using the target within a longer utterance, or combining with previously learned targets to support generalization (distributed practice); and (4) instructions for both AB and her parents regarding a home practice activity. Activities were selected to be naturalistic, developmentally appropriate, engaging, and motivating. The parents observed the entire session, and were aware of strategies used to elicit targets so they could support home practice. Strategies included discussion of how the sound(s) and word(s) were produced, slow and clear visual and auditory modeling, many opportunities to repeat the target, and provision of specific feedback regarding the speech movement (e.g., "You used your round lips for /o/'!"). Additionally, Prompts for Restructuring Oral Muscular Phonetic Targets (PROMPT)[4] was employed to cue and stimulate articulatory movement and inhibit unnecessary movements through tactile-kinesthetic input.

A meeting was held at AB's school to discuss her delays in receptive and expressive language. Her treating SLP, an SLP from an agency specializing in augmentative and alternative communication (AAC), the parents, classroom teacher, special-education teacher, and principal of the school attended. It was decided that AB would be placed in a language-impaired class for grade 1, taught by a teacher and educational assistant in a small group setting. AB was also prescribed a voice-output AAC device and the classroom teacher was trained to facilitate its use.

Table 20.1 Scores over time on the *Goldman–Fristoe 2 Test of Articulation*

Age	Raw score[a]	Standard score	Percentile
5.1 years	65	<40	<1
5.6 years	47	46	<1
6.0 years	27	69	2
6.7 years	17	81	5
6.11 years	9	92	13

[a]Number of errors.

20.6 Outcome

Following her 16, twice weekly sessions, AB had a consolidation period over the summer. Over the next year and a half, AB received 30 more weekly sessions, with consolidation periods over the summer and winter when it was more difficult for the family to attend therapy. Goals were regularly reviewed and altered based on progress.

When AB was 6.11 years old, a meeting was held at her school and included the teacher of the language–impaired class, the treating SLP, the school SLP, and the SLP who specialized in AAC. All participants acknowledged significant gains in AB's speech skills, to the point that she could make herself understood in most situations without the use of the AAC device, using increasingly clear words and phrases accompanied by gestures. The SLP who prescribed the AAC device would now work with the classroom teacher to use the device to enhance AB's participation in literacy activities, as this was an area of need. Delays in expressive and receptive language were determined to be impacting AB's communication abilities more than her speech. The school SLP continued to consult with the classroom teacher to support AB's language skills and AB was referred for school-based speech therapy services. AB's parents supported the transition. ▶ Table 20.1 illustrates the progression of AB's speech testing scores over time.

20.7 Key Points

- It is crucial to involve parents and professionals to assist the child with an SSD in becoming an effective communicator and involved participant in his or her daily activities and to support generalization of newly acquired speech skills.
- Application of the principles of motor learning to therapy, including types and frequency of feedback, massed, and distributed practice, can facilitate success and progress.[2,3]
- Multisensory and hierarchical cueing is considered a valuable component of therapy for children with SSDs with motor involvement.[1,2]

Suggested Reading

[1] Namasivayam A, Pukonen M, Hard J, et al. Motor speech treatment protocol for developmental motor speech disorders. Dev Neurorehabil. 2015; 18(5): 296–303

References

[1] Hayden DA, Square PA. Motor speech treatment hierarchy: a systems approach. Clin Commun Disord. 1994; 4(3):162–174
[2] McCauley RJ, Strand EA. Treatment of children exhibiting phonological disorder with motor speech involvement. In: Strand EA, Caruso AJ, eds. Clinical Management of Motor Speech Disorders in Children. New York, NY: Thieme; 1999:187–208
[3] Maas E, Robin DA, Austermann Hula SN, et al. Principles of motor learning in treatment of motor speech disorders. Am J Speech Lang Pathol. 2008; 17(3): 277–298
[4] Hayden DA. PROMPT: A tactually grounded treatment approach to speech production disorders. In: Stockman I, ed. Movement and Action in Learning and Development: Clinical Implications for Pervasive Developmental Disorders. San Diego, CA: Elsevier–Academic Press; 2004:255–297

21 Treatment of Childhood-Onset Fluency Disorder in a High-School Student

Risa Battino

21.1 Introduction

Childhood-onset fluency disorder is a speech disorder characterized by disfluencies or interruptions in the flow of speech. Core stuttering behaviors, including blocks, repetitions, and prolongations, are often accompanied by a variety of secondary behaviors. In addition, negative attitudes and emotions associated with stuttering often negatively impact overall quality of life.

Though about 1% of the population identify as people who stutter, stuttering continues to be misunderstood. Many speech-language pathologists express discomfort working with this population due to their own lack of knowledge and training in this area. Furthermore, speech-language therapy, which focuses on increasing fluency and teaching "speech tools" while ignoring the emotional impact of disfluency, is often ineffective.

21.2 Clinical History and Description

JS was a 17-year-old female high-school student who reportedly began stuttering in early childhood. At the time of initial evaluation, she was enrolled in an 11th–grade regular education class; she repeated the third grade. JS was previously evaluated in elementary school and diagnosed with a fluency disorder and mild language deficits. Speech and language therapy was recommended at that time. She was enrolled in speech and language therapy through both elementary and middle school, but did not receive services in high school. She was reportedly reluctant to resume therapy in high school due to a negative experience, but has expressed desire to attend speech and language therapy outside of school.

21.3 Clinical Testing

JS was initially reluctant to engage in conversation. As the session progressed and she acclimated to the environment, JS more readily engaged in conversation with the clinician. She demonstrated appropriate use of eye gaze to regulate interaction and often used gestures to enhance verbal output and facilitate listener comprehension. However, she frequently looked away from the clinician during moments of dysfluency and formulation of complex ideas. Based on analysis of conversational and reading samples, JS demonstrated various types of disfluencies, including blocks, sound repetitions, reformulations, and fillers, which were accompanied by concomitant behaviors. In addition, she used word substitutions and reformulations to avoid difficult words and sounds.

The Stuttering Severity Instrument-4 (SSI-4) was administered to formally assess JS's fluency (see ► Table 21.1). Percent syllables stuttered was calculated for two 300-syllable speaking samples (storytelling and conversation) and a reading sample to determine the frequency score. Duration score was calculated by averaging the duration, in seconds, of JS's three longest stuttering events (6.2 seconds). The physical concomitant portion was based on clinical observation of four subcategories, which were subjectively scored on a 5-point scale (0 indicating *none*, 5 indicating *severe and painful-looking associated behaviors*). JS exhibited consistent lip/jaw tension, and occasional hand movements and eye gaze aversion. JS received a total overall score of 35, which places her in the 89th to 95th percentile, indicative of a severe fluency disorder.

The Overall Assessment of the Speaker's Experience of Stuttering (OASES) was administered to assess different aspects of JS's experiences with stuttering (► Table 21.2). JS exhibited strong negative reactions to her stutter and these thoughts and feelings interfered with communication, often preventing her from saying what she wanted to in a variety of situations. Though she continued to have a strong drive to communicate, she often changed words to hide her stuttering. JS's negative emotional reactions to stuttering included anger, shame, anxiety, and embarrassment. Although she reported vast knowledge about her stuttering behaviors and the factors that influenced overall severity, she indicated less awareness of general speech

Table 21.1 Scores from the Stuttering Severity Instrument-4 (SSI-4)

Subscale	Description	Task score
Frequency	Percent syllables stuttered (PSS) (average for two speaking tasks) = 20.2% PSS (reading task) = 28.75%	17
Duration	Average duration = 6.2 seconds	12
Physical concomitants	Distracting sounds = 0, facial grimaces = 3, head movements = 2, movements of the extremities = 1	6
Total overall score	**Percentile**	**Severity**
35	89–95	Severe

Table 21.2 Scores from the Overall Assessment of the Speaker's Experience of Stuttering (OASES)

Scale	Raw score	Items answered	Impact scores	Impact rating
General information	49	15	3.3	Moderate/severe
Reactions to stuttering	77	25	3.08	Moderate/severe
Communication in daily situations	70	20	3.5	Moderate/severe
Quality of life	58	19	3.05	Moderate/severe
Overall impact	254	79	3.2	Moderate/Severe

production, treatment options, and self-help groups. JS exhibited significant physical tension and struggle during both stuttered and fluent speech, which often affected her self-image, confidence, perception of how others see her, and her choice of words and speaking situations. Of note, JS reported differences in the degree of difficulty she experienced communicating across contexts. She reported that her stuttering intensified when there was more "pressure" (both in terms of audience size and time considerations) or when she was requesting items (asking for information, ordering food, etc.). She experienced difficulty talking with less familiar people and indicated that she avoided some social situations (e.g., using the telephone, telling stories/jokes, ordering food) to prevent stuttering.

Overall, JS had difficulty accepting stuttering and felt that many aspects of her life had been affected by her disfluency. Her thoughts and experiences negatively impacted her satisfaction with communication, self-esteem, overall attitude toward life, and confidence in herself, resulting in some limitations in her ability to participate in daily activities. Overall, stuttering had a moderate-to-severe impact on JS's life.

21.4 Questions and Answers for the Reader

1. Like JS, children who stutter often experience negative emotional reactions to stuttering, which can interfere with their participation in various activities of daily life. In treatment, the following goals may be considered to address these thoughts and feelings and encourage participation across settings.
   a) JS will increase her knowledge of basic stuttering facts.
   b) JS will demonstrate desensitization by using pseudo-stuttering in the therapy room.
   c) JS will decrease the stresses in her life that cause her to stutter.
   d) JS will identify incidences of avoidance and solve problems to develop a plan to decrease this avoidance.
   e) a, b, and c.
   f) a, b, and d.
   Answer: f is correct. Education leads to empowerment. By increasing a child's knowledge about stuttering in general, they can educate others (parents, teachers, peers) about stuttering and learn to advocate for themselves. Using voluntary/pseudo-stuttering can help a child desensitize to the fear and anticipation of stuttering moments. This helps decrease negative emotions associated with moments of disfluency and

may also lead to decreased avoidance. Children avoid situations due to the anticipation and fear of stuttering. When they successfully avoid, this maintains only the fear and can result in increased struggle and avoidance. Breaking that cycle can help decrease fear and allow the child to participate in daily life activities.
c is incorrect. While stress may aggravate or exacerbate stuttering, it does not *cause* stuttering.
e is incorrect.

2. Many children, such as JS, have negative experiences in speech therapy that lead to a reluctance to attend sessions. Which factors may contribute to this negative experience?
   a) Speech pathologists, as a group, are not empathetic.
   b) Speech therapy is not the correct type of intervention for children who stutter.
   c) Many speech pathologists have decreased knowledge about stuttering and reduced confidence in their ability to treat people who stutter.
   d) Speech therapy focuses solely on "speech tools."
   e) c and d.
   Answer: e is correct. Speech-language pathologists often report difficulty working with students who stutter due to decreased understanding of stuttering treatment, stuttering in general, and the effect of stuttering on academic achievement. This may result from limited or no experience working with persons who stutter during clinical training, no fluency course in graduate school, and limited exposure to people who stutter. This decreased understanding and confidence may result in therapy that is not individualized to the client. It is important for speech-language pathologists to consider the individual and the entirety of the disorder. Therapy that aims to improve overall communication should include goals that target both the emotional and physical manifestations of stuttering. Therapy that focuses solely on techniques to reduce stuttering behaviors is missing a critical component and can result in unrealistic criteria for success.
a is incorrect. This is a gross generalization. While it is possible that individual speech-language pathologists may fit this description, this broad statement is not true across all members of the discipline and does not represent a primary complaint among people who stutter.
b is incorrect. Childhood-onset fluency disorder is a diagnostic classification that falls under the scope of practice for speech-language pathologists. While concomitant developmental disabilities might exist and be treated by professionals from other disciplines, speech-language pathologists take a primary role in the treatment and management of stuttering.

3. It is important for students who stutter and SPLs to educate teachers about the impact stuttering can have on academics. All of the following statements show ways in which stuttering can affect a child's ability to be successful in school **except**:

    a) Students who stutter may be unwilling to read aloud in class.
    b) Students who stutter are not as smart as children who do not stutter, and therefore are unable to complete their schoolwork at the same level as students who do not stutter.
    c) Students who stutter may be reluctant to engage in conversation with peers resulting in isolation from classmates.
    d) Students who stutter may provide incorrect answers to questions in class to avoid saying words/phrases that they anticipate stuttering on.

    Answer: b is correct. Students who stutter have the same range of academic and cognitive strengths and weaknesses as the general population. There is no correlation between stuttering and intelligence.

    a is incorrect. Students who stutter are often unwilling to read aloud in class due to fears that they will stutter in front of their classmates. They have feelings of embarrassment and fear that their classmates and teachers will interpret their stuttering as difficulties with decoding. They fear looking "stupid" in front of classmates and teachers. If the teacher is unaware of the student's communication difficulties and fears, this can result in miscommunication between the student and teachers, resulting in lower grades, especially in the area of class participation.

    c is incorrect. Children who stutter are often reluctant to participate fully in conversation and group discussion with peers, especially when the pressure increases due to increased audience size. This can result in withdrawal from social interactions, avoidance of school events, and missed opportunities for social–emotional growth and sharing of ideas with peers.

    d is incorrect. Owing to feelings of shame and embarrassment, students who stutter may prefer to provide an incorrect response to questions or indicate that they have not completed an assignment instead of stuttering on the correct answer. This results in incorrect perception by peers and teachers of the child's work ethic, knowledge, and abilities, and may result in lower grades.

21.5 Description of Disorder and Recommended Treatment

JS presented with a childhood-onset fluency disorder and, furthermore, stuttering had a negative impact on her quality of life and ability to participate in daily activities. Weekly speech and language therapy sessions were recommended to improve overall communication. Therapy focused on stuttering–modification techniques, as well as avoidance reduction and cognitive restructuring. Goals included increasing her knowledge about speech production and general stuttering facts, identifying negative thoughts and feelings associated with stuttering, identifying situational avoidances, desensitization using pseudo-stuttering, and identifying moments of disfluency and secondary behaviors during moments of disfluency. Family involvement was encouraged and JS was instructed to share information learned in therapy with her parents.

21.6 Outcome

Over the course of the year, JS learned about the etiology of stuttering, developed an understanding of the anatomy of the speech mechanism, identified negative feelings related to stuttering, and identified roadblocks in her ability to communicate in a variety of settings. In addition, she engaged in therapy activities designed to help her face her identified speaking fears. She also worked on strategies to reduce the frequency and severity of stuttering using stuttering–modification techniques. JS improved her overall communication ability and made progress in her ability to discuss feelings and beliefs about stuttering and communication. The amount and severity of JS's disfluencies decreased; specifically, decreased use of secondary behaviors (increased eye contact and decreased hand tapping during moments of disfluency), shorter duration of disfluencies, and decreased tension were observed. After 6 months, the SSI-4 and OASES were administered to assess progress. JS obtained a score of 4 on the physical concomitant scale (previously 6), a score of 16 on the frequency scale (previously 17), and a score of 8 on the duration scale (previously 12). She also demonstrated increased knowledge about stuttering and reported transferring some of her negative thoughts into more constructive concepts. Her scores on the OASES placed her in the mild-to-moderate range for General Information, moderate range for Reactions to Stuttering, moderate range for Communication in Daily Situations, and moderate range for Quality of Life. Though she has made progress, JS continued to exhibit significant disfluencies and struggled with feelings of embarrassment and shame.

21.7 Key Points

- Stuttering is a complex disorder, which includes both physical and emotional factors. Both aspects should be taken into consideration during evaluation and when determining whether a child is a good candidate for speech and language therapy.
- Stuttering therapy should be individualized to the client and should include goals that target both stuttering behaviors and emotional challenges. Treatment goals often include speech–modification techniques to decrease the frequency and severity of disfluencies as well as goals that focus on improving self-esteem and confidence, learning to manage stuttering, and decreasing the impact of disfluency on overall quality of life.
- Many children have negative experiences with stuttering therapy that lead to doubts about its effectiveness. There is no simple cure, and for many school-aged children who stutter, complete fluency is not a realistic goal. Therefore, it is important to determine appropriate criteria for success.

Suggested Readings

[1] Chmela K, Reardon NA. The School-Age Child Who Stutters: Working Effectively with Attitudes and Emotions. Memphis, TN: Stuttering Foundation; 2001

[2] Coleman C, Yaruss JS. A comprehensive view of stuttering: implications for assessment and treatment. SIG 16 Perspectives on School-Based Issues. 2014; 15(2):75–80

[3] Guitar B. Stuttering: An Integrated Approach to Its Nature and Treatment. 4th ed. Baltimore, MD: Lippincott Williams & Wilkins; 2014

22 Language-Based Learning Disability and Literacy in a School-Aged Student

Megan Dunn Davison

22.1 Introduction

This case highlights the complexity of a school-aged student with language-based learning disability in integrating language and literacy in the academic setting. In the Common Core State Standards for English Language Arts, grade-level standards for writing are included in an integrated model of literacy—a model that recognizes that effective communication requires skills across four modalities: reading, writing, speaking, and listening. Language is the foundation of each of these modalities. Students are expected to use written language to offer and support opinions, demonstrate understanding of academic subjects, and convey real and imagined experiences and events often relying on decontextualized language. For students with language-based learning disabilities, reading and writing are particularly challenging academic skills.

22.2 Clinical History and Description

AD was a 9.2-year-old girl in the third grade. She was referred for speech-language pathology consultation in the second grade to address academic difficulties resulting from decoding and spelling weaknesses and expressive language deficits identified by her classroom teacher. AD's parents also expressed concern regarding her academic difficulties, particularly her struggle with reading and math homework. She had an individualized education plan (IEP) in place and received teacher consultant services twice weekly in the classroom and speech-language intervention twice weekly individually. AD also received testing accommodations including a separate, small-group setting with test questions provided orally.

22.3 Clinical Testing

A battery of tests was administered to gain additional information regarding AD's language and literacy difficulties. Results are presented in ▶ Table 22.1.

As shown in ▶ Table 22.1, weaknesses were observed in decoding and reading comprehension. As reported by the speech-language pathologist, during the assessment, AD often guessed words in passages based on a few letters (e.g., airplane/alphabet; rainbow/rain boots; instant/insect). The combination of decoding weakness and a tendency toward guessing words in passages greatly impacted her ability to use semantic and syntactic context to determine the meaning of a sentence (Woodcock Reading Mastery Tests-Revised [WRMT-R]: passage comprehension). Similar difficulty was noted on theGray Oral Reading Tests-5 (GORT-5), as the vocabulary in the passages became less familiar (e.g., jay/jar; peach/perched; found/flown).

Table 22.1 Clinical testing results

	Standard score[a]	Percentile rank[b]	Descriptive rating
Comprehensive Test of Phonological Processing-2 (CTOPP-2)			
Elision	9	37	Average
Blending words	7	16	Low average
Phoneme isolation	8	25	Average
Memory for digits	6	9	Below average
Non–word repetition	7	16	Low average
Rapid digit naming	9	37	Average
Rapid letter naming	10	50	Average
Woodcock Reading Mastery Tests-Revised (WRMT-R)[c]			
Visual–auditory learning	82	12	Borderline average
Word identification	91	28	Average
Word attack	80	9	Below average
Passage comprehension	68	2	Poor
Gray Oral Reading Tests-5 (GORT-5)			
Rate	8	25	Average
Accuracy	7	16	Low average
Fluency	8	25	Average
Comprehension	9	37	Average

[a]Mean of 10; standard deviation of ±3 or mean of 50; standard deviation of ±15.

[b]Mean of 50.

[c]Norms based on grade level—all other norms based on age.

Because accuracy scores on the GORT-5 are impacted by repetitions as well as errors in productions, and the ceiling is achieved by decoding performance only, AD reached ceiling just at the point where her decoding weaknesses affected comprehension.

Classroom artifacts were also collected to examine her written language performance on curriculum-based reading and writing assignments (▶ Fig. 22.1). Her underlying language difficulties directly impacted the length, accuracy, and semantic and syntactic complexity of written language.

22.4 Questions and Answers for the Reader

1. Which of the following best describes the areas of weakness for a student with a language-based learning disability?
   a) Decoding key vocabulary words.
   b) Following two-step directions.
   c) A spectrum of difficulties related to language, reading, spelling, and/or writing.
   d) Expressive language.

   Answer: c is correct. Language-based learning disabilities include a spectrum of difficulties related to reading, spelling, and/or writing across the curriculum.

   a is incorrect. Although students with language-based learning disabilities will likely have difficulty in decoding single words and words within text due to limited phonological, semantic, and syntactic understanding, decoding is only one of several areas of difficulty.

   b is incorrect. Most students will be able to follow simple, two-step directions. However, the more complex the directions, the more difficult it is for students with language-based learning disabilities. For example, note the difference in semantic and syntactic complexity between the following: "If there is a star circle it" compared to "If there is a moon circle it unless it is next to a star."

   d is incorrect. Students with language-based learning disabilities will have difficulty with expressive language, but this describes only one piece of the spectrum of difficulties students will likely demonstrate.

2. Children who have difficulties with reading and conversational speech:
   a) Do not often have difficulty with writing.
   b) Also have difficulty with spelling.
   c) Do not have difficulty with spelling.

Fig. 22.1 Writing sample from classroom assignment: After reading *Jesse's Favorite Holiday*, write about your favorite holiday and why.

d) Often have difficulties with spelling and writing due to the underlying phonological, semantic, and syntactic deficits of language.

Answer: d is correct. Language-based learning disabilities include a spectrum of difficulties related to reading, spelling, and/or writing. It is important to recognize the many different facets that language can impact in academic success and how each of these modalities is required to meet curriculum-based standards.

a is incorrect. Students with language-based learning disabilities often demonstrate difficulties with written language.

b is incorrect. Students with language-based learning disabilities often have difficulties with spelling, and also a range of related difficulties with decoding, reading comprehension, and written language.

c is incorrect. Students with language-based learning disabilities often exhibit difficulties with spelling.

3. Which of the following are effective strategies for a teacher and speech-language pathologists to use in collaboration to increase academic outcomes in students with language-based learning disabilities?
   a) Providing a workshop on language techniques for teachers.
   b) Requesting a speech-language pathologist to determine whether strategies in therapy sessions are being used in the classroom to formally evaluate students.
   c) Focusing on the writing process, including self-regulation and cognitive strategies in both speech-language therapy sessions and classroom activities.
   d) Providing teachers with evidence-based research articles.

   Answer: c is correct. Best practice in speech-language pathology includes generalization of skills and strategies across contexts, including speech-language sessions and the classroom; therefore, speech-language pathologists and teachers may best support students by collaboratively supporting the same instructional strategies.

   a is incorrect. Opportunities to share specific language techniques and strategies may be useful for developing a collaborative relationship between teachers and speech-language pathologists; however, when considering instructional strategies that students can use across a variety of subjects and classes, it is important for students to learn strategies that can carry over to all types of learning situations.

   b is incorrect. Informal observations may occur by each professional in each respective setting, but it will not be the sole responsibility of the speech-language pathologist nor would formal assessments be required as part of the IEP.

   d is incorrect. Although sharing resources with teachers will be a part of cross-professional training and development, collaborative teaching directly impacts the student.

4. For a student in first or second grade who has difficulty in decoding as a result of a language-based learning disability, the most appropriate early-intervention strategy would focus on efforts to increase the student's:
   a) Naming skills through vocabulary–building exercises.
   b) Phonological abilities, including phonological awareness and phonological memory.
   c) Production of target language structures through drill.
   d) Social skill practice through storytelling and narratives.

Answer: b is correct. The ability to manipulate and understand sounds is key to decoding; therefore, targeting phonological abilities will help support decoding of key vocabulary words.

a is incorrect. Naming may be an area of weakness; however, building the foundational skills for decoding is an important first step to facilitate decoding of both familiar and unfamiliar words.

c is incorrect. Language structures, including grammatical markers, prefixes, and suffixes, etc., may be an area of weakness and can be targeted by first teaching foundational phonological abilities (e.g., blending, segmenting, and elision).

d is incorrect. Narrative development may be an area of weakness and will be a focus of intervention along with targeting phonological skills related to decoding.

22.5 Description of Disorder and Recommended Treatment

AD presented with a language-based learning disability. Language-based learning disabilities include a spectrum of difficulties related to reading, spelling, and/or writing. Students with language-based learning disabilities often have difficulty understanding and employing both spoken and written language, which undermines their academic success. Specifically, limited language skills impede comprehension and communication, which are the basis for most academic outcomes. Most students with language-based learning disabilities demonstrate weakness across multiple areas of language that specifically relate to literacy. Potential difficulties include errors in phoneme production (particularly when sounding out words in oral reading activities), use of nonspecific language to express ideas or opinions in spoken and written language, difficulty retelling stories, difficulty with topic maintenance, and difficulty creating written sentences or limited sentences with grammatically complete information.

Table 22.2 TWA + PLANS

TWA	PLANS
Think before reading	1. Do **Pick** goals
Think about:	• **List** ways to meet goals
• The author's purpose	• **And**
• What you know	make **Notes**
• What you want to learn	• **Sequence** notes
Think **While** reading	
Think about:	2. Write and say more
• Reading speed	• Test goals
• Linking knowledge	
• Rereading parts	
Think **After** reading	
Think about:	
• The main idea	
• Summarizing information	
• What you learned	

Source: Adapted from Harris et al.; 2008.[1]

The focus of intervention for AD was improved reading comprehension and writing using a cognitive apprenticeship model of reading and writing instruction, also known as self-regulated strategy development. This model highlights the underlying cognitive processes that connect what is being read to writing. Self-regulated strategy development is implemented by using steps to develop background knowledge, discussing the strategy goals and significance, modeling the strategies, having the student memorize the strategy, supporting continued strategy practice, and providing opportunities for the student to engage in independent practice. Using a mnemonic device, TWA + PLANS (see ▸ Table 22.2), and an outline, AD learned how to Think before reading, While reading, and After reading while taking notes to write a summary paragraph, including the main idea and three supporting details after reading a grade-level science or social studies text. She employed PLANS to Pick goals, List ways to meet goals, And make Notes and Sequence notes, to further support writing a complete essay.

After following these steps, AD reviewed her essay to see whether her selected writing goals were met. A completed written essay using TWA + PLANS is shown in ▸ Fig. 22.2.

22.6 Outcome

In the previous academic year, goals of literacy intervention included identifying the main idea and supporting details in short (two to three) paragraphs and phonological decoding principles, which were met. However, when text became longer

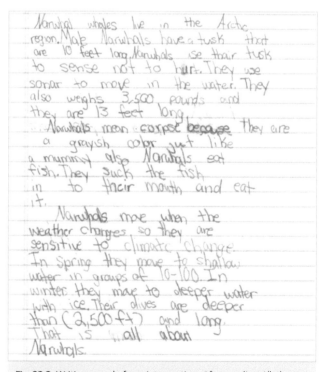

Fig. 22.2 Writing sample from intervention: After reading *All about Narwhals*, write three things that you learned.

and included many detailed points or dialogue, AD's decoding decreased and her accuracy in identifying the main idea decreased. In addition, written language was a particular area of weakness when paired with a reading assignment, which is often required in daily classroom activities and homework. Therefore, the focus of intervention was improved reading comprehension and writing using TWA + PLANS. AD was motivated using this strategy and demonstrated increased accuracy and length of written language. At the start of the academic year, AD required verbal prompts and maximal clinician support to identify and implement the steps of TWA + PLANS. Over the course of the academic year, as AD's knowledge and familiarity with this strategy increased, the level of support and verbal prompts provided gradually decreased. Currently, AD independently identifies all steps of TWA + PLANS and requires minimal support to implement the strategy to identify and write the main ideas and supporting details from grade-level text in a three- to four-paragraph essay.

22.7 Key Points

- School-aged children are expected to participate in academic discourse in both spoken and written modalities using decontextualized language.

- Underlying language deficits can significantly impact literacy, including decoding, reading comprehension, spelling, and written language.
- Using a cognitive apprenticeship model, such as self-regulated strategy development, speech-language pathologists can help support students comprehensive development of the writing process through supported reading and writing.

Suggested Readings

[1] Graham S, McKeown D, Kiuhara S, Harris KR. A meta-analysis of writing instruction for students in elementary grades. J Educ Psychol. 2012; 104(4): 879–896

[2] Harris KR, Graham S, Mason LH. Improving the writing performance, knowledge, and motivation of struggling writers in second grade: The effects of self-regulated strategy development. Am Educ Res J. 2006; 43:295–340

[3] Graham S, Harris KR. Strategy instruction and the teaching of writing: A meta-analysis. In: MacArthur C, Graham S, Fitzgerald J, eds. Handbook of Writing Research. New York, NY: Guilford; 2006:187-207

References

[1] Harris KR, Graham S, Mason LH, Friedlander B. Powerful Writing Strategies for All Students. Baltimore, MD: Brookes; 2008.

23 Global Language Impairment in a Preschooler with Autism

Jennifer C. Friberg and Savannah P. Little

23.1 Introduction

Global language impairment is common in autism, with delays observed in pragmatics, semantics, syntax, and morphology development. Young children with autism may display lack of joint attention, eye gaze, expression, use of gestures, and a general lack of flexibility with language. Because these deficits impact on how language is employed to listen and to verbally communicate, these language disorders are termed global impairments.

23.2 Clinical History and Description

BW was a 39-month-old female child who was recently evaluated by a pediatrician for suspicion of autism. She was eventually given a diagnosis of autism due to specific observable behaviors (repetitive motions) and what was considered to be significant communication concerns. BW had never been evaluated by a speech-language pathologist (SLP). BW's mother reports that she "isn't a good communicator," struggling to make her wants and needs known with "meltdowns" when she is not understood.

23.3 Clinical Testing

Clinical testing began with classroom observation. BW had difficulty establishing joint attention, disengaging with most tasks that involved social interaction with other peers or adults. She tended to fixate on her favorite objects (e.g., a flashlight) for extended periods of time. BW followed simple, one-step directions that referenced classroom routines, but needed verbal cueing from peers and the teacher to do so. BW was observed to request during this observation, saying "pencil" when asked what she needed during art time. BW's verbal output was restricted to one- to two-word utterances, containing mostly nouns and verbs in common word categories (e.g., animals, food words). The MacArthur Bates Communicative Development Inventory[1] questionnaire was sent home for BW's mother to complete. This questionnaire confirmed that similar word usage was employed at home.

Following classroom observation, play-based assessment quantified BW's communication skills in social contexts. A language sample was collected during snack time, which revealed difficulties with vocabulary and grammar. Her vocabulary lacked diversity; a 0.26 type-token ratio (TTR) was observed. TTR is a measurement of lexical diversity in a child's spontaneous speech. TTR is calculated by dividing the total number of different words used by the total number of words a child says in a given language sample. TTR scores can range from 0 to 1, and the higher the ratio, the higher the degree of word varia-

tion in a child's natural speech. BW's TTR was considered low. BW used verbal language to request or refuse. No commenting or use of social words (e.g., hello, please) was noted. BW's language was characterized by one- to two-word utterances, with a mean length of utterance of 1.47. BW also struggled to take turns or display appropriate proximity with peers. Her gross motor skills appeared intact, but some fine motor deficits were evident (e.g., inability to grasp snack crackers in a pincer grasp).

The Preschool Language Scales, 5th Edition,[2] was also administered. Her standard scores were as follows:
- Auditory comprehension = 68.
- Expressive communication = 63.
- Total communication = 65.

This assessment was completed over the course of 2 weeks in 5- to 15-minute increments to minimize the potential for attentional and/or behavioral issues to negatively affect her score. Even with this testing approach, BW was not compliant or attentive for all parts of testing; thus, results from this standardized assessment may represent a minimal estimate of BW's communication skills.

23.4 Questions and Answers for the Reader

1. Joint attention is considered critical for language development and use because:
   a) Shared attention between a speaker and the listener is the foundation for successful communication and learning.
   b) Joint attention allows for children to focus intently on an object of personal interest in isolation.
   c) Joint attention is a skill that is innate in all children and is therefore something that does not need to be taught to any child.
   d) After learning vocabulary and grammar, children develop joint attention skills that allow them to participate in conversations with adults and peers.

   Answer: a is correct. If a child lacks joint attention skills, she or he is not able to actively attend to another person. Children learn language primarily through exposure to language via conversation, direct labeling, and/or observations of others using language. Thus, a child who lacks joint attention misses out on important opportunities to learn language due to social disengagement.

   b is incorrect. Joint attention necessitates shared focus with a social partner and cannot occur in isolation.

   c is incorrect. Joint attention develops by engaging with others socially. For children with autism, this skill often has to be directly taught so that intervention can be most effective.

d is incorrect. Joint attention is the driving force behind vocabulary or grammar acquisition and, as such, must be established in the first year of life for a child to acquire language competency that eventually allows for conversational skills to develop.

2. Social skills instruction to increase pragmatic language functioning in children with autism is thought to be most effective when it occurs:
   a) Primarily with other children with autism or other disabilities.
   b) Across naturalistic settings in and out of the classroom over the course of each day.
   c) When children are engaged in 1:1 intervention with the SLP.
   d) Via consultative intervention only.

Answer:b is correct. As social situations arise throughout the day, teaching pragmatic language skills to support these interactions as they occur is important. Additionally, if pragmatic language skills are modeled in varied settings, with a range of communication partners throughout the day, children with autism are better able to generalize these skills to use them independently.

a is incorrect. Children with autism should be exposed to neurotypically developing peers as language models to encourage age-appropriate social interactions/pragmatic language use.

c is incorrect. Intervention such as this represents a social/conversational environment that does not mirror the natural contexts where children with autism need to use social language skills. The best outcomes for facilitating social language occur when SLPs and others take advantage of teachable moments in the context of commonplace social experiences.

d is incorrect. Consultation is often a component of intervention to provide training and support for other individuals (e.g., teachers, parents, teacher's aids) seeking to engage socially with a child with a pragmatic language disorder. That said, it is rarely the only service delivery model that should be used, as direct teaching and support from the SLP is necessary to facilitate the social language skills vital to effective communication.

3. BW's annual review is approaching at school, and her case manager recommends reassessment. She specifically asks for results from at least one standardized test. Considering BW's previous assessment history, how might you proceed?
   a) Administer a standardized test as specified in the examiner's manual, making no accommodations for BW.
   b) Administer a standardized test as specified in the examiner's manual, but calculate her standard scores using norms for a child 1 year younger so that you can account for her language disorder.
   c) Use dynamic assessment to administer the standardized test to BW, making accommodations for her as needed (e.g., modifying questions, materials, cues) to gather data to inform intervention planning.
   d) Administer a standardized test as specified in the examiner's manual but report age–equivalent scores only (no standard scores) to allow a different perspective of BW's functional language skills.

Answer:c is correct. Dynamic assessment allows the SLP to modify the content, instructions, materials, etc. of the test being administered to observe language use by individualizing the testing experience for a child who is less responsive to the structured environment necessary for administration of an assessment in a standardized fashion. Data collected via dynamic assessment are typically very supportive of intervention planning.

b is incorrect. Because standard scores are calculated by comparing a test taker to his or her peers, the practice of comparing a child with a disorder to a chronologically younger peer is not valid and should never be used.

a is incorrect. As BW's eligibility for services is not in question, the need to administer a standardized test with no accommodations is questionable, as data collected in this manner will likely yield data that underestimate BW's language competency. Rather, other forms of assessment should be considered to maximize the value of the information collected.

d is incorrect. Age-equivalent scores are considered to be "developmental" scores rather than scores of relative standing. Thus, age-equivalent scores do not allow for comparisons of a student's performance within or across tests. Additionally, because of how they are computed, age-equivalent scores are considered to be inaccurate and should not be used to describe a child's competency in language or any other developmental area.

23.5 Description of Disorder and Recommended Treatment

BW presented with a language disorder that impacted receptive, expressive, and pragmatic language skills. These deficits, which impacted her ability to encode, decode, and effectively engage with others to share information, were consistent with her medical diagnosis of autism. The Individuals with Disabilities Education Act[3] and the Diagnostic and Statistical Manual of Mental Disorders-5th Edition (DSM-5)[4] both define the spectrum of behaviors observed in autism. Both entities identify autism as a disorder characterized by significant verbal, nonverbal, and social communication deficits; stereotypical and repetitive activities and motor movements; insistence on sameness and adversity to environmental change; and abnormal sensory processing, which results in unusual responses to sensory stimuli.

Intervention for BW focused on play-based approaches within classroom settings to improve pragmatic and expressive language skills. Treatment predominantly followed a social interactionist approach to improve and expand vocabulary, follow classroom and home routines, improve joint attention, and increase functional communication (i.e., expression of wants, needs, feelings, and preferences). For work on mastery of rote concepts such as shapes, colors, letters, and numbers, a behavioral approach was implemented with a focus on stimuli (material to be taught), responses (verbal communication from BW), and positive reinforcement (from the SLP) to teach concepts while reducing problem behaviors. ▶ Fig. 23.1 illustrates the interaction and overlap between these approaches, which,

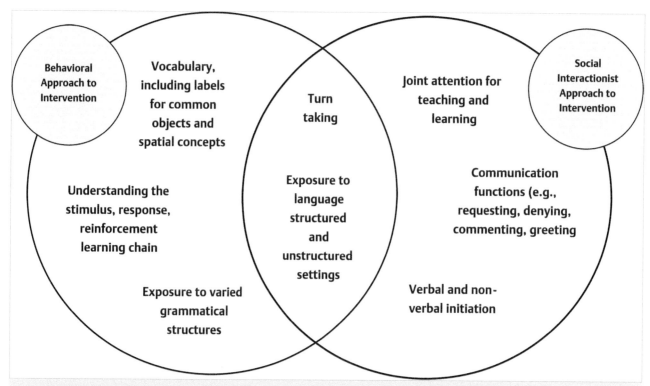

Fig. 23.1 Integration of potential treatment priorities by theoretical approach. This figure illustrates the similarities and differences in the types of skills targeted when different theoretical approaches are used as part of a language intervention plan. Optimally, these different approaches will be complimentary, with social and behavioral learning integrating for functional, generalized communication across academic and social contexts.

when implemented together, should lead to increased language competency in social and academic settings.

Additionally, BW's teachers and parents were trained on the approaches used as part of treatment to support generalization of skills and concepts from language intervention across home and school environments.

23.6 Outcome

After 3 months of treatment, BW made observable classroom improvements. She followed most daily classroom routines (i.e., bathroom, snack time) with verbal directions and visual aids (e.g., matching picture cards with a schedule board). She frequently verbalized two– to three-word utterances 50% of the time to comment and to state her likes/dislikes to her teachers and classmates. BW interacted more appropriately with her classmates by taking turns. Parallel play was emerging in structured activities. Although problem behaviors persisted, their frequency and severity decreased, leading to successful social interaction with her peers.

BW's parents reported that she employed more diverse language at home, incorporating some pronouns, more adjectives, and different verb tenses into conversational speech. They also reported that her behavioral outbursts decreased, as they are now able to understand more of her communication attempts and needs, and have successfully implemented approaches suggested by the teacher and SLP at home.

BW was evaluated by the school occupational therapist (OT), physical therapist, and school psychologist and was eligible for special education services and occupational therapy. BW's

teacher reported that she improved in her developmental play skills, such as completing puzzles, sorting colors, and identifying shapes. She manipulated writing and coloring pencils with OT-developed accommodations. Supports will be implemented as long as needed in an effort to allow BW to function as independently as possible within her home and school settings.

23.7 Key Points

- BW's language was consistent with a global language delay because she struggles to use expressive, receptive, and pragmatic language to meet her needs.
- Assessment for BW was difficult due to her lack of joint attention. A variety of approaches and measures were needed to triangulate observations and form a clear picture of BW's strengths and weaknesses, relative to communication.
- Treatment for BW's language disorder incorporated a variety of approaches to serve different needs: teaching, socializing, and generalizing.
- BW's problem behaviors and repetitive actions impacted her ability to learn, socialize, and function within her classroom. Pairing the social interactionist and behavioral models in her therapy sessions helped decrease her problem behaviors and increase her language abilities.

Suggested Readings

[1] Burton KD, Wolfberg P, Eds. Learners on the Autism Spectrum: Preparing Highly Qualified Educators and Related Practitioners. 2nd ed. Shawnee Mission, KS: AAPC Publishing; 2014

[2] Prelock PA, McCauley RJ, Eds. Treatment of Autism Spectrum Disorders: Evidence-Based Intervention Strategies for Communication and Social Interaction. Baltimore, MD: Brookes Publishing; 2012

References

[1] Fenson L, Marchman VA, Thal DJ, Dale PS, Reznick JS, Bates E. MacArthur-Bates Communicative Development Inventories. Baltimore, MD: Brookes Publishing; 2007

[2] Zimmerman IL, Steiner BS, Pond RE. Preschool Language Scales. 5th ed. San Antonio, TX: Pearson; 2011

[3] Individuals with Disabilities Education Act, 20 U.S.C. § 1400 (2004)

[4] American Psychiatric Association. Diagnostic and Statistical Manual of Mental Disorders. 5th ed. Washington, DC: American Psychiatric Association; 2013

24 Voice Care for the Child Who Is Post–Airway Reconstruction: Special Challenges

Lisa N. Kelchner, Susan Baker Brehm, and Barbara Weinrich

24.1 Introduction

Caring for children who have a voice disorder secondary to airway reconstruction requires specific knowledge of the repaired anatomy and physiology, its potential for successful behavioral manipulation and change, and the capacity of the child and his/her family to participate in the recommended treatment. The larynx may be so scarred that the source of vibration involves structures other than the true vocal folds (TVFs). Often, these children have complex medical histories, and during their early years, voice quality is not a priority. However, as the child develops and his/her overall health becomes more stable, voice quality essential to effective communication and educational achievement increases in importance. Collaborative assessment and treatment that includes speech-language pathology, pediatric otolaryngology, educators, and family members is essential for these children.

24.2 Clinical History and Description

JD, a 12-year-old girl, was born at 27 weeks and required 3 weeks of endotracheal intubation and subsequent tracheotomy for long-term airway management. At age 3 years, she underwent airway reconstruction (anterior costal cartilage graft) and was decannulated 2 months later. Her parents described her postsurgical voice as weak and airy. Her medical history included bronchopulmonary dysplasia and asthma. She was followed by an otolaryngologist and speech-language pathologist for voice, reflux, and airway protection issues until age 5 years. Her parents reported that her only remaining complaint was her voice and difficulty being understood. She looked forward to college and eventually becoming a teacher. All other developmental milestones were adjusted or typical, and she had no persistent health issues other than a very occasional episode of asthma.

24.3 Clinical Testing

Pediatric Voice Handicap Index (pVHI): The pVHI,[1] a parent-proxy voice handicapping index, was administered to JD's mother, who recorded the following scores for her daughter: Functional—17/28, with the highest scores related to being understood in a noisy environment, being asked to repeat herself, and voice difficulties restricting personal, educational, and social activities; Physical—9/36, with the highest scores relating to running out of air while speaking and using excessive strain/yell; and Emotional—6/28, with the highest scores for frustration and embarrassment.

The Consensus Auditory Perceptual Evaluation of Voice (CAPE-V)[2] is a 100-mm visual analog scale clinicians use to rate the perceptual qualities of overall severity (OS), roughness (R), breathiness (B), strain (S), pitch (P), and loudness (L). The higher number rating is equivalent to increased severity. Ratings for JD were: OS = 60; R = 40; B = 55; S = 40; P = 57 (low); L = 58 (soft). Intermittent ventricular fold phonation was detected perceptually.

Acoustic measures were obtained utilizing a Computerized Speech Laboratory (CSL; Model 4500; PENTAX Medical). Initially, JD was asked to sustain /a/ for 5 seconds. Visual inspection of a narrow-band spectrogram of the vowel revealed a type 2 acoustic signal, as depicted in ▶ Fig. 24.1. Some variability in the voice signal was noted with bursts of both type 1 and type 3 signal productions. Intensity level of a sustained vowel was 63 dB/SPL, which is within a normal-to-low range for this production. JD's maximum phonation time was 7 seconds, which is a shorter duration than expected, indicating limitations in respiratory support and/or laryngeal valving. However, generally, if a patient can sustain a vowel for 5 seconds, conversational phrasing is not impacted.

Aerodynamic measures were obtained utilizing the Phonatory Aerodynamic System (PAS; Pentax Medical). The system consists of an airflow mask connected to a pneumotach to obtain measures of airflow characteristics during speech. Mean airflow rate was 196.6 mL/s. Estimated subglottic pressure (Psub) is quantified through an intraoral pressure tube. Average peak airflow during a syllable train of /pa-pa-pa.../ was 13.13 cm H_2O, which was higher than average given JD's age.

Laryngeal imaging was performed using both rigid and flexible endoscopes. JD's left TVF was scarred along the posterior portion and the mobility of the left cricoarytenoid (CA) joint was restricted. The right TVF appearance and CA joint motion appeared normal. A large posterior gap was noted with difficulty maintaining closure of the anterior two-thirds of the TVFs during brief periods of sustained phonation. ▶ Fig. 24.2, a still

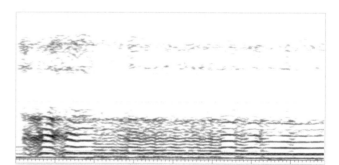

Fig. 24.1 Baseline narrow-band spectrogram. Note the presence of subharmonics between harmonics. Voice sample was a sustained /ah/.

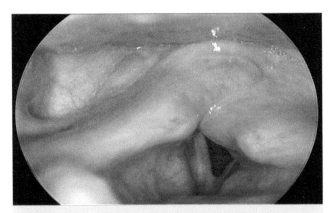

Fig. 24.2 JD's baseline endoscopy. Note the scarred, thin left TVF.

photo from JD's endoscopic exam taken while the TVFs were abducted, shows the scarred and shortened left TVF and healthy right TVF. In an effort to improve glottic closure, a tendency for moderate-to-severe compression of the ventricular folds was observed such that intermittent ventricular phonation was noted, indicating a mixed phonation source. Of note, discreet stroboscopic ratings were not made due to issues of acoustic fidelity and signal tracking (predominant type 2 signal). During brief periods of more periodic signal and improved tracking, a mildly reduced mucosal wave across the surface of the right TVF was observed.

Direct examination under anesthesia included palpation of the joints and close inspection of the TVFs. Restricted mobility of the left CA joint and scarring of the posterior portion of the left TVF were confirmed. The subglottic airway was patent.

24.4 Questions and Answers for the Reader

1. A type 2 signal indicates:
   a) Harmonics in this voice signal are not at all distinguishable.
   b) Harmonics can be clearly viewed, but subharmonics are also observed.
   c) The interpretation of the acoustic measures (e.g., average F_0; frequency range) associated with this voice signal are reliable.
   d) The equipment on which you captured and analyzed the signal needs to be checked.

Answer: b is correct. Using a narrow-band spectrogram, the presence of harmonics is definitely detectable but the presence of subharmonics indicates the presence of noise in the voice signal. In this case, the multiple sources of vibration and incomplete glottis closure (resulting in increased air turbulence) are generating the noise in this child's voice signal.

a is incorrect. Using a narrow-band spectrogram to visualize and analyze the sustained vowel voice segment, inability to distinguish any harmonics would be seen on a type 3 voice signal.

c is incorrect. Using a narrow-band spectrogram, the presence of the subharmonics calls into question the reliability of the interpretation of acoustic values. If acoustic values are reported, they should note they were done so in this context.

d is incorrect. If you are collecting and analyzing voice signal data using standard protocols and appropriate settings, identifying a voice signal as type 2 is not an indication of any equipment issue. Type 2 signals are often associated with varying degrees of dysphonia.

2. What do the reported airflow measures tell you about the work of voicing this young woman must use on a daily basis to be understood?
   a) That she is having to force her voice to be heard and understood.
   b) They are of little value since she has a unilateral restricted arytenoid joint mobility.
   c) They are a direct indication of the degree of scarring of the left TVF.
   d) They are always found in someone who also has a type 2 voice signal.

Answer: a is correct. Although 196 mL/s is considered within an appropriate average airflow range for her age, it is on the high end of the normal. It suggests that she is not able to adequately valve the larynx during phonation. It may be why her maximum sustained phonation is short. Likewise, her elevated average estimated subglottal pressure is indicative of hyperfunction during speech production. This corresponds to the report of vocal and general fatigue during conversation.

b is incorrect. Using standard protocols and procedures, collecting airflow measures on individuals with suspected or reported incomplete glottic closure is appropriate and helpful in quantifying the degree of laryngeal incompetence and effort used during connected speech.

c is incorrect. Although scarring can impact glottic closure and phonatory function, there is no reported correspondence of presence of scarring on the TVFs and alteration of airflow measures.

d is incorrect. Although both type 2 signals and elevated airflow values may be found in the same individual, type 2 signals may be found in individuals with normal or restricted airflow measures.

3. What does the presence of mixed voice source mean?
   a) There is no such thing. There can be only one source of vibration within the larynx: the TVFs.
   b) The individual has a unique talent that allows him/her to switch between glottic and supraglottic phonation.
   c) The individual is also using an augmentative or amplification device to generate speech.
   d) To accomplish voicing, the individual uses such effort that other laryngeal structures, such as the ventricular folds, are compressed and as such are in the phonatory airstream and able to vibrate.

Answer: d is correct. The use of supraglottal structures as a sound source during phonation is often observed when there is incomplete closure of the TVFs and this is what we refer to as an individual having a mixed sound source. In some instances, all structures (supraglottic and TVFs) may vibrate simultaneously or you can have periods where one vibration source dominates. It often has to do with the degree of impairment and subsequent effort. In some children post–airway reconstruction, the TVFs are so scarred that they are unable to vibrate at all and only supraglottic structures are used.

a is incorrect. In most typical healthy larynges, only the TVFs vibrate during sustained phonation and connected speech. In a damaged, repaired, or otherwise structurally altered larynx, other structures can be compressed and vibrate on the phonatory airstream.

b is incorrect. Although some individuals and certain performers can control and switch between true and ventricular fold vibration, that is not what we refer to in this instance. In this case, a mixed voicing source is an unintended consequence of the original airway injury and subsequent reconstruction.

c is incorrect. If an individual also uses an augmentative communication device and amplification, it is termed as such and they are not referred to as having a mixed phonation source.

24.5 Description of Disorder and Recommended Treatment

At the time of evaluation, JD and her parents were sufficiently concerned and wanted to pursue options for voice therapy, especially given her nearing her teenage years. It is not unusual for parents of children with a history of complex airway conditions to wait until the child is older before seeking treatment. JD's parents expressed a particular concern that her voice was low and rough for a female. JD also complained of vocal fatigue during conversation and was tired of people asking her to repeat herself. Voice therapy was recommended with the long-term goal of improving voice quality using behavioral therapy techniques and possible surgical intervention in the form of injection augmentation.

Behavioral therapy included use of techniques intended to reduce laryngeal tension and regional hyperfunction and maximize closure of the TVF edges during sustained phonation. Therapeutic strategies included general voice use and hygiene counseling, semi-occluded vocal tract(SOVT) exercises, modified vocal function exercises (e.g., sustained /o/ and /i/ on limited pitches), and amplification for noisy environments, particularly in school.

24.5.1 Voice Use and Vocal Hygiene

Vocal behaviors were identified for modification and/or reduction. These behaviors consisted primarily of straining to project her voice in noisy environments, but also included frequent throat clearing, minimal water intake, and moderate caffeine intake. Using a daily record form (yes/no response) to monitor vocal hygiene behaviors, JD and her family noted these behaviors in an effort to appropriately alter the behavior. These tasks were discussed in each session, and progress toward modification/reduction of each behavior was noted. A personal amplifier was introduced early on in treatment to reduce the need to strain in the classroom and noisy environments.

24.5.2 Semi-Occluded Vocal Tract Exercises

SOVT Exercises[3] were utilized to increase vocal efficiency and minimize laryngeal tension and hyperfunction, while maximiz-

ing vocal fold closure. During each session, lip buzzes were used as warm-up exercises in an effort to improve breath support and engage the vocal folds, thereby improving and increasing the amplitude of the mucosal wave of the TVFs. This exercise also helped isolate the TVFs as the primary source of vibration. Initially, a comfortable note was used, followed by slow glides extending up and down the pitch range. Nasal consonants were used in the semi-occluded exercises, with emphasis on abdominal support and reduction of pressed voice, which increases a light, buzzing voice. This maneuver also diminished ventricular fold compression and overall laryngeal effort during therapy tasks. Straw phonation included straws of various sizes placed between the lips and phonating /o/ for pitch glides, followed by musical notes for simple tunes. Flow phonation techniques[4] included cup bubble blowing and gargling sounds followed by voicing /m-m-m/, /m/ + vowel syllables, words with initial nasal phoneme, and continuous speech tasks using efficient voicing. A marked contrast in vocal quality was evident after the fourth week when JD was able to use less tension, suggesting there was more engagement of the TVFs and less lateral-medial compression of the ventricular folds.

24.5.3 Modified Vocal Function Exercises

After JD was consistently successful in reducing ventricular fold vibration, four steps of vocal function exercises[5] were implemented to improve the tone focus to an anterior, oral position and improve breath support for sustained tones. First, the vowel /i/ was produced with a nasal tone for as long as possible. Initially, JD was able to comfortably sustain phonation for only 7 seconds. The next two steps entailed lip buzzes that were used to glide up (stretching the vocal folds) and glide down (contracting the vocal folds). Last, three notes were chosen (low pitch-comfortable pitch-high pitch) to produce /o/ as softly as possible for as long as possible. Maximum tone clarity was emphasized. The sustained tones were all timed and recorded on a daily record form. Over the course of therapy, JD was able to increase her times to an average of 13 seconds. The ability to sustain phonation was an indicator of improved glottic closure and control of respiratory support. Transfer from sustained vowels to improved function to conversational speech in all settings was a challenge. Phrasing and breath control to support increasingly longer segments of connected speech were practiced in and outside of therapy sessions. Intelligibility of connected speech in quiet during therapy improved from 50% to 75%. With amplification, her intelligibility in noisier environments improved to 90%.

24.6 Outcome

After 2 months of using the above-mentioned therapeutic strategies during weekly sessions and with a consistent home program, JD made moderate progress to reduce overall laryngeal hyperfunction, eliminating a "mixed" voice source and increasing sustained TVF phonation. She also improved her loudness. On repeat pVHI, her functional score was 12/28, with the highest scores still related to being understood in a noisy environment; the score for physical dropped 3 points to 6/36, with the highest scores relating to still using excessive strain at times; and emotional fell to 2/28, demonstrating fewer issues with frustration and embarrassment.

The repeat CAPE-V revealed changes in perceptual ratings of OS = 50; R = 25; B = 55; S = 40; P = 30 (low); L = 35 (soft). Ratings related to breathiness and strain remained the least changed, and JD continued to complain of vocal fatigue and not being understood well in the classroom without amplification (and she expressed an interest in stopping the use of the amplifier due to social concerns). Acoustic measures revealed a greater degree of type 1 and 2 signals, with no type 3 signals captured during sustained phonation. Airflow volume measures (mean airflow rate = 170 mL/s) remained elevated within the normal range but reduced from JD's baseline. Psub was 9.35 cm H_2O indicating a reduction from baseline, revealing slight improvement. Repeat stroboscopic examination revealed less ventricular compression and improved glottic closure; however, the combination of reduced left joint motion and posterior left TVF scarring resulted in a persistent large posterior gap during glottic closure. Based on these residual deficits, the treating team, JD, and her parents wished to proceed with augmentation injection of the posterior left TVF to assist with closure of the posterior gap. Augmentation provided improved closure, resulting in increased loudness and improved intelligibility.

24.7 Key Points

- Intelligibility in noise and perceived effort are key outcome measures in voice therapy, especially in individuals with structural airway changes.

- Despite chronic dysphonia due to underlying structural and physiologic alterations, a coordinated medical/surgical and behavioral intervention can benefit the pediatric patient.
- A variety of voice therapy techniques and recommendations for voice use and care are often needed in the treatment of pediatric voice disorders.

Suggested Readings

[1] Kelchner LN, Brehm SB, de Alarcon A, Weinrich B. Update on pediatric voice and airway disorders: assessment and care. Curr Opin Otolaryngol Head Neck Surg. 2012; 20(3):160–164

[2] Kelchner L, Baker-Brehm S, Weinrich B. Pediatric Voice: A Modern, Collaborative Approach to Care. San Diego, CA: Plural Publishing; 2014

[3] Brehm SB, Weinrich B, Zieser M, et al. Aerodynamic and acoustic assessment in children following airway reconstruction: an assessment of feasibility. Int J Pediatr Otorhinolaryngol. 2009; 73(7):1019–1023

References

[1] Zur KB, Cotton S, Kelchner L, Baker S, Weinrich B, Lee L. Pediatric Voice Handicap Index (pVHI): a new tool for evaluating pediatric dysphonia. Int J Pediatr Otorhinolaryngol. 2007; 71(1):77–82

[2] Kempster GB, Gerratt BR, Verdolini Abbott K, Barkmeier-Kraemer J, Hillman RE. Consensus auditory-perceptual evaluation of voice: development of a standardized clinical protocol. Am J Speech Lang Pathol. 2009; 18(2):124–132

[3] Titze IR. Voice training and therapy with a semi-occluded vocal tract: rationale and scientific underpinnings. J Speech Lang Hear Res. 2006; 49(2):448–459

[4] Gartner-Schmidt JL. Flow phonation. In: Stemple J, Fry L, Eds. Voice Therapy: Clinical Studies. 3rd ed. San Diego, CA: Plural Publishing; 2010:84–92

[5] Stemple J, Glaze L, Klaben B. Clinical Voice Pathology: Theory and Management. 4th ed. San Diego, CA: Plural Publishing; 2010

25 Autism Spectrum Disorders and Word Associations

D. Battaglia

25.1 Introduction

Individuals with autism spectrum disorders (ASD) demonstrate impairments in two major areas: social communication (both linguistic and nonlinguistic) and behavioral/sensory interests.[1] The Centers for Disease Control[2] state that 1 in 68 children are diagnosed with ASD. More specifically, ASD affects 1 in 42 boys and 1 in 189 girls.[2] Individuals with ASD, therefore, are not attending to the environment, nor associated language, in the same way as their typical counterparts. These signs and symptoms can have deleterious effects on language acquisition and word association.[3]

25.2 Clinical History

JB was an endearing 30-month-old boy who had just been diagnosed with ASD. Both parents were consistent and reliable informants. His prenatal and birth history were unremarkable. Hearing tested at birth was within normal limits. JB's parents became concerned at approximately 15 months of age when JB was still not talking. They further reported that he seemed to understand everything they said, although he had several tantrums and "needed" things to be the same. JB did not seem to enjoy engaging with his family members other than for fleeting moments. His parents, therefore, sought further evaluation.

25.3 Clinical Testing

The Toddler module of the Autism Diagnostic Observation Scale, Second Edition (ADOS-2)[4] was administered prior to the arrival of the speech-language pathologist (SLP). The diagnostic report indicated that, while response to joint attention bids were, at times, present (though fleeting), engagement during items such as a pretend birthday party, functional and symbolic play, free play, and response to name yielded a score that fell within the moderate-to-severe range of concern. These findings aligned with guidelines put forth by the Diagnostic Statistical Manual, Fifth Edition.[1] That is, JB demonstrated persistent deficits in social-emotional reciprocity, nonverbal communication for social interactions, and developing and maintaining relationships. Stereotyped mannerisms, such as noncontextual vocalizations, reported need for sameness, and routine, as well as toe-walking, were also reported. Genetic evaluation confirmed no chromosomal anomalies precluding ASD. Cumulatively, with parent report and interprofessional discussion, a diagnosis of ASD was confirmed.

Language and communication evaluations were conducted by the SLP. Evaluation included administration of the Rossetti Infant-Toddler Language Scale,[5] the Preschool Language Scales, Fifth Edition (PLS-5),[6] behavioral observation, and parent interview. The PLS-5 revealed the following: standard score of 69 with a percentile rank of 2 in the auditory comprehension domain, and a standard score of 60 with a percentile rank of 1 was obtained in the expressive communication domain. Collectively, the total language standard score resulted in a standard score of 69 with a percentile rank of 1. During play, JB was not observed to imitate facial expressions. He did not discriminate between a speaker's mouth or eyes, although he showed awareness of a speaker by way of fleeting eye contact and occasional approaches for physical proximity. He would cry to get attention and would produce verbal approximations for either attention or to obtain a desired item. He reached for objects in play and occasionally smiled at himself in the mirror. Based on these interactions and observations, JB achieved a score of 3 to 6 months on the age performance profile.

JB initially noticed the arrival of the SLP, although he did not greet the SLP as noted by lack of initiation of eye gaze, vocalization, or hand wave. He walked around the perimeter of the room, seemingly inattentive, while the SLP gathered information regarding developmental speech, language, and communication milestones from the parents. Three times during the intake, JB approached the SLP, smiled, initiated eye contact, and then walked away, returning to toe-walking the perimeter of the room. These observations appeared to be self-stimulatory and confirmed findings in the diagnostic report. He was engaging in vowel-like, noncontextual vocalizations, such as "ah-ah-ah-eee-eee-eee." He was observed once to grab his father's hand, pulling him to the kitchen, and pointing to a cookie. During this time, he spontaneously looked at his father and approximated "ooooh" to request the item, demonstrating JB's inconsistent ability to initiate joint attention for purposes of requesting.

25.4 Questions and Answers for the Reader

1. A diagnosis of ASD requires impairments in which two areas:
   a) Social communication skills and behavioral sensory interests.
   b) Social skills and communication skills.
   c) Communication skills and aggression.
   d) Sensory stimulation and behavior.

Answer: a is correct. The DSM-5[1] defines ASD as a collection of deficits falling under both social communication *and* behavioral sensory interests. Examples of deficits in social communication may include but are not limited to deficits in social reciprocity, reduced sharing of interest, and/or impairments in social use of eye contact. Examples of restrictive/repetitive sensory interests may include but are not limited to excessive adherence to routines, highly fixated interests, and/or hypo- or hyperreactivity to sensory stimulation.

b is incorrect. Social and communication skills are considered together as one of the two minimum characteristics to diagnose ASD.

c is incorrect. The term "communication skills" is incomplete. Further, aggression is a singular example of a maladaptive behavior and is not an indicator, on its own, of ASD.

d is incorrect. Sensory stimulation is one component of the diagnostic criteria, considered under behavioral and sensory interests. No mention of social communication here deems this choice incomplete.

2. Rocking, humming, hand-flapping, and toe-walking are all examples of:
   a) Noncompliance.
   b) Passive-aggressive behavior.
   c) Self-stimulatory behavior.
   d) Oral-stimulatory behavior.

Answer: c is correct. Self-stimulatory behavior falls under the umbrella of behavioral/sensory interests. These behaviors (among others, such as tantrums, persistent need for sameness, and self-injury) are particularly monitored when considering a potential diagnosis of ASD.

a is incorrect. Noncompliance may be a function of escape maintained or attention-seeking behavior. However, this sign, in isolation, is insufficient for a diagnosis of ASD.

b is incorrect. This response is irrelevant to a diagnosis of ASD. Further, passive-aggressive behaviors are not mentioned JB's case.

d is incorrect. The behaviors in the example are not described as those restricted to the craniofacial area.

3. A little boy is 28 months old and newly diagnosed with ASD. His SLP has been working on eye contact as a treatment objective. This SLP feels this goal is particularly important, as it will help him fast map words to referents,[7] thereby expanding his lexicon. In other words, this child will associate what he sees and experiences with the words he is hearing, by way of a shared experience. This child will currently respond to bids for eye contact. The SLP is now working on having him initiate eye contact. Collectively, these objectives are targeting:
   a) Articulation.
   b) Attending to details.
   c) Joint attention.
   d) Expressive language.

Answer: c is correct. Joint attention is the triadic engagement between a child, caregiver, and external entity. Joint attention is socially motivated, and facilitates word learning and subsequent word association.

a is incorrect. Articulation focuses solely on how sounds are produced from an oral-motor perspective.

b is incorrect. Attending to details is one element, of many, involved in joint attention and word association.

d is incorrect. While expressive language is a long-term goal of joint attention, it is too broad of a response, in light of choice c.

25.5 Description of Disorder and Recommended Treatment

Joint attention is triadic in nature, in that there are three entities involved (e.g., the caregiver, the child, and the object of mutual attention).[8,9] During joint attention engagement, one of the two individuals initiates by gesturing, vocalizing, or both, toward an object of interest. Both individuals look at the entity, and look at one another. If the caregiver is the initiator, he or she may label the object (e.g., "bottle"). If the child is the initiator, he or she may not know the label, and point, seeking social engagement and a verbal model from the caregiver. Joint attention is instrumental in word learning and subsequent word associations. Multiple joint attention experiences, with several exposures to similar referents, serve to further expand representations of a particular item. Hence, exposure to a green, red, and yellow "apple" on different occasions serve to expand the referent-label relationship of "apple."

Young children with ASD may attend to the environment. Accordingly, these individuals may atypically perceive and organize items in the lexicon (i.e., mental dictionary), leading to atypical word associations. These atypical associations may be due to awkward initial learning experiences,[10] causing children with ASD to fast map inappropriate referents to their underlying concepts.[11] For example, a child who hears the word "apple" from his caregiver for the first time, while looking at a dog, may label the dog as an "apple," based solely on this initial learning experience. If a child with ASD stores a newly acquired word according to a first exposure, or a part of the visual presentation rather than the underlying integrated semantic concept, he or she may associate words qualitatively differently than typically developing children. Over time, these associations may become increasingly rigid, rather than expanded and integrated, which is symptomatic of ASD.

Upon initial diagnosis, JB received 40 hours of early intensive behavioral intervention to target speech, language, and communication, as well as other areas of daily functioning (e.g., independent eating, toileting). A large body of evidence, spanning minimally three decades, supports applied behavior analysis (ABA) as the most effective intervention method for individuals with ASD.[11,12,13,14] More specifically, early intensive behavior intervention not only has been shown to improve skills in the domains of cognition, language, and adaptive skills, but also has demonstrated maintenance of these skills over time.[15]

One of the main tenets of a well-coordinated ABA intervention is that the objectives must be socially significant.[11] JB's age, social interest in others, observed desire to communicate wants and needs, and reduced expressive language were considered. A set of treatment objectives focused on eye contact, joint attention, verbal imitation, and expressive language were immediately implemented. Using multiple exemplars of the same stimuli while varying context and directions facilitated word association during treatment sessions. Biweekly meetings and regularly scheduled cotreatment sessions facilitated stimulus control, maintenance, and generalization of skills across all service providers.

25.6 Outcome

Within 12 months of this early intensive behavioral intervention program, JB began spontaneously approximating for desired items and activities. Over time, these requests for tangible items and activities were communicated both verbally and consistently. His older siblings (4-year-old twins) were trained by the SLP and, subsequently, incorporated into therapy sessions as "peers." Acquisition of novel words continued at an accelerated rate between sessions, as his siblings were able to generalize and maintain new words that JB approximated within therapy sessions. By age 4, JB was included for a part-time preschool program, with support. During that time, his articulation improved significantly, and his vocabulary was minimally behind that of his typical peers. While he continued to demonstrate behavioral issues (e.g., toe-walking), JB was easily redirected by multiple members of the intervention team. He was, and continued to be, quite social and endearing; traits that enhanced his learning during initial treatment sessions focused on eye contact and joint attention and word association. JB's parents reported that quality of life for all family members improved dramatically with JB's improved communication skills.

25.7 Key Points

- During the initial evaluation, JB demonstrated several stereotypic behaviors. Despite these behaviors, he also demonstrated social interest in others, evidenced by a noncontingent social smile and spontaneous eye contact.
- When therapy ensued, JB demonstrated interest in learning new words, as evidenced by pointing and vocalizing "oooh." Verbal imitation goals provided successive approximations toward high-frequency words JB could practice regularly and independently with several different family members, friends, and interprofessional service providers.
- The inherent interest in people and spontaneous communication provided a more steeply sloped learning curve for JB than other individuals with ASD, who are not socially motivated by, nor interested in, communicating with others.

Suggested Readings

[1] Jones EA, Carr EG. Joint attention in children with autism: theory and intervention. Focus Autism Other Dev Disabil. 2004; 19(1):13–26

[2] Wong C, Kasari C. Play and joint attention of children with autism in the preschool special education classroom. J Autism Dev Disord. 2012; 42(10): 2152–2161

References

[1] American Psychiatric Association. Desk Reference to the Diagnostic Criteria from DSM-5. Arlington, VA: American Psychiatric Association; 2013

[2] Centers for Disease Control and Prevention. 2017. Available at: https://www.cdc.gov/ncbddd/autism/data.html. Last accessed October 23, 2017

[3] American Speech-Language-Hearing Association. Autism (Practice Portal). 2017. Available at: www.asha.org/Practice-Portal/Clinical-Topics/Autism/. Last accessed October 22, 2017

[4] Lord C, Rutter M, DiLavore PC, Risi S, Gotham K, Bishop SL. Autism Diagnostic Observation Schedule. 2nd ed. (ADOS-2) Manual (Part I): Modules 1–4. Torrance, CA: Western Psychological Services; 2012

[5] Rosetti L. The Rossetti Infant-Toddler Language Scale. East Moline, IL: LinguiSystems; 1990

[6] Zimmerman IL, Steiner BS, Evatt Pond R. Preschool Language Scales. 5th ed. San Antonio, TX: Pearson; 2011

[7] Carey S. The child as word learner. In: Halle M, Bresnan J, Miller JGA, Eds. Linguistic Theory and Psychological Reality. Cambridge, MA: MIT; 1978

[8] Adamson LB, Chance SE. Coordinating attention to people, objects, and language. In: Wetherby AM, Warren SF, Reichle J, Eds. Communication and Language Intervention Series. Vol. 7. Transitions in Prelinguistic Communication. Baltimore, MD: Brookes; 1998:15–37

[9] Wetherby AM, Prizant BM, Schuler AL. Understanding the nature of communication and language impairments. In: Wetherby M, Prizant BM, Eds. Autism Spectrum Disorders: A Transactional Developmental Perspective. Baltimore, MD: Brookes; 2000:109–141

[10] Baron-Cohen S, Baldwin DA, Crowson M. Do children with autism use the speaker's direction of gaze strategy to crack the code of language? Child Dev. 1997; 68(1):48–57

[11] Cooper JO, Heron TE, Heward WL, Eds. Applied Behavior Analysis. 2nd ed. Upper Saddle River, NJ: Pearson; 2007

[12] Lovaas OI. Behavioral treatment and normal educational and intellectual functioning in young autistic children. J Consult Clin Psychol. 1987; 55(1): 3–9

[13] McEachin JJ, Smith T, Lovaas OI. Long-term outcome for children with autism who received early intensive behavioral treatment. Am J Ment Retard. 1993; 97(4):359–372, discussion 373–391

[14] Weiss MJ. Differential rates of skill acquisition and outcomes of early intensive behavioral intervention for autism. Behav Interv. 1999; 14:3–22

[15] Howard JS, Sparkman CR, Cohen HG, Green G, Stanislaw H. A comparison of intensive behavior analytic and eclectic treatments for young children with autism. Res Dev Disabil. 2005; 26(4):359–383

26 Combined Modality Fluency Therapy in a Teenager with Severe Stuttering

Kenneth Logan

26.1 Introduction

Fluency therapy can be challenging when clients have a long-standing history of stuttering. This case describes the utility of concurrent standard behavioral fluency-management strategies and altered auditory feedback (AAF) via the Speech Easy device (Janus Development Group). The clinical activities described in this case occurred in the context of a research study.

26.2 Clinical History and Description

T was a 16-year-old male with a history of severe stuttering, which was characterized primarily by lengthy word-initial disfluencies, most of which involved audible sound prolongation or cessation of articulatory movements during speech-sound production (i.e., inaudible prolongation or "blocking"). Many of T's stuttering-related disfluencies featured noticeably excessive physical tension in speech-related muscles, along with extraneous limb and torso movements. Onset of stuttering symptoms reportedly occurred at the age of 3 years, following a period of ostensibly typical speech development. Family history was significant for a sibling with developmental stuttering. T had worked with several speech-language pathologists over a span of 9 years in public school settings, which, he said, resulted in "some improvement" in communicative functioning. T reported stuttering most severely during group conversations and oral reading, and least severely during one-on-one conversations with family members or friends. Although T reported feeling embarrassed about his disfluent speech, he stated that he seldom used word substitution or circumlocution to cope with or conceal anticipated instances of stuttering-related disfluency. He restricted his participation in verbal interactions, particularly at school, because of his fluency difficulties, and he expressed a desire to "get rid of stuttering."

26.3 Clinical Testing

Clinical testing took place during two 60-minute sessions, which occurred over a 2-week period. The research protocol began with completion of the informed consent process and then proceeded to the following activities:

- Review of a written case history form that the client and his mother completed.
- Completion of stuttering-related, self-rating instruments:
  - Perceptions of Stuttering Inventory (PSI),[1] which provided information about the presence of behaviors related to the anticipation of stuttering, stuttering-related "struggle" when speaking, and the expectancy of stuttering.
  - S-24 scale,[2] which provided information about T's attitude toward communication.
  - Overall Assessment of the Speaker's Experience of Stuttering (OASES),[3] which provided information about T's knowledge of stuttering, stuttering-related experiences, and the impact of stuttering on overall functioning and quality of life.
  - Self-Rating of Stuttering form (SROS; Logan, unpublished clinical tool), an informal instrument, which uses twelve 7-point rating scales to collect information about stuttering experiences during the preceding week. (The SROS was administered weekly during treatment, as well.)
- Elicitation of two 300- to 500-syllable conversational speech samples in response to a set of questions about T's developmental history, communication concerns, and goals.
- Narrative and oral reading speech samples in conjunction with the Stuttering Severity Instrument-4 (SSI-4),[4] which yielded a stuttering severity rating based on T's stuttering frequency, duration of stuttering "events," and use of "distracting" physical behaviors that accompany stuttering events.
- Basic audiological examination and informal oral mechanism screening.

T attended a third preintervention session that focused on introducing the SpeechEasy device (Comfort Fit model, Janus Development Group) and completing device programming, fitting, and introductory speaking activities as indicated by the manufacturer. The SpeechEasy is an electronic device similar to a hearing aid in appearance. Unlike a hearing aid, however, it alters auditory feedback when talking via simultaneous presentation of delayed auditory feedback (DAF) and frequency-altered feedback (FAF). In this case, the SpeechEasy device was programmed so that T heard his speech at a 70-ms delay and at 0.5 octaves above his habitual (unaltered) vocal frequency.

The effects of DAF and FAF have been studied, separately and in combination, by a number of investigators (for reviews, see Lincoln et al.[5] and Logan[6]). Both types of AAF appear to facilitate speech fluency in people who stutter in the laboratory setting[5]; however, data are limited on long-term outcomes in real-world settings. Findings from studies that used AAF as a sole form of treatment in real-world settings are mixed. For example, Van Borsel et al.[7] reported that speakers with severe stuttering significantly reduced stuttering frequency following prolonged exposure to DAF. In contrast, Pollard et al.[8] found that, although a group of adults who stuttered showed improved fluency immediately after being fitted with a SpeechEasy device, fluency improvement was not maintained. In many studies, considerable individual variability in response to AAF has been reported.[5,8]

One aim of the present research project was to investigate how clients approach stuttering management when provided behavioral, rate-based stuttering-management strategies along with access to AAF. In addition to overall treatment outcomes, we were also interested in examining how the two approaches were used when attempting to improve speech fluency and reduce stuttering-related disability. Client preference for one approach over the other was also of interest, as was the client's approach to stuttering management over time and across situations.

26.4 Questions and Answers for the Reader

1. A client reports that he/she seldom uses word substitution or circumlocution to conceal anticipated instances of stuttering. Which of the following describes how a clinician most likely would regard this information?
   a) Unfavorably, because word substitution and circumlocution are evidence-based strategies for treating stuttering.
   b) Unfavorably, because use of word substitution and circumlocution would limit the effectiveness of the SpeechEasy device.
   c) Favorably, because it will provide the client with opportunities to practice modification of stuttering-related disfluency.
   d) Favorably, because the clinician now can teach the client how to use word substitution and circumlocution properly as primary strategies for stuttering management.

   Answer: c is correct. The use of word substitution and circumlocution reduces the frequency of overt stuttering in one's speech and thus the number of chances one would have to implement stuttering-management strategies.

   a and d are incorrect. Neither word substitution nor circumlocution is regarded as evidence-based treatment for stuttering.

   b is incorrect. There is no clear association between use of word substitution and circumlocution and AAF effectiveness.

2. Given T's history, which of the following best describes how a clinician would regard his goal to be "rid of stuttering"?
   a) It is feasible to attain this goal following a 10-week course of fluency therapy.
   b) It is feasible to attain this goal because most adolescents outgrow stuttering before they reach adulthood.
   c) It is feasible to attain this goal following a 10-week course of fluency therapy, but only if the client is able to overcome feelings of embarrassment about stuttering.
   d) It is more productive for the client to focus on reducing stuttering-related disability in the near term.
   e) a, b, and c.

   Answer: d is correct. Outcome research indicates that certain contemporary treatments for stuttering are effective at both improving speech fluency and reducing stuttering-related activity limitations and participation restrictions. The notion of being "rid of stuttering" implies that stuttering will be cured. At present, none of the treatments for stuttering offer a reliable cure for the impairment that underlies the disorder. Also, given the length of time the client's stuttering has persisted, his current stuttering severity, and the limited benefit he has gained from previous therapy, it is unlikely he will be "rid" of stuttering in the near term. Accordingly, and e are incorrect.

   a and e are incorrect?

b is incorrect. Research data indicate that the odds of "recovering" from stuttering diminish substantially in cases like this, where stuttering has persisted from early childhood beyond age 12.

c is incorrect. Embarrassment is not a primary cause of stuttering.

3. Given that T achieved only modest improvement in fluency functioning through previous participation in fluency therapy, which of the following options would be a plausible rationale for developing a new treatment plan that combines rate-based stuttering-management techniques with use of AAF?
   a) Use of AAF may facilitate the client's ability to maintain a targeted speaking rate over a long period of time.
   b) Listeners may be less likely to respond negatively to the client's stuttering after noticing that he is wearing an assistive device.
   c) Training in rate-based techniques may help the client supplement the fluency-facilitating effects associated with AAF.
   d) Both a and c.

   Answer: d is correct (i.e., both a and c).

   a is plausible because DAF (a component of AAF) reduces articulation rate. Thus, the client might be able to sustain a targeted speaking rate longer and more consistently when given continuous access to a DAF signal compared to receiving no DAF signal at all.

   c is plausible as well. AAF devices have been found to enhance fluency, even without explicit training in rate-management strategies. However, long-term maintenance of fluency gains under AAF has not been demonstrated consistently. Thus, it is plausible that the client's outcome with the AAF device may be better if he has access to behavioral strategies that supplement the fluency-enhancing properties of AAF.

   b is incorrect. It is much less plausible than either a or c because the client history makes no mention of listeners' reactions to stuttering as being a critical factor in the client's response to past intervention. Also, if negative listener reactions were a significant factor in the client's disability, there is no guarantee that a listener would notice an AAF device or understand its purpose. Thus, it would be better to target negative listener behaviors by teaching the client how to address the behaviors directly.

26.5 Description of Disorder and Treatment Activities

Results from clinical testing yielded a detailed picture of T's communicative functioning. His SSI-4 scores across the two testing sessions suggested a stuttering severity rating of *severe* to *very severe*. The percent of syllables stuttered was relatively stable during conversation, narration, and oral reading (i.e., 24%–27% of syllables were stuttered during these tasks). T's communication attitudes, as measured by the S24 scale, were more negative than the attitudes of other adults who stutter (i.e., 0.42 standard deviations more negative than the S24's reference group of adults who stutter) and also adults who do not stutter (i.e., 2.20 standard deviations more negative than the S24's mean score for a reference group of typical adults). T exhibited many stuttering-related symptoms as indicated by his responses on the PSI's avoidance and struggle subscales (the client identified 55% of the 20 items on each subscale as being characteristic of him) and expectancy subscale (the client identified 35% of the 20 subscale items as being characteristic of him). T's responses on both the OASES and the SROS suggested that he viewed his stuttering as being moderately severe and as having a moderately negative impact on his overall functioning and quality of life.

Treatment activities followed procedures that were specified in the research protocol for the larger study. The protocol called for ten one-1 sessions (one session per week for 10 weeks) with a certified speech-language pathologist. Activities in the intervention protocol were based on principles associated with traditional fluency shaping and stuttering modification interventions (e.g., Shames and Florance[9] and Van Riper[10]). Treatment activities were compiled in a workbook so that the order, content, and scope of intervention were consistent across participants. T received a copy of the workbook to facilitate home-based practice. Primary goals included the following:

1. Development of the ability to regulate/monitor articulatory movements in ways that improve speech continuity. T and the clinician spent portions of the first three sessions reviewing basic information about speech production and stuttering and conducting activities that focused on improved identification and description of features of his stuttering and associated coping and avoidance strategies. During all sessions, T used regulated articulation rate (i.e., "prolonged speech"), such that over 10 weeks of training, he progressed from saying very slow (2 seconds per syllable) short phrases to longer, slightly faster (1 second per syllable) phrases and sentences, to narrative and conversational speech that he produced at a typical, but still self-monitored, articulation rate. While using a regulated articulation rate, T was also encouraged to attend to proprioceptive and kinematic aspects of articulation, particularly at transitions between syllable boundaries and between syllable onsets and rimes, and in syllables immediately preceding points of anticipated stuttering-related disfluency. T used the Speech-Easy device during about 20% of practice time. When wearing the device, he was encouraged to speak at an articulation rate that was slow enough to eliminate the echo heard when using typical articulation rate under DAF and to talk along with the signal. The workbook also included a suggested schedule of activities for practicing with the SpeechEasy device at home on a daily basis.

2. **Development of skills for reducing the severity of residual stuttering instances**. Use of regulated articulation rate resulted in substantial reduction of stuttering frequency during practice activities. Nonetheless, T experienced residual stuttering during these activities and in spontaneous speech. The treatment protocol included activities in weeks 6 to 10 that addressed strategies for modifying anticipated or actual stuttering-related disfluency. These strategies were based on principles from Van Riper's desensitization → cancellation → pullout → preparatory set sequence,[10] and, as such, essentially involved having T apply principles of regulated articulation (described earlier) to repair or modify situational instances of stuttering.

26.6 Outcome

T was reassessed in a clinical testing session that took place 1 week after completion of the 10-week treatment protocol (posttreatment assessment) and again 6 months later (6 months posttreatment). Both reassessments featured readministration of pretreatment clinical tests. T reported that he had not been attending formal stuttering therapy since completing the treatment phrase of the study. Analysis of reassessment results indicated the following:

1. Reduced stuttering severity, as measured by scores on the SSI-4 and the PSI. Pretreatment severity was rated as *severe* to *very severe*, whereas posttreatment severity was *mild* (though close to *moderate*); and 6-month posttreatment severity was *moderate*. He improved in stuttering frequency, stuttering duration, and physical concomitants over time. The extent of T's improvement in stuttering severity was consistent with findings from past treatment outcomes in severe stuttering (e.g., Boberg and Kully[11]).
On the PSI, a comparison of pretreatment versus 6-month posttreatment responses indicated that the number of speech-related struggle behaviors T identified decreased by 64%, and the number of avoidance behaviors decreased by 45%. In contrast, the number of expectancy behaviors identified increased by 71% from pretreatment to posttreatment (which may reflect increased self-monitoring of speech), but then returned to baseline levels at 6-months posttreatment (which may reflect reduced stuttering frequency, improved ability to manage anticipated stuttering, and/or a return to baseline levels of speech monitoring).

2. Modest improvements in self-perception of quality of life and stuttering-related disability. The total score on the OASES improved by 22%, from 2.85 at pretreatment to 2.33 at 6-months posttreatment. In other words, T's overall perception of stuttering impact shifted from the upper end of the moderate range to the lower end of the moderate range. This reduction resulted from less severe reactions to stuttering, where the OASES score decreased from the lower end of the moderate/severe range at pretreatment to the lower end of the moderate range at 6-months posttreatment. Improved knowledge about speech production and stuttering occurred as well. Responses on the OASES Communication in Daily Situations subscale, however, indicated that T continued to report moderate difficulty communicating in a range of life situations. His responses on the SROS instrument were generally consistent with the SSI-4 Stuttering Prediction Instrument and OASES data. His SROS responses from the pretreatment and treatment sessions were averaged and then compared to the 6-month posttreatment responses. Consistent with the OASES data, T reported modest improvements in stuttering frequency and severity (reductions of 0.7 scale points), and more substantial improvement in avoiding speech (a reduction of 1.5 scale points) and attempting to hide stuttering from others (a reduction of 2.6 scale points).

3. T's approach to and perceptions of stuttering management. In an oral interview at 6-months posttreatment, T reported that his ability to "work out of" stuttering blocks improved significantly since pretreatment and that he regularly applied the recently learned behavioral strategies (primarily "pullout" and "preparatory set") to modify/repair instances

of stuttering. He stated that he actively attempted to manage nearly every time he talks, and focused on stuttering management most during social interactions with friends or when meeting new people. He reported that he felt "less afraid" of stuttering than he did prior to commencing treatment, that his verbal participation increased over the past year, and that he became less apt to "give up on" attempts to speak since completion of treatment.

The role of the SpeechEasy device was difficult to determine. The SpeechEasy device was incorporated into the 10-week-long clinical phase and, during that time, T was assigned home-based activities to promote device usage. At the posttreatment assessment, T reported the SpeechEasy device as helping "just a little." Still, he reported using it several times per week, mainly at school, with usage patterns varying from brief and situational to extended use over several hours. It is possible that these experiences facilitated his ability to apply behavioral fluency-management strategies. However, at the 6-month posttreatment assessment, he reported that in the 6 months following treatment, he relied on behavioral strategies much more often than the SpeechEasy device. He reported that SpeechEasy use gradually tapered off to approximately once per week, and at the 6-month posttreatment assessment, he had not worn the device for approximately 3 months. His summative perception of the device was that "it helped a little, but not enough to make me wear it regularly." Overall, he reported feeling satisfied with the speech-related changes to date. He indicated that he was unsure of whether he would ever "get rid of stuttering," but remained motivated to continue working at "getting control over it."

26.7 Key Points

- People who stutter, including individuals who stutter severely, can realize and appreciate improvement in communicative functioning following treatment that develops skills in self-regulating articulatory movements and modifying instances of stuttering-related disfluency.
- Feelings, attitudes, and beliefs about stuttering often change more slowly than speech behaviors such as stuttering frequency.

- The process of successful stuttering management is ongoing, such that it continues well after the completion of formal fluency therapy.
- The clinical activities described were part of a research protocol. In a clinical setting, a clinician could elect to conduct additional treatment sessions and/or introduce additional treatment strategies, based on ongoing assessment of performance, treatment preferences, and communication goals.

26.7.1 Acknowledgments

The activities described in this case study were funded in part by a research grant from the Janus Development Group to the author.

Suggested Readings

[1] Bothe AK, Davidow JH, Bramlett, RE, Ingham RJ. Stuttering treatment research 1970-2005. I: Systematic review incorporating trial quality assessment of behavioral, cognitive, and related approaches. Am J Speech-Lang Pat. 2006; 15 (4):321–341

References

[1] Woolf, G. The assessment of stuttering as struggle, avoidance, and expectancy. Brit J Disord Commun. 1967; 2:158–171
[2] Andrews G, Cutler J. Stuttering therapy: The relation between changes in symptom level and attitudes. J Speech Hear Disord. 1974; 39(3):312–319
[3] Yaruss JS, Quesal RW. Overall Assessment of the Speaker's Experience of Stuttering (OASES). Minneapolis, MN: Pearson; 2008
[4] Riley GD. Stuttering Severity Instrument (4th Ed.). Austin, TX: Pro-Ed; 2009
[5] Lincoln M, Packman A, Onslow M. Altered auditory feedback and the treatment of stuttering: A review. J Fluency Disord. 2006; 31(2):71–89
[6] Logan KJ. Fluency Disorders. San Diego, CA: Plural Publishing; 2015
[7] Van Borsel J, Reunes G, Van den Bergh N. Delayed auditory feedback in the treatment of stuttering: Clients as consumers. Int J Lang Comm Dis. 2003; 38 (2): 119–129
[8] Pollard R, Ellis JB, Finan D, Ramig PR. Effects of the SpeechEasy on objective and perceived aspects of stuttering: A 6-month, phase I clinical trial in naturalistic environments. J Speech Lang Hear Res. 2009; 52:516–533
[9] Shames GH, Florance CL. Stutter-Free Speech: A Goal for Therapy. Columbus, OH: Charles E. Merrill; 1980
[10] Van Riper C. The Treatment of Stuttering. Englewood Cliffs, NJ: Prentice-Hall; 1973
[11] Boberg E, Kully D. Long-term results of an intensive treatment program for adults and adolescents who stutter. J Speech Hear Res. 1994; 37:1050-1059

27 Pediatric Feeding and Swallowing Impairment in a Child with a Craniofacial Disorder

Tina M. Tan

27.1 Introduction

Pediatric speech-language pathologists (SLPs) practicing in a variety of clinical settings encounter a wide range of disorders that impact the normal progression of feeding and swallowing skills starting in infancy and beyond. This case describes the process of diagnosis and the clinical management required when working with a child with a craniofacial disorder.

27.2 Clinical History and Description

JL was a 4-week-old female infant who presented with failure to thrive and increased difficulty breathing at a tertiary medical center. JL was diagnosed shortly after birth with Pierre Robin sequence with cleft palate and moderate-to-severe retro-micrognathia. She had been discharged home from the neonatal intensive care unit on full oral feeds. Shortly after discharge, she was seen by her pediatrician. Her pediatrician referred her to the aerodigestive clinic due to failure to gain weight, noisy and labored breathing, feeding difficulties, and "choking" with feeds. Physical examination revealed respiratory distress with suprasternal, substernal, and intercostal retractions as well as inspiratory noise with breathing. Her weight was well below the first percentile. JL was admitted directly to the pediatric intensive care unit from the aerodigestive clinic. Nasogastric tube feedings were initiated for supplemental nutrition and hydration, as it was clear that the baby was not meeting nutritional requirements.

27.3 Clinical Testing

JL was referred for speech pathology consultation for a clinical feeding and swallowing evaluation. She was evaluated during a normally scheduled feeding. Her parents were present at the bedside, which allowed for the acquisition of a detailed history of feeding skills prior to admission. JL had been taking expressed breast milk with use of a commercially available, specialized bottle and nipple designed for babies with cleft palate. This bottle contains a one-way valve within the nipple, which allows for extraction of milk from the nipple utilizing compression only without generation of negative pressure (suction). JL was using this bottle system with a level 1 or "slow flow" nipple. JL was consuming approximately 45 to 60 mL per feeding. Feedings were characterized by loud, noisy breathing; fast rate of breathing; and intermittent coughing. Additionally, she fell asleep quite frequently during feeding. It was rare that she consumed beyond 60 mL.

An examination of the oral peripheral mechanism revealed a cleft of the hard and soft palates and a small, recessed mandible. Upper and lower lips were intact without a cleft. Infant oral reflexes were present including rooting and nonnutritive suck

on the clinician's gloved finger. Transverse tongue and phasic bite reflexes were elicited bilaterally. Nonnutritive sucking movements were rhythmical, but weak without suction, as is expected with cleft palate. JL exhibited increased work of breathing (WOB) with stimulation. Suprasternal and clavicular retractions were noted during the oral examination. Noisy breathing, consistent with stertor and stridor, was also noted intermittently due to laryngomalacia, which was diagnosed by the otolaryngologist.

Clinical evaluation then proceeded with observation of feeding. JL was held in her mother's arms in a semi-upright position. She was observed to root, opening her mouth to allow intraoral placement of the bottle nipple. Initiation of sucking was observed, although latch was weak. Reduced extraction of fluid from the nipple was suspected, given the small amounts consumed during feeding. Anterior spillage of bolus was noted. Difficulty with coordination of the suck, swallow, and breathe sequence was apparent as evidenced by rapid swallows without detection of a breath in between. JL demonstrated these rapid suck–swallow bursts for approximately five to eight sucks. "Catch-up breathing" with nasal flaring, increased WOB, and retractions were noted following these sucking bursts. Elevated heart rate and respiratory rate were observed during feeding. As feeding progressed, increased upper airway congestion was audible and one episode of desaturation to 90% was observed via pulse oximetry. The SLP intervened during feeding to determine whether a change in positioning or other strategies were useful to improve feeding/swallowing performance; no significant changes were noted. Given the presentation during the clinical feeding and swallowing assessment, parental report, underlying medical diagnosis, and failure to gain weight, an instrumental assessment of swallowing via videofluoroscopic swallow study (VFSS) was recommended.

VFSS was conducted. JL was seated semi-upright, swaddled, and well supported in a tumble form feeding seat. Lateral views were obtained. Thin liquid barium was provided via bottle/nipple. Oral preparatory and oral phase functions were moderately impaired. Anterior spillage of bolus, increased suck-to-swallow ratio (due to poor extraction of fluid from nipple), spreading of bolus through oral cavity, and premature spillage of the bolus into the oropharynx prior to pharyngeal swallow initiation were observed. Delayed onset of the pharyngeal swallow was also noted, with delayed laryngeal vestibule closure. Initially, bolus penetration into the laryngeal airway entrance with full and spontaneous clearance was observed. As the study progressed, these episodes became increasingly frequent and eventually led to aspiration during the swallow. A cough was not elicited in response to aspiration (e.g., "silent"). Spontaneous clearance of the aspirate was not noted. JL became increasingly disorganized with respect to coordination of sucking, swallowing, and respiration as the study progressed, which was likely secondary to fatigue. Additionally, as the study progressed, increased hypopharyngeal residue was noted in the valleculae and pyriform sinuses. Side-lying position, a slower flow nipple, a change in bottle type (assisted extraction of fluid from feeder), and removal of the nipple from the mouth every two to three sucks to "pace" the feeding was attempted with no success at eliminating aspiration or improving swallow function. Additionally, a thickened liquid was attempted; however, the baby was unable to extract it from the nipple.

27.4 Questions and Answers for the Reader

1. How will this baby receive necessary nutrition and hydration?
   a) Baby will continue to take full oral feeds.
   b) Baby will continue to receive nasogastric tube feedings until her feeding and swallowing difficulties improve. At that time, she will resume full oral feeds.
   c) Baby will require long-term nonoral means of nutrition and hydration (e.g., G-tube) to ensure adequate weight gain and growth.

   Answer: c is correct. This baby will require G-tube placement to meet nutrition and hydration needs and to ensure appropriate weight gain and growth. Given the underlying medical diagnosis, her airway obstruction, failure to thrive, energy expenditure during feeding, and results of the VFSS, full oral feeding is not realistic at this time. The feeding and swallowing difficulties are expected to persist for an extended period of time, which would necessitate a G-tube.

   a and b are incorrect. Upon initial consult with the aerodigestive team, this baby was already struggling to meet her nutrition/hydration needs solely by mouth; therefore, it is unrealistic to consider that this will change in the near future. Discoordination and aspiration documented during VFSS will likely further compromise her respiratory function. Repeated "negative" oral feeding experience/practice could lead to future oral aversion. With continued oral feeding, failure to thrive will persist and may result in poor candidacy for future surgical and medical management for her underlying condition. As her feeding and swallowing difficulties are related to an underlying syndrome, it is not expected that these issues are acute in nature and will resolve with time. For that reason, a G-tube will be needed as a nasogastric tube would be utilized when the feeding difficulties are acute and are expected to be short term.

2. How will positive oral experiences, development of oral motor skills, normal oral sensation, and developmental feeding skills be promoted if the baby does not eat by mouth?
   a) The baby will benefit from pleasurable stimulation to the face, mouth, and intraorally. Additionally, a pacifier may be provided to promote nonnutritive sucking practice. Small volume oral feeds for therapeutic and developmental purposes such as dips of formula or breast milk on a pacifier/gloved finger or small oral feeds (e.g., < 2–5 mL) may be considered by the SLP and medical team.
   b) No intervention is necessary. Once oral feeds are reintroduced, the baby will return to eating without difficulty.
   c) The baby cannot be fed by bottle but can be fed baby foods from a spoon to promote developmental oral motor, sensory, and feeding skills.

Answer: a is correct. A baby who will not be fed by mouth will benefit from experiencing pleasurable and developmentally appropriate facial and oral stimulation, which would normally be provided during breast- and bottle-feeding. Furthermore, the baby would benefit from intraoral stimulation via pacifier and age-appropriate teething toys to facilitate normalized oral sensation and gag reflex. Without this, the chances of developing oral hypersensitivity and/or an oral aversion are increased (especially in the presence of "unpleasant" medical procedures, which will be done near the mouth and face). Whenever possible, providing practice swallowing small amounts of formula or expressed milk would be highly desirable to further promote normalized oral sensation. This would also allow the baby to practice oral motor skills required for bolus formation and A-P transport. Therapeutic feedings allow the baby opportunities to develop swallowing skills such as coordinating oral and pharyngeal stages and integrating respiration with swallowing. Limiting the volume or amount of these feedings would hopefully minimize aspiration episodes or complications from aspiration, but allow the baby to experience oral feeding without stress under controlled, optimal conditions. Ultimately, the decision to pursue these types of feedings should be made by the medical team in conjunction with the SLP, not solely by the SLP.

b and c are incorrect. If the baby is not eating by mouth and is not provided with alternative opportunities to experience pleasurable sensation to the face, mouth, and intraorally, there is increased likelihood that oral hypersensitivity or oral aversion will develop. This may result in gagging, refusal, or negative response to oral feeding when attempting to reintroduce after an extended period of time, as critical windows for skill development may be missed. The role of therapy in this case is to facilitate development of oral motor and oral sensory skills, which are age appropriate to keep them as close as possible to the normal developmental trajectory. Caregiver and parent training to support this is essential. Spoon-feeding of baby foods would not be recommended at this time given this baby's young age. Likely, her oral motor skills could not support this and we would further risk the possibility of an aspiration episode or promotion of unpleasant oral feeding experience.

3. Given the underlying medical diagnosis, what might the planned medical or surgical interventions be for this child? How will these interventions impact upon the feeding and swallowing treatment plan?
   a) Babies with Pierre Robin sequence do not usually require any medical or surgical management.
   b) This child will require cleft palate surgery only when she is older.
   c) There are a number of surgical procedures that this baby may undergo including procedures to improve airway patency (e.g., tracheostomy, distraction osteogenesis of the mandible) prior to cleft palate repair.

Answer: c is correct. Owing to the posterior position of the mandible and the tongue, babies with Pierre Robin sequence often experience airway obstruction. If obstruction is severe enough, establishment of a patent airway often needs to be addressed surgically. This is typically done well in advance of cleft palate repair. These procedures will have impact upon oral feeding abilities immediately postoperatively and beyond due to pain, healing, and changes in the anatomy. In the long term, remediation of the airway obstruction will typically result in increased oral feeding success, given increased ease of respiration and ability to integrate respiration into the sucking and swallowing sequence. In this baby's case, the decision to pursue the G-tube was made largely due to the fact that her airway obstruction was quite significant, and was primarily impacting upon her oral feeding abilities and the ability to maintain an patent airway, especially during sleep. Knowing that mandibular osteogenesis surgery was highly probable, the team wanted to ensure appropriate weight gain for surgery, for healing, and until turning of the distractors was complete with improved airway patency. Timing of initiation of "therapeutic oral feeds" in this baby's case and/or swallow reassessment were coordinated with the baby's medical team and planned procedures to optimize outcomes and provide positive oral feeding experience. a and b are incorrect. Certainly, if a cleft of the palate is present, this will be repaired once the baby is older (e.g., 10–12 months). However, as noted earlier, if the airway obstruction is significant, babies with Pierre Robin sequence will require surgical procedures to correct this. In less severe cases, other therapeutic and medical managements may be recommended such as positioning (in prone or side lying) or use of CPAP to alleviate obstructive sleep apnea.

27.5 Description of Disorder and Recommended Treatment

Characterized by retrognathia, micrognathia, glossoptosis, and U-shaped cleft palate, feeding problems, respiratory difficulties, and airway obstruction are common in babies with Pierre Robin sequence (see ▶ Fig. 27.1). Feeding plans must account for not only proper nutrition and hydration but also promotion of developmental oral motor, oral sensory, and feeding skills. Additionally, it is essential that the feeding plan is developed within the context of the overall medical presentation and planned interventions. In JL's case, nonoral nutrition was necessary based on significant respiratory difficulties, failure to gain weight, and the presence of oropharyngeal swallow dysfunction. Additionally,

JL was scheduled to undergo future surgical procedures including mandibular osteogenesis to alleviate upper airway obstruction (performed during this admission) and cleft palate surgery (around 11–12 months of age). With these procedures pending, maximum growth and nutrition during this period were of critical importance.

27.6 Outcome

G-tube placement and mandibular osteogenesis were performed. To promote developmental oral feeding skills in preparation for future oral feeding, the medical team agreed to allow therapeutic oral feedings consisting of dips of expressed breast milk on pacifier and gloved finger. Once mandibular osteogenesis was complete, 5 mL of expressed breast milk was introduced one time per day via specialized cleft palate feeder with a preemie-level nipple. Given that oropharyngeal swallow discoordination, difficulty in coordination of the suck, swallow, breathe sequence, and aspiration appeared to occur more readily with fatigue on VFSS, small volumes were provided for positive oral feeding experience while minimizing aspiration risk. Feeding treatment and management focused on parent training and monitoring of tolerance while JL consumed small oral feedings. Her parents became quite skilled at providing these therapeutic feedings, utilizing upright positioning, removing the bottle every two to three sucks, and providing prolonged breaks in between sucking bursts. The parents were also trained to identify overt and clinical signs or symptoms suggestive of aspiration and to stop feeding when they were observed or when JL exhibited stress cues during the feeding.

JL successfully took these therapeutic oral feeds for several months. At 4 months of age, a repeat VFSS was conducted to assess candidacy for advancement of oral feedings and introduction of spoon-feeding of purees. She maintained a level of oral stage impairment as expected with known cleft palate and a degree of discoordination between oral and pharyngeal stages of swallowing. However, airway protection was adequate with no episodes of aspiration. Slow advancement of oral feeding was recommended. She continued to progress with bottle-feeds. Amounts were gradually increased over several weeks and months. Additionally, purees were introduced, which allowed for increased flavor and texture exposure. Her family worked with the nutritionist to slowly decrease reliance of

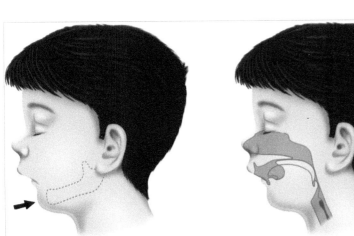

Fig. 27.1 Micro- and retrognathia resulting in posterior tongue position and obstruction of the upper airway.

G-tube feedings as oral feedings increased. She was eventually weaned from the G-tube shortly after undergoing cleft palate repair around 12 months of age.

27.7 Key Points

- Specialized equipment is necessary when feeding an infant or child with a craniofacial disorder.
- Oropharyngeal swallow and related respiratory functions may be altered following surgical procedures given changes in anatomy. Clinicians should review the possible impact of these procedures when considering therapeutic options including the timing of instrumental reassessment of swallowing.
- When primary nutrition and hydration is required via nonoral means, it is necessary to provide children with oral sensory and oral motor stimulation to promote developmental oral sensorimotor feeding skills, allow for "swallow practice" (whenever medically appropriate), and prepare them for future oral feedings.
- Feeding and swallowing impairment in children with craniofacial anomalies requires a team approach, including plastic surgery, otolaryngology, gastroenterology, pulmonology, SLPs, and dietitians. Many other professions may be integral to the team including social workers, occupational/physical therapists, and nurses. However, it is critical to include the parents as an essential member of the team.

Suggested Readings:

[1] Evans KN, Sie KC, Hopper RA, Glass RP, Hing AV, Cunningham ML. Robin sequence: from diagnosis to development of an effective management plan. Pediatrics. 2011; 127(5):936–948

[2] Miller CK. Feeding issues and interventions in infants and children with clefts and craniofacial syndromes. Semin Speech Lang. 2011; 32(2):115–126

28 Selective Mutism: A Pragmatic Approach

Suzanne Hungerford

28.1 Introduction

Typically, children with selective mutism (SM) speak normally at home, but do not speak in certain social situations outside the home, particularly school. It is generally considered to be an anxiety disorder; however, other risk factors have been identified, including bilingualism, developmental delay, an inhibited temperament, environmental stressors, and the presence of a speech or language disorder.

28.2 Clinical History and Description

At age 7, KL was referred to a university speech clinic by her school principal and mother. They reported that KL had never spoken in school, but did speak normally at home. She did not communicate by any means at school except for an occasional head nod, and her teacher became particularly concerned when KL started urinating herself in the classroom. She rarely used the bathroom at school and did not eat or drink when other children were around.

KL spoke to no one at school, but did her schoolwork if it did not involve speaking and got average grades. Her mother reported that when around unfamiliar people, she would slump over, avoid eye contact, put her head down, and become unresponsive. However, she did interact and play with familiar classmates in school, albeit nonverbally.

28.3 Clinical Testing

Case history information was gathered through a written case history form and an interview with KL's mother. She reported

KL had a normal birth history, met developmental milestones, and had no significant illnesses or injuries. She said KL appeared to hear well and spoke normally at home to her sisters and parents. English was the only language spoken in the home. Through the clinical interview, a matrix was created to clarify the people and environments in which she spoke (▶ Table 28.1). During the assessment, KL's mother provided the clinicians with home audio recordings of KL reading aloud, which her teacher used to assess reading fluency. These recordings revealed mild articulation errors (f/θ and w/r).

Approaching the assessment room, KL walked slowly and then sat slowly in a chair. She did not make eye contact with the clinician; she lowered her head, looked down, and held her hands stiffly at her side. She made very little spontaneous movement and did not respond verbally or nonverbally to attempts to engage verbally or nonverbally in any social interaction or activity. Hearing screening and speech/language testing requiring interaction could not be accomplished.

The Social Skills Improvement System (SSIS) was used to obtain information about KL's social skills and behaviors. The SSIS is a checklist based on observational data. The teacher and the parent forms were administered and both suggested KL had severe deficits in social interaction and significant internalization (e.g., anxiety; ▶ Table 28.2). Additionally, a pragmatic language checklist was used to describe KL's deficits in verbal and nonverbal interaction in the clinic and to track changes in behavior over time (▶ Table 28.3). Severe deficits were observed not only in all verbal aspects of pragmatics, but also in nonverbal aspects, including physical proximity, body posture, body movement, gestures, facial expression, and eye gaze.

Table 28.1 Discriminative stimuli for speaking: baseline

	Home (only family present)	Home (nonfamily present)	Classroom	Hallway	Playground	Mall	Grandma's
Mom	X					X (when she thinks no one else can hear)	X (when she thinks no one else can hear)
Dad	X						
Sister 1	X			X (when no one else is around)			X (when she thinks no one else can hear)
Sister 2	X			X (when no one else is around)			X (when she thinks no one else can hear)
Grandma	X (only on the telephone)						X (whispers answers to questions)
Teacher							
Peers							

X, contexts in which KL spoke.

Table 28.2 Results of the Social Skills Improvement System (SSIS): parent and teaching ratings

	Teacher rating	Parent rating
Social skills		
Communication	Below average	Below average
Cooperation	Average	Average
Assertion	Below average	Below average
Responsibility	Average	Below average
Empathy	Below average	Below average
Engagement	Below average	Below average
Self-control	Below average	Below average
Total	Standard score = 62; percentile rank = 1	Standard score = 63; percentile rank = 1
Problem behaviors		
Externalizing	Average	Average
Bullying	Average	Average
Hyperactivity/inattention	Average	Average
Internalizing	Above average	Above average
Total	Standard score = 104; percentile rank = 67	Standard score = 111; percentile rank = 80

Low scores in social skills indicate the child has fewer social skills; high scores in problem behaviors indicates the presence of more problem behaviors.

28.4 Questions and Answers for the Reader

1. Which of the following statements about KL's case are most likely true?
   a) KL's SM was most likely caused by childhood abuse or trauma.
   b) Since KL made average or good grades in school, the disorder was not educationally relevant.
   c) KL was initially not a good candidate for cognitive behavior therapy.
   d) KL was most likely simply refusing to speak.

Answer: c is correct. Cognitive behavior therapy is an intervention based on active collaboration with the therapist and patient, and requires active patient participation in the therapeutic process. The therapist and the patient work together to actively solve problems and evaluate distortions in thinking that lead to maladaptive emotions and behaviors. Since KL initially had no means of communication with the therapist, this active therapeutic process was not possible; thus, a behavioral approach was used.

a is incorrect. Research indicates that childhood abuse is not a common cause of SM. The disorder is most often attributed to social anxiety. Social phobia is frequently reported in family members of people with SM.

b is incorrect. Many Common Core Learning Standards include oral communication skills, such as "ask and answer questions about what a speaker says in order to clarify comprehension," and "speak audibly and express thoughts, feelings, and ideas clearly." Children learn language and academic content by using language to engage with others in the academic environment.

d is incorrect. Children with SM are not simply refusing to speak. It is generally believed that children with SM find it impossible to speak in certain social situations because of overwhelming anxiety.

2. Which of the following best describes the role of the speech-language pathologist in the assessment and treatment of individuals with SM?
   a) Because this is a psychiatric problem, SM is outside the scope of practice of speech-language pathologists.
   b) The speech-language pathologist's role is to monitor the child's progress with communication and make a referral for treatment if no progress is made in a year.
   c) Speech-language pathologists, using evidence-based treatments, can effectively treat SM.
   d) Speech-language pathologists can only work in the context of interprofessional teams in the assessment and treatment of SM.

Answer: c is correct. Speech-language pathologists, with appropriate training in relevant evidence-based practices, can be effective in the treatment of children with SM.

a is incorrect. The American Speech Language Hearing Association scope of practice documents indicate that speech-language pathologists may work with individuals whose communication disorder is of psychiatric etiology.

b is incorrect. Early intervention of SM is more effective; the longer the duration of SM, the poorer the prognosis.

d is incorrect. Because of the complex nature of SM, it is preferable to assess and treat children with SM using interprofessional teams. Ideally, teams should include a physician (who may prescribe medications), the classroom teacher, a clinical or educational psychologist, and a speech-language pathologist. In KL's case, the parent did not follow through on a referral to a psychiatrist, and in KL's small, rural private school, there were no school professionals willing or able to treat her at school. When an interprofessional team cannot be established, a trained speech-language pathologist can and should provide evidence-based therapy for this pragmatic communication disorder.

3. Which of the following is true?
   a) A "silent period" is a normal stage of second language learning; therefore, SM cannot be diagnosed in children who are nonnative speakers of the ambient language.
   b) Children who have articulation or language delays or disorders cannot be diagnosed with SM.
   c) Children with developmental disabilities such as autism, fragile X, or intellectual disability cannot be diagnosed with SM.
   d) None of the above.

Answer: d is correct. Research indicates that articulation or language disorders and second language learning are risk factors for the development of SM. Additionally, SM has been documented in a wide variety of populations, including those with other developmental disorders such as autism spectrum disorder. The emergence of SM appears to depend on a variety of temperamental, developmental, and environmental factors. While social anxiety appears to be at the core of SM, the population is heterogeneous in other ways.

Table 28.3 Assessment of the pragmatic aspects of language

	Rating (0 = inappropriate; 1 = emerging; 2 = appropriate)		
Verbal aspects	Time 1	Time 2	Time 3
a) Speech acts	0		
1. Speech act pair analysis (takes both speaker and listener role)			
2. Variety of speech acts (comments, asserts, requests, etc.)	0		
a) Topic	0		
3. Selection (appropriate selection of discourse topic)			
4. Introduction (introduction of new topics)	0		
5. Maintenance (maintenance of topic across discourse)	0		
6. Change (change of topic in discourse)	0		
a) Turn-taking	0		
7. Initiation (initiation of speech acts)			
8. Response (responds to speaker's speech acts)	0		
9. Repair/revision (to conversation breakdowns)	0		
10. Pause time (between words, sentences, turns)	0		
11. Interruption/overlap (in discourse)	0		
12. Feedback to speakers (verbal and nonverbal indicators)	0		
13. Adjacency (utterances occur immediately after partner's utterance)	0		
14. Contingency (utterances semantically related)	0		
15. Quantity/conciseness (of verbal output)	0		
a) Lexical selection/use across speech acts	0		
16. Specificity/accuracy (of content)			
17. Cohesion (unity/connectedness of discourse)	0		
a) Stylistic variation	0		
18. Varying of communicative style			
Paralinguistic aspects			
a) Intelligibility and prosodics	0		
19. Intelligibility			
20. Vocal intensity	0		
21. Vocal quality	0		
22. Prosody	0		
23. Fluency	0		
Nonverbal aspects			
a) Kinesics and proxemics	0		
24. Physical proximity			
25. Physical contacts	0		
26. Body posture	0		
27. Foot/leg and hand/arm movements	0		
28. Gestures	0		
29. Facial expression	0		
30. Eye gaze	0		

Source: Prutting and Kirchner 1987.[4]

a is incorrect. Some children newly immersed in an unfamiliar language environment will go through a silent period. Most children will emerge from this silence and begin to speak the new language as it becomes more familiar to them; however, very anxious or inhibited children may "get stuck" in this period, and the silence and reticence to speak become habitual, eventually becoming SM.

b is incorrect. Articulation and language disorders appear to be risk factors for the development of SM. Communication disorders may make an anxious or inhibited child self-conscious about speaking, which may contribute to the development of SM.

c is incorrect. SM can be found in children with and without other developmental disorders.

28.5 Description of Disorder and Recommended Treatment

Children with SM typically find it challenging to speak in the face of severe anxiety in certain social situations. SM is a relatively rare disorder and presents certain challenges to parents, teachers, and therapists. Although often thought of as "treatment resistant," emerging data suggest that behavioral interventions (e.g., using reinforcement, shaping, stimulus fading, systematic desensitization) and cognitive behavior therapy (a type of psychotherapy that aims to change a person's maladaptive thinking, emotions, and behaviors) can be effective in treating the disorder. Other general therapy recommendations include use of "defocused" communication, reduced speaking pressure, and errorless learning.

Like some other children with SM, KL presented with a global disorder of verbal and nonverbal social interaction (pragmatics) manifested in specific contexts. Therapy began targeting early developing social interaction behaviors that precede verbal interaction, and worked up to oral communication in a hierarchical manner. The early developing skills targeted included joint attention behaviors (body and gaze orientation to others), shared affect, gestural communication, and reciprocal play. Reciprocal social interaction was initiated through hand-over-hand manipulation so that KL could engage in craft activities (e.g., gluing objects) and games that required nonverbal turn-taking. Hand-over-hand assistance was slowly extinguished and independent participation in these nonverbal activities was eventually obtained. Desensitization was used to increase KL's tolerance for noise making. Toy musical instruments were used, for example, to participate in a "band" with the clinician. Speech was shaped through reinforcement of noncommunicative vocalization of voiceless phonemes and then consonant–vowel combinations in gamelike activities. Real words were eventually shaped and were slowly transferred from noncommunicative contexts to communicative contexts. Clinicians sought to maintain a relaxed and supportive atmosphere and moved slowly and in small increments through behaviors that varied in novelty, communicative load, loudness, and modality (e.g., written and spoken communication).

28.6 Outcome

Once KL was speaking, pragmatic aspects of discourse were targeted in therapy. These included appropriate loudness of speech, quantity of conversational output, conversational adjacency and contingency, lexical specificity, and use of a variety of speech acts (e.g., asking, commenting, asserting). Skills obtained in the clinical context were then carefully generalized to the school setting through the use of stimulus fading; KL and the clinician met and talked in the school library before school began, and over time, teachers and, students were slowly integrated into the interaction.

Standardized testing was now possible, and revealed KL's language skills were within normal limits; composite standard scores on the CELF-4 ranged from 90 to 104; the standard score on the PPVT-4 was 100. KL no longer demonstrated articulation errors, and she participated in and passed a hearing screening.

Two and a half years after the initiation of therapy, KL interacted and spoke to her teachers and classmates in and out of the classroom. She no longer engaged in the immobile body posturing when in new social situations. She readily smiled and laughed. When the therapist called the school 6 months after discharge, her teacher reported her social and communicative behaviors were indistinguishable from those of her peers, except that she was "rather bossy."

28.7 Key Points

- SM is an anxiety disorder in which children speak normally at home, but do not speak much, or at all, outside the home. It is not due to any (other) communication disorder that prevents speech production (e.g., apraxia of speech, dysarthria).
- It is psychiatric in its etiology, but SM is a profound pragmatic communication disorder. Communication disorders of psychiatric etiology are within the speech-language pathologist's scope of practice.
- Using evidence-based practices, SM can be effectively treated by psychiatrists, psychologists, behavior therapists, speech-language pathologists, and interprofessional teams.
- The problem can be much more pervasive than mutism, and clinicians may need to initially target nonverbal reciprocal interaction behaviors and production of speech sounds in noncommunicative contexts.

Suggested Readings

[1] Bergman RL, Gonzalez A, Piacentini J, Keller ML. Integrated Behavior Therapy for Selective Mutism: a randomized controlled pilot study. Behav Res Ther. [serial online]. 2013; 51(10):680–689

[2] Lang C, Nir Z, Gothelf A, et al. The outcome of children with selective mutism following cognitive behavioral intervention: a follow-up study. [serial online]. Eur J Pediatr. 2016; 175(4):481–487

[3] Toppelberg CO, Tabors P, Coggins A, Lum K, Burger C. Differential diagnosis of selective mutism in bilingual children. J Am Acad Child Adolesc Psychiatry. [serial online]. 2005; 44(6):592–595

[4] Prutting CA, Kirchner DM. A clinical appraisal of the pragmatic aspects of language. J Speech Hear Disord. 1987; 52(2):105–119

29 School-Based Swallowing and Feeding Treatment: Oral Phase Dysphagia Secondary to Cerebral Palsy and Moebius Syndrome

Emily M. Homer and Katie C. Miranda

29.1 Introduction

Moebius syndrome is a nonprogressive craniofacial/neurological disorder that manifests primarily in facial paralysis. Individuals with Moebius syndrome cannot smile or frown, and do not have lateral eye movements. Respiratory problems, speech and swallowing disorders, visual impairments, sensory integration dysfunction, sleep disorders, and weak upper body strength may also be present.

29.2 Clinical History and Description

ML was a 7-year-old boy referred to the school district for multidisciplinary evaluation at 2 years, 6 months due to a diagnosis of Moebius syndrome, cerebral palsy, and global developmental delays. An initial screening revealed the student was "at risk" with regard to vision, hearing, sensory, fine motor, gross motor, speech, health, dysphagia, social/emotional/behavioral, and preacademic/readiness. Parent interview revealed a maternal family history of hearing loss, maternal and paternal history of depression, and a paternal aunt with mental disability. According to the parents, ML's birth and developmental history included a full-term pregnancy; however, prenatal care was not obtained for the first 6 to 7 months of pregnancy due to lack of health care. ML's delivery was uneventful. Developmental milestones, however, were significantly delayed. Medical history was unremarkable: no reported major accidents or illnesses requiring hospitalization. No daily medications were reported at the time of the evaluation. ML's parents reported difficulty chewing and expressed concern regarding his feeding. However, ML was currently receiving all nutrition and hydration orally.

29.3 Clinical Testing

Multidisciplinary Special Education Evaluation: The evaluation process to qualify for special education services included academic testing as well as language, motor, and self-help assessments. Components of the eligibility evaluation for special education services met the requirements described in the Individual with Disabilities Education Act (IDEA). Academic testing indicated a severe developmental delay.

Speech and Language Testing: ML was assessed by a speech-language pathologist (SLP) to determine communicative functioning, including assistive technology needs as well as swallowing and feeding. Formal and informal assessment, parent interviews, and student observations were conducted. Although ML was nonverbal, he used a combination of eye gaze and vocalizations during the evaluation to indicate pleasure and/or dislike. Mean length of utterances was not obtained due to his lack of verbal communication. Articulation, fluency, and voice were also not assessed due to lack of verbal responses. The Communication subtest of the Developmental Assessment of Young Children (DAYC) was completed and confirmed that ML displayed global language deficits of greater than two standard deviations from the mean. He exhibited deficits in his ability to understand and use vocabulary, comprehend oral information, follow oral directions, use short-term memory, and use appropriate social language skills. Assistive technology assessment indicated that ML may benefit from augmentative communication strategies to increase functional communication and interaction with others.

Swallowing and Feeding: An examination of the oral peripheral mechanism was attempted, but due to ML's age and disability, he was unable to fully cooperate. Therefore, structures were observed during play, and the ML's parents were queried for additional information. ML was not observed to drool during the evaluation; however, his parents reported that ML frequently drooled and grinded his teeth. His parents also reported that ML used a sippy cup or straw to draw liquids. ML routinely overstuffed his mouth when eating with no choking or coughing observed. His parents also reported that ML pocketed food and swallowed solid foods without chewing. A videofluoroscopic swallow study (VFSS) was conducted, which indicated no aspiration or penetration. It was recommended that an oral peripheral mechanism be attempted again once rapport and cooperation were established.

Occupational Therapy/Physical Therapy: Occupational therapy evaluation revealed delays in self-help and fine motor skills. Upper extremity functioning, postural control, and mobility skills were decreased. Physical therapy evaluation revealed delayed gross motor skill development at the 6- to 8-month level. ML was dependent on others for transfers and general mobility; he demonstrated severe gross motor deficits. Results of the Developmental Profile 3 indicated moderate-to-severe deficits in all areas of development, including physical, adaptive behavior, social-emotional, cognitive, and communication skills.

Based on the multidisciplinary evaluation, ML met criteria for the classification of Other Health Impairment. Along with special education instruction, he was eligible to receive speech and language pathology, assistive technology, occupational therapy, physical therapy, adaptive physical education, and health services. He was referred to the swallowing and feeding team for comprehensive evaluation of his oral phase dysphagia.

Once in school, the school-based swallowing and feeding team conducted a clinical evaluation to determine how to safely feed ML at school. An oral mechanism examination was reattempted. ML presented with low tone in the cheeks and lips. Tongue cupping was observed, indicating possible ankyloglossia (tongue-tie); however, the SLP was unable to assess for tongue-tie secondary to ML's lack of cooperation. High palatal arch and impaired dentition were noted. During oral intake, mild tongue and jaw protrusion were observed. ML exhibited a decreased rotary chew with munching pattern. He utilized his preferred sippy cup from home or a straw to draw liquids. Impaired lip rounding was observed with open cup drinking and, as a result, he was unable to drink from an open cup unassisted. Anterior loss of solids and liquids was also noted.

29.4 Questions and Answers for the Reader

1. Michael, a 6-year-old male student with Down syndrome, has oral phase dysphagia. He needs the following to be safe during meals at school: to have his food soft and bite-sized, to be supervised one-on-one during all meals and snacks, alternate one drink per three bites of food with cueing, and thin liquids in a low-flow cup. A swallowing and feeding plan is established for him and the classroom staff are trained. What should the school-based swallowing and feeding team SLP do to assist with the implementation of a student's swallowing and feeding plan?
   a) Train the classroom staff/feeders on implementing the swallowing and feeding plan. Staff need to be trained on all areas of the plan, including texture modification of the student's cafeteria meal.
   b) Share the swallowing and feeding plan with the teacher and tell her to put it in an easily accessed location.
   c) Have the parents demonstrate how to feed the student at school.
   d) Train the teacher so that she can train her paraprofessionals.
   e) Write the swallowing and feeding plan on the student's individual education plan (IEP).

Answer: a is correct. It is important that the classroom staff completely understand how to follow the student's plan and that they have demonstrated correct implementation when observed by the team SLP.

b is incorrect. Although is it important to share the swallowing and feeding plan with the classroom teacher, it is not sufficient to give her/him a copy to file. Classroom staff will need to be trained on how to implement the plan.

c is incorrect. It is often helpful for parents to demonstrate how the student eats at home; however, the school must feed the student according to what the district swallowing and feeding team has determined to be safe. As a member of the team, the parents should be aware of the student's plan, which they may want to implement at home. The parents may choose not to be trained on the plan but the training should be offered to them.

d is incorrect. Teachers must know how to safety feed all of the students in their classroom; however, they should not be responsible for training the paraprofessionals who may be the primary feeders. The team SLP and/or occupational therapist (OT) should do the training of at least three classroom staff members.

e is incorrect. The IEP describes the student's disorder and indicates what services the student will receive, including goals and objectives. The swallowing and feeding plan is a separate and more detailed description of how the student should be fed safely at school. The entire contents of the swallowing and feeding plan will not be on the IEP.

2. Mary is a 12-year-old student in the severe/profound special needs class. Her swallowing and feeding evaluation indicated low tone in her cheeks and lips and overstuffing if left alone. Her swallowing and feeding plan included minced and moist food modification, swallowing before taking another bite, and one-on-one supervision during all meals and snacks. Monitoring and consulting is part of a comprehensive swallowing and feeding procedure. What service should the school-based SLP swallowing and feeding team member provide now that a safe feeding plan has been established?
   a) Check on the student once a month to make sure the plan is still effective.
   b) Consult with the classroom staff on a regular basis by observing the student eating and providing suggestions when indicated.
   c) Send written reminders to the teachers and paraprofessionals on how to feed the student correctly.
   d) Once the classroom staff is trained, tell the teachers to contact the swallowing and feeding team if there are any concerns.
   e) Remind teachers that the plan should be follow when possible.

Answer: b is correct. The team should work closely with the classroom staff to ensure that the plan continues to be correct and that it is being implemented with fidelity. The team should be available to classroom staff to answer questions, demonstrate techniques, and guide them with implementation. The frequency of the monitoring will depend on the student and the therapist.

a is incorrect. For some students, once a month monitoring may be recommended; however, every child is different and some will need more frequent monitoring and more active participation by the SLP and other team members.

c is incorrect. Although sending a written reminder might be one way the team communicates with teachers, it should not be the only method. Swallowing and feeding training takes a hands-on approach, with the SLP meeting with classroom staff on a regular basis.

d is incorrect. The team cannot wait for a teacher to contact them with a concern. Professionals with training in swallowing and feeding must provide ongoing monitoring and consultation services to the classroom staff.

e is incorrect. The plan must always be followed. The words "when possible" make this answer unacceptable.

3. Jenna, a 3-year-old student, was identified during her multidisciplinary evaluation as having a developmental delay with a swallowing and feeding disorder. The district should:
   a) Refer the parents to an outpatient clinic for swallowing and feeding services.
   b) Talk to the parents and request a physician's script to be able to address the swallowing and feeding at school.

c) Refer the student to the school-based swallowing and feeding team for an evaluation of the student's feeding skills.

d) Inform the teacher that the student may have some trouble eating the cafeteria meal and to watch her.

e) Put the results in the evaluation report and recommend that the student bring her lunch from school since the cafeteria meal may need to be modified.

Answer: c is correct. The evaluation team identifies the concern of a swallowing and feeding disorder and recommends referral to the school-based team. The core team, made up of an SLP, OT, and nurse, then evaluates the student's skills and determines how to safely feed the student at school. The evaluation includes a parental interview, clinical evaluation (observation of the student eating at school) and, if there is a concern of aspiration, a referral for VFSS.

a is incorrect. School districts have the responsibility to provide health services (of which swallowing and feeding is included) when they are necessary for the child to stay in school; therefore, they cannot refer the student to a private clinic without providing the services.

b is incorrect. It is important for a district to communicate with both the parents and the physician when a student has a swallowing and feeding disorder; however, it is not a requirement for the district to have a physician's script to set up a swallowing and feeding plan. If they have a script from the physician, they must consider it but ultimately follow the recommendations of the school swallowing and feeding team.

d is incorrect. The teacher should not be responsible for determining what is safe feeding for a child with a swallowing and feeding disorder.

e is incorrect. School districts have a responsibility to provide a safe environment for their students. Parents cannot be required to provide the student's lunch for it to meet safe guidelines. The student is eligible for either a free or reduced school meal or the parent has the option to purchase the cafeteria meal. The district should modify the meal if it is required for the child to be healthy and safe at school and to participate in her curriculum.

29.5 Description of Disorder and Recommended Treatment

ML's IEP targeted increased functional communication, oral motor skills, and diet tolerance/advancement. The following goals were added to ML's IEP:

- Improving functional communication skills/initiation of interactions with peers and adults by making requests, labeling, and/or terminating during structured activities/meal using assistive technology strategies (i.e., visuals, voice output devices, switches, etc.) with cueing at 60% proficiency for 8 out of 10 sessions.
- Performing three to four repetitions of oral motor exercises to improve strength, coordination/mobility, and sensation of articulators for swallowing and vocalizations with maximum assist three times per day.
- Giving feeding and swallowing compensatory strategies; tolerating least restrictive diet as evidenced by no signs/

symptoms of aspiration, as progress is made, advancing diet to include one new food item per week.

The school district's assistive technology team recommended ML utilize augmentative communication strategies/equipment to request, comment, and terminate during structured activities, such as meal time. The following augmentative and alternative communication strategies were trialed: a picture exchange system to request highly preferred toy/food items; single message voice output device to request "more" for desired foods, music, activities; multichannel voice output device to participate in educational activities and circle time, such as counting, days of the week, months of the year, and repetitive lines of a story.

The following oral motor exercises were incorporated into therapy:

- Facial/labial massage to improve sensation.
- Lip tapping with gloved hand and lip pulls with trimmed Toothette to improve lip rounding.
- Tongue pulls with trimmed Toothette to improve lingual retraction.

Because of his history of poor postural control and scoliosis, the SLP consulted with his physical therapist regarding optimal positioning during meals. It was recommended that ML be fitted with an adapted Rifton chair. He was seated at 90 degrees upright at a toddler table. ML's back brace was also utilized to support his trunk when sitting at a table. Occupational therapy also recommended a low-flow training cup to improve tongue retraction/lip rounding and facilitate open cup drinking, teaspoon/fork with adapted grip, and suction bowl.

The SLP recommended soft, bite-sized solids and thin liquids. A safe swallowing and feeding plan was established based on information gathered from the interdisciplinary swallowing and feeding team. Feeding techniques/precautions included the following:

- One teaspoon per bite/sip.
- One bite/sip at a time.
- Use of utensils as student preferred finger foods.
- Maintain upright position 30 minutes after meal.
- Drink after every three to four bites.
- Direct supervision by classroom staff/feeders was required for all meals and overstuffing/rapid intake needed to be monitored. It was recommended that staff provide verbal and tactile prompts as needed to slow rate.
- Staff/feeders ensured that ML's mouth was clear of residue after every bite (▶ Fig. 29.1).

All recommendations were included in a written swallowing and feeding plan. Classroom staff/feeders were educated regarding recommendations and demonstrated proficiency in implementation, including texture modification. They were also educated regarding signs/symptoms of aspiration, such as coughing, choking, watery eyes, wet vocal quality, lethargy, and labored breathing.

As part of federal requirements for school cafeteria programs and because ML required a modified cafeteria meal at school, a prescription for meal modification form was completed and signed by a physician. The school's cafeteria manager and

Student: Date of Birth: Date of Plan:
School: Teacher:

Swallowing and Feeding Case Manager: (name of case manager). If there are any questions regarding this student's feeding plan, please contact the Case Manager (SLP) at the following: Location(s):

Case History and Presenting Concerns:

Feeding Recommendations:

Positioning:

Equipment:

Tube Fed: ☐ tube fed/nothing by mouth   ☐ tube and oral fed
(amount fed orally:)

Diet/Food Prep (according to the IDDS:

Food Consistency:

    ☐ Liquidized   ☐ Pureed ☐ Minced and moist   ☐ Soft and bite sized   ☐ Regular

Liquid Consistency:

    ☐ Extremely Thick (pureed) ☐ Moderately thick (liquidized) ☐ Mildly thick
    ☐ Slightly thick   ☐ Thin

Other recommendations:

Feeding Plan Techniques/Precautions:

Amount of food per bite (be specific to amount and size):

Food placement:

Keep student in upright position ___ minutes after meal.

Offer a drink after ___ bites

Additional precautions/comments:

Swallowing and Feeding Plan Training

I, the undersigned, have read and been trained on implementing the swallowing and feeding plan for (student name). I agree to implement the swallowing and feeding plan as specified.

Name   **Position**   **Date**

_____   _____ _____

_____   _____ _____

_____   _____ _____

I understand that I am responsible for the implementation of the swallowing and feeding plan in my classroom.

Signed: _____ (classroom teacher) **Date:** _____

Fig. 29.1 Students eat safely: swallowing and feeding plan.

staff were notified regarding ML's modifications to ensure compliance.

29.6 Outcome

ML received speech and language therapy, including assistive technology and swallowing/feeding intervention three times a week for 20 minutes per session. Therapy sessions took place in the ML's self-contained classroom; classroom staff were also trained regarding strategies to continue therapeutic tasks throughout the school day. ML progressed using a small jelly switch to activate cause/effect toys and adapted computer software. He also used a two-cell, static-display (pictured icons) voice output device to request "more" and terminate (e.g., "all done") during structured language activities and meals. ML consistently activated switches and voice output devices with increased accuracy and improved timing; however, he continued to require multisensory prompts and cues.

With implementation of oral motor exercises and use of a low-flow cup, ML exhibited improved tone/sensation, tongue retraction, and lip rounding. Anterior loss of solids and liquids improved, but persisted. He no longer used the preferred sippy cup at school, which required a sucking action, and increasingly attempted an open cup. ML ate lunch in the cafeteria and had a modified school lunch tray prepared for him. Classroom staff prepared the modified meal tray at a blending station in the cafeteria to meet the recommendations of the swallowing and feeding plan and sat with him throughout his meal to ensure compliance with the feeding plan. ML did not exhibit any signs or symptoms of aspiration or penetration and received adequate hydration/nutrition at school. The SLP continued to address functional communication and dysphagia goals per ML's IEP for the entire school year.

29.7 Key Points

- Swallowing and feeding concerns should be considered during a multidisciplinary evaluation to qualify for special education services. Clinical evaluation of swallowing and feeding may be done once the student is enrolled in school. If a student does not qualify for special education services, then the student's swallowing and feeding concerns may be addressed through a 504 plan.
- School-based SLPs work on many areas, including assistive technology, swallowing, and feeding. The identification and management of swallowing and feeding should be a part of the student's overall communication and special education program. Therapeutic intervention to improve oral motor and functional feeding skills may often be done while working on communication. Training classroom staff to implement both communication and swallowing strategies simultaneously may be effective in carryover of skills.
- Addressing swallowing and feeding disorders in a school system should be done utilizing a team approach and a district-approved procedure to provide consistency, accountability, and clarification of roles and responsibilities, resulting in safe feeding at school.
- When addressing swallowing and feeding in the school setting, it is essential that a safe swallowing and feeding plan be established, that classroom staff/feeders are trained on implementation of the plan, and that there is ongoing monitoring of the plan's implementation.

Suggested Readings

[1] American Speech-Language-Hearing Association. Clinical topics/pediatric dysphagia. 2007. Available at: http://www.asha.org/Practice-Portal/Clinical-Topics/Pediatric-Dysphagia

[2] Benfer KA, Weir KA, Bell KL, Ware RS, Davies PS, Boyd RN. Oropharyngeal dysphagia and gross motor skills in children with cerebral palsy. Pediatrics. 2013; 131(5):e1553–e1562

[3] Benfer KA, Weir KA, Bell KL, Ware RS, Davies PS, Boyd RN. Validity and reproducibility of measures of oropharyngeal dysphagia in preschool children with cerebral palsy. Dev Med Child Neurol. 2015; 57(4):358–365

[4] Homer E, Ed. Management of Swallowing and Feeding in Schools. San Diego, CA: Plural Publishing; 2016

[5] Overland L. A sensory-motor approach to feeding. Perspect Swallowing Swallowing Disord (Dysphagia). 2011; 20:60–64

30 Early Identification and Early Intervention in the Birth-to-Three Population

Nancy Lewis

30.1 Introduction

Early identification of speech-language delays/disorders and other developmental conditions through early and regular developmental and behavioral screening is critical. The identification of delays during these screenings should result in timely referral to early intervention (EI) to ensure a thorough evaluation and subsequent initiation of appropriate specialized services.

30.2 Clinical History and Description

CJ was a 2-year, 9-month-old boy referred to EI at 26 months of age due to a delay in expressive language skills and severe speech sound disorder (SSD). He was full-term and the first-born child to his 44-year-old mother. Delivery was prolonged, yet otherwise unremarkable. Newborn hearing screening and metabolic screening were unremarkable.

CJ's mother reported that she first became concerned when CJ was around 12 months of age as he was still babbling with no intelligible single words and often batted at his ears. The American Academy of Pediatrics recommends the administration of standardized developmental screening at 9, 18, and 24 or 30 months with an autism-specific screening at 18 and 24 months. According to CJ's mother, his pediatrician used "developmental forms," but did not discuss any results. When she expressed concern regarding CJ's communication delays and the persistent batting of his ears, the pediatrician informed her that CJ had fluid in his ears, but no infection and no further action was taken.

At 24 months of age, CJ's mother learned of EI through a colleague, who also recommended that CJ be evaluated by an audiologist. The audiologist referred CJ to an ear, nose, and throat physician who immediately placed bilateral tubes in CJ's ears and referred him to a local EI agency.

30.3 Clinical Testing

Developmental testing occurred at 26 months of age upon enrollment in EI. The EI team administered the Hawaii Early Learning Profile, a curriculum-based assessment, and CJ met eligibility criteria of a 25% or more delay in the domains of communication, cognition, gross motor, fine motor, and self-help. He passed a vision screening. Audiology testing revealed that CJ oriented to speech stimuli at 20 dB. Sound-field testing indicated that CJ responded to narrow-band noise stimuli at 500 to 4,000 Hz in the borderline normal hearing range. Tympanometry indicated reduced middle ear admittance bilaterally.

Upon enrollment in EI, the Goldman–Fristoe Test of Articulation-Third Edition (GFTA-3) was administered.[1] At 33 months of age, given the severity of CJ's SSD, the Khan–Lewis Phonological Analysis-Third Edition (KLPA-3) was administered as part of a comprehensive evaluation for public school developmental preschool (part B services).[2] The KLPA-3 is a norm-referenced, in-depth analysis of phonological process usage in individuals ages 2,0–21,11. Designed as a companion tool to the GFTA-3, the KLPA-3 provides an analysis of the GFTA-3 target words for any sound changes and allows for the identification of phonological processes used to produce those sound changes. Though single-word measures of speech production have limitations and should not be used in isolation, such measures have utility when assessing children with unintelligible speech as a means of identifying the target word.

CJ obtained a standard score of 70 on the KLPA-3 corresponding to the second percentile and an age equivalence of less than 24 months. The percent of occurrence for the Core Phonological Processes chart revealed the frequency of occurrence of the 12 *Core Phonological Processes* (▶ Fig. 30.1). In addition, CJ's speech sound production was characterized by the use of 6 of the 12 Supplemental Phonological Processes and nine Other Phonological Processes. CJ's speech sound production contained excessive use of multiple phonological processes producing a process-per-word average of 2.55.

CJ's phonetic inventory is shown in ▶ Fig. 30.2. The phonetic inventory is a visual display of the sounds a child does and does not produce regardless of the accuracy, relative to the target, in word-initial, word-medial, and word-final position. Each table is arranged horizontally by manner of production and vertically by place of production. Voiced and voiceless cognates are side by side. On the KLPA-3, when a sound is produced accurately as the target, that phoneme is circled. When there is a sound change from the target sound, a tally mark is placed in the appropriate cell. For example, if the target word "five" is produced as "dive," a tally mark would be placed in the word-initial /d/ cell (target /f/ became /d/) and the word-final /v/ would be circled (correct production of target). The organization of the phonetic inventory by place, manner, and voicing displays clinically relevant trends in a child's speech repertoire, such as overuse of a particular type of sound or complete omission of other types of sounds, at a glance.

30.3.1 KLPA-3 Summary

The summary of consonants analysis in Fig. 30.3 reveals the following:

- Excessive use (greater than 15% of the time) of 9 of the 12 Core Phonological Processes: Deaffrication, stopping of fricatives and affricates, stridency deletion, vocalization, palatal fronting, velar fronting, cluster simplification, syllable reduction, final devoicing.
- Use of 6 of the 12 Supplemental Phonological Processes: Stopping of other, affrication, gliding of other, deletion of initial consonant, medial devoicing, initial devoicing.

KLPA™
KHAN-LEWIS
PHONOLOGICAL ANALYSIS

ANALYSIS FORM

Linda M. L. Khan and Nancy P. Lewis

Name: __CJ__ ☐ Female ☑ Male

Grade/Ed. Level: _____ School/Agency: __Early Intervention__

Language(s) Spoken in the Home: __English__

Examiner: __NL__

Reason for Testing: __Unintelligible speech__

AGE CALCULATION

	Year	Month	Day
Test Date			
Birth Date			
Age	2	9	15

Reminder: Do not round up to next month or year.

KLPA-3 SCORE SUMMARY

*Total Raw Score	Standard Score	Confidence Interval ☐90% ☑95%	Percentile Rank	Age Equivalent
93	70	67 – 73	2nd	< 2;0

* Raw score equals total number of occurrences of scored phonological processes.

PERCENT OF OCCURRENCE FOR CORE PHONOLOGICAL PROCESSES

	Phonological Process	Number of Occurrences	Total Possible Occurrences	Percent of Occurrences
Manner	Deaffrication (DF)	6	of 8 =	75 %
	Gliding of liquids (GL)	3	of 20 =	15 %
	Stopping of fricatives and affricates (ST)	11	of 48 =	23 %
	Stridency deletion (STR)	9	of 42 =	21 %
	Vocalization (VOC)	15	of 15 =	100 %
Place	Palatal fronting (PF)	12	of 12 =	100 %
	Velar fronting (VF)	8	of 23 =	35 %
Reduction	Cluster simplification (CS)	11	of 23 =	48 %
	Deletion of final consonant (DFC)	2	of 36 =	6 %
	Syllable reduction (SR)	4	of 25 =	16 %
Voicing	Final devoicing (FDV)	9	of 35 =	26 %
	Initial voicing (IV)	1	of 33 =	3 %

VOWEL ALTERATIONS

Notes: • vowel prolongation
• addition of /ə/

DIALECTAL INFLUENCE

☐ Yes ☑ No

Notes:

OVERALL INTELLIGIBILITY

☐ Good ☐ Fair ☑ Poor

Notes:

Unintelligible > 75% of time to unfami[liar] Listener

Fig. 30.1 KLPA-3 summary of standard scores and percent of occurrence of the core phonological processes for CJ at age 2,9.

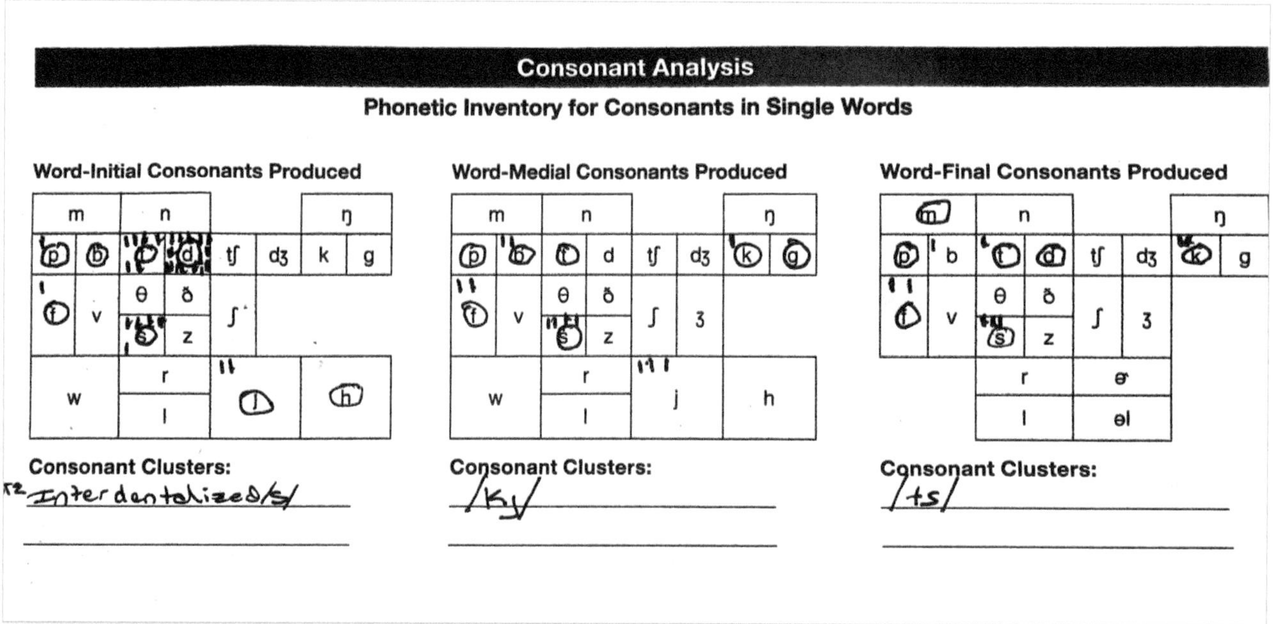

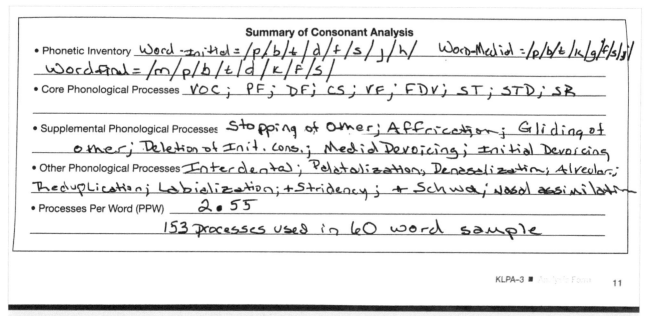

Fig. 30.2 KLPA-3 phonetic inventory of consonants in single words for CJ at age 2,9.

Fig. 30.3 KLPA-3 summary of consonants analysis: phonetic inventory, core phonological processes, other phonological processes, and process per word (PPW).

- Use of nine Other Phonological Processes: Interdentalization, palatalization, denasalization, alveolarization, reduplication, labialization, addition of stridency, addition of schwa, nasal assimilation.
- Extremely limited phonetic repertoire consisting primarily of labial and alveolar stop consonants, with infrequent instances of fricative sounds.
- Vowel elongation.

30.4 Questions and Answers for the Reader

1. Early and regular developmental and behavioral screening is recommended by the American Academy of Pediatrics (AAP) at:
   a) Every well-child check appointment.

b) Developmental screening at 9, 18, and 24 or 30 months and autism-specific screening at 18 and 24 months.

c) The AAP does not recommend screening and instead relies on ongoing surveillance by pediatricians.

d) The AAP does not have a recommendation regarding autism-specific screening.

Answer: b is correct. In 2006, the AAP adopted a set of guidelines for developmental and autism screening.[5]

a is incorrect. Though some pediatricians may screen children at every well-child visit, the current AAP guidelines call for a periodicity schedule of developmental screening at 9, 18, and 24 or 30 months with specific autism screen at 18 and 24 months.

c is incorrect. The AAP recommends surveillance by pediatricians at every well-child check visit and developmental/behavioral screening at 9, 18, and 24 or 30 months. The AAP supports the concept that early childhood screening is an essential component of health supervision and provides a foundation for monitoring and supporting healthy physical, cognitive, and psychosocial development.

d is incorrect. The AAP guidelines include a periodicity schedule for administration of an autism-specific tool at ages 18 and 24 months.

2. EI is a federally mandated service for children and their families who:
   a) Are determined eligible for services by demonstrating delays, typically at least by 25%, in one or more developmental domain.
   b) Qualify by being at 100% below the federal poverty level.
   c) Use English as the primary language in the home.
   d) Are located in metropolitan areas near EI programs.

Answer: a is correct. This response is correct. EI providers complete a comprehensive, multidisciplinary assessment to determine the eligibility for services. States determine the percent of delay that a child must demonstrate in one or more developmental domains to be determined eligible.

b is incorrect. Income level is not part of the eligibility criteria for EI services. EI programs provide services to families across the income spectrum.

c is incorrect. Primary home language of English is not part of the eligibility criteria for EI services. EI programs provide services to eligible families regardless of the primary home language.

d is incorrect. Geographic location is not part of the eligibility criteria for EI services. EI programs provide services to eligible families regardless of residence.

3. According to the DSM-V, SSDs are defined as:
   a) Persistent difficulty with speech sound production.
   b) Disturbance causes limitations in effective communication that is interfering.
   c) Onset in early developmental period.
   d) Not attributable to congenital or acquired conditions.
   e) All of the above.

Answer: e is correct. The DSM-V definition for SSD includes criteria of the four components listed above. SSD is a persistent condition that interferes with communication via multiple speech sound production errors. It presents in early childhood without a known congenital or acquired cause.

4. A phonological approach to assessment of SSDs in children resulting in unintelligible speech involves:
   a) A quick screening of a child's speech production to identify correct production of individual, early developing sounds.
   b) An in-depth analysis of a child's speech production system to identify the phonological processes, phonetic environment, and phonetic inventory that capture the rules that are governing speech sound errors and the sound repertoire available to a child.
   c) A spontaneous speech sample in which the target productions are not able to be identified.
   d) A methodology that enables clinicians to design treatment plans at a phonological systems level to impact change in an efficient manner.
   e) b and d.

Answer: e is correct. A phonological approach to assessment provides the clinician with in-depth information regarding a child's speech production system and enables the clinician to integrate the results into treatment plans.

a is incorrect. A phonological approach to assessment of SSDs in children is an in-depth analysis of the rules and patterns that govern a child's multiple speech production errors. The approach involves identifying the phonological processes or patterns that the child employs that contribute to reduced speech intelligibility.

b is one of the correct answers. A phonological approach to assessment of SSDs in children requires the collection of a preponderance of evidence including phonological process usage, phonetic environment of patterns of errors, and the phonetic inventory of available sounds.

c is incorrect. When a child presents with SSD, typically there is reduced speech intelligibility, oftentimes unintelligible speech production the majority of the time. Phonological assessment requires the examiner to compare the child's speech production to the intended target word or phrase, a task that is often not possible with children presenting with highly unintelligible speech.

d is one of the correct answers. The summary from a phonological assessment provides the information needed to determine phonological treatment goals and objectives and to identify treatment stimuli.

30.5 Description of Disorder and Recommended Treatment

EI, a federally mandated service, is operated in states as a comprehensive, coordinated interagency system that provides multidisciplinary interventions for infants and toddlers with or at risk for developmental delays. EI is designed to serve children under the age of 3 and their families. Communication difficulties are among the most widely reported developmental delays in this age group. Speech-language pathologists (SLPs) and audiologists play an essential role in the early identification of developmental concerns to ensure linkage to services. Communication delays may present in various ways; however, SSDs are highly prevalent and are identified in approximately 15.6% of 3-year-old children. The majority of children receiving EI services qualify with a communication delay. The DSM-V[3] provides the following criteria for SSD: (1) persistent difficulty with speech sound production; (2) disturbance causes limitations in effective communication that is interfering; (3) onset in early developmental period; and (4) not attributable to congenital or acquired conditions. SSD includes the conditions formally referred to as articulation disorders and phonological disorders.

CJ presented with a severe SSD characterized by frequent use of multiple phonological processes, both typical and atypical, along with a limited phonetic repertoire. Through his EI program, CJ received weekly visits from a certified SLP and bimonthly visits from a developmental specialist. Initially, a sound-by-sound articulation treatment approach was used as demonstrated by the goal: "Correct production of initial /p/ and /b/." After 6 months of EI services, CJ's speech remained highly unintelligible with a high frequency of multiple phonological processes usage and speech sound errors.

When CJ transitioned from EI services to the public school developmental preschool services, the treating SLP used a systems-level phonological approach to intervention. Broad diversity exists in the literature regarding approaches to target selection, intervention, and service delivery.[4] Though the importance of a systematic approach to target selection is indisputable, some advocate for a *developmental* approach by building on early-to-develop, stimulable sounds, while others advocate for a paradoxically distinct *complexity* approach that promotes the prioritization of late-developing, nonstimulable sounds.

Treating children with SSD presents challenges. Assessment relies on the accurate transcription of unintelligible speech and a deep analysis of the rules, or phonological processes that impact the sound changes. Furthermore, clinical decisions include:
- Service delivery:
  - Individual or group.
  - Dosage:
    - Number of days per week.
    - Length of session.
    - Duration of treatment.
- Target selection:
  - Where to begin.
- Impact on intelligibility:
  - Developmental or complex strategy.
- Treatment approach
- Method of feedback
- Discharge decisions

In summary, a phonological approach to intervention with children with SSDs is based on the rule-governed nature of the phonological system. Phonological processes describe patterns of errors within a phonetic environment. Treatment goals may target entire classes of sounds (e.g., decreasing the use of stopping of fricatives and affricates), word structure (e.g., decreasing deletion of final consonants), and/or distinctive features such as voicing errors (e.g., decreasing final devoicing) rather than targeting correct production of individual sounds toward a percent of accuracy. The research on phonological remediation reports generalization of accurate production to sounds that are not targeted directly, thereby increasing the likelihood of improved speech intelligibility while decreasing the time achieving this goal.

After review of CJ's comprehensive evaluation for speech-language services within the part B special education preschool program, a developmental approach to treatment was recommended. Initial targets included the decrease of Stopping. Typically, stopping involves the sound change from fricatives and affricates to stop consonants. In CJ's case, he used stopping not only for fricative and affricates, but also on nasals and glides. Stopping of other sounds is considerably less common than stopping of fricatives and affricates and has a negative impact on intelligibility. In spite of the consistent occurrence of Stopping, CJ's phonetic inventory included instances of fricative productions in word-initial, word-medial, and word-final positions. Treatment methodology benefited from CJ's fricative productions in his phonetic repertoire to influence the decrease of stopping.

30.6 Outcome

At 3 years of age, CJ qualified for services through the public school part B special education services based on his severe SSD. He participated in a 4-day per week developmental preschool program designed for children with severe SSDs and received individual therapy for 30 minutes, 4 days a week. The SLP collaborated with the special education preschool teacher to integrate opportunities for CJ to practice his speech/language goals within classroom activities. CJ also received follow-up audiological services every 3 months to monitor hearing acuity and middle-ear function.

KLPA-3 was administered after 6 months of intervention. ▶ Table 30.1 demonstrates the change in the quantitative metrics. CJ demonstrated a 25% reduction in the raw score, a metric based on the number of occurrences of the 12 Core Phonological Processes. CJ's KLPA-3 standard score and percentile rank continued to qualify him for speech/language services. The process-per-word measure was sensitive to the improvement in CJ's overall speech intelligibility.

Qualitative measures such as the percent of occurrence of individual phonological processes decreased for the Core Phonological Processes, and CJ used fewer overall Supplemental/Other Phonological Processes. The phonetic inventory included an increase in the use of fricatives in all word positions, the use of the initial nasals /m/ and /n/ (previously absent in phonetic inventory), and the use of word-initial affricates.

Table 30.1 KLPA-3 scores at onset of treatment (36 months of age) and after 6 months of treatment (42 months of age)

KLPA-3 scores	Prephonological treatment	Post-6-month course of treatment
Raw score	93	70
Standard score	70	75
Percentile rank	2nd	5th
Process per word	2.55	1.91

At 42 months, CJ's mother reported that he had recently demonstrated a significant gain in his overall speech intelligibility. Family members and his preschool teachers were better able to understand CJ's speech production. As well, CJ's expressive language skills improved, and he appeared more confident and willing to engage with others at school and at home.

30.7 Key Points

- SLPs and audiologists play an essential role in the promotion of developmental monitoring as well as early and regular developmental and behavioral screening that improve early identification practices.
- EI for children with speech, language, and/or hearing delays/disorders relies on the early identification efforts of health care providers and early childhood professionals, including SLPs and audiologists.
- SSDs are reported in 15.6% of 3-year-olds, and communication concerns, in general, surface early as parental concerns.
- A phonological analysis is a critical component of a comprehensive evaluation for children with unintelligible speech.
- Though approaches to treatment vary, a phonological approach to the remediation of SSDs instructs clinicians to target aspects of a child's phonological system that can lead to improved speech intelligibility.

References

[1] Khan L, Lewis N. Khan–Lewis Phonological Analysis. 3rd ed. San Antonio, TX: Pearson; 2015

[2] Goldman R, Fristoe M. Goldman–Fristoe Test of Articulation. 3rd ed. San Antonio, TX: Pearson; 2015

[3] American Psychiatric Association. Diagnostic and Statistical Manual of Mental Disorders. 5th ed. Arlington, VA: American Psychiatric Publishing; 2013

[4] Baker E, McLeod S. Evidence-based practice for children with speech sound disorders: part 1 narrative review. Lang Speech Hear Serv Sch. 2011; 42(2): 102–139

[5] Council on Children with Disabilities, Section on Developmental Behavioral Pediatrics, Bright Futures Steering Committee, Medical Home Initiatives for Children with Special Needs Project Advisory Committee. Identifying infants and young children with developmental disorders in the medical home: an algorithm for developmental surveillance and screening. Pediatrics. 2006; 118(1):405–420

31 Treatment of Pragmatic Language Disorders in Preschool and School-Age Children

Jessie L. Ginsburg

31.1 Introduction

CJ was a 3-year-old boy who was referred for speech and language therapy after being diagnosed with a social communication disorder by a psychologist at a state-funded agency. At 3 years of age, children typically begin preschool and are expected to interact with peers and participate in preacademic activities. Strong social communication skills are needed to build and maintain friendships, as well as form the foundation for academic success.

31.2 Case Description

CJ was a 3-year-old male born at 38 weeks via cesarean section following an unremarkable pregnancy. He lived with his biological parents and English was the only language spoken in his home. CJ said his first word at 12 months, walked at 15 months, and combined words at 30 months. At CJ's 3-year checkup, his pediatrician recommended speech and language evaluation due to concerns with his language development. A psychologist from a state-funded agency diagnosed CJ with a social communication disorder. At 3.6 years, CJ's parents enrolled him in a private preschool 5 days per week, where he reportedly followed directions and participated in classroom activities without difficulty. His teachers observed repetitive behaviors that led his parents to seek a developmental evaluation through the local school district.

31.3 Clinical Testing

At 3.6 years, a speech-language pathologist (SLP) in CJ's school district assessed his language using the Preschool Language Scale, fifth Edition (PLS-5), and diagnosed him with an expressive language disorder (▶ Table 31.1). CJ's parents brought him to a private clinic where an SLP performed an informal assessment of his play using the Floortime Observation Checklist. This assessment revealed that CJ demonstrated difficulties with continuous interaction, answering questions, problem solving, perspective taking, and emotional thinking.

Table 31.1 Preschool Language Scale, Fifth Edition

	Standard score	Percentile rank
Auditory comprehension	97	42nd
Expressive communication	84	14th

At 3.8 years, a school psychologist assessed CJ's cognitive skills and his performance qualified him to receive special education services based on the criteria of autism. CJ's parents rejected the services offered as the school district was unable to provide transportation to and from therapy.

Two months later, CJ's parents obtained a developmental evaluation for CJ through a state-funded agency. A psychologist assessed him using the Vineland Adaptive Behavior Scales, Second Edition (VABS-II). He scored in the fifth percentile in the socialization domain, indicating significant deficits in social skills. The psychologist also assessed CJ using the Autism Diagnostic Observation Schedule, Second Edition (ADOS-2). Based on the results of that assessment, the psychologist diagnosed CJ with low-to-moderate level of autism.

31.4 Questions and Answers for the Reader

1. What major deficit area(s) should be addressed in CJ's treatment goals?
   a) Receptive and expressive language.
   b) Expressive language and auditory processing.
   c) Pragmatics.
   d) Expressive language and pragmatics.

Answer: d is correct. CJ's score of 84 on the expressive communication subtest of the PLS-5 was below average, and, therefore, expressive language should be addressed in treatment. CJ was diagnosed with autism spectrum disorder, which suggests he has deficits in his social use of language. Accordingly, improving CJ's pragmatic language should be a primary goal in his treatment.

a is incorrect. CJ did not show deficits in his receptive language on the PLS-5, nor did his teachers or parents have concerns with his language comprehension.

b is incorrect. CJ's auditory processing skills had not been assessed.

c is incorrect. CJ's pragmatic language should be targeted in therapy; however, it is not the only deficit area that should be targeted.

2. In addition to individual speech and language therapy, what other type of therapy would you recommend for CJ?
   a) Occupational therapy.
   b) Physical therapy

c) Social skills groups.

d) Vision therapy.

Answer: c is correct. Social skills groups should be recommended to address CJ's pragmatic language deficits.

a is incorrect. While it may be appropriate to recommend an evaluation for occupational therapy, it would not be within an SLP's scope of practice to recommend therapy sessions.

b is incorrect. CJ's parents did not voice concerns regarding CJ's motor development.

d is incorrect. CJ's parents did not voice concerns regarding his vision or visual processing.

3. What role(s) should CJ's parents play in therapy?

a) Participate in coaching sessions with the SLP.

b) Target CJ's goals in the home.

c) Demonstrate an understanding of the SLP's therapy approach.

d) All of the above.

Answer: d is correct. Parent education and training is key to the success of CJ's treatment. The SLP must educate CJ's parents on her therapy approach, CJ's goals, and how to target his goals at home. The SLP should also demonstrate strategies and provide parents with the opportunity to participate in therapy sessions. Parent education and training helps ensure CJ's generalization of new skills.

a is incorrect. Participating in coaching sessions is a key element; however, it is not the only role that CJ's parents should play in his treatment.

b is incorrect. Targeting CJ's goals in the home is crucial; however, it is not the only role that his parents should play in his treatment.

c is incorrect. Demonstrating an understanding of the SLP's therapy approach is important; however, it is not the only role that CJ's parents should play in his treatment.

4. What other professional should CJ's SLP communicate with on a regular basis?

a) Teacher.

b) Audiologist.

c) Occupational therapist.

d) Physical therapist.

Answer: a is correct. It is important for CJ's SLP to collaborate with his teacher to improve his treatment outcome. CJ's teacher should be made aware of his treatment goals and should be taught strategies that she can use to target his goals in the classroom.

b is incorrect. CJ has no history of hearing loss or ear infections.

c is incorrect. CJ has not been assessed by an occupational therapist.

d is incorrect. CJ does not receive physical therapy.

Table 31.2 Diagnostic Evaluation of Language Variation

Domain	Scaled score	Percentile rank
Pragmatics	7	5th

31.5 Description of Disorder and Recommended Treatment

CJ began receiving individual speech and language therapy sessions at a private clinic two times per week at the age of 3.6 years. Treatment focused on improved expressive and pragmatic language skills, with a strong emphasis on parent education and training. Therapy goals included answering WH-questions, engaging in multistep symbolic play schemas, and conversational turn taking. CJ's teachers were continuously informed of his treatment goals and were also taught strategies to employ in the classroom. The SLP recommended an occupational therapy evaluation; however, due to difficulties with scheduling, his parents decided they would have him assessed at a later date.

At 3.9 years, CJ was placed in a social skills group in the private clinic with one other peer. Five months later, an additional peer was added to the group. Throughout this time, CJ continued to receive individual speech and language therapy in the private clinic one to two times per week.

31.6 Outcome

At 4.6 years, the CELF-P (Clinical Evaluation of Language Fundamentals Preschool) was readministered. CJ tested in the average range in all subtests of the CELF-P, scoring in the 55th percentile. These results suggested that he no longer demonstrated deficits in the area of expressive language. He used appropriate grammar, answered age-appropriate WH-questions, and had a typical mean length of utterance for his age.

At 5 years, CJ's social language was assessed via the Developmental Evaluation of Language Variation (DELV). He scored in the fifth percentile on the pragmatics subtest with significant difficulties with social use of language (▶ Table 31.2). CJ's language was also reassessed using the CELF for school-age children. He scored within the average range on all subtests with the exception of the pragmatics profile, in which he scored in the first percentile (▶ Table 31.3).

Table 31.3 Clinical Evaluation of Language Fundamentals, Second Edition

Subtest	Scaled score	Percentile rank
Sentence comprehension	15	95th
Linguistic concepts	8	25th
Word structure	9	37th
Word classes	10	50th
Following directions	11	63rd
Formulated sentences	10	50th
Recalling sentences	7	16th
Understanding spoken paragraphs	7	16th
Pragmatics profile	3	1st

CJ is currently 5.7 years. He recently completed a 12-week integrated day program for children with autism in the neuropsychiatric department of a local hospital. The program consisted of five children and three special education teachers. During the program, CJ received intensive speech therapy and occupational therapy, and was followed by a psychologist and neurologist. He showed great gains in his expressive language and cognitive skills. The program's occupational therapist recommended that he continue occupational therapy to improve sensory processing, although he showed considerable improvement in this area. Professionals in the program recommended he continue attending social skills therapy to improve pragmatic language. CJ is currently participating in two social skills groups per week in a private clinic. These group sessions target conversational skills such as topic maintenance, continuous interaction, and appropriate commenting. These sessions also target cognitive and play skills necessary for successful social interaction, including turn taking, problem solving, perspective taking, and emotional thinking.

31.7 Key Points

- SLP collaboration with parents and teachers is critical to the success of a child's speech and language treatment. Parents and teachers should be educated regarding a child's treatment goals and trained in the strategies they can use to target these goals in home, at school, and in other environments. This education and training is crucial to ensuring a child's generalization of skills across settings.
- Children on the autism spectrum may test in the average range for receptive and expressive language, but show significant deficits in their use of social language. Assessments of pragmatic language and play skills are critical to obtain baseline measurements and show progress in treatment.
- Social skills groups are key in treating pragmatic language disorders.

Suggested Readings

[1] Greenspan S, Wieder S. The Child with Special Needs: Encouraging Intellectual and Emotional Growth. Reading, MA: Perseus Books; 1998

[2] Greenspan S, Wieder S. Engaging Autism: Using the Floortime Approach to Help Children Relate, Communicate, and Think. Philadelphia, PA: Da Capo Press; 2009

32 Cognitive-Linguistic Deficits in Pediatric Acquired Brain Injury

Shayne Kimble

32.1 Introduction

This case study outlines the evaluation and treatment of a pediatric client with a cognitive-linguistic disorder secondary to acquired brain injury. Acquired brain injuries in pediatrics can be caused from a variety of situations, including motor vehicle accidents or nonaccidental traumas (i.e., abuse). They can vary from patient to patient, where different clinical symptoms are shown based on neuropathophysiology.

32.2 Clinical History and Description

AB was a 9-year-old, right-handed male admitted to inpatient rehabilitation following an unrestrained motor vehicle accident. At the time of the accident, AB had no significant past medical history. He was in the third grade, where he made "good" grades with no previous history of therapy services or intervention. He lived at home with both parents and one sister.

Upon arrival to the acute care facility, a magnetic resonance imaging of the brain revealed an extensive shear injury and multiple contusions. After AB was medically stable, he was transferred to an inpatient rehabilitation facility for evaluation. He presented in a minimally conscious state with a G-tube in place for all hydration and nutrition. The term "minimally conscious" is applicable when "vegetative/unresponsive patients show minimal signs of consciousness, but are unable to reliably communicate."[1] The term is further subcategorized into two groups, MCS(+) and MCS(−). The difference between the two states is contingent on the level of behavioral responses produced by the patient, higher (i.e., following commands) versus lower level behaviors (i.e., localizes to noxious stimulation).

32.3 Clinical Testing

AB was evaluated at bedside with both parents present to serve as informants. He was evaluated to determine current functional status with regard to cognitive-linguistic and swallowing skills. Although the purpose of this chapter is focused on cognitive-linguistic skills, a clinical bedside swallow examination was completed during initial evaluation where the patient continued to be NPO (nil per os) secondary to, but not limited to, no volitional cough/volitional purposeful oral-motor movements. An interdisciplinary evaluation was completed by physical therapy, occupational therapy, and speech-language pathology, and each discipline administered portions of the JFK-Coma Recovery Scale (CRS).[2] The purpose of this numeric scale is to assist with differential diagnosis, prognostic assessment, and treatment planning in patients with disorders of consciousness. The scale has six assessment domains, including consistent movement to command, object recognition, object manipulation, oral reflexive movement, and eye opening with stimula-

tion. AB presented with eyes opening without stimulation (CRS Arousal Scale: 2), no auditory startle or localization (CRS Auditory Function Scale: 0), a visual startle (CRS Visual Function Scale: 1), flaccid with no other motor responses (Motor Scale: 0), oral reflexive movements (CRS Oro-Motor/Verbal Function Scale: 1), and no nonfunctional (intentional) communication (CRS Communication Scale: 0). AB's mother reported some minimal vocalizations, but none were observed during the evaluation. AB presented with a left visual fixation, which was consistent throughout the evaluation.

32.4 Questions and Answers for the Reader

1. Based on the diagnosis of the patient, which assessment would be best to be included in your evaluation?
   a) Test of Language Development Primary (TOLD-P).
   b) Comprehension of Spoken Language (CASL).
   c) Goldman–Fristoe Test of Articulation (GFTA).
   d) Pediatric Test of Brain Injury (PTBI).[3]

Answer: d is correct. The PTBI may be better suited secondary to the content corresponding with deficits generalized from brain injuries. Skills such as memory, orientation, and organizational language skills are typically affected by acquired brain injuries; therefore, these should be assessed during an initiation evaluation in the inpatient rehabilitation setting. Of course, a standardized assessment should only be one key portion of your complete evaluation, but can be a valuable tool.

a, b, and c are incorrect. Although some information may be beneficial for the academic and back-to-school setting, some subtests of developmental language/articulation assessments may assess skills that are not typically affected by an acquired brain injury (i.e., morphology/phonology).

2. What member would drive the care of this patient on the inpatient rehabilitation acquired brain injury team for a patient similar to this?
   a) Orthopedic surgeon.
   b) Neurologist.
   c) Physical medicine and rehabilitation physician (PM&R).

Answer: c is correct. Although team members may vary from facility to facility along with their roles, the most common individuals are PM&R, pediatrician, clinical psychologist, physical therapist, occupational therapist, speech-language pathologist, social worker, care coordinator, nurse, child life specialist, recreational therapist, nutritionist, school specialist, and orthotics doctor.

a is incorrect. The orthopedic surgeon, at times, is an important consult on the brain injury team as the patient may have sustained a variety of trauma to the musculoskeletal system.

This team member may make some decisions within the care of their field, but may not drive the care for the patient holistically.

b is incorrect. Again, like the orthopedic surgeon, the neurologist is a key consult when making decisions regarding the neurological system, but may not drive the care in the specific setting.

3. Which of the following is not a disorder of consciousness?
   a) Coma.
   b) Minimally conscious state.
   c) Vegetative state.
   d) Mild traumatic brain injury.

Answer: d is correct. Mild traumatic brain injury is typically the term given for a concussion. Although it is believed that individuals with mild traumatic brain injuries, or concussions, may go through disorders of consciousness quickly and progressively, it itself is not a disorder of consciousness.

a is incorrect. A person who presents at this level of disorder of consciousness usually presents with no behavioral evidence or arousal and demonstrates no voluntary response to stimuli. This individual may present with no arousal/eye-opening, impaired spontaneous breathing, and impaired brainstem reflexes.[1]

b is incorrect. A person who presents at this level of consciousness is a severely altered consciousness with behavioral evidence present for self- or environmental awareness. This individual may present with spontaneous eye opening, some reproducible behavioral signs of awareness, response to verbal directions, and object localization and manipulation.[4]

c is incorrect. A person who presents at this level of consciousness is similar to the coma state, but with preserved capacity for spontaneous or stimulus-induced arousal. This individual may present with arousal/eye-opening and no purposeful behaviors, and may grimace to pain/localize to sounds inconsistently.[4]

4. Which of the following is not a type of attention?
   a) Metacognition.
   b) Focused.
   c) Alternating.
   d) Sustained.
   e) Selective.
   f) Divided.

Answer: a is correct. Metacognition is not a type of attention but is a cognitive domain that is typically assessed by speech-language pathologists to gain further insight into self-awareness.

b is incorrect. Focused attention is the ability to perceive and respond to internal and external stimuli.[4]

c is incorrect. Alternating attention is the shift of focus between tasks.[4]

d is incorrect. Sustained attention is the ability to maintain attention to complete tasks.[4]

e is incorrect. Selective attention is the ability to maintain attention in the presence of competing distractions.[4]

f is incorrect. Divided attention is the ability to respond simultaneously to multiple task demands.[4]

32.5 Description of Disorder and Recommended Treatment

AB presented initially as minimally conscious (−) with a cognitive-linguistic disorder and oropharyngeal dysphagia. The patient presented with no functional communication skills upon evaluation and received continuous feeds via G-tube. Patient was showing some emerging skills such as a visual startle and eye opening without stimulation. When treating acute, acquired brain injuries, it is important for the clinician to adapt and engage in critical thinking, given that the child's status may change rapidly. Regular reassessment is required for driving modification of treatment goals, as a patient one day may be unable to answer basic yes/no questions, but the next day being able to answer complex "WH" questions. As AB progressed in therapy, the team's goals and intervention were frequently altered. AB was seen initially three times daily for 30 minutes for 10 weeks.

Week 1–4: During initial therapy sessions, basic cause/effect relationships were trialed. AB utilized a one-cell device with a picture of his sister, which would play a message read by his sister when selected. This meaningful reward was used to target intentional active movements of his upper extremities. Physical prompts were given initially as other rewards were integrated into the cause/effect select such as bubbles, familiar music, pleasant smells, and deep pressure. During this time, dysphagia was targeted in regard to rebuilding motor plan for oro-motor skills such as labial seal around a dry spoon/jaw grading when presented with a dry spoon. Patient continued intensive dysphagia therapy to further target coordination of the swallow.

Week 5–6: As AB progressed, higher level goals were incorporated. Basic two-step sequential motor directions were targeted to improve receptive language skills, reduce impulsivity, and increase attention. As these increased, commands then incorporated verbal output (expressive language) and more difficult directions. Following directions targeted multiple language skills and higher executive functioning skills. As the ability to follow directions increased, it is important to note at this time that AB received a Modified Barium Swallow Study where the patient was cleared for a regular diet and thin liquids.

Week 7–10: As AB's language skills improved, his goals were expanded to target following commands, organizational language, memory, and other executive functioning skills. Functional therapy tasks included following written recipes during baking activities, following visual directions during Lego building activities, creating age-appropriate narratives, and concrete/abstract divergent naming. Functional and engaging activities are necessary to aid attention and to promote carryover of skills.

32.6 Outcome

The CRS was administered weekly by each discipline (▶ Table 32.1). As AB progressed and demonstrated emerging cognitive-linguistic skills, the team administered the PTBI to further assess more specific cognitive-linguistics deficits. His scores over time are shown in ▶ Table 32.2.

Table 32.1 JFK Coma Recovery Scale-revised scores

Date	Total scores
Week 1	4
Week 2	5
Week 3	8
Week 4	12
Week 5	17
Week 6	22
Week 7	23

At week 10, the rehabilitation team determined that AB was ready to return to home, school, and outpatient therapy. He was reassessed with the PTBI; his numeric score increased concurrently with his classification on all subtests administered (▶ Table 32.2). Overall, AB made significant improvement in all therapies. He was discharged walking with contact guard, completing all activities of daily living with minimal assistance, eating regular diet with thin liquids, and independently communicating basic wants and needs.

Table 32.2 Pediatric test of brain injury

Date	Orientation	Following directions	Naming	Word fluency	What goes together	Digit span	Story re-tell immediate	Yes/no/maybe	Picture recall	Story retell delayed
Week 7	Low	Very low	Very low	Very low	Very low	Very low	Very low	Very low	Very low	Very low
Week 10	Moderate	Moderate	Moderate	Low	Low	Low	Low	Low	Low	low

32.7 Key Points

- A team approach is necessary for the treatment of acquired brain injuries. Teams must be in constant discussion with each other for treatment planning.
- Patients with acquired brain injuries typically made high-velocity changes, so the clinician must be flexible to change and always critically thinking during care.

Suggested Readings

[1] ASHA. Pediatric traumatic brain injury. Available at: http://www.asha.org/PRPSpecificTopic.aspx?folderid=8589942939&section=Resources

References

[1] Reyst H, Brain Injury Association of America. The Essential Brain Injury Guide 5.0. Vienna, VA: Brain Injury Association of America; 2016

[2] Bruno MA, Vanhaudenhuyse A, Thibaut A, Moonen G, Laureys S. From unresponsive wakefulness to minimally conscious PLUS and functional locked-in syndromes: recent advances in our understanding of disorders of consciousness. J Neurol. 2011; 258(7):1373–1384

[3] Giacino JT, Kalmar K, Whyte J. The JFK Coma Recovery Scale-Revised: measurement characteristics and diagnostic utility. Arch Phys Med Rehabil. 2004; 85(12):2020–2029

[4] Hotz G, Helm-Estabrooks N, Nelson NW, Plant E. Pediatric Test of Brain Injury. Baltimore, MD: Paul H. Brookes; 2010

33 A Holistic Approach to Treating a Preschool-Aged Child Who Stutters

Brooke Leiman

33.1 Introduction

Early detection and intervention is critical when treating a child who stutters. By intervening close to the onset of stuttering, we can increase the likelihood that the child outgrows stuttering and reduce the frequency, severity, and impact of stuttering for those who stutter into adulthood.

33.2 Clinical History and Description

KE was a 4-year, 6-month-old boy seen for evaluation of stuttering. He was born full-term and with no reported complications during pregnancy or birth. KE was delayed in achieving linguistic milestones and was diagnosed with mixed receptive/expressive language disorder at 3 years old. He received speech/language therapy for approximately 1 year, targeting receptive and expressive language skills. KE did not have difficulty feeding or swallowing, and his hearing was within normal limits in both ears. At the time of referral, he was enrolled in a half-day special education preschool that focused on supporting language development. KE was a monolingual English speaker.

Parent interview revealed that KE's mother began noticing disfluencies in her son's speech 6 months prior to the assessment. His disfluencies began suddenly, but varied from day to day. According to his mother, KE's disfluencies presented as part word repetitions (e.g., be-be-because) and blocks (i.e., no sound). She reported that he frequently covered his mouth when he was disfluent and avoided eye contact. KE did not give up on words when he started to stutter and did not avoid any specific speaking situations. When KE stuttered, his parents and older sister typically responded by telling him to "slow down" or "think about what you want to say." KE's sister demonstrated developmental disfluencies when she was 3 years old, but these issues resolved approximately 3 months later. Formal fluency evaluation was indicated due to the following concerns/risk factors:

- Male.
- 6 months post-onset of stuttering.
- Coexisting speech/language disorder.
- Negative reactions to stuttering (e.g., covering mouth, losing eye contact).
- Parental concern.

33.3 Clinical Testing

KE appeared at ease as he accompanied the speech/language pathologist and his mother to the testing room. He engaged in pretend play with a farm and picnic set. During play, he relied heavily on one- to three-word utterances and often waited for the adult to begin speaking prior to participating in conversation. KE demonstrated appropriate eye contact with both the clinician and his mother. He was able to answer a variety of "WH" questions (e.g., what toy are you playing with?), but had difficulty responding to questions about past events (e.g., what did you eat for breakfast?).

Comprehensive speech/language assessment was completed approximately 3 months ago, suggesting that KE required support in the following areas:

- Expanding length and complexity of utterances.
- Improving age-appropriate grammatical structures.
- Following directions including spatial and quantitative concepts.
- Answering open-ended questions.

The Stuttering Severity Instrument, Fourth Edition (SSI-4),[1] was used to rate the severity of KE's observable stuttering and was based on two speaking samples. KE received a score for frequency (i.e., percent syllables stuttered), duration (i.e., average length of three longest stuttering events), and physical concomitants. Physical concomitant behaviors refer to maladaptive reactions to stuttering, which include distracting sounds, facial grimaces, head movements, and movements of the extremities. KE received an overall score of 19, suggestive of a moderate fluency disorder. Although the SSI-4 indicated moderate stuttering, it is important to consider the variable nature of stuttering. KE's frequency and severity of stuttering reportedly fluctuated over time and across situations.

The first SSI-4 speaking sample was collected while KE was engaged in a picture description task with his mother. The sample contained 274 syllables. Stuttering-like disfluencies included monosyllabic whole word repetitions (e.g., can-can-can), part word repetitions (e.g., h-h-hey), prolongations (e.g., mmme), and a mixed-type disfluency, which contained a block (i.e., no sound) followed by a part word repetition. Stuttering-like disfluencies were present in 4.01% of total syllables in the speaking sample. Nonstuttered (typical) disfluencies are disfluencies that occur when attempting to formulate a thought or find a word. KE demonstrated nonstuttered disfluencies in the form of phrase repetitions (e.g., I want-I want the cookie) and multisyllabic whole word repetitions (e.g., because-because). Nonstuttered disfluencies were present in less than 1% of the total syllables produced in the sample and were not included in the SSI-4 frequency count. Overall, stuttering-like disfluencies made up 85% of all disfluencies (▶ Table 33.1).

Table 33.1 First speaking sample: 274 syllables (picture description)

Stuttering-like disfluencies			Nonstuttered disfluencies		
Type	Total No.	No. per 100 syllables	Type	Total No.	No. per 100 syllables
Whole word repetition (monosyllabic)	4	1.46	Phrase repetition	1	0.36
Part word repetition	1	0.36	Whole word repetition (multisyllabic)	1	0.36
Prolongation	5	1.82			
Mixed type	1	0.36			
	11	4.01		2	0.73

Table 33.2 Second speaking sample: 73 syllables (dialogue)

Stuttering-like disfluencies		
Type	Total No.	No. per 100 syllables
Whole word repetition (monosyllabic)	1	1.37
Mixed type	1	1.37
	2	2.74

Table 33.3 Stuttering Severity Instrument-4 (SSI-4)[1]

Subtest	Task performance	Task score
Frequency	First speaking sample: 4.01 Second speaking sample: 2.74	8
Average duration of three lengthiest stuttering events	~2 seconds	8
Physical concomitants	1. Distracting sounds (e.g., increased pitch): barely noticeable to casual observer 2. Facial grimacing (e.g., nostril flaring): not noticeable unless looking for it	3

Total score: 19
Percentile rank: 41–60
Severity rating: moderate

The second SSI-4 speaking sample was collected while KE and his mother played with a picnic set. The sample contained 73 syllables. The developers of the SSI-4 encourage samples to be at least 150 syllables. However, after engaging KE in several different play activities, this 73-syllable sample was the largest sample collected. Stuttering-like disfluencies included monosyllabic whole word repetitions and were present in 2.74% of total syllables in the speech sample. No nonstuttered disfluencies were observed in this sample (▶ Table 33.2).

The average of KE's three lengthiest stuttering moments was approximately 2 seconds in duration. During the assessment, KE's stuttering was sometimes accompanied by increased pitch. This behavior was rated as "barely noticeable to casual observer" on the SSI-4 rating scale. KE also demonstrated flaring of the nostrils, which was rated as "not noticeable unless looking for it." KE's mother noted that, at onset, KE covered his mouth and averted eye contact when he stuttered. These behaviors were not observed during the assessment and were not included in the SSI-4 scoring (▶ Table 33.3).

In addition to using the two speaking samples to arrive at an SSI-4 score, the data were also used to calculate a weighted measure of disfluencies. Ambrose and Yairi[2] developed a weighted measure to differentiate between young children who demonstrate developmental disfluencies and those with a diagnosis of childhood-onset fluency disorder. The equation is ([part word repetitions + single syllable repetitions] × mean number of repetition units) + (2 × dysrhythmic phonation). A weighted score 4 or higher indicates the presence of a disorder. More specifically, scores between 4.00 and 9.99 indicate mild stuttering, scores between 10.00 and 29.99 indicate moderate stuttering, and scores above 30.00 indicate severe stuttering. When the two speaking samples were combined, KE received a weighted measure of 7.07 ([(0.29 + 1.44) × 1.75] + (2 × 2.02) = 7.07), corresponding with mild stuttering.

Although the scores and severity ratings obtained via the SSI-4 and the weighted measure are informative, the two speaking samples are merely a snapshot of the disorder on one day and in one environment. The parent and child interview helped provide the clinician with a full profile of KE, including what stuttering looks/sounds like in other environments, the cognitive/emotional components of KE's stuttering, his ability to effectively communicate on a daily basis, and the impact stuttering has on his quality of life. Information obtained in the parent interview can be found in the Clinical History and Description section.

In addition to the parent interview, KE was asked a series of questions about talking (e.g., "Tell me about your talking," "When does talking feel hardest"). Due to KE's coexisting mixed receptive/expressive language disorder, comprehending and formulating answers to these types of question was difficult for him. The clinician simplified questions and provided multiple choice answers to choose from; however, KE often did not respond or would provide off-topic responses. As a result, the clinician relied heavily on parent report and observations.

A questionnaire was also provided to KE's teacher; however, it was not returned.

33.4 Questions and Answers for the Reader

1. Which of the following factors is *not* considered a risk factor for persistent stuttering?
   a) Severity of stuttering.
   b) Gender.
   c) Time since onset.
   d) Family history.

Answer: a is correct. Although initial severity of stuttering may result in the decision to quickly intervene, it does *not* predict chronicity.[3]

b is incorrect. Males are more likely to continue to stutter into adulthood and, therefore, gender is considered a risk factor. Females not only outgrow stuttering more than males but also outgrow it earlier.[3] By the time children are school-aged, three to four times more males stutter than females.[4]

c is incorrect. Children who stutter for more than 6 to 12 months are more likely to continue to stutter into adulthood and, therefore, time since onset is considered a risk factor.[5] Children who are stuttering for over 6 months should be evaluated by a speech/language pathologist to ensure they receive intervention as close to the onset of stuttering as possible.

d is incorrect. Children who have a family history of stuttering, especially a family history of persistent stuttering, are at an increased risk for stuttering into adulthood.[6] Therefore, family history is considered a risk factor. If a child is stuttering and has a family history, they should be evaluated by a speech/language pathologist to determine whether intervention is necessary.

2. Which of the following should be considered when making a differential diagnosis during a stuttering evaluation?
   a) Formal analysis of speaking samples.
   b) Child interview.
   c) Parent or teacher report/questionnaire.
   d) All of the above.

Answer: a is incorrect. Although a clinician must formally analyze speaking samples to qualify a child for services in most settings, a clinician cannot make a diagnosis or develop a treatment plan based solely on these samples. Due to the variability of stuttering, it is possible for children to stutter less frequently or severely in their samples than they typically stutter. In addition, speaking samples often do not provide information about how children are responding to stuttering or how stuttering is impacting them.

b is incorrect. Although the interview is a helpful way of gathering information about stuttering and often provides insight into the emotional and cognitive components of the disorder, formal analysis of speaking samples is often required to qualify a child for services. In addition, young children often may not have the self-awareness or the willingness to share their feelings about stuttering, especially with an unfamiliar person. Interviewing parents and teachers can supplement the information that the child is unable or is not ready to provide.

c is incorrect. Parent and teacher interviews/questionnaires are a beneficial way of gathering information about stuttering. However, the child's perspective and formal analysis of speaking samples are also necessary to qualify a child for services and ensure the clinician is considering the whole picture.

d is correct. A comprehensive stuttering assessment must include (but is not limited to) (1) formal analysis of speaking samples, (2) child interview/questionnaires, (3) parent interview/questionnaires, and (4) teacher interview/questionnaires. Formal speech/language assessment is also recommended to make a differential diagnosis and to determine whether there is a coexisting communication disorder.

3. True or false: KE's disfluencies are characterized as language formulation disfluencies because of his diagnosis of mixed receptive/expressive language disorder.
   a) True.
   b) False.

Answer: a is incorrect. KE was diagnosed with childhood-onset fluency disorder because of the types of disfluencies, the frequency of disfluencies, the physical tension/struggle behaviors, and KE's negative reactions to stuttering. Despite his coexisting diagnosis of mixed receptive/expressive language disorder, KE did not demonstrate the profile of a child with solely language formulation disfluencies.

b is correct. Although KE demonstrated some language formulation disfluencies, the majority of his disfluencies were considered stuttering-like (e.g., monosyllabic whole word repetitions, part word repetitions, prolongations, and blocks). In addition, the presence of physical concomitant behaviors such as pitch increase, loss of eye contact, nostril flaring, and covering of his mouth all assisted in making the differential diagnosis.

4. Treatment for preschool-aged children who stutter:
   a) Should always follow an operant approach (e.g., Lidcombe Program).
   b) Should always follow an indirect approach (e.g., Demands and Capacities, Palin PCI, etc.).
   c) Should be individualized based on the child's and family's needs.
   d) Should never acknowledge stuttering moments.

Answer: a is incorrect. Although an operant approach to preschool stuttering therapy is one approach that has been supported by research, evidence is based on group averages and does not reflect what is appropriate for all children.[7] Treatment should be individualized to meet the child's and family's needs and therefore there is no specific approach that should *always* be used with every child who stutters.

b is incorrect. An indirect approach to preschool stuttering therapy is another approach that has been supported by research.[7–9] However, the clinician must consider the child's and family's specific needs when determining the best approach.

c is correct. Stuttering is a multidimensional disorder and each child who stutters has a unique set of factors that contribute to the onset of stuttering as well as how it impacts them. As a result, the development of a treatment plan should be individualized to meet the needs of both the child and family.

d is incorrect. Stuttering is a disorder with a neurological basis.[10,11] Although stuttering can certainly have an emotional impact on a child, the initial onset of childhood-onset fluency disorder is not psychologically based. Bringing awareness to a disfluent moment would not cause a child to become a child who stutters. In fact, acknowledging stuttering moments in a neutral and accepting way can be beneficial and support the child in building a healthy attitude toward communication.

33.5 Description of Disorder and Recommended Treatment

The focus of the assessment was to determine whether KE had a fluency disorder and whether therapy was warranted. The results of informal and formal testing indicated KE had a mild-to-moderate childhood-onset fluency disorder (stuttering) characterized by monosyllabic whole word repetitions, part word repetitions, prolongations, and blocks. KE also demonstrated a slight increase in pitch and nostril flaring. He did not appear overtly aware of his disfluencies and did not show signs of frustration during the assessment. Although not observed during the assessment, his mother reported that he sometimes covered his mouth and averted eye contact when he stuttered. The type, frequency, and duration of disfluencies as well as the physical concomitant behaviors helped differentiate between typical language formulation disfluencies and KE's diagnosis of childhood-onset fluency disorder.[2,12]

Based on this evaluation, KE was determined to be an ideal candidate for therapy. It was recommended that he receive services one time weekly, to address stuttering, in addition to his current speech/language therapy to address his receptive/expressive language development. KE's prognosis in therapy was good due to his family's willingness to be active participants in the therapy process and client compliance. At the time of the assessment, it was suggested that an indirect approach be used to address stuttering. This type of approach is supported by research to be an effective way to eliminate or greatly reduce the frequency and severity of stuttering in preschool-aged children.[7-9] An indirect approach focuses on making changes to the child's environment to enhance fluency and build healthy communication attitudes. Ongoing evaluation would determine whether/when a more direct approach should be added to KE's treatment plan.

33.6 Outcome

KE's mother and father were both encouraged to attend therapy sessions, so the clinician could provide feedback specific to their unique interaction styles. Due to the father's work schedule, only the mother was able to arrange to be present for sessions. The clinician suggested that the father participate by sending weekly videos of his home "therapy time" with KE. Therapy began by providing information about stuttering to the parents, including information on the neurological components of the disorder, the different types of stuttering, the different ways KE

was reacting to this stuttering, and how the environment may contribute to the disorder.

The clinician introduced KE's mother to the concept of "special time," 5-minute play sessions completed three times a week per parent that would act as their therapy time. Once KE's special time routine was established, KE's mother was introduced to the following interaction strategies: (1) reducing questions, (2) speaking at KE's speech/language level, (3) following KE's lead during play, and (4) slowing the pace of communication by adding pauses.[9] During sessions, the clinician modeled the special time targets and provided an opportunity for KE's mother to practice and receive feedback.

In addition to introducing interaction targets, a portion of each session was dedicated to teaching strategies aimed at promoting healthy communication attitudes. The clinician approached topics such as (1) how to respond to stuttering moments, and (2) reducing interruptions among family members. Following the completion of the parent training program, KE no longer covered his mouth when he stuttered. When KE's mother spoke openly about stuttering with him, he responded by smiling. He occasionally praised himself for sticking with a disfluent word. However, KE's observable stuttering continued and his mother began noticing tension around his eyes. In addition, on several occasions, KE stated "I can't say that word" or skipped a word altogether when he was struggling. Due to these negative reactions (e.g., word avoidances, voicing frustration), a more direct therapeutic component was introduced in therapy. Direct therapy involved (1) providing kid-friendly terms to talk about stuttering, (2) "playing around" with different types of stuttering on purpose, (3) monitoring/catching stuttering moments, (4) contrast drills aimed at "playing around" with tension, and (5) practicing how to release tension by stretching or bouncing out of stuttering moments.

Reassessment was completed approximately 1 year after the initial assessment. Informal and formal testing indicated mild-to-moderate childhood-onset fluency disorder characterized by monosyllabic whole word repetitions. Part word repetitions and prolongations were also present but at a low frequency. KE demonstrated a slight increase in pitch during stuttering moments, but no other forms of physical tension or frustration were observed. His parents shared that the speaking samples collected during the assessment were representative of what they are seeing at home and reports from school. When compared to the previous assessment, KE continued to demonstrate a mild-to-moderate fluency disorder. However, his physical concomitant behaviors decreased. KE demonstrated increased ability and willingness to talk about stuttering, but required more practice to increase his comfort speaking about stuttering with those not in his family. KE's mother reported feeling better equipped to respond to her son's stuttering moments and reported less concern about KE's future if he continues to stutter. Since KE and his peers were getting older, his mother reported that she wondered how other children would respond to her son when he stuttered. Future sessions will focus on building KE's comfort responding to peers questions/teasing related to stuttering.

33.7 Key Points

- Childhood-onset stuttering has a neurological basis and, as a result, must be approached differently than communications disorders such as an articulation disorder. The child has not developed or learned a "bad habit," rather there are subtle differences in the structure and functioning of the speech/language areas of the child's brain.[10,11]
- Although many children go through temporary periods of disfluency during speech and language development, there is a distinct difference between developmental disfluencies and the disfluencies of a child who stutters. Identifying these differences is critical in determining whether a child might benefit from early intervention.
- Even in young children, stuttering is a multidimensional disorder and the clinician must take a holistic approach, including consideration of the child's observable stuttering, their reactions to stuttering, the reactions of others in their environment, and the impact stuttering is having on their willingness and ability to participate in daily roles and situations.[13]
- Evaluation of a child who stutters should be ongoing. Treatment goals and approaches must be adjusted as stuttering and/or the child's reactions (or the reactions of others) to stuttering change.

Suggested Readings

[1] Rustin L, Cook F. Parental involvement in the treatment of stuttering. Lang Speech Hear Serv Sch. 1995; 26(2):127–137

[2] Yaruss JS, Reardon-Reeves NA. Early Childhood Stuttering Therapy: A Practical Guide. McKinney, TX: Stuttering Therapy Resources; 2017

References

[1] Riley GD, Bakker K. Stuttering Severity Instrument: SSI-4. Austin, TX: Pro-Ed; 2009

[2] Ambrose NG, Yairi E. Normative disfluency data for early childhood stuttering. J Speech Lang Hear Res. 1999; 42(4):895–909

[3] Yairi E, Ambrose NG. Early childhood stuttering I: persistency and recovery rates. J Speech Lang Hear Res. 1999; 42(5):1097–1112

[4] Craig A, Hancock K, Tran Y, Craig M, Peters K. Epidemiology of stuttering in the community across the entire life span. J Speech Lang Hear Res. 2002; 45 (6):1097–1105

[5] Yairi E, Ambrose NG, Paden EP, Throneburg RN. Predictive factors of persistence and recovery: pathways of childhood stuttering. J Commun Disord. 1996; 29(1):51–77

[6] Ambrose NG, Cox NJ, Yairi E. The genetic basis of persistence and recovery in stuttering. J Speech Lang Hear Res. 1997; 40(3):567–580

[7] de Sonneville-Koedoot C, Stolk E, Rietveld T, Franken MC. Direct versus indirect treatment for preschool children who stutter: The RESTART randomized trial. PLoS One. 2015; 10(7):e0133758

[8] Kelman E. Practical Intervention for Early Childhood Stammering: Palin PCI Approach. London: Routledge; 2017

[9] Yaruss JS, Coleman C, Hammer D. Treating preschool children who stutter: description and preliminary evaluation of a family-focused treatment approach. Lang Speech Hear Serv Sch. 2006; 37(2):118–136

[10] Chang SE, Zhu DC. Neural network connectivity differences in children who stutter. Brain. 2013; 136(Pt 12):3709–3726

[11] Beal DS. The advancement of neuroimaging research investigating developmental stuttering. Perspect Fluen Fluen Disord. 2011; 21(3):88–95

[12] Tumanova V, Conture EG, Lambert EW, Walden TA. Speech disfluencies of preschool-age children who do and do not stutter. J Commun Disord. 2014; 49:25–41

[13] Yaruss JS, Quesal RW. Stuttering and the International Classification of Functioning, Disability, and Health: an update. J Commun Disord. 2004; 37(1):35–52

34 Language and Cognitive Deficits Associated with Landau–Kleffner Syndrome

Barbara Culatta and Carol Westby

34.1 Introduction

Landau–Kleffner syndrome (LKS)[1] is a childhood neurological disorder characterized by nighttime seizures and sudden or gradual development of aphasia. This chapter reports the case of a child diagnosed at age 4 years with LKS.[1] The case raises clinicians' awareness about the negative impact that seizures can have on language functioning and highlights that initial observations of language disturbances are often not immediately diagnosed correctly. This diagnosis is further complicated by the fact that seizures can occur when children are asleep.

34.2 Clinical History and Description

DG was a 7-year-old boy when he was referred for a language evaluation to a university speech and language clinic. His mother reported that shortly before his fourth birthday he was not responding well to comments and commands. She initially felt that he was being oppositional. His language abilities began to decay further, and at age 4 years, DG lost the ability to communicate orally and was not following commands or making appropriate verbal responses to people's comments. An initial evaluation ruled out autism spectrum disorder; he was eventually diagnosed with LKS. An aggressive regime of steroids and subsequent anticonvulsant medications eventually controlled his seizures.

34.3 Clinical Testing

DG underwent a comprehensive language evaluation at the age of 7 years. Using the International Classification of Functioning, Disability and Health (ICF) framework,[2] the evaluators assessed DG's language capacity and performance. *Capacity* refers to the ability to execute a skill or task in a standardized environment; *performance* refers to the use of those skills in naturalistic contexts.

34.3.1 Assessing Capacity

DG scored significantly below average on the overall and subtest standard scores (SS) on the Comprehensive Assessment of Spoken Language (CASL[3]; SS = 55 composite; SS = 60 basic concepts; SS = 53 syntax; SS = 65 paragraph comprehension; and SS = 56 pragmatics).

Vocabulary: DG understood many concrete and common words. He exhibited difficulty understanding spatial, temporal, and quantity terms (e.g., first/last; alike/same; couple/less/none; under/below/round/outside) and less common words such as "stretch" and "measure". DG exhibited difficulty with semantic associations, synonyms, and generic category words (e.g., he did not know the word "pet"). DG was not able to define words.

Grammar/morphology: DG communicated primarily in simple sentences. He made relevant comments and asked appropriate questions about events he experienced. He produced grammatical errors in signaling tenses ("my mom has a cockatiel" when she had one when she was young), subject/verb agreement ("it can moves and turn"), copula verbs ("what's he's eating?"), and irregular past tense verbs ("he growed up."). Omissions of conjunctions interfered with DG's ability to convey connected ideas.

Narrative skills: On the Paris and Paris narrative task, DG responded to a few questions about the pictured story that required comprehension of particular story grammar elements (i.e., initiating event, problem, solution, character reactions), but his score of 6 fell approximately two SDs below the mean for first grade. On the Narrative Language Measures assessment that required DG to retell a narrative, he commented on a few pictures presented in a sequence but did not express or convey relationships between the pictures. He also had difficulty answering questions about story grammar elements. Without picture support, DG could not relate any of the actions in the stories, and he exhibited difficulty responding to questions about simple stories presented orally, particularly when explicit picture support did not accompany the passage.

34.3.2 Assessing Performance

DG responded to simple questions, comments, and commands in reference to familiar and contextualized events. When language was decontextualized, abstract, or presented at a text level, DG failed to respond or produced irrelevant remarks. He had difficulty completing multistep directions and understanding explanations (e.g., he failed to respond to indirect requests embedded into simple explanations). DG exhibited difficulty making inferences from texts. When discussing texts in therapy sessions, even ones at a kindergarten or preschool level, DG answered a few explicit questions but no questions that required inferences. DG was not able to engage in conversations about texts in the classroom setting even though he was placed in a grade that was 1 year below his chronological age.

With respect to social and conversational interactions, DG had difficulty recalling words to express his thoughts and ideas and retelling life events and experiences in an organized and detailed fashion. When asked to retell experiences, or when spontaneously attempting to relate experiences, he included a few phrases or sentences about a salient action or two and needed question prompts. DG occasionally engaged in topically related turn-taking exchanges when a conversational topic was concrete, familiar, or related to the immediate context. When engaged in a conversation, DG answered some questions, but tended to make tangential and irrelevant remarks. He rarely elaborated on the partner's utterances. He also had difficulty relating compelling events that happened in the recent past, tending to produce fragmented comments. For example, when asked about a recent trip to California to see his neurologist, he produced the following:

Adult: Didn't you just get back from California?
DG: Yeah. Then got white cap and purple glue. Bad car!
Adult: Why?
DG: Because two doors in front and no doors in back. We had a bad car, a very bad car. Small car; but it doesn't fit. Hurts my leg.

34.4 Questions and Answers for the Reader

1. Which of the following features is particularly important in the diagnosis of LKS?
   a) Feeding problems and oral motor apraxia.
   b) Gradual sensorineural hearing loss.
   c) Gradual or sudden loss of language after normal language development.
   d) Delayed development of morphology and syntax.

Answer: c is correct. Gradual or sudden loss of language after normal language development is a hallmark feature of LKS.

a is incorrect. Children with LKS may have an oral motor apraxia, but so may many other children with speech impairments who do not have LKS.

b is incorrect. A child with LKS may appear to have hearing loss because they have poor language comprehension, but typically there is no impairment at the level of the ear or auditory nerve.

d is incorrect. Children with LKS are highly likely to exhibit deficits in morphology and syntax, but so do many other children with language impairments and, unlike other children with language impairments, children with LKS had typical morphological and syntactic skills before the onset of the condition.

2. Which of the following tasks/activities assesses capacity?
   a) Negotiating the rules of a game.
   b) Participating in a class discussion about a science experiment.
   c) Telling a friend about a movie you saw.
   d) Giving definitions of words.

Answer: d is correct. Giving a definition for a word is a skill; knowledge of the meaning of a word does not ensure that the word will be used functionally in naturalistic contexts.

a, b, and c are incorrect. They are examples of performance of language skills in naturalistic contexts.

3. How can a clinician best address World Health Organization's (WHO) ICF framework when setting goals and determining a focus for intervention?
   a) Consider the client's needs both in acquiring capacity (skills) and in functioning (performance in natural contexts).
   b) Draw upon a set of specified diagnostic categories.
   c) State how the individual performs on standardized tests and construct goals based on these test results.
   d) Fit goals with Common Core State Standards (CCSS).

Answer: a is correct. ICF is based on addressing both an individual's capacity and functioning.

b is incorrect. The ICF provides codes for functioning not for diagnosis of the cause of the disability.

c is incorrect. Standardized tests measure only capacity. Goals should be based on both a student's capacity *and* performance levels.

d is incorrect. Fitting goals with CCSS is compatible with the ICF because a number of the CCSS address academic capacity skills and performance in academic settings. However, academic capacity/performance is only one aspect of functioning. When using the ICF framework, the speech-language pathologist should address capacity and performance in a variety of life areas—not only academic areas.

4. Which of the following is an example of a higher-level (macrostructure) aspect of language?
   a) Answering factual questions about a specific event mentioned in a story.
   b) Graphically representing the organization of a text and retelling the text from the representation.
   c) Decoding targeted words in a text.
   d) Segmenting multisyllable words into their components.

Answer: b is correct. Text organization is the text macrostructure; retelling the text from the graphic representation indicates an understanding/awareness of the macrostructure.

a is incorrect. Answering a factual question does not require comprehension of the text as a whole. One need understand only a single sentence to answer many factual questions.

c and d are incorrect. Decoding and segmenting syllables are lower-level microstructure skills.

34.5 Description of Disorder and Recommended Treatment

DG had deficits at both microstructure (lower vocabulary and morphosyntactic skills) and macrostructure levels (higher organizational/inferential skills). He also had difficulties with both capacity (specific skills) and performance (using his skills and knowledge in naturalistic contexts). Therefore, the therapy focused on basic skills (microstructure and capacity levels) while always considering ways to develop higher skills (macrostructure and inferencing) and impact performance (functioning) in social and academic contexts.

Therapy goals were established with CCSS and academic and social functioning in mind. Themes in informational texts were linked to hands-on experiences and content in narrative texts, which, in turn, provided foundations for personal event narratives. To develop vocabulary, syntax, and discourse organization at the capacity level, language/literacy activities were embedded into experiences within interesting topics (e.g., making and flying kites while talking about wind pressure pushing against the kite and connecting to the text *Gilberto and the Wind*; bringing in bugs and snails and comparing and contrasting them: daddy long legs with spiders; slugs with snails). Expository and narrative text structures were mapped. Attention was given to recognizing how character thoughts and feelings could influence their plans and actions and to highlighting important information needed to make inferences. Character emotions and goals/plans in fictional narratives were linked to DG's personal life experiences. Language use at a performance level was facilitated by reminiscing about these experiences in therapy and then having DG relate these experiences to others.

34.6 Outcome

Outcomes after a 3-year period again considered DG's gains according to ICF's distinction between capacity and performance.

34.6.1 Capacity Outcomes

By age 11 years, DG made significant gains in lower-level, capacity-based language skills as illustrated by improved standard scores on formal testing (Comprehensive Assessment of Spoken Language [CASL], Woodcock–Johnson Test of Achievement,[4] and the Wechsler Intelligence Scale for Children [WISC] [5]).

Vocabulary: On vocabulary measures on the CASL and WISC, DG scored within the average and low average range. Despite these scores, he continued to exhibit considerable difficulty acquiring abstract and relational (spatial, temporal, quantity) terms and needed a great deal of specific, direct instruction to acquire new vocabulary. To acquire academic vocabulary, emotional and mental state words, multiple meaning words, and figurative language encountered in texts, DG required exposure to many examples with the meaning explicitly highlighted.

Syntax and morphology: DG scored in the average range on the Sentence Comprehension and Grammatical Morphemes subtests of the CASL. However, in social and academic contexts, such as retelling texts or generating stories, DG had difficulty producing complex syntactic constructions. Although he was able to use "because" to signal cause/effect relationships in sentence-combining tasks and when referring to personal experiences, he was not observed to use causal "because" or *so* when generating cause/effect or problem/solution texts from a graphic representation, and he did not spontaneously use "but" when comparing and contrasting objects and events.

Text comprehension: DG made gains in text comprehension. On the CASL, his oral comprehension scaled score was 91, indicating no impairment. On the WISC verbal comprehension subtest, his scaled score of 80 (18th percentile) was judged to be within the average range. However, DG also performed below average on the Nonliteral Language and Pragmatic Judgment subtests of the CASL that require inferring, a higher-level skill. In regard to informal assessments, DG could retell simple, well-organized stories by including story grammar elements in response to guiding questions. He was able to coconstruct stories and fill in story grammar elements on a graphic representation. However, he exhibited difficulty answering inferential questions about the relationship between characters' internal states and their plans and goals. Without support, he was unable to map or retell informational texts (i.e., problem/solution, cause/effect, compare/contrast, or sequence structures)

and scored below proficiency in comprehension of informational texts on the state-level criterion referenced test.

34.6.2 Performance Outcomes

DG made gains in higher-level and performance aspects of language, but these gains were smaller than those related to capacity-based skills. By age 11 years, DG continued to exhibit marked difficulties in higher-level areas of language.

DG's performance deficits were particularly marked in conversation and narrative situations. He had difficulty participating in collaborative discussions in the classroom (knowing what to say). He continued to have difficulty clearly conveying personal experiences. To comprehend DG's stories, listeners needed prior background knowledge about what happened. DG could retell personal experiences when his listener shared his knowledge and gave him scaffolding support for putting events in a temporal and causal sequence. His interactions with peers continued to be limited to making comments about shared, concrete events or initiating conversations about his own favorite topics. Although DG made progress in telling scaffolded personal stories (a capacity skill), he did not know when to tell his stories or how to respond to stories told by others, lacking the ability to perform storytelling in life situations. He could make more than one-sentence contributions in conversations with peers when an adult mediated the exchange by suggesting a particular personal story that could fit a theme.

Because of his overall scores on standardized tests, DG no longer qualified for special education services at school. Formal testing measured primarily DG's lower-level linguistic and cognitive capacity; it included few tasks that measured higher-level discourse capacity skills and did not reveal the severity of his difficulties in performing in naturalistic social and academic contexts. DG's poor working memory (1st percentile on standardized testing), deficits in abstract language/reasoning and discourse skills, slow processing speed, and attentional issues markedly contributed to his restricted functioning in real-life contexts. His mother was concerned about his poor social interactions and difficulty keeping friends.

34.7 Key Points

- LKS is a rare neurological condition that results in loss of language skills in children who had been developing normally. The first indication of the language problem is usually auditory verbal agnosia.
- It is important to identify ways to address capacity while also arranging for targeted skills to impact performance.
- Clinicians and teachers should work to support capacity level in contexts that also support or are likely to influence performance.
- Higher-level tasks require clinicians, teachers, and parents to support use of skills across contexts, content, and texts.
- The relationship between essential skills and the ultimate requirement to apply skills to functioning in authentic contexts must be maintained during therapy.

- Gains in capacity, as measured by standardized tests, may not predict performance in authentic contexts or the ability to use language in functional ways in natural contexts.

Suggested Readings

[1] Besag FM. Cognitive and behavioral outcomes of epileptic syndromes: implications for education and clinical practice. Epilepsia. 2006; 47 Suppl 2:119–125

[2] Dempsey L, Skarakis-Doyle E. Developmental language impairment through the lens of the ICF: an integrated account of children's functioning. J Commun Disord. 2010; 43(5):424–437

[3] Westby C, Culatta B. Telling tales: personal narratives and life stories. Lang Speech Hear Serv Sch. 2016; 47(4):260–282

References

[1] Landau WM, Kleffner FR. Syndrome of acquired aphasia with convulsive disorder in children. Neurology. 1957; 7(8):523–530

[2] World Health Organization (WHO Workgroup for development of version of ICF for Children & Youth). International Classification of Functioning Disability and Health - Children and Youth Version (ICF-CY). Geneva, Switzerland: World Health Organization; 2007

[3] Carrow-Woolfolk E. The Comprehensive Assessment of Spoken Language. San Antonio, TX: Pearson; 1999

[4] Woodcock RW, Shrank FA, McGrew KS, Mather N. Woodcock-Johnson IV Tests of Achievement. Rolling Meadows, IL: Riverside; 2014

[5] Wechsler D. Wechsler Intelligence Scale for Children. 5th ed. Bloomington, MN: Pearson; 2014

35 Feeding and Language Therapy in a Child with Congenital Cytomegalovirus and Traumatic Brain Injury

Debra L. Kerner

35.1 Introduction

This case illustrates the challenges across multiple areas of communication related to a complex medical history, including feeding difficulties and language deficits as well as cognitive and auditory challenges. An evidence-based rationale is provided for treatment approaches.[1-3,4,5-6]

35.2 Clinical History and Description

MD was an 8.6-year-old boy born at 35 weeks via emergency C-section due to nonresponse from ultrasound stimuli. At birth, he weighed 5.4 lb and was 18 in. long. Complications following birth included congenital cytomegalovirus, grade 2 intraventricular hemorrhage (IVH), hypotonia, liver failure, low platelets, high bilirubin, profound hearing loss, as well as patent ductus arteriosus (PDA). He also had a history of retinopathy, nystagmus, and retinitis, and wore corrective lenses. Before he was 12 months old, he had multiple surgeries, including 14 blood transfusions, PDA repair, gastrostomy button (G-button) insertion due to poor feeding, and bilateral cochlear implantation. His G-button was employed for medications and occasionally for hydration, as needed. MD consumed liquids, purees, and mechanical soft foods for caloric intake orally. He was nonverbal and used ProLoQuo2Go as his primary means of communication. He also occasionally used minimal sign language. MD attended a private school that focused on education for children with disabilities. He received private occupational therapy, physical therapy, and hippotherapy in addition to speech therapy as well as group speech therapy, music therapy, and occupational therapy at school.

35.3 Clinical Testing

An initial evaluation by this clinician, conducted at age 6.4 years, revealed his overall functioning was age equivalent to 12 to 18 months in all areas of communication. Using the San Diego Occupational Therapy Feeding Skills checklist and Morris and Klein feeding checklist, his feeding skills were age equiva-

lent to 6 to 8 months. His augmentative and alternative communication (AAC) device had yet to be introduced at his initial evaluation and he only communicated via sign language characterized by less than 30 signs recognized by familiar communicative partners only.

At the next evaluation, age 8.2 years, MD was not appropriate for standardized testing due to his cognitive level as well as his communication skills. The Peabody Picture Vocabulary Test, Fourth Edition, was attempted, but was discontinued. A Functional Communication Profile Revised (FCP-R) was administered (▶ Table 35.1). The Rossetti Infant-Toddler Language Scale was also completed to assess overall communication skills (▶ Table 35.2). Although this test was not appropriate for his chronological age, it did provide meaningful clinical information given his poor cognitive function across all communicative domains. His overall scores in all areas confirmed inconsistent skills. He scored at 15 to 18 months for interaction attachment, 15 to 18 months for pragmatics, 21 to 24 months for play, 24 to 27 months for gestures, 30 to 33 months for language comprehension, and 18 to 24 months for language expression.

Table 35.1 Functional communication profile

Domain assessed	Normal	Mild	Moderate	Severe	Profound
Sensory				x	
Motor			x		
Behavior			x		
Attentiveness			x		
Receptive language					x
Expressive language					x
Pragmatic/social					x
Speech					x
Voice	x				
Oral				x	
Fluency	x				

Table 35.2 Rossetti Infant-Toddler Language Scale

Age (mo)	Interaction attachment	Pragmatics	Gesture	Play	Language comprehension	Language expression
9–12	2/4	2/3	5/5	4/6	12/12	5/8
12–15		3/5	3/5	3/6	7/9	8/13
15–18	2/3	2/3		4/4	5/6	4/7
18–21		1/4	1/4	1/3	4/5	3/5
21–24			2/5	2/3	2/4	3/8
24–27			2/4	1/3	3/4	2/5
27–30				2/3	2/3	1/6
30–33				0/3	2/4	1/6
33–36				0/3	1/5	0/6

Using several feeding checklists and guidelines, MD's overall feeding skills were 12 to 14 months. He consumed thin liquids and ground, mashed, and mechanical soft solids. He developed compensatory strategies when eating nonpureed foods, including a nondissociated munch chew where he suckled food on the surface of his tongue, pooled the bolus on the anterior surface, and suckled the food behind his front central incisors. Boluses were also held intraorally for an extended period of time to promote bolus breakdown. He was learning to transfer food laterally to the center of mouth when it was placed on the back molars and his lips were active during chewing. He swallowed liquids from a cup with a sucking movement without anterior spillage, although he struggled at times with multiple swallows. He was also learning to independently feed himself finger foods.

AAC evaluation was completed using a variety of checklists, including the AAC Needs Assessment Checklist (Van Tatenhove). MD performed at Brown's stage 2; MD could demonstrate relational functions (greetings, recurrence, rejection, cessation of activities, commenting, directives, and associative). He also used semantic relationships, including agent-action, action-object, locatives, and attributes. MD navigated multiple screens to request desired items/activities as well as to comment spontaneously on events occurring in structured activities.

35.4 Questions and Answers for the Reader

1. MD eats purees and mechanical soft foods that he can swallow without mastication. Of the four stages of swallowing, in which stage does he exhibit the most difficulty and why?
   a) Oral stage.
   b) Oral transit stage.
   c) Pharyngeal stage.
   d) Esophageal stage.

Answer: a is correct. This is the initial phase where the food is triturated (chewed and moistened) and then the tongue carries the food to the postcanine region and rotates laterally, placing the food onto the occlusal surface of the lower teeth for food processing. During this stage, the tongue and soft palate together move cyclically in coordination with jaw movement. Tongue motions are coordinated with buccal movement to keep food on the occlusal surfaces of the lower teeth. The hyoid bone also moves constantly during feeding and helps control the movements of the jaw and tongue. When food is placed in the mouth, the mouth closes and the buccal muscles tighten to prevent remnants of food from pocketing in the lateral buccal sulci. Chewing mixes the food and saliva and prepares the bolus for the swallow. a is correct because MD is not able to masticate his food and thus moves immediately into the transport stage once food enters the oral cavity.

b is incorrect. When a portion of the food is ready to be swallowed, food is placed on the tongue surface and propelled back through the fauces to the oropharynx. The tongue tip rises touching the alveolar ridge, while the posterior tongue drops to open the back of the oral cavity; the tongue surface then moves upward, squeezing the chewed food back along the palate and into the pharynx. The duration of bolus aggregation in the oropharynx ranges from a fraction of a second to about 10 seconds in normal individuals eating solid food. MD is able to manipulate his jaw and tongue, and is able to propel boluses to the oropharynx without difficulty.

c is incorrect. This is the most complex phase of swallowing and also the most rapid sequential activity that occurs within a second involving (1) food passage, propelling the food bolus through the pharynx, and upper esophageal sphincter (UES) to the esophagus, and (2) airway protection, insulating the larynx and trachea from the pharynx during food passage to prevent food from entering the airway. The soft palate closes the nasopharynx to ensure food does not enter the nasal cavity simultaneously, while the vocal folds close and the larynx moves upward, which results in tilting of the epiglottis and closure of the larynx enabling the trachea to be protected from food. The three pharyngeal constrictor muscles contract from top to bottom to transport the bolus into the esophagus. MD does not demonstrate difficulty with this phase.

d is incorrect. This is the last phase of the swallowing process where the bolus enters the esophagus, which is from the lower part of the UES to the lower esophageal sphincter (LES). The LES is also tensioned at rest to prevent regurgitation from the stomach and relaxes during the swallow to allow the bolus to pass into the stomach, while the larynx is lowered and the vocal folds open, allowing the patient to take a breath. MD does not demonstrate difficulty with this.

2. Given MD's medical history and aversion for attempting foods with different textures, what approach is most likely to yield favorable outcomes in feeding therapy?
   a) Purely behavioral approach.
   b) Combination of variety of approaches.
   c) Purely sensory approach.
   d) No approach (e.g., let him develop the skills independently).

Answer: a is incorrect. Purely behavioral feeding programs use preferred foods, toys, books, or television to reinforce children for eating challenging foods. This approach does not account for the sensory and motor challenges MD demonstrates. Also, this type of program encourages children who have compromised motor skills to swallow purees only and can often be at risk for choking at the introduction of solids.

b is correct. One singular approach for feeding therapy is likely inappropriate for MD. He responded well to both structured and behavioral approaches to therapy. It is important to consider auditory stimuli, environmental surroundings, gustatory and olfactory sensitivities, as well as tactile, vestibular, and proprioceptive input during mealtimes when considering therapeutic approaches. He required direct teaching of oral motor skills as well as a modified behavioral approach for feeding. He made great progress when working in conjunction with occupational therapy for feeding and progressed 6 months in a span of 12 months with his overall feeding skills.

c is incorrect. Using a strictly sensory approach encourages children to smell, feel, play, and taste the food. However, this approach does not help MD with his limited motor skills to develop the skills needed to eat safely.

d is incorrect. Without direct intervention, he would not gain the skills needed to become a more proficient eater, and due to his disabilities could be at risk for malnutrition or becoming even a more picky eater.

3. What language therapy approach would be appropriate for MD?
   a) No specific approach.
   b) Core vocabulary approach.
   c) Applied behavior analysis.
   d) Play-based therapy.

Answer: a is incorrect. Not using specific evidence-based therapeutic approaches is neither efficacious nor productive and could result in lack of reimbursement from insurance. It is also within our scope and sequence as practicing speech-language pathologists to use evidence-based therapy approach(es) for therapy.

b is incorrect. Core vocabulary is not appropriate because it is intended for children with inconsistent speech disorder when the underlying deficit is a phonological planning deficit and not a cognitive-linguistic deficit. Since MD is nonverbal, it is not an appropriate therapy approach.

c is incorrect. Although evidence based, it is not appropriate to use for MD. Applied behavior analysis (ABA) principles for feeding often have a significant negative impact, especially in the context of poor motor skills. ABA is also very time intensive for the family (25–40 h/wk).

d is correct. Play-based assessment involves knowledge of communication skills for each level of play. Play-based therapy is effective for young children as they are often highly energetic with decreased attention. Play-based therapy allowed MD to lead activities and for opportunities to model therapeutic tasks. Therapy incorporated videos to maintain motivation and attention as well as his ProLoQuo2Go.

4. Initially, how should MD's ProLoQuo2Go be programmed and what type of vocabulary should be employed?
   a) Combination of core and fringe vocabulary of 20 icons per screen.
   b) Core words only.
   c) Full vocabulary screen with 1 × 1 icons that consisted of 64 icons.
   d) Program words as needed or as staff/parents requested.

Answer: a is correct. Due to his visual deficits as well as his language skills, MD required a limited amount of stimuli on the screen including core vocabulary. His high-frequency words were used initially with the intention of expanding this list as his communication skills improved. Personal and motivating fringe vocabulary was also programmed.

b is incorrect. Although core vocabulary is a necessity, not incorporating fringe vocabulary limits requesting personal items/actions, which is often motivating. If personal words are used often, this fringe vocabulary must be considered when programming.

c is incorrect. Providing comprehensive vocabulary with small icons to an emergent language learner can be overwhelming. Additionally, MD's visual and motor deficits may also be problematic and, furthermore, he is unlikely to utilize these icons based on his current language skills.

d is incorrect. This approach does not incorporate evidence-based core vocabulary critical to language development. Programming vocabulary based on only the needs of his surroundings is unlikely to yield improved vocabulary.

35.5 Description of Disorder and Recommended Treatment

MD presented with several communication disorders that, when combined, created a unique challenge for treatment. He was diagnosed with traumatic brain injury, resulting from IVH grade 2 at birth, hearing impairment, receptive and expressive language disorder, and feeding difficulties. He also presented with significantly impaired cognitive function as well as autism-like characteristics, including difficulty with socioemotional reciprocity, abnormal eye contact and body language when engaging with others, and deficits in developing relationships with others.

With regard to feeding, treatment focused on improved tolerance of foods with different textures as well as gaining necessary skills for chewing and eating a variety of foods. Using a combination of approaches and strategies, improved oral phase skills emerged. With regard to language, a combination treatment approach was executed involving play-based therapy with a focus on movement and cause/effect. This approach created an opportunity for MD to develop natural and spontaneous language using his AAC device. Following the hierarchy of Brown's stages of development, recommended treatment was systemic and followed the natural progression of language for his cognitive level. Classroom themes were incorporated in therapy to help promote communicative opportunities.

35.6 Outcome

The prognosis for MD to improve feeding was fair, secondary to limited follow-through outside of therapy. He made steady progress for 10 months during feeding therapy, progressing from strictly purees to a combination of purees and mechanical soft foods. He required assistance to place the foods on his occlusal molars and begin mastication versus using the phasic bite and suck pattern. He also improved in self-feeding with finger foods and drank from a cup without anterior spillage. Follow-through for therapeutic feeding suggestions was minimal among both school staff and MD's family.

Significant progress was also noted in MD's communicative efficacy. At the start of therapy, MD's overall communication skills were determined to be between 12 to 18 months. Within 24 months of therapy, his overall communication skills increased to a range spanning 8 to 33 months. Competency with the ProLoQuo2Go required methodical and consistent routine as well as play-based activities that maintained MD's interest and created natural communicative opportunities. He was extremely motivated by electronics, so videos and video modeling were often used during treatment. He was able to formulate two- to three-word utterances (Brown stage 2) and navigate multiple screens. Increased core vocabulary and progress toward Brown stage 3 were targeted in continued therapy.

35.7 Key Points

- AAC assessment is vital for nonverbal clients to determine the ideal mode of communication.

- Formal diagnoses of medical conditions are not always indicative of function. Thorough assessment of competencies, interests, and communication skills is critical to determine appropriate intervention strategies.
- A thorough understanding of typical development of feeding skills is necessary to determine appropriate therapeutic strategies. Developmental feeding skills are not always commensurate with chronological age.

Suggested Readings

[1] Sharp WG, Jaquess DL, Morton JF, Herzinger CV. Pediatric feeding disorders: a quantitative synthesis of treatment outcomes. Clin Child Fam Psychol Rev. 2010; 13(4):348–365

[2] American Speech-Language-Hearing Association. Augmentative and alternative communication: knowledge and skills for service delivery [Knowledge and Skills]. Available at: http://www.asha.org/policy/KS2002–00067/. doi:10.1044/policy.KS2002–00067

[3] Van Tatenhove G. Normal Language Development, Generative Language & AAC 2007;1–11. Available at: http://www.texasat.net/Assets/1–normal-language–aac.pdf

References

[1] Morris SE, Klein MD. Pre-Feeding Skills: A Comprehensive Resource for Mealtime Development. 2nd ed. Austin, TX: Pro-Ed; 2000

[2] Fernando N, Potock M. Raising A Healthy, Happy Eater: A State-by-Stage Guide to Setting Your Child on the Path to Adventurous Eating. New York, NY: The Experiment; 2015

[3] Rowell K, McGlothlin J. Helping Your Child with Extreme Picky Eating. Oakland, CA: New Harbinger; 2015

[4] ASHA Pediatric Feeding History and Clinical Assessment Form (Infant 6 months and older). Available at: http://www.asha.org/uploadedFiles/Pediatric-Feeding-History-and-Clinical-Assessment-Form.pdf

[5] AAC Needs Assessment Checklist by Gail M. Van Tatenhove PA. 2016. Available at: http://praacticalaac.org/praactical/aac-assessment-forms/

[6] Typical Developmental Feeding Skills. Available at: http://sandiegooccupationaltherapy.com/wp-content/uploads/2012/01/TypicalDevelFeeding.pdf

[7] ASHA Traumatic Brain Injury Deficits. Available at: http://www.asha.org/public/speech/disorders/TBI/#deficits

36 Psycholinguistic Approach to Assessment and Treatment of Complex Speech-Language Impairment in a School-Age Child

Toby Macrae, Emily Berteau, and Kaitlin Lansford

36.1 Introduction

Children with complex speech-language impairment may have deficits in one or more levels of speech processing (e.g., input processing, stored linguistic knowledge, and/or output processing). A psycholinguistic approach may be employed to identify levels of deficits in these children and, therefore, provide specific targets for treatment.

36.2 Clinical History and Description

HH, a 6.11-year-old girl, received speech therapy services since she was approximately 4 years old when she was diagnosed with a speech-sound disorder (SSD). Although some therapeutic gains were achieved, she recently plateaued and full speech-language reassessment was completed.

36.3 Clinical Testing

As a framework for testing and intervention, a seven-step evidence-based practice (EBP) decision-making process[1] was employed to evaluate the evidence regarding a psycholinguistic approach to assessment and treatment of speech-language impairment. Specifically, the following clinical question was posed (step 1), using the PICO (population, intervention, comparison, outcome) format: Does the psycholinguistic approach (I) result in improved speech-language performance (O) in comparison to baseline performance or alternative treatment approaches (C) in children with speech-language impairment (P)? Several research articles supporting this approach to speech-language assessment and treatment were identified and critically evaluated (steps 2–5).[2–4] Based on the supporting evidence, this approach was determined to be appropriate for this complex case of speech-language impairment (step 6).

According to the psycholinguistic model, children may have deficits in input processing, stored linguistic knowledge, and/or output processing.[5] Comprehensive testing attempts to identify precise deficit levels in speech processing. Identifying the level of breakdown has implications for skills to be targeted in treatment. Assessment of input, storage, and output in this case included the following:

- Hearing screening: pure-tone audiometry involving presentation of 500, 1,000, 2,000, and 4,000 Hz at 20 dB.
- Auditory discrimination: informal (discriminating between recordings of participant's own correct and incorrect productions of speech sounds in words) and formal (Speech Assessment and Interactive Learning System [SAILS])[6] assessments.
- Overall expressive and receptive language: Clinical Evaluation of Language Fundamentals, Fourth Edition (CELF-4).[7]

- Expressive vocabulary: Expressive Vocabulary Test, Second Edition (EVT-2).[8]
- Receptive vocabulary: Peabody Picture Vocabulary Test, Fourth Edition (PPVT-4).[9]
- Phonological processing (including phonological awareness, phonological memory, and rapid naming): Comprehensive Test of Phonological Processing (CTOPP)[10] and portions of the Phonological Awareness Test, Second Edition (PAT-2).[11]
- Nonsense word repetition (NWR): Syllable Repetition Task (SRT).[12]
- Real and nonsense word decoding: Test of Word Reading Efficiency, Second Edition (TOWRE-2).[13]
- Speech motor control: Oral and Speech Motor Protocol (OSMP).[14]
- Speech-sound production: Goldman–Fristoe Test of Articulation, Second Edition (GFTA-2).[15]
- Token-to-token inconsistency: Word Inconsistency Assessment from the Diagnostic Evaluation of Articulation and Phonology, American Edition (WIA).[16]

36.4 Questions and Answers for the Reader

1. Which area(s) of speech processing (input, storage, and/or output) are assessed via auditory discrimination tasks?
   a) Input only.
   b) Input and storage.
   c) Storage only.
   d) Output.

Answer: b is correct. Auditory discrimination tasks involve listening to the stimuli presented (input) and calling upon stored knowledge of the perceptual features of sounds and words.

a is incorrect. Successfully discriminating between correctly and incorrectly produced sounds requires the listener to have well-formed categorical representations for those sounds in long-term memory.

c is incorrect. Auditory discrimination tasks necessarily involve auditory input and therefore involve more than just storage.

d is incorrect. These tasks require the child to point to a happy face if the sound was produced correctly or a sad face if the sound was produced incorrectly, and thus do not involve speech output.

2. In which area(s) of speech processing (input, storage, and/or output) did HH have difficulties?
   a) Input.
   b) Storage.
   c) Output.
   d) All of the above.

Answer: d is correct. HH showed difficulty with auditory discrimination (input and storage), auditory memory (storage), and speech-sound production (storage and output), for example, reflecting deficits in all levels of speech processing.

a is incorrect. HH showed difficulty with tasks that involved more than just input.

b is incorrect. HH showed difficulty with tasks that involved more than just storage.

c is incorrect. HH showed difficulty with tasks that involved more than just output.

3. Rapid naming involves many of the same skills as which of the following?
   a) Auditory discrimination.
   b) Speech-sound production.
   c) Fluent reading.
   d) Reading comprehension.

Answer: c is correct. Rapid naming involves rapidly processing visual as well as phonological information, skills that are also required for fluent reading.

a is incorrect. Rapid naming involves speech output, whereas auditory discrimination does not.

b is incorrect. Rapid naming involves, among other things, rapidly processing visual information, whereas speech-sound production does not.

d is incorrect. Reading comprehension is closely related to oral language abilities, including vocabulary, whereas rapid naming is closely related to processing visual and phonological information.

36.5 Description of Disorder and Recommended Treatment

Based on this assessment strategy, HH presented with deficits in input, storage, and output. With regard to input, although HH passed the hearing screening, she had difficulty with both informal and formal assessments of auditory discrimination. Auditory discrimination tasks tap input as well as some aspects of storage (e.g., stored knowledge of the perceptual qualities of sounds and words). HH was required to point to a happy or sad face representing correctly and incorrectly produced sounds within words; sounds that she had difficulty producing were targeted. She had difficulty discriminating between her correct and incorrect productions of /kr/ (50% accurate), /kw/ (50% accurate), /fl/ (50% accurate), /sl/ (50% accurate), /ð/ (8% accurate), and /v/ (50% accurate) in the initial position in words. She also had difficulty discriminating between other speakers' correct and incorrect productions of /r/ (60% accurate) and /θ/ (75% accurate) in the initial position in words. With regard to storage, HH scored 101 on the PPVT-4, suggesting age-appropriate receptive vocabulary. Her standard score of 89 on the EVT-2 confirmed age-appropriate expressive vocabulary, which reflects aspects of both storage and output. With regard to output, HH's total functional score of 106 on the OSMP suggested some difficulty with functional speech motor tasks (e.g., loudness variation). In addition, HH scored more than two SDs below the mean for children aged 6.6 to 6.11 years from Robbins and Klee[14] (the oldest age group tested) on three of the five diadochokinetic tasks (rapidly alternating speech movements)

on the OSMP. HH's standard score of 73 on the GFTA-2 revealed difficulties with speech-sound production. This task also involved aspects of storage, as it requires access to stored representations for words, including phonological representations.

HH obtained subtest scaled scores of 6 for recalling sentences and 5 for formulated sentences on the CELF-4, suggesting difficulties listening to and accurately repeating spoken sentences and formulating semantically and grammatically correct sentences. HH's difficulties with these subtests may be attributable, at least in part, to auditory memory deficits. With regard to phonological processing, HH had difficulty with rapid naming with standard scores of 79 on the rapid naming composite and 57 on the alternate rapid naming composite on the CTOPP. Rapid naming involves some of the same skills as reading fluently (i.e., rapidly processing visual as well as phonological information) and has been shown to be one of the strongest predictors of later reading fluency.[17] HH received mostly age-appropriate scores on the phonological awareness tasks on the CTOPP and the PAT-2. She had some difficulty identifying medial and final phonemes in words on the PAT-2. HH received a standard score of 88 on the phonological memory composite on the CTOPP, revealing low average phonological memory. She also had difficulty with phonological memory on the NWR task (SRT). NWR tasks involve aspects of input, storage, and output. The majority of HH's consonant substitutions on this task (7/8) reflected different manner classes to the consonant targets, revealing auditory-perceptual encoding difficulties.[18,19] In addition, HH had difficulty repeating nonsense words of increasing syllable length (two syllables: PCC [percent consonants correct] = 100%; three syllables: PCC = 72%; four syllables: PCC = 56%), revealing difficulties with phonological memory.[18,19] HH used a typical number of consonant additions in her NWRs, in comparison to similarly aged children with speech-language impairment,[18] revealing normal speech motor planning/programming. This finding was used to rule out a diagnosis of childhood apraxia of speech (CAS). Although HH's WIA score was 44%, suggesting some difficulty producing words consistently, increased token-to-token inconsistency has been seen in children with typical speech development and children with non-CAS SSDs.[20] Lastly, HH received standard scores of 73 for real words and 78 for nonsense words on the TOWRE-2, suggesting poor single-word decoding.

A psycholinguistic approach does not prescribe a specifically designed therapy program, but rather emphasizes the importance of implementing treatment tasks that address the particular skill deficit. Deficits in input, storage, and output were identified as targets, and given the importance of reading for academic success, decoding was identified as a primary target for treatment. The Lindamood Phoneme Sequencing Program for Reading, Spelling, and Speech, Fourth Edition (LiPS-4)[21] was used to target phonemic awareness, decoding, and spelling directly as well as other deficits secondarily. Phonemic awareness was also targeted directly using tasks that required HH to identify medial and final consonants in words. With regard to input, HH's auditory discrimination difficulties were targeted by bringing HH's attention to the perceptual qualities of and differences among sounds produced in isolation and in words during LiPS activities. Particular attention was paid to minimal pair words that differed by a target sound that HH had difficulty producing and her error sound, when she also misperceived this difference (e.g., /ʃ/ and /s/ in "shoe" and "Sue"). With regard to output, HH's speech-sound production difficulties were targeted by focusing on HH's use of the correct sound in spoken words during LiPS activities. Particular attention was paid to minimal pair words that differed by a target sound and HH's error. If incidental treatment of these difficulties during the LiPS was ineffective, they were targeted directly using the SAILS perceptual training program and formal speech-sound intervention (e.g., minimal pair therapy). HH's auditory memory difficulties were targeted recalling details from and answer questions about spoken sentences.

36.6 Outcome

Step 7 in Gillam and Gillam's[1] EBP decision-making process involves evaluating the outcome of a particular approach to treatment. Data were collected to determine the effectiveness of treatment. HH's performance in real and nonsense word decoding and spelling in the LiPS treatment activities was tracked each session and shown in ▶ Fig. 36.1 and ▶ Fig. 36.2, respectively. With regard to both decoding and spelling accuracy, HH showed variable performance over approximately 4 months of treatment. CV (consonant-vowel) and VC (vowel-consonant) word shapes were the initial focus, CVC shapes were then targeted throughout treatment, and complex shapes were introduced toward the end of treatment. Sessions of low accuracy were limited; sessions of 60% or higher for reading and

70% or higher for spelling predominated. Furthermore, new objectives were introduced during most (72%) sessions, including new letters and sounds and new decoding and spelling conventions (e.g., "e" at the end of a word makes the vowel say its name; when two vowels go walking, the first one does the talking). HH maintained encouraging levels of accuracy as new skills were targeted. The DIBELS nonsense word fluency probes were administered approximately weekly as an independent measure of reading fluency. HH had a slightly increased total number of letter sounds decoded correctly and words read completely as treatment concluded (ranges: 22–32 and 5–9, respectively) in comparison to the beginning and middle stages of treatment (ranges: 19–26 and 4–7, respectively). HH continued to exhibit difficulty decoding words fluently. Treatment is ongoing and will continue to target decoding and spelling skills. Improving self-monitoring and self-correction strategies, accuracy, and consistency will be prioritized from session to session. Once accuracy and consistency improve, focus will shift to decreasing response latency in an attempt to improve reading fluency.

HH's performance on phonemic awareness tasks involving identification of medial and final sounds is shown in ▶ Fig. 36.3. HH steadily increased in the accuracy and these tasks were discontinued. The DIBELS phoneme segmentation fluency probes, which required HH to segment as many spoken words into component sounds as possible in 1 minute, were also administered weekly. These probes served as a measure of generaliza-

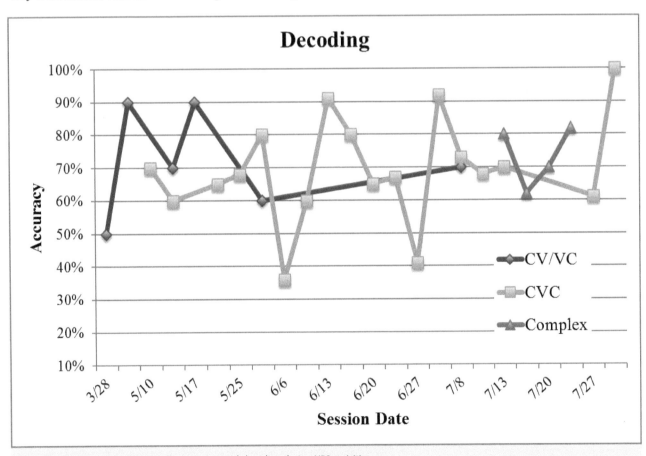

Fig. 36.1 Accuracy of single real and nonsense word decoding during LiPS activities.

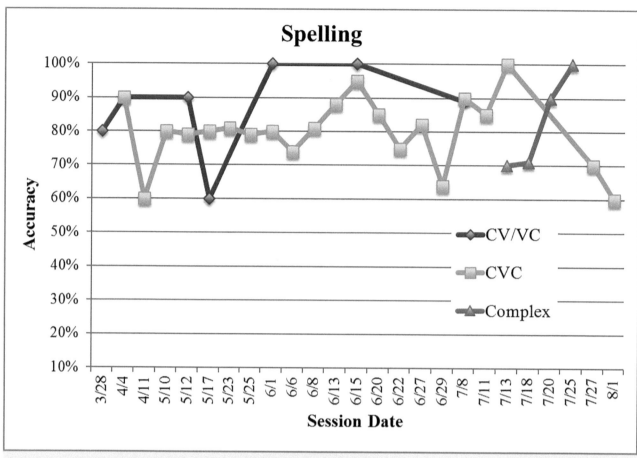

Fig. 36.2 Accuracy of single real and nonsense word spelling during LiPS activities.

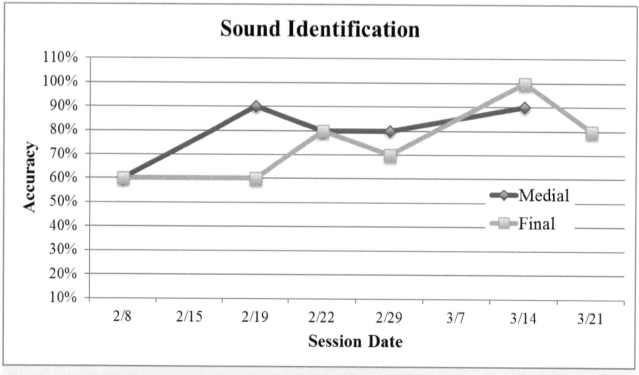

Fig. 36.3 Accuracy of medial and final sound identification in spoken words.

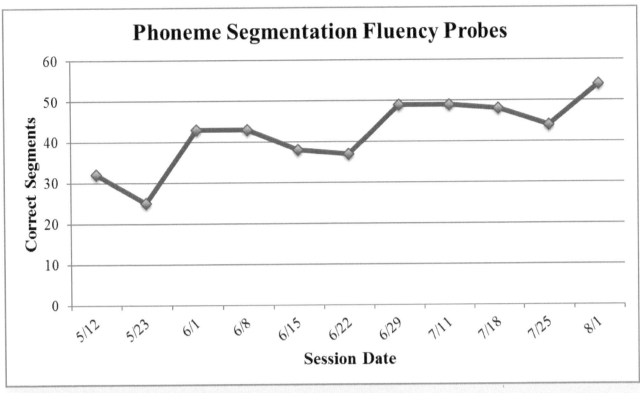

Fig. 36.4 Number of phonemes accurately segmented from spoken words within 1 minute.

tion from sound identification to the more advanced skill of segmenting words. HH's performance on these probes is shown in ▶ Fig. 36.4. HH showed steady improvements in segmentation fluency throughout treatment. HH's performance on auditory memory activities was tracked each session. HH performed consistently throughout treatment, but only once scored above 70%. This skill will continue to be targeted in treatment with an emphasis on teaching HH strategies to improve auditory memory, for example, visualizing items or characters to be recalled.

36.7 Key Points

- Making evidence-based decisions about treatment approaches for children with speech-language impairment is a methodical process that involves creating a clinical question, finding and evaluating evidence that pertains to the question, making a decision by integrating the evidence, and evaluating outcomes.[1]
- A psycholinguistic approach to speech-language assessment and treatment involves identifying deficits in input processing, stored linguistic knowledge, and/or output processing and targeting these deficits in treatment.[5]
- A psycholinguistic approach may be appropriate for some children with complex speech-language impairment, although speech-language pathologists should not always expect to see rapid gains in all areas.

References

[1] Gillam SL, Gillam RB. Making evidence-based decisions about child language intervention in schools. Lang Speech Hear Serv Sch. 2006; 37(4):304–315

[2] Pascoe M, Stackhouse J, Wells B. Phonological therapy within a psycholinguistic framework: promoting change in a child with persisting speech difficulties. Int J Lang Commun Disord. 2005; 40(2):189–220

[3] Pascoe M, Stackhouse J, Wells B. Children's Speech and Literacy Difficulties: Book 3. Persisting Speech Difficulties in Children. Chichester, UK: Wiley; 2006

[4] Waters D, Hawkes C, Burnett E. Targeting speech processing strengths to facilitate pronunciation change. Int J Lang Commun Disord. 1998; 33 Suppl: 469–474

[5] Stackhouse J, Wells B, Eds. Children's Speech and Literacy Difficulties 1: A Psycholinguistic Framework. London, UK: Whurr; 1997

[6] Rvachew S. Speech Assessment and Interactive Learning System [Computer software]. Montréal, QC: McGill University; 2011

[7] Semel E, Wiig E, Secord W. Clinical Evaluation of Language Fundamentals. 4th ed. San Antonio, TX: Pearson; 2006

[8] Williams KT. Expressive Vocabulary Test. 2nd ed. Bloomington, MN: Pearson; 2007

[9] Dunn L, Dunn D. Peabody Picture Vocabulary Test. 4th ed. Bloomington, MN: Pearson; 2007

[10] Wagner R, Torgesen J, Rashotte C. Comprehensive Test of Phonological Processing. Austin, TX: Pro-Ed; 1999

[11] Robertson C, Salter W. The Phonological Awareness Test. 2nd ed. East Moline, IL: LinguiSystems; 2007

[12] Shriberg LD, Lohmeier HL, Campbell TF, Dollaghan CA, Green JR, Moore CA. A nonword repetition task for speakers with misarticulations: the Syllable Repetition Task (SRT). J Speech Lang Hear Res. 2009; 52(5):1189–1212

[13] Torgesen JK, Wagner RK, Rashotte CA. Test of Word Reading Efficiency. 2nd ed. Austin, TX: Pro-Ed; 2012

[14] Robbins J, Klee T. Clinical assessment of oropharyngeal motor development in young children. J Speech Hear Disord. 1987; 52(3):271–277

[15] Goldman R, Fristoe M. Goldman–Fristoe Test of Articulation. 2nd ed. San Antonio, TX: Pearson; 2000

[16] Dodd B, Hua Z, Crosbie S, Holm A, Ozanne A. Diagnostic Evaluation of Articulation and Phonology (U.S. ed.). San Antonio, TX: Pearson; 2006

[17] Norton ES, Wolf M. Rapid automatized naming (RAN) and reading fluency: implications for understanding and treatment of reading disabilities. Annu Rev Psychol. 2012; 63:427–452

[18] Lohmeier HL, Shriberg LD. The Syllable Repetition Task (Technical Report No. 17). Madison, WI: University of Wisconsin-Madison; 2011

[19] Shriberg LD, Lohmeier HL, Strand EA, Jakielski KJ. Encoding, memory, and transcoding deficits in Childhood Apraxia of Speech. Clin Linguist Phon. 2012; 26(5):445–482

[20] Macrae T, Sosa AV. Predictors of token-to-token inconsistency in preschool children with typical speech-language development. Clin Linguist Phon. 2015; 29(12):922–937

[21] Lindamood PC, Lindamood PD. Lindamood Phoneme Sequencing Program for Reading, Spelling, and Speech. 4th ed. Austin, TX: Pro-Ed; 2011

37 Treatment of Communication and Feeding Disorders in a Complex Pediatric Patient with a Neurogenic Disorder

Alicia Morrison-Fagbemi

37.1 Introduction

Medically complex pediatric cases require clinicians to develop specialized person-centered intervention plans that involve family and caregivers. This case describes a pediatric patient with a neurogenic syndrome resulting in both feeding and communication deficits. The treatment approach used in this case highlights the pedagogy of neurogenic communication etiologies, dynamic assessment, and best practices in treatment.

37.2 Clinical History and Description

LG was a 15-month-old male child born following a full-term, uncomplicated pregnancy. No anoxic events during birth were reported. LG weighed 7.8 lb with normal APGAR (appearance, pulse, grimace, activity, and respiration) scores. LG demonstrated feeding difficulties characterized by dyscoordination of systems within the first 2 postpartum months. At 3 months of age, motor delays and ocular delays were noted. No accidents, illnesses, or hospitalizations were reported. Following genetic testing, LG was diagnosed with Mowatt–Wilson's syndrome affecting motor movement and language development. Beyond physical impairments of gross and fine motor control, LG presented with limited verbal repertoire characterized by isolated open vowels with minimal nonverbal communication.

37.3 Clinical Testing

LG was referred for an outpatient speech and language assessment by early intervention to develop and support the Individ-

ualized Educational Program. Clinical testing included both formal and informal measures of communication ability. The communication matrix was used to evaluate LG's communication abilities and to support goal derivation. The communication matrix is an online assessment tool designed to identify how a child is communicating, and to provide a framework for determining communication goals. It was designed primarily for speech-language pathologists and educators to use to document communication skills in children with severe or multiple disabilities, including children with sensory, motor, and/or cognitive impairments. The online version also provides a parent design so that the parent and professionals working with the child can access the profile to describe communication in the home (▶ Fig. 37.1; www.communicationmatrix.org).

The Communication Matrix Profile describes four major aspects of communication: (1) four reasons for communicating, (2) seven levels of communication, (3) 24 specific messages (e.g., "I want that"), and (4) nine categories of behaviors used to communicate (e.g., simple gestures). The profile is a matrix providing a visual representation of communication behaviors and messages employed. Informal measures were collected during play; LG presented at level 1 (preintentional behavior). Promisingly, LG demonstrated joint attention skills during paired communication with voice and simple sign language, indicating receptiveness to alternative means of communication.

Informal evaluation of feeding skills was completed during a typical morning meal; LG was presented with applesauce, mashed potatoes, and cereal. Two incidences of gagging with apple sauce were observed, followed by arching and crying. He refused mash potatoes by turning his head away and crying. Approximately 10 minutes following the meal, LG began cough-

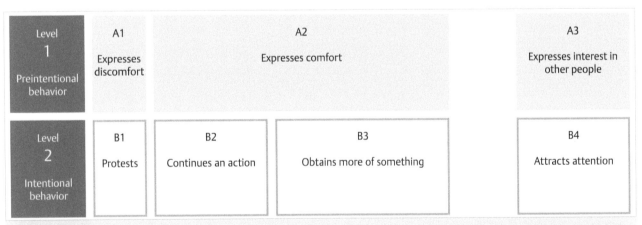

Fig. 37.1 LG's online assessment confirms goal formulation based on his use of precursory means of communication at only a level 2 communication stage (represented by the gray box). The yellow box represents LG's ability to express discomfort, demonstrate comfort and regulation with family members, and attention to others. These target domains provide a framework for activities to communicate likes and dislikes, and pairing language to these areas. In addition, the image displays how the child demonstrated joint attention skills during paired communication with voice and simple sign language, indicating receptiveness to alternative means of communication. (The Communication Matrix is a service of the Design to Learn Projects at Oregon Health & Science University, 2017 Charity Rowland, PhD.)

ing and vomiting. He was then given a bottle, which appeared to resolve this discomfort. When seated on his mother's lap, LG arched his head and neck backward. He coughed and turned away from pureed food. He appeared unhappy and/or uncomfortable during feeding, and fell asleep at one point during the feeds. He tolerated about 1 oz of pureed food per meal as noted by his mother. Thin liquids were bottle fed by the parent. An upright, slight tilt was recommended to ensure safe liquid intake. His mother reported that he does not cough on liquids. Advancing from the bottle to flexible weighted straw sippy cups was recommended.

The family was encouraged to follow up with their physician to obtain a modified barium swallow and nutrition evaluation. Modified barium swallow (MBS) indicated oral dysphagia characterized by decreased mastication and oral aversion to solids. Laryngeal elevation and epiglottal inversion was within normal limits. No pharyngeal residue was noted. No laryngeal penetration or aspiration was observed.

37.4 Questions and Answers for the Reader

1. Given the unknown etiology of a rare genetic disorder, what is an appropriate starting point for the family and child?
   a) Discuss natural language development and reevaluate in 3 months.
   b) Discuss alternative and augmentative communication immediately, stating that early intervention is needed immediately.
   c) Provide information on a total communication approach that involves use of voice paired with gestures, simple sign language, and exploration of augmentative and alternative communication (AAC) needs.
   d) Provide information related to language development and the supportive communication strategies a parent can provide with their child to foster speech and language skills.
   e) c and d.

Answer: e is correct (c and d). The optimal starting point involves a total communication approach that incorporates multiple modalities and parent counseling. A total communication approach promotes voice, gestures, facial expression, sign language, and simple augmentative communication aids to support comprehensive learning.

a is incorrect. It does not provide the family with the support of communication needs for their child. Discussing language development is important to educate the family; however, the child needs early intervention. Reevaluation is not appropriate at this time.

b is incorrect. Multiple communication strategies are critical to promote speech and voice as well as enhance communication.

2. When considering use of augmentative means of communication, which answer describes a good starting point for intervention?
   a) Picture cue representation of abstract objects.
   b) Simple speech generation devices to indicate simple requests to continue an activity or request recurrence of an activity.

   c) Pair all communication exchanges with not only gesture and simple sign language, but also voice.
   d) b and c.

Answer: d is correct (both b and c). A total communication approach is appropriate. And, as such, pairing voice with a simple augmentative communication device set the foundation knowledge for use of a dynamic language display for AAC, while use of voice also promotes but does not suffocate the chance of the individual to express simple needs and wants with open vowel productions. Simple sign language gestures also promote fast communication expression during direct cause/effect tasks (e.g., requesting "more" or "give me").

a is incorrect. Picture cue representation of an abstract item is the first step in communication. Communication symbols are built from concrete to abstract development when discussing AAC. Concrete items have stronger connections to the meaning of the intended message.

3. Given the MBS results, what is the first step of feeding intervention?
   a) Begin with solids and promote rotary movement.
   b) Allow for natural feeding skills to develop over time.
   c) Begin to work to address his aversion of food by addressing the smell/touch of various stimuli within a close range without intake to promote comfort and supportive feeding experience.
   d) Test for food allergies to address why the individual is arching during feeding in discomfort.
   e) c and d.

Answer: e is correct (c and d). In therapeutic feeding, it is critical to address the aversion and fear of food. Creating tolerance of smell and the proximity to food is stage one (sequential oral sensory [SOS] approach). It is important for a physician to rule out food allergies to address the causes of physical body arching and/or discomfort during eating. Routine follow-up is required to ensure safety of the swallowing mechanism. Consultation with both the nutritionist and gastroenterologist is also likely indicated.

a is incorrect. The child is not appropriate for this level of intervention based on his current deficits.

b is incorrect. Natural feeding skills are impaired and require intervention to improve to maintain appropriate nutrition.

4. When considering ongoing treatment and goal derivation for the child, what should be considered for speech and language?
   a) Speaking with the family to educate them on the treatment trajectory and school transition.
   b) Reassessing communication skills with a reevaluation of milestones met utilizing informal measures with the communication matrix.
   c) Exploring options of AAC for high-tech devices and apps that may be the preferred communication options for the individual.
   d) Ensure that social closeness and pragmatic skills are nurtured into the intervention plan.
   e) All of the above.

Answer: e is correct. All of the strategies are required to ensure the appropriate evaluation of intervention planning. It is important to maintain dynamic assessment, encourage plan development in intervention, goal derivation, and action plans for the family. The family is critical to the therapeutic process, and family support, advocacy, and school transition are prioritized. It is also important to remember that pragmatics is an integral part of intervention in individuals who utilize AAC; peers and social closeness must be promoted and encouraged.

37.5 Description of Disorder and Recommended Treatment

LG presented with a moderate-to-severe neurogenic communication disorder characterized by severe language and feeding impairment. He also presented with gross and fine motor deficits that may affect his ability to employ sign language as well as dynamic, high-tech augmentative communication devices. His treatment plan included intervention targeting both communication and feeding simultaneously. A total communication approach paired with low-tech alternative/augmentative communication device was recommended. A major focus was also placed on family education and counseling; they were informed of speech and language milestones as well as strategies to include alternative means of communication including sign language, gesture, and pragmatic functions to promote language expression. Although augmentative/alternative communication strategies were considered in LG's treatment plan, they were not employed to replace speech and/or voice production. Treatment was provided four times a week for 30-minute sessions. Two sessions were dedicated to feeding therapy and two sessions were devoted to speech and language development and augmentative communication intervention.

37.6 Outcome

After six treatment sessions, LG developed a language system that was multimodel. At 3 years of age, he was able to use low-tech communication, gestural language, and nonverbal commu-

nication. LG gained skill in the use of an iPad with predesigned icons to support communication. LG's speech was limited to approximations of sounds to indicate "more," paired with a sign. He steadily developed preliteracy skills through the use of word combinations in pairs as he accessed the device to communicate. Ongoing reassessment utilized the communication matrix online system to mark progress and alter therapy goals.

LG's feed skills improved; however, oral preparatory deficits persisted. Currently, LG tolerates a range of foods and textures and has advanced to straw drinking with weighted support. Gluten and dairy allergies were diagnosed; diet change was initiated and regular consultations with a nutritionist support the family. Routine follow-up with the swallowing specialist and gastroenterologist are planned.

37.7 Key Points

- It is important to utilize a multimodal total communication approach and person-centered intervention when planning intervention and goal advancement. Family involvement in all aspects of assessment and goal planning is critical to support therapeutic progress.
- The speech-language pathologist is critical in family and caregiver education.
- A hierarchical approach should be employed when assessing communication to support appropriate development of language milestones.

Suggested Readings

[1] Stremel-Campbell K, Rowland C. Prelinguistic communication intervention: birth-to-2. Top Early Child Spec Educ. 1987; 7(2):49–58

[2] Rowland C, Schweigert P. Tangible symbols, tangible outcomes. Augment Altern Commun. 2009; 16(2):61–78

[3] Rowland C, Schweigert P. Cognitive skills and AAC: Where we've been, what we know and the questions we should ask. In: Light J, Beukelman D, Reichle J, Eds. Communicative Competence for Individuals Who Use AAC. Baltimore, MD: Paul Brookes; 2003

38 Language Assessment in a Child with Minimal Verbal Skills

Kristen E. Muller and Nancy C. Brady

38.1 Introduction

This case involves communication assessment and recommended treatment for an individual with an intellectual and developmental disabilities and minimal verbal skills.

JZ is an 11-year-old boy with a diagnosis of fragile X syndrome and autism spectrum disorder (ASD).

38.2 Clinical History and Description

JZ was an 11-year-old boy diagnosed with ASD and fragile X syndrome when he was 2.6 years old. At the time of evaluation, he was able to produce the word "no" and sign "please," "more," and "eat." He had TouchChat on his iPad, but his parents and teachers reported that he never used it. JZ's classroom teacher reported that he often attended to a "work task" for about 3 minutes and would then get up and run around the room. However, his teacher reported that he was easily redirected to return to his seat. JZ did not interact with his peers at school unless they had an item that he wanted. JZ was described as "pretty easygoing" by his mother, unless an unexpected change in his schedule arose or if he could not have a toy that he really liked. In these scenarios, JZ hit his head, legs, and torso, and banged his wrists together. JZ's mom expressed concerns that JZ was safe and able to communicate basic wants and needs.

38.3 Clinical Testing

Assessment of JZ's language employed the communication matrix, Peabody Picture Vocabulary Test, Fourth Edition (PPVT-IV), and Communication Complexity Scale (CCS). The communication matrix is a parent-report measure that presents profiles of how individuals with complex communication needs request and reject items and activities, comment, and ask questions. JZ's communication matrix profile indicated that he communicated consistently at the "unconventional communication" level; he used body movements, vocalizations, facial expressions, and simple gestures to communicate. JZ was beginning to communicate at the conventional communication level characterized by pointing, nodding or shaking his head, waving, or looking from a person to a desired object. These behaviors were emerging, but not yet mastered. Behaviors at this level are typically employed to intentionally communicate.

On the PPVT-IV, JZ obtained a raw score of 12, indicating he correctly responded to 12 pictures. His standard score was 20 (average range: 85–105) and percentile rank was 0.1. The CCS describes three levels of communication. The first level is preintentional communication (scores 2–5). Communication at this level includes changing behaviors in response to toys or activities. For example, an individual might look at an object or reach toward the object. The second level is intentional nonsymbolic communication (scores 6–10). Communication at this level consists of behaviors that clearly refer to an object or event and are directed to a communication partner. For example, an individual might try to open a jar of bubbles, but then hand the bubbles to someone to request help. The third level is intentional symbolic communication (scores 11 and 12). Communication at this level consists of speech, signs, or symbols used via an augmentative communication device. JZ's top three scores across 12 different activities were 9, 9, and 8. When averaged together, the three top scores resulted in an overall score of 8.67. This score indicated that JZ communicated intentionally with a variety of gestures and vocalizations, but was not yet using symbolic communication such as words, signs, or symbols.

38.4 Questions and Answers for the Reader

1. A child sees a toy they want that is out of reach. The child looks at the toy, then at their mom, and back at the toy while vocalizing. What kind of communicative act is this?
   a) Preintentional communication.
   b) Intentional nonsymbolic communication.
   c) Intentional symbolic communication.
   d) Augmentative and alternative communication (AAC).

Answer: b is correct. Triadic eye gaze with vocalization is intentional communication with a communication partner, but it is not yet symbolic because it does involve spoken or augmentative language.

a is incorrect. Preintentional communication involves behaviors that are purposeful, but not directed toward another person.

c is incorrect. Intentional symbolic communication includes the use of words, either spoken verbally or with AAC.

d is incorrect. AAC involves the use of communication methods such as pictures, gestures, sign, and speech-generating devices that supplement spoken speech.

2. A 7-year-old boy with a diagnosis of autism is new on your caseload. His mom and teacher report that he is able to have short conversations with adults and peers about preferred topics. His mother's main concerns are that her son is not making friends and is not keeping up with his peers in school. Which of these assessments would you use for this student?
   a) The CCS.
   b) The social communication questionnaire (SCQ).
   c) The communication matrix.
   d) A language sample.

Answer: d is correct. A language sample allows you to look at the mean length of utterance, total number of words, and number of different words. The CCS and communication matrix are appropriate for individuals who are minimally verbal, meaning they have 30 or fewer spoken words. The SCQ is an autism screener, and this student already has a diagnosis of ASD.

a is incorrect. The CCS is appropriate for individuals who are minimally verbal, meaning they have 30 or fewer spoken words.

b is incorrect. The SCQ is an autism screener, and this student already has a diagnosis of ASD.

c is incorrect. The communication matrix is appropriate for individuals who are minimally verbal, meaning they have 30 or fewer spoken words.

3. You are evaluating a 10-year-old girl with cerebral palsy who communicates using AAC software on her iPad. Her mother reports that she uses the iPad to communicate at home and in the community and can say about 15 different words. What additional assessment would you use if you wanted to learn more about how and why this girl communicates at home?
   a) The communication matrix.
   b) The Mullen Scales of Early Learning.
   c) The PPVT-IV.
   d) The Goldman–Fristoe Test of Articulation.

Answer: a is correct. The communication matrix is a parent report that would allow you to see how she communicates in different settings.

b is incorrect. The Mullen Scales of Early Learning is a standardized assessment that examines early intellectual development. A caregiver questionnaire would provide more information about naturalistic communication in the home.

c is incorrect. The PPVT-IV is a standardized receptive language assessment. This would provide information of word knowledge, but not about their communication at home.

d is incorrect. The Goldman–Fristoe Test of Articulation is an articulation assessment and would not provide information about naturalistic communication at home.

4. A child and teacher are playing with a ball toy. The teacher puts a ball in the ball toy and the child looks at the ball toy, then looks at the teacher, and vocalizes while clapping her hands. What is the function of this communication act?
   a) Behavior regulation.
   b) Joint attention.
   c) Asking a question.
   d) Refusing.

Answer: b is correct. This behavior is joint attention, because the child is making a social exchange with the teacher as if to say "this is fun." The child is not requesting or rejecting, which would be behavior regulation.

a is incorrect. Communication acts that involve requesting or rejecting an item or activity are behavior regulation acts. This act is a social exchange rather than a request or protest.

c is incorrect. This communication act is shared social enjoyment, rather than asking a question.

d is incorrect. This communication act is shared social enjoyment, rather than refusing an object or activity.

38.5 Description of Disorder and Recommended Treatment

Based on the assessment, JZ primarily used intentional non-symbolic communication (e.g., gestures, eye gaze, vocalizations) to express wants and needs. These communication acts were directed at a communication partner, but may be more difficult for partners to interpret than symbolic communication (i.e., speech, signs, or symbols). For example, communicating with unfamiliar communication partners or creating novel utterances is typically facilitated with symbolic communication. Therefore, one goal for JZ was to increase potential communicative effectiveness by introducing symbolic forms of communication. A second goal was to continue to encourage his use of nonsymbolic communication in appropriate contexts such as with family and caregivers.

The focus of treatment was functional communication by building upon JZ's existing skills and teaching symbolic communication with an AAC device. Communication partners were prompted to reinforce his verbal and sign communication acts by honoring his requests (e.g., if he signs more, give him more or if he says "no," then stop the activity) and providing verbal or gestural praise (e.g., nice job telling me "no," high five, or thumbs up). New AAC skills were taught by providing core vocabulary words and modeling their use to request, comment, protest, and ask questions. Incidental teaching strategies were used to promote communication opportunities in natural contexts. For example, favorite toys were placed on a shelf that he could not reach. When he requested the toy with gestures or vocalizations, communication partners modeled a symbolic request by selecting the toy on his AAC device. Intervention was provided in multiple settings (e.g., classroom, lunchroom, home, community) to optimize generalization. Family members, teachers, and paraprofessionals were coached on how to support communication goals throughout his day.

38.6 Outcome

Over time, JZ began to make independent requests and comments using his AAC device and/or speech. His device was updated regularly as his vocabulary expanded and environments changed. Five months after the initial assessment, his communication was reassessed using the CCS and communication matrix. JZ's top three scores on the CCS were 9, 11, and 11. When averaged together, the three top scores resulted in an overall score of 10.33. JZ's communication matrix profile indicated that he consistently communicated at the conventional communication level and had emerging skills at the concrete symbol level. These scores were suggestive of significant progress in therapy and the emergence of more symbolic communication.

38.7 Key Points

- Early, preverbal communication can be measured with assessments such as the CCS and the communication matrix.
- Individuals who are minimally verbal communicate using preintentional and intentional presymbolic communication acts, such as eye gaze, gestures, and vocalizations.
- Intervention goals include progressing to more advanced forms of communication including symbolic communication and promoting communication across environments.

Suggested Readings

[1] Abbeduto L, Brady N, Kover ST. Language development and fragile X syndrome: profiles, syndrome-specificity, and within-syndrome differences. Ment Retard Dev Disabil Res Rev. 2007; 13(1):36–46

[2] Brady N. Augmentative and alternative communication for children with Down syndrome or fragile X syndrome. In: Roberts J, Chapman R, Warren S, Eds. Speech and Language Development and Intervention in Down Syndrome and Fragile X Syndrome. Baltimore, MD: Paul H. Brookes; 2008:255–274

[3] Brady NC, Fleming K, Thiemann-Bourque K, et al. Development of the communication complexity scale. Am J Speech Lang Pathol. 2012; 21(1):16–28

[4] Rowland C, Fried-Oken M. Communication matrix: a clinical and research assessment tool targeting children with severe communication disorders. J Pediatr Rehab Med. 2010; 3:319–329

39 A Profound Phonological Disorder in a Preschooler

Jennifer St. Clair

39.1 Introduction

Children with profound phonological disorders are unintelligible to both familiar and unfamiliar listeners. These children typically produce speech containing only a few vowels and consonants. They often have difficulty producing multiple classes of sounds and regularly omit parts of syllable/word shapes.

39.2 Clinical History and Description

BM was a 4-year, 2-month-old male. Pregnancy and his birth history were remarkable for delivery at 35 weeks via cesarean section. He weighed 5 lb, 5 oz, but was not hospitalized following birth. BM crawled at 5 months, walked at 11 months, and ran at 15 months. His first word was noted at 19 months. At the time of testing, BM's parents reported that he combined words "rarely" and usually used "one word at a time." His parents reported that BM understood "almost all" of what was said to him. He typically used gestures and "grunting" to communicate his needs and wants. He had a reported vocabulary of 15 words and he was only 50% intelligible.

39.3 Clinical Testing

Assessment was completed in a university clinic setting and conducted by graduate student clinicians under the supervision of a speech-language pathologist. The assessment included parent interview, oral-motor examination, and administration of the Preschool Language Scales-5 (PLS-5) and Hodson Assessment of Phonological Patterns-3 (HAPP-3) as well as a spontaneous language sample.

Oral-motor examination revealed no abnormalities. BM obtained an average standard score of 102 on the Auditory Comprehension subtest of the PLS-5. The Expressive Communication subtest was attempted, but aborted due to increased frustration exhibited by BM. For example, after one, typically unintelligible attempt at answering a given item, he refused to repeat his response. Testing was ceased on this subtest because the examiners felt the score would be influenced by BM's unintelligibility; his scores would not be representative of his ability. The HAPP-3 revealed > 40% occurrence in the following areas: consonant sequences/clusters (115%), postvocalic singletons (94%), liquids (100%), stridents (100%), and velars (100%). These scores were consistent with a severity rating of "profound."

A spontaneous language sample revealed a mean length of utterance of 1.2, with an estimated 20% intelligibility to unfamiliar listeners. His phonemic inventory consisted of the vowels /i/, /o/, /ɪ/, and /ʌ/ and the consonants /h/, /m/, /t/, and /p/. He was able to follow all age-appropriate verbal directions and appeared to understand all that was said to him by both the examiners and his parents. He exhibited immediate frustration when the listener failed to understand what he said or when he was asked to repeat himself.

39.4 Questions and Answers for the Reader

1. What diagnosis is most appropriate for BM?
   a) Expressive language disorder.
   b) Phonological disorder.
   c) Childhood apraxia of speech (CAS).
   d) Receptive language disorder.

Answer: b is correct. He exhibited difficulties with classes of sounds that affect word shape and intelligibility.

a is incorrect. Although an expressive language disorder cannot be ruled out at this point, there is not enough evidence to support this diagnosis. He was unable to complete the expressive portion of the PLS-4 due to frustration and unintelligibility. Expressive language should be reassessed at a later time when intelligibility has increased and frustration decreased.

c is incorrect. He exhibited none of the hallmarks of CAS. He did not exhibit groping, inconsistency, or significant difficulty with vowels.

d is incorrect. His scores were within the average range for auditory comprehension. In addition, at no time did his parents or evaluators indicate difficulty with receptive language.

2. What type of therapy would be most appropriate?
   a) Hodson's cycles approach.
   b) Traditional articulation approach.
   c) Core vocabulary approach.
   d) All of the above.

Answer: a is correct. Expressive language disorder is correct because of the severity and number of potential targets. A Hodson's cycles approach would target multiple sounds at a time by targeting the missing classes of sounds. Syllable shape would also be potential targets. Targets would be rotated on a weekly basis, which would lead to greater overall intelligibility at a more rapid pace than targeting one phoneme at a time.

b is incorrect. A traditional articulation approach would target each individual phoneme until mastery, which would be a very slow approach, given the number of potential targets and his level of frustration.

c is incorrect. Core vocabulary approach is typically used for clients with inconsistent errors. BM's errors are consistent, so this would not be appropriate for him.

d is incorrect. For the reasons listed above for answer b and c.

3. What two targets should be addressed first?
   a) Liquids and velars.
   b) Velars and stridents.
   c) Final consonant deletion (FCD) and liquids.
   d) FCD and consonant sequences/clusters.

Answer: d is correct. Targeting these two first will create the greatest change in intelligibility. Since he exhibited frustration quickly, giving him success quickly is paramount. intelligibility increases the most if the word/syllable shape is correct, even if the phonemes are produced incorrectly.

b is incorrect. Velars and stridents will not impact intelligibility as effectively as FCD and consonant sequences/clusters.

c is incorrect. Liquids are not appropriate targets for his age.

a is incorrect. Liquids are not appropriate targets for his age.

4. Are familiar or unfamiliar listeners more valuable when determining intelligibility?
   a) Familiar listener percentage is more valuable.
   b) Unfamiliar listener percentage is more valuable.
   c) They are both equally important.
   d) Neither is important; the test scores are the only important aspect.

Answer: c is correct. One is not more important than the other. They both give valuable information in determining the diagnosis and severity. Both scores provide a more accurate picture of actual severity. These scores also help when showing progress.

a is incorrect. If the percentage for familiar listeners was the only one taken into consideration, the outcomes are typically skewed toward more intelligible.

b is incorrect. If the percentage for unfamiliar listeners was the only one taken into consideration, the outcomes are typically skewed toward less intelligible.

d is incorrect. Test scores alone should never be considered. Additional information must be considered to accurately capture performance.

39.5 Description of Problem and Recommended Treatment

BM was found to have a profound phonological disorder characterized by difficulty in the word/syllable shapes, containing final consonants and consonant sequences/clusters as well as the classes of liquids, velars, and stridents. He was 50% intelligible to familiar listeners and 20% intelligible to unfamiliar listeners. His phonemic inventory consisted of the vowels /i/, /o/,

/ɪ/, and /ʌ/ and the consonants /h/, /m/, /t/, and /p/. Frustration was high when listeners did not understand him. No evidence of receptive or expressive language disorders was observed.

It was recommended that BM receive 90 minutes of therapy per week. A Hodson's cycles approach (minimum of 3, 10-week cycles) was recommended in a small group setting.

39.6 Outcome

BM received five cycles (10 weeks each) following a modified Hodson's cycles approach. Every week a different target (e.g., consonant sequences/clusters, FCD, liquids, velars, and stridents) was addressed. These targets were rotated based on previous testing. On the 10th week of each cycle, the HAPP-3 was administered to assess progress and determine targets for the following cycle(see ▶ Table 39.1). The percentage of occurrence reflecting progress across the five cycles is reflected in.

Therapy was child-directed, following a modified Hodson's cycles approach. Each session followed the following schedule:
• Listening time (BM listened, through amplification, to a list of target words).
• Pretest (assessment of BM's productions of the target words).
• Activity time (BM-directed therapy using age-appropriate toys, working with the target words as much as possible).
• Phonological awareness focus (group reading from a book containing multiple examples of BM's target).
• Listening time (BM listened, through amplification, to a list of target words).
• Posttest (assessment of BM's productions of the target words).

At the end of therapy, at the age of 5 years, 8 months, BM was 90% intelligible to unfamiliar listeners and 100% intelligible to familiar listeners. He had no expressive or receptive language difficulties. The PLS-5 was readministered at 5 years, 6 months and BM achieved scores in the average range in auditory comprehension (standard score [SS] = 108) and expressive communication (SS = 98). At discharge from therapy, BM had residual errors on /r/ and /l/.

Table 39.1

	Percentages of occurrence					
Dates of administration	10/6 Pretherapy	12/5 End of cycle 1	3/2 End of cycle 2	6/3 End of cycle 3	8/26 End of cycle 4	12/4 End of cycle 5
Consonant sequences/clusters	115	104	104	84	55	38
Postvocalic singletons (FCD)	94	90	80	50	30	10
Liquids	100	100	100	80	75	60
Velars	100	90	95	80	60	25
Stridents	100	95	80	60	45	20
Severity rating	Profound	Profound	Severe	Severe	Moderate	Mild

Performance on HAPP-3 at the end of each 10-week cycle.

39.7 Key Points

- Poor expressive language scores in phonologically disordered children are not always indicative of an expressive language disorder.
- When picking targets, it is important to focus on what will make the biggest impact on intelligibility.
- Upon reaching 100% intelligibility, children who were severely phonologically impaired may still have residual errors on /r/ and /l/.

Suggested Readings

[1] Crosbie S, Holm A, Dodd B. Intervention for children with severe speech disorder: a comparison of two approaches. Int J Lang Commun Disord. 2005; 40 (4):467–491

[2] Hodson BW. Enhancing phonological patterns of young children with highly unintelligible speech. ASHA Lead. 2011; 16:16–19

[3] Hodson B, Paden E. Targeting Intelligible Speech: A Phonological Approach to Remediation. 2nd ed. Austin, TX: Pro-Ed; 1991

[4] Rudolph JM, Wendt O. The efficacy of the cycles approach: a multiple baseline design. J Commun Disord. 2014; 47:1–16

40 Childhood Motor Speech Disorders in a Child with 7q11.23 Duplication Syndrome

Shelley L. Velleman, Myra J. Huffman, and Carolyn B. Mervis

40.1 Introduction

Childhood apraxia of speech (CAS) and childhood dysarthria (CD) often co-occur, especially in children with neurodevelopmental syndromes, making differential diagnosis and intervention challenging.

40.2 Clinical History and Description

DC was a female child enrolled in a longitudinal study of children with 7q11.23 duplication syndrome, a genetic disorder characterized by CAS, symptoms of CD (e.g., low muscle tone), and social anxiety at the age of 2.2 years. DC lived with her mother, one younger brother, and two older half-brothers. Her mother was a supportive advocate for DC and sought opportunities to ensure that her communication, developmental, and educational needs were met. Her speech, language, and cognitive abilities were evaluated five times between the ages of 2.2 and 8.9 years.

40.3 Clinical Testing

At the age of 2.2 years, the Mullen Scales of Early Learning[1] was the only formal assessment administered. DC's visual reception (nonverbal reasoning) and receptive language T-scores were in the average range for children her age. However, her fine motor T-score was borderline and her expressive language T-score was at floor level (< 1st percentile). Based on her mother's responses on the MacArthur–Bates Communicative Development Inventory: Words and Sentences,[2] DC's spontaneous (nonimitated) expressive vocabulary included seven items: two spoken words and five manual signs (< 1st percentile).

Speech samples were collected during free play with her mother and an interactive play/diagnostic therapy session. DC vocalized rarely. When she did speak, it was typically quiet, although she was loud at times. She was noted to be hypersensitive to touch in the oral area and to avoid contact with certain food textures. Her mother reported that DC occasionally silently mouthed long sequences of syllables. She displayed a tendency to rest her tongue on her lower lip, occasionally skewed to the right. She also presented with an asymmetric lip retraction (i.e., smile), and although she was able to achieve lip closure, she was not able to retract or protrude them adequately for tense vowels (e.g., [i] and [u]). She produced four recognizable word approximations: "mmhmm" (for "yes"), "uh-oh," "mommy," and "meow." She was not stimulable for other words or most other syllables, although she did imitate some sound effects (e.g., the voiceless bilabial fricative [ɸ] as a pouring noise) and the syllable [bæ], once each. Most of DC's utterances were

either a consonant (mostly [m]) or a vowel. In addition, she used prosody overlaid on long nasalized vowels, protest vocalizations ([ʔʌʔʌʔ]), fake crying, grunts, a few signs, gestures, and other body language to communicate. Her phonetic repertoires at the age of 2.2 years are shown in ▶ Table 40.1.

Despite these limitations, DC laughed appropriately, nodded her head yes, pointed to objects both to express interest and to request, followed simple directions, took turns in conversations, and engaged in simple pretend play. At times, she combined two signals (e.g., gesture and vocalization) to communicate a more complex message. When a book was handed to her, DC turned it right-side up and pointed at individual pictures.

Table 40.1 Phonetic repertoires at age 2.2 years

	Initial	Medial	Final
Consonants	m, ʔ	m, ʔ	ʔ
Vowels	ɪ, ə, ʌ, æ, ʊ		

40.4 Questions and Answers for the Reader

1. Appropriate communication sample analyses for a 2- to 3-year-old include:
   a) Phonetic repertoires.
   b) Phonotactic repertoire.
   c) Functional use of prosody.
   d) Functional use of other communication modalities.
   e) All of the above.

Answer: e is correct. For a communication sample evaluation to be complete, all of a to d should be included.

a is correct, but incomplete. Typically developing English-learning children are expected to have about 10 consonants by age 2 years,[3] about half of which occur in final as well as initial position.[4] They should have about 12 different consonants by age 3 years.[3] Failure to develop a sufficient number of phones raises red flags about possible delay or disorder.

b is correct, but incomplete. Having the sounds expected for one's age is not enough; one must also be able to combine them flexibly into a variety of syllable and word shapes. According to Stoel-Gammon,[4] all typically developing English-learning 2-year-olds have CV (consonant-vowel) and CVC syllables; most have CVCV and CVCVC words as well. About half have at least some consonant clusters. By 42 months, at least some clusters should be used, even if they are not accurate (e.g., [tw] instead of [tɹ]).[5]

c is correct, but incomplete. Prosody is the first aspect of speech that young infants recognize and produce. By 18 months, their pitch patterns already match those of the ambient language[6] and they use some aspects of intonation to mark grammatical functions,[7] although their intonation is not yet adultlike even at age 3 years.[8]

d is correct, but incomplete. Communicative gestures, facial expressions, and other body language (leading, mime, etc.) typically precede or coemerge with the onset of meaningful words. In fact, they appear to lay the groundwork not only for words but also for two-word combinations.[9] For children with speech delay, nonoral signals are vital communication tools to supplement the spoken word. Children who lack communicative intent are at risk of social-pragmatic disorders, such as autism spectrum disorder.

2. Primary symptoms of CD include the following:
   a) Poor transitions between consonants and vowels.
   b) Groping of articulators.
   c) Imprecise consonant closures.
   d) Phonotactic errors more predominant than phonetic errors.
   e) Mis-stressed multisyllabic words.

Answer: c is correct. The imprecision results from low muscle tone, which leads to difficulty achieving complete consonant closures and may result in frication of stops, for example.[10]

a is incorrect. This is a symptom of CAS, resulting from impaired motor planning and programming.

b is incorrect. This is a symptom of CAS, resulting from impaired motor planning and programming.

d is incorrect. This is a symptom of CAS, resulting from impaired motor planning and programming.

e is incorrect. This is a symptom of CAS, resulting from impaired motor planning and programming.

3. Primary symptoms of CAS include the following:
   a) Choppiness due to segregated syllables or words.
   b) Decreased volume.
   c) Frication of stops.
   d) Poor quality of phonation.
   e) Decreased ability to produce prolonged vowel sounds.

Answer: a is correct. This is a result of impaired motor planning and programming. It appears that each sound, syllable, or word (depending upon the degree of impairment) is planned individually, with inappropriate pauses between productions of the units, as the next chunk of speech is planned.[11]

b is incorrect. This is a symptom of CD, resulting from low muscle tone.[10] Of course, some children may speak quietly for other reasons.

c is incorrect. This is a symptom of CD, resulting from low muscle tone.[8]

d is incorrect. This is a symptom of CD, resulting from poor neural coordination of muscle contractions.[10]

e is incorrect. This is a symptom of CD, resulting from low muscle tone.[12]

4. Therapy recommendations for speech–sound disorders, including motor speech disorders, include all of the following except:
   a) Many trials per session.
   b) Nonspeech oral motor exercises.
   c) Delayed, inconsistent feedback to ensure skill mastery.
   d) Consistent feedback for new skills.
   e) Variable stimuli and random trials to ensure skill mastery.

Answer: b is correct. It is *not* a recommended approach for speech–sound intervention. Research has shown that neurological control for speech is distinct from neurological control for nonspeech functions, such as chewing and blowing. The developmental progressions of these two functions also differ. There is no current research evidence supporting the use of nonspeech oral motor activities to improve speech production.[13,14]

a is incorrect. It *is* a recommended strategy. More motor practice yields more complete learning.[15]

c is incorrect. It *is* a recommended strategy. Delayed, inconsistent feedback encourages the child to rely more and more on his/her own self-monitoring and feedback systems, which yields more complete learning.[16]

d is incorrect. It *is* a recommended strategy. When a skill is initially being taught, the learner needs more consistent feedback until his/her own self-monitoring and feedback systems begin to develop.[16]

e is incorrect. It *is* a recommended strategy. Real communication situations are varied and unpredictable. Therefore, to be able to generalize new skills functionally, we must practice them with variable stimuli and with trials of different sorts intermixed.[17,18]

40.5 Description of Disorder and Recommended Treatment

At the age of 2.2 years, DC's speech disorder was profound. However, communicative intent was a relative strength. Intervention included modeling simple vocalizations, including emotion words ("ow, ooh, wow, haha") and key words and phrases ("mine, no, stop it, more, go") in predictable routines (book reading, songs, daily activities). Continued use of manual sign and the addition of picture communication were also encouraged to decrease frustration and increase conventional communication. Occupational therapy was recommended to determine the potential efficacy of tactile cues such as those provided in the Prompts for Restructuring Oral Muscular Phonetic Targets (PROMPT) approach[19] despite her tactile defensiveness.

40.6 Outcome

DC was reevaluated at the age of 3.2 years following 1 year of intervention. On the Mullen Scales, visual reception (nonverbal reasoning) and receptive language T-scores continued in the average range and her expressive language T-score, although at the first percentile, was no longer at floor. Again, she was observed playing with her mother as well as in a diagnostic therapy session. DC's lips were sometimes parted and sometimes closed as she chewed with a mostly rotary chew. She cleared a spoon full of pudding with her lips but did not lick off pudding from around her lips. She sipped juice from a straw with no leakage. She engaged in pretend and cause–effect play and made excellent eye contact. DC's linguistic progress was striking: she now produced approximately 40 different recognizable imitated and spontaneous words. Many, but not l-break/>all, vocalizations were whispered or quite quiet. She produced one two-word utterance, "baby hand." DC's consonant and vowel repertoires also had expanded considerably, as shown in ▶ Table 40.2.

Table 40.2 Phonetic repertoires at age 3.2 years

	Initial	Medial	Final
Consonants	b, p, d, t, g, k	p, d, k, ?	b, p, d, t, k, ?
	n	m, n	m, n
	w, j	f, s, ʃ	f
	f, dʒ, tʃ		
Vowels	i, ɪ, e, ɛ, æ, u, ʊ, o, ɑ, ʌ		
	ɑɪ, ɑʊ		

However, she continued to demonstrate weak lip-rounding for [w] and word productions were inconsistent. Although her syllable shapes were predominantly CV (consonant + vowel), she produced quite a few final consonants (i.e., CVC syllable shapes) as well. Most of DC's words were one to two syllables in length. Two-syllable words tended to be produced with a slight pause between syllables (e.g., [gɑ.di] for "doggie;" [bɑ.dɛ] for "bottle"). She produced one internal consonant sequence (CVCCVC) twice, in the word "backpack," which appeared to be articulated with careful effort. DC also demonstrated the ability to incorporate prosodic elements into one-word utterances to express communicative intent such as questions, comments, and commands.

DC's symptoms suggested a combination of at least two motor speech disorders. Symptoms of CD included slow speech, low muscle tone in her lips, asymmetry of the lips and tongue, and some delays in feeding skills. Symptoms of CAS included a limited phonotactic repertoire, segregated syllables, inconsistency, and effortful speech. However, due to her limited expressive vocabulary, neither diagnosis was made at age 3.2 years. DC's social interaction and play skills, however, were strong.

At the age of 3.2 years, adults were encouraged to expand DC's utterances, provide her fill-in-the-blank prompts ("The wheels on the bus go ___"), and model simple complete grammatical utterances in a repetitive manner (e.g., "Look, there's a dog. He's a big dog. The dog is running fast. Wow, he's a fast dog!"). It was also suggested that DC be given choices between a desired object or activity and an undesirable one, ideally with the two objects held near the adult's face to encourage her to take advantage of visual modeling of the correct word.

DC was next evaluated at the age of 4.2 years. The Verbal Motor Production Assessment for Children (VMPAC)[20] was attempted, but she was not compliant. Her score on the Assessment of Phonological Patterns-3 (HAPP-3)[21] fell below the first percentile. DC spoke words and phrases in a slow and effortful, but prosodically natural, manner. She demonstrated groping, inconsistency, vowel distortions, atypical error patterns, and poor control of voicing. Coarticulation and reduction across words within phrases were also noted (e.g., [tɝ-nəigɑn] for "Turn the heaton;" [wʌ dɪ?nʌnʌms] for "Wantit num-nums"). Although she was resistant to tactile cues on her face, she responded well to gestural cues and to tactile cues performed on the examiner or in the air. A diagnosis of CAS, with symptoms of CD, was made.

At the age of 5.7 years, DC produced multisyllabic words with equalized stress and complete sentences with atypical pauses. Inconsistency, atypical patterns, vowel deviations, effort, and groping all persisted, confirming the diagnosis of CAS. Symptoms of dysarthria also persisted, including immature chewing, imprecise consonant production, inability to move the tongue laterally, persistent breathiness, decreased pitch range, and

decreased velar control with nasal leakage. She completed the VMPAC with difficulty, scoring within the severe range in all areas: global motor control (general and specific movement systems supporting speech production), focal oral motor control (volitional movement control of the jaw, lips/face, and tongue), sequencing (nonspeech and speech movement sequencing), connected speech and language control (words, phrases, and sentences), and speech characteristics (pitch control, vocal resonance, vocal quality, loudness, prosody, and rate). On the Goldman–Fristoe Test of Articulation-2 (GFTA-2),[22] she achieved a standard score of 75, at the fourth percentile for her age. Her HAPP-3 score again fell below the first percentile. The Comprehensive Test of Phonological Processing-2 (CTOPP-2)[23] was given to assess her reading readiness. She scored at the sixth percentile on phonological awareness and third percentile on phonological memory. Syllable control practice,[24,25] articulatory gesture practice (e.g., *Moving across Syllables* by Kirkpatrick et al.[26]), and backward buildups in conjunction with explicit practice of word stress, sentence stress, and pausing within sentences[24] were recommended.

DC was most recently reevaluated at the age of 8.9 years. Although she continued to progress in all areas, she had not caught up to her peers in most areas. Her General Conceptual Ability (GCA; similar to IQ) on the Differential Ability Scales-II (DAS-II)[27] was in the borderline range, with nonverbal reasoning within the low average range and verbal skills in the borderline range. Her standard scores for receptive vocabulary as measured by the Peabody Picture Vocabulary Test-4 (PPVT-4)[28] and expressive vocabulary as measured by the Expressive Vocabulary Test-2 (EVT-2)[29] were in the low average range. On the Clinical Evaluation of Language Fundamentals-5 (CELF-5),[30] DC's performance varied widely as a function of the subtest; she scored in the average range on the formulated sentences and recall of sentences subtests, in the borderline range on sentence comprehension, and in the low range on word structure, linguistic concepts, and following directions. On the CTOPP-2, DC demonstrated some gains, with phonological awareness and phonological memory now both at the 14th percentile (low average range). On the Wechsler Individual Achievement Test-III (WIAT-III),[31] DC's single-word reading and passage reading accuracies were within the average to low average range for children her age. Her pseudoword decoding, oral reading rate, and reading comprehension were considerably weaker, with standard scores in the borderline range. On the VMPAC, DC continued to score in the severe range in all areas except speech control, on which she demonstrated improvement except for control of prosody, which affected her intelligibility. DC now exhibited some inappropriate compensatory strategies for cueing her articulators; she self-cued her tongue to move using her left index finger on her teeth or her fist pressed into her cheekbone. She occasionally stabilized her jaw by biting her lip and speaking through this gesture, which resulted in distorted speech. Her eyes widened when her jaw moved in an apparently unplanned direction. Her sentences were longer and more grammatically appropriate than previously observed, but syntactic as well as speech–sound errors persisted. Her score on the GFTA-2 fell to below the first percentile relative to children her age. She continued to have difficulty contrasting front ([d] and [t]) with back consonants ([g] and [k]) and moving from continuant (e.g., [s], [f]) to stopping sounds (e.g., [t], [p]) and back again in sentences. Given the severity and atypicality of her speech–sound disorder, it was recommended that DC continue to receive intensive speech-language therapy to improve consistency and accuracy of speech–sound production. Suggestions included achieving stable oral postures for speaking tasks without using overt compensatory self-cueing strategies by practicing simple repetitive sequences (e.g., [babababababa]) with smooth direct jaw-opening and jaw-closing movements, increasing her flexible use of prosodic features in conversation, and mastering consistent use of age-appropriate speech sounds in words. Intensive systematic phonics instruction with additional instruction focused on reading comprehension also was strongly advised.

40.7 Key Points

- CAS and CD often co-occur, especially in children with neurodevelopmental syndromes.
- Although progress in therapy is expected with appropriate intervention, CAS is a long-term disorder associated with language and literacy difficulties as well as oral motor, motor speech, and speech deficits.
- Appropriate compensatory strategies must be taught as these children tend to develop inappropriate strategies that draw unfortunate attention to themselves.

40.8 Acknowledgments

This case is part of a larger dataset on 7q11.23 duplication syndrome research supported by the Simons Foundation (238896) and the National Institute of Child Health and Human Development (R37 HD29957). We acknowledge the child and her mother, as well as the current and former members of the Neurodevelopmental Sciences Laboratory at the University of Louisville for their participation in this project.

Suggested Readings

[1] Lewis BA, Freebairn LA, Hansen AJ, Iyengar SK, Taylor HG. School-age follow-up of children with childhood apraxia of speech. Lang Speech Hear Serv Sch. 2004; 35(2):122–140

[2] Velleman SL, Mervis CB. Children with 7q11.23 duplication syndrome: speech, language, cognitive, and behavioral characteristics and their implications for intervention. Perspect Lang Learn Educ. 2011; 18(3):108–116

[3] Wetherby AM, Prizant B. Communication and Symbolic Behavior Scales Developmental Profile. Baltimore, MD: Brookes; 2002

[4] Dale PS, Hayden DA. Treating speech subsystems in childhood apraxia of speech with tactual input: the PROMPT approach. Speech Lang Pathol. 2013; 22:644–661

References

[1] Mullen EM. Mullen Scales of Early Learning. Circle Pines, MN: American Guidance Service; 1995

[2] Fenson L, Marchman VA, Thal DJ, Dale PS, Reznick JS, Bates E. MacArthur-Bates Communicative Development Inventories: User's Guide and Technical Manual. 2nd ed. Baltimore, MD: Brookes; 2007

[3] McIntosh B, Dodd B. Two-year-olds' phonological acquisition: normative data. Speech Lang Pathol. 2008; 10(6):460–469

[4] Stoel-Gammon C. Phonolical skills of 2-year-olds. Lang Speech Hear Serv Sch. 1987; 18:323–329

[5] Smit AB, Hand L, Freilinger JJ, Bernthal JE, Bird A. The Iowa articulation norms project and its Nebraska replication. J Speech Hear Disord. 1990; 55(4):779–798

[6] Hallé PA, de Boysson-Bardies B, Vihman MM. Beginnings of prosodic organization: intonation and duration patterns of disyllables produced by Japanese and French infants. Lang Speech. 1991; 34(Pt 4):299–318

[7] Branigan G. Some reasons why successive single word utterances are not. J Child Lang. 1979; 6(3):411–421

[8] Loeb DF, Allen GD. Preschoolers' imitation of intonation contours. J Speech Hear Res. 1993; 36(1):4–13

[9] Iverson JM, Goldin-Meadow S. Gesture paves the way for language development. Psychol Sci. 2005; 16(5):367–371

[10] Pennington L, Parker NK, Kelly H, Miller N. Speech therapy for children with dysarthria acquired before three years of age. Cochrane Database Syst Rev. 2016; 7(7):CD006937

[11] ASHA. Childhood Apraxia of Speech [Technical Report]. Rockville Pike, MD: American Speech-Language-Hearing Association; 2007

[12] Thoonen G, Maassen B, Gabreels F, Schreuder R. Validity of maximum performance tasks to diagnose motor speech disorders in children. Clin Linguist Phon. 1999; 13(1):1–23

[13] Forrest K. Are oral-motor exercises useful in the treatment of phonological/articulatory disorders? Semin Speech Lang. 2002; 23(1):15–26

[14] McCauley RJ, Strand E, Lof GL, Schooling T, Frymark T. Evidence-based systematic review: effects of nonspeech oral motor exercises on speech. Am J Speech Lang Pathol. 2009; 18(4):343–360

[15] Edeal DM, Gildersleeve-Neumann CE. The importance of production frequency in therapy for childhood apraxia of speech. Am Speech-Lang Pathol. 2011; 20(2):95–110

[16] Maas E, Robin DA, Austermann Hula SN, et al. Principles of motor learning in treatment of motor speech disorders. Am J Speech Lang Pathol. 2008; 17(3):277–298

[17] Skelton SL. Concurrent task sequencing in single-phoneme phonologic treatment and generalization. J Commun Disord. 2004; 37(2):131–155

[18] Skelton SL, Hagopian AL. Using randomized variable practice in the treatment of childhood apraxia of speech. Am J Speech Lang Pathol. 2014; 23(4):599–611

[19] Hayden D. The PROMPT model: use and application for children with mixed phonological-motor impairment. Adv Speech-Lang Pathol. 2006; 8(3):265–281

[20] Hayden D, Square P. Verbal Motor Production Assessment for Children (VMPAC). San Antonio, TX: Psychological Corporation; 1999

[21] Hodson BW. Hodson Assessment of Phonological Patterns (HAPP-3). 3rd ed. East Moline, IL: LinguiSystems; 2004.

[22] Goldman R, Fristoe M. Goldman-Fristoe Test of Articulation-Second Edition (GFTA-2). Circle Pines, MN: American Guidance Service; 2000

[23] Wagner RK, Torgeson JK, Rashotte CA, Pearson NA. Comprehensive Test of Phonological Processing-2 (CTOPP-2). Austin, TX: Pro-Ed; 2013

[24] Velleman SL. Resource guide for Childhood Apraxia of Speech. Florence, KY: Cengage; 2003

[25] Thomas DC, McCabe P, Ballard KJ. Rapid syllable transitions (ReST) treatment for childhood apraxia of speech: the effect of lower-dose frequency. J Commun Disord. 2014; 51:29–42

[26] Kirkpatrick J, Stohr P, Kimbrough D. Moving across syllables. Tucson, AZ: Communication Skill Builders; 1990

[27] Elliott CD. Differential Ability Scales-II. San Antonio, TX: Psychological Corporation; 2007

[28] Dunn LM, Dunn DM. Peabody Picture Vocabulary Test-4 (PPVT-4). Minneapolis, MN: Pearson Assessments; 2007

[29] Williams KT. Expressive Vocabulary Test-2. Minneapolis, MN: Pearson Assessments; 2007

[30] Wiig EH, Semel EM, Secord WA. Clinical Evaluation of Language Fundamentals-5. San Antonio, TX: Pearson; 2013

[31] Wechsler D. Wechsler Individual Achievement Test-III. San Antonio, TX: Pearson; 2009

41 Prioritizing Clinical Decisions in a Complex Medical Case

Erin Embry

41.1 Introduction

Often in clinical practice, speech-language pathologists are faced with individuals who present with multiple cooccurring impairments, complicating the process related to differential diagnosis and the selection of priority intervention goals. This case report highlights the challenges of that process for a 65-year-old woman who experienced a left middle cerebral artery cerebrovascular accident (MCA CVA) (▶ Fig. 41.1) and provides systematic, clinical decision-making guidelines based on evidence-based approaches.

41.2 Clinical History and Description

BR was a 65-year-old woman admitted to an urban center emergency department with bilateral pleural effusion. She was treated with diuretics and Coumadin on admission. The following day, she was found unresponsive with aphasia, left gaze preference, right facial droop, and right-sided posturing upon noxious stimulation. A computed tomography of the head showed no bleed but an early left MCA CVA. BR was within the appropriate time window for tissue plasminogen activator, a protein used to break down blood clots. However, due to her high National Institutes of Health Stroke Scale (NIHSS) score of 28 (▶ Fig. 41.2), she was deemed to not be a candidate.

A percutaneous endoscopic gastrostomy (PEG) tube, as opposed to a nasogastric tube, was placed to deliver nutrition due to inconsistent alertness. Magnetic resonance imaging revealed a patchy subacute hemorrhage and peripheral laminar necrosis in the parietal and frontal lobe white matter within an evolving large left MCA infarct with midline shift. After 2 weeks in acute care, BR was medically stable. Following a fiberoptic endoscopic evaluation of swallow (FEES) at bedside, she was advanced to a soft chewable diet with thin liquids. Her impairments were primarily associated with the oral preparatory and oral phases of the swallow. She was still largely nonverbal with a dense right hemiparesis. BR was then transferred to the inpatient rehabilitation unit for intensive speech, occupational, and physical therapy.

Prior to admission, BR's past medical history included newly diagnosed atrial fibrillation and congestive heart failure as well as a history of mild depression, smoking, and social alcohol use. Her discharge plan was to return home with her husband and continued care, as needed.

41.3 Clinical Testing

Given the size of the CVA, in conjunction with premorbid diffuse white matter necrosis, BR presented with multiple issues related to communication, cognition, and swallowing. Even though BR was reportedly tolerating a soft diet with thin liquids safely, overall oral intake was limited and a subsequent clinical swallowing evaluation was performed upon admission to the rehabilitation unit to assess any potential change in swallow function. An oral motor examination was discontinued as BR was unable to follow basic commands. Evidence of oral motor apraxia was observed for nonspeech tasks. At rest, BR presented with significant right-sided facial/labial asymmetry. Dentition was natural and complete. Intake of food/liquids was more spontaneous; BR was trialed with pureed and soft chewable solids only due to oral motor weakness and reduced range of motion. Labial containment was adequate; mild delays noted in bolus formation and propulsion and improved in timeliness with an increased number of trials; a seemingly timely reflexive swallow and adequate hyolaryngeal rise with all textures. Minimal oral residue with soft solids was noted in the right lateral sulci post swallow, likely due to sensory impairment. It was recommended that BR remain on her current diet with a calorie count and continued tube feed supplements as needed.

Comprehensive evaluation of speech, language, and cognition was performed to establish baseline measures and to implement a basic system for communication. Given BR's limited responses to single-step commands and reduced verbal output, nonstandardized measures were used to evaluate basic expressive and receptive language skills in lieu of formal testing.

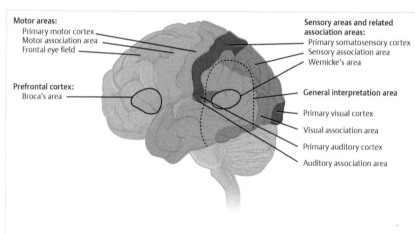

Motor areas:
Primary motor cortex
Motor association area
Frontal eye field

Prefrontal cortex:
Broca's area

Sensory areas and related association areas:
Primary somatosensory cortex
Sensory association area
Wernicke's area

General interpretation area

Primary visual cortex

Visual association area

Primary auditory cortex

Auditory association area

Fig. 41.1 Motor cortex and sensory cortex of the brain and surrounding areas.

N I H
STROKE
SCALE

Patient Identification. ___ ___-___ ___ ___-___ ___ ___

Pt. Date of Birth ___ ___/___ ___/___ ___

Hospital _____(___ ___-___ ___)

Date of Exam ___ ___/___ ___/___ ___

Interval: [ ] Baseline   [ ] 2 hours post treatment   [ ] 24 hours post onset of symptoms ±20 minutes   [ ] 7-10 days
[ ] 3 months   [ ] Other_____(___ ___)

Time: ___ ___:___ ___   [ ] am [ ] pm

Person Administering Scale _____

Administer stroke scale items in the order listed. Record performance in each category after each subscale exam. Do not go back and change scores. Follow directions provided for each exam technique. Scores should reflect what the patient does, not what the clinician thinks the patient can do. The clinician should record answers while administering the exam and work quickly. Except where indicated, the patient should not be coached (i.e., repeated requests to patient to make a special effort).

Instructions	Scale Definition	Score
1a. Level of Consciousness: The investigator must choose a response if a full evaluation is prevented by such obstacles as an endotracheal tube, language barrier, orotracheal trauma/bandages. A 3 is scored only if the patient makes no movement (other than reflexive posturing) in response to noxious stimulation.	0 = **Alert;** keenly responsive. 1 = **Not alert;** but arousable by minor stimulation to obey, answer, or respond. 2 = **Not alert;** requires repeated stimulation to attend, or is obtunded and requires strong or painful stimulation to make movements (not stereotyped). 3 = Responds only with reflex motor or autonomic effects or totally unresponsive, flaccid, and areflexic.	_____
1b. LOC Questions: The patient is asked the month and his/her age. The answer must be correct - there is no partial credit for being close. Aphasic and stuporous patients who do not comprehend the questions will score 2. Patients unable to speak because of endotracheal intubation, orotracheal trauma, severe dysarthria from any cause, language barrier, or any other problem not secondary to aphasia are given a 1. It is important that only the initial answer be graded and that the examiner not "help" the patient with verbal or non-verbal cues.	0 = **Answers** both questions correctly. 1 = **Answers** one question correctly. 2 = **Answers** neither question correctly.	_____
1c. LOC Commands: The patient is asked to open and close the eyes and then to grip and release the non-paretic hand. Substitute another one step command if the hands cannot be used. Credit is given if an unequivocal attempt is made but not completed due to weakness. If the patient does not respond to command, the task should be demonstrated to him or her (pantomime), and the result scored (i.e., follows none, one or two commands). Patients with trauma, amputation, or other physical impediments should be given suitable one-step commands. Only the first attempt is scored.	0 = **Performs** both tasks correctly. 1 = **Performs** one task correctly. 2 = **Performs** neither task correctly.	_____
2. Best Gaze: Only horizontal eye movements will be tested. Voluntary or reflexive (oculocephalic) eye movements will be scored, but caloric testing is not done. If the patient has a conjugate deviation of the eyes that can be overcome by voluntary or reflexive activity, the score will be 1. If a patient has an isolated peripheral nerve paresis (CN III, IV or VI), score a 1. Gaze is testable in all aphasic patients. Patients with ocular trauma, bandages, pre-existing blindness, or other disorder of visual acuity or fields should be tested with reflexive movements, and a choice made by the investigator. Establishing eye contact and then moving about the patient from side to side will occasionally clarify the presence of a partial gaze palsy.	0 = **Normal.** 1 = **Partial gaze palsy;** gaze is abnormal in one or both eyes, but forced deviation or total gaze paresis is not present. 2 = **Forced deviation,** or total gaze paresis not overcome by the oculocephalic maneuver.	_____

Fig. 41.2 National Institutes of Health Stroke Scale.

N I H
STROKE
SCALE

Patient Identification. ___ _. ___ _. ___ ___ ___

Pt. Date of Birth ___ ___ / ___ / ___ ___

Hospital _____ (___ _. ___)

Date of Exam ___ ___ / ___ / ___ ___

Interval: [ ] Baseline   [ ] 2 hours post treatment   [ ] 24 hours post onset of symptoms ±20 minutes   [ ] 7-10 days
[ ] 3 months   [ ] Other _____ (___ ___)

3. Visual: Visual fields (upper and lower quadrants) are tested by confrontation, using finger counting or visual threat, as appropriate. Patients may be encouraged, but if they look at the side of the moving fingers appropriately, this can be scored as normal. If there is unilateral blindness or enucleation, visual fields in the remaining eye are scored. Score 1 only if a clear-cut asymmetry, including quadrantanopia, is found. If patient is blind from any cause, score 3. Double simultaneous stimulation is performed at this point. If there is extinction, patient receives a 1, and the results are used to respond to item 11.	0 = **No visual loss.** 1 = **Partial hemianopia.** 2 = **Complete hemianopia.** 3 = **Bilateral hemianopia** (blind including cortical blindness).	_____
4. Facial Palsy: Ask – or use pantomime to encourage – the patient to show teeth or raise eyebrows and close eyes. Score symmetry of grimace in response to noxious stimuli in the poorly responsive or non-comprehending patient. If facial trauma/bandages, orotracheal tube, tape or other physical barriers obscure the face, these should be removed to the extent possible.	0 = **Normal** symmetrical movements. 1 = **Minor paralysis** (flattened nasolabial fold, asymmetry on smiling). 2 = **Partial paralysis** (total or near-total paralysis of lower face). 3 = **Complete paralysis** of one or both sides (absence of facial movement in the upper and lower face).	_____
5. Motor Arm: The limb is placed in the appropriate position: extend the arms (palms down) 90 degrees (if sitting) or 45 degrees (if supine). Drift is scored if the arm falls before 10 seconds. The aphasic patient is encouraged using urgency in the voice and pantomime, but not noxious stimulation. Each limb is tested in turn, beginning with the non-paretic arm. Only in the case of amputation or joint fusion at the shoulder, the examiner should record the score as untestable (UN), and clearly write the explanation for this choice.	0 = **No drift;** limb holds 90 (or 45) degrees for full 10 seconds. 1 = **Drift;** limb holds 90 (or 45) degrees, but drifts down before full 10 seconds; does not hit bed or other support. 2 = **Some effort against gravity;** limb cannot get to or maintain (if cued) 90 (or 45) degrees, drifts down to bed, but has some effort against gravity. 3 = **No effort against gravity;** limb falls. 4 = **No movement.** UN = **Amputation** or joint fusion, explain: _____ 5a. **Left Arm** 5b. **Right Arm**	 _____ _____
6. Motor Leg: The limb is placed in the appropriate position: hold the leg at 30 degrees (always tested supine). Drift is scored if the leg falls before 5 seconds. The aphasic patient is encouraged using urgency in the voice and pantomime, but not noxious stimulation. Each limb is tested in turn, beginning with the non-paretic leg. Only in the case of amputation or joint fusion at the hip, the examiner should record the score as untestable (UN), and clearly write the explanation for this choice.	0 = **No drift;** leg holds 30-degree position for full 5 seconds. 1 = **Drift;** leg falls by the end of the 5-second period but does not hit bed. 2 = **Some effort against gravity;** leg falls to bed by 5 seconds, but has some effort against gravity. 3 = **No effort against gravity;** leg falls to bed immediately. 4 = **No movement.** UN = **Amputation** or joint fusion, explain: _____ 6a. **Left Leg** 6b. **Right Leg**	 _____

Rev 10/1/2003

The following baseline data were obtained for receptive language skills: responses to simple yes/no questions pertaining to self/environment (via pointing to written word or head nod) = 2/10 (20%); following simple one-step directions = 3/10 (30% with visual cue only); identification of body parts = 0/5; and identification of real, functional objects in field of two = 1/10 (10%). The following baseline data were obtained for expressive language skills: automatized sequences (e.g., days of week, ABCs, Happy Birthday, etc.) = 0/5, although evidence of melody to support songs and rhythm was emerging; patient spontaneously responded "Oh God" in response to failed attempts at various tasks; repetition of CV/CVC words with visual prompt = 0/5; and required hand-over-hand assist to initiate pointing of picture representations of basic wants and needs.

In addition to difficulty with CV/CVC word repetition, BR could not imitate more reflexive vocalizations such as coughing, sighing, or throat clearing. Further, significant articulatory groping was observed when attempting to produce speech. Although assessment of BR's cognitive functioning was limited due to language and speech impairments, overall sustained attention to structured tasks was reduced and BR required cues for redirection after an average of 25 seconds. Significant inattention to the left visual field was also observed. Insight into current impairments was beginning to emerge as BR exhibited a high level of frustration with failed attempts to communicate.

41.4 Questions and Answers for the Reader

1. What is the significance of a score of 28 on the NIHSS? What does this mean in terms of prognosis?

Answer: The NIHSS is a standardized protocol used by physicians to quantify the severity and functional impacts of stroke. The score integrates components of the neurologic exam including cranial nerves (visual), motor, sensory, cerebellar, inattention, language, and loss of consciousness. Scores greater than 15 to 20 are considered more severe and are associated with less than 20% good or excellent outcome.[1]

2. BR presents with multiple cooccurring impairments. How would you determine the priority for evaluation and treatment for a patient who presents with deficits in swallowing and all modalities of communication?

Answer: Safety is a priority in patient care and guides both the evaluation and treatment process. In the acute care stages, if swallowing is compromised and puts him/her at risk for either aspiration or inadequate nutrition and/or hydration, the most immediate need is to determine the cause of the problem and implement a plan of care that allows the patient to safely tolerate the least restrictive textures while meeting hydration and nutrition needs. If the patient is medically stable, the next step in the process shifts to establishing the most effective method for the patient to communicate basic wants and needs to his/her caregivers and hospital staff. Approaches are highly variable and based on individual patient needs. More often than not, both the evaluation and treatment processes typically address individual and overlapping skills simultaneously in an attempt

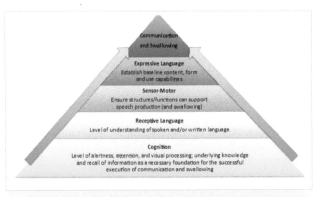

Fig. 41.3 Assessment and treatment hierarchy for complex patients.

to obtain a differential diagnosis, keeping in mind that the clinical presentation at this stage may rapidly evolve. For a patient who is essentially nonverbal with limited communicative intent, the clinician must proceed with an awareness of the underlying cognitive processes that support each domain. Remediation of these skills will be based on a hierarchal approach, beginning with comprehension (written and/or reading) and progressing to a focus on motor speech production and language expression (spoken and/or written) (▶ Fig. 41.3).

3. A swallow study (FEES) was initially performed while BR was on the acute care unit, but not repeated on the rehabilitation unit. Why was instrumental assessment of swallowing not repeated?
   a) A minimum of 2 weeks in between testing is required.
   b) BR's swallow difficulties were primarily limited to the oral preparatory/oral phase and decisions to advance her diet could be safely determined based on clinical findings.
   c) It was unlikely that the patient made any functional gains in 2 weeks.
   d) BR could not tolerate a follow-up FEES secondary to decreased alertness and/or arousal.

Answer: b is correct. Per the FEES performed while on the acute care unit, BR's primary impairments were associated with the oral preparatory and oral phases of swallow, while the pharyngeal phase was determined to be within functional limits with no observed penetration or aspiration. The risk for aspiration with more viscous textures is significantly reduced and, as a result, the clinician can proceed with a certain level of confidence that any dietary advancement can be safely recommended without additional instrumental assessment.

a is incorrect. Although a clinician should always consider patient safety and endurance levels and then carefully determine the actual need and/or benefits for a follow-up examination within that time frame, there is no contraindication to performing a second FEES within 2 weeks (like there may be for videofluoroscopy).

c is incorrect. BR was medically stable and transferred to the inpatient rehabilitation unit. Progress was slow due to the size and location of the stroke, but improvement in swallow function was reported and BR remained in the acute phase when spontaneous neurological gains were a strong possibility.

d is incorrect. This information was not explicitly reported, although a transfer from the acute care unit to an inpatient rehabilitation unit typically requires patients to be able to tolerate a minimum of 3 hours of therapy daily.

4. Based on BR's presentation, what recommendation(s) would you provide to the team and caregivers as the most effective approach to facilitate communication?
   a) Alternative/augmentative communication.
   b) Framing questions in yes/no format.
   c) Framing questions in choice format.
   d) Gestures and/or visual choices.
   e) Writing information down.

Answer: All of the above are correct. Continuing to provide BR with a multimodal approach to communication in the acute care phase is beneficial as it offers a variety of opportunities that may not have initially been successful during the evaluation, but have the potential to evolve as her status becomes more stable. It is important to note that while each of these approaches has merit, they should be based on her strengths and introduced systematically. Based on the initial evaluation, BR would likely achieve the highest level of success responding to structured yes/no questions followed by choice questions to indicate her basic wants and needs. These responses would be strengthened if coupled with visual cues such as gestures and the use of real/pictured objects. Written supports might also be beneficial, although her level of comprehension of written words has yet to be determined and, therefore, cannot be used in isolation. However, alternative forms of communication such as a basic picture board would be another potential supplemental approach until verbal expression improves. Independence with this approach would be challenging due to the coexisting ideational and motor apraxia that limits accuracy with pointing.

41.5 Diagnosis and Recommended Treatment

BR presented with multiple impairments: mild oropharyngeal dysphagia characterized by difficulty managing hard solids due to oral motor weakness and oral apraxia and global aphasia with a cooccurring severe verbal apraxia. Evidence of cognitive impairments in the area of attention and executive functioning was also noted. Differential diagnosis of speech versus language versus cognitive impairments proved difficult in the initial stages, although given reported ideational and motor apraxia by physical and occupational therapy, it was suspected that motor impairments were greater than language impairments, which were likely more impaired than cognition. In addition, due to oral motor weakness, dysarthria was likely present, although it could not yet be determined secondary to limited verbal output. BR consistently exhibited frustration with unsuccessful attempts to communicate, spontaneously responding with "Oh God" in these instances. Given BR's presentation, all basic wants and needs were to be anticipated and facilitated by staff and family.

Since BR was safely tolerating a solid diet with thin liquids and receiving supplemental nutrition/hydration via PEG tube as needed, the focus of treatment shifted to attempting to establish a basic system of communication between her and her family and hospital staff. The presence of cognitive impairments coupled with severe motor apraxia impacted BR's initiation and coordination for both speech production and pointing and limited BR's candidacy for a basic picture board to independently communicate. Therefore, a multimodal approach that focused first on improving auditory comprehension using functional pictures and stimulus items representing target sound classes in the initial position of words was implemented while simultaneously training with a basic picture and yes/no communication board for daily interactions. Treatment for improved speech production was based on principles of motor learning infused with traditional apraxia remediation approaches with the intended consequence that oral sensorimotor swallow function would also improve. Training of compensatory, postural, and/or therapeutic swallow techniques was not an option.

Patient and family education, counseling, and training were ongoing as the discharge plan was to return home with family support and additional hired care and therapy as needed.

41.6 Outcome

By the end of her 4-week stay in acute inpatient rehabilitation, BR was tolerating a mechanical soft diet with thin liquids and her feeding tube was removed. Comprehension of verbal direction, object identification, and social conversation in highly contextual situations had improved but was still impaired for noncontextual situations and abstract information. Verbal output minimally increased but was limited to single words that were imprecise due to both altered speech rate and precision. Repetition of CV/CVC words was inconsistent at 20% and accuracy of yes/no responses doubled to 40% using a combination of verbal, gestural, and written responses.

The most salient barrier to therapeutic progress, however, was depression resulting in a lack of motivation and reduced participation in all therapies. Cotreatments were scheduled to maximize therapy and to promote more opportunities for positive social interactions. BR was resistant to using a communication board other than a laminated yes/no response board. Her family was trained on modification of communication approaches to simultaneously promote yes/no responses while reducing frustration levels. BR was an avid dog lover and pet therapy was incorporated in therapy sessions when possible. Despite all efforts, the entire team agreed that BR did not meet her full potential for success while in rehab and she was discharged home with her family. Additional hired supports and continued therapy were provided by both a home care agency and private therapists.

41.7 Key Points

- Individuals who experience a stroke present differently depending on their health history, activity level, educational background, and severity of the infarct.
- When faced with a patient with multiple therapeutic needs with regard to cognitive-communication and swallow function, as with any evaluation and treatment plan, safety is the primary target for intervention.

- Progress for individuals who present with cooccurring impairments is often slow. The frequency and structure of treatment sessions, types of stimulus items selected, the nature of the feedback, and patient motivation are key prognostic indicators to help patients regain and/or compensate for deficits.

Suggested Readings

[1] Teasell R, Hussein N. Evidence-based review of stroke rehabilitation: clinical consequences of stroke. Last updated November 2013. http://www.ebrsr.com/sites/default/files/chapter2_clinical-consequences_final_16ed.pdf

[2] Maas E, Robin DA, Austermann Hula SN, et al. Principles of motor learning in treatment of motor speech disorders. Am J Speech Lang Pathol. 2008; 17(3): 277–298

[3] Wambaugh JL, Duffy JR, McNeil MR, et al. Treatment guidelines for acquired apraxia of speech: a synthesis and evaluation of the evidence. J Med Speech-Lang Pathol. 2006; 14(2):15–34

[4] Alexander MP, Lovreso F. A specific treatment for global aphasia. In: 21st Clinical Aphasiology Conference Proceedings. Austin, TX: Pro-Ed; 1993:277–289

References

[1] Adams HP, Jr, Davis PH, Leira EC, et al. Baseline NIH Stroke Scale score strongly predicts outcome after stroke: a report of the Trial of Org 10172 in Acute Stroke Treatment (TOAST). Neurology. 1999; 53(1):126–131

42 Transfeminine Voice Training

Christie Block

42.1 Introduction

This case report outlines an approach to feminine voice training by addressing the gender expression needs of a transgender woman.

42.2 Clinical History and Description

Z is a 27-year-old transgender woman who sought to increase the feminine features of her voice. She was assigned male at birth, has identified as female since early childhood, and has gender dysphoria (i.e., distress resulting from the mismatch between sex assignment and gender identity). She felt that her voice was not congruent with her gender identity and was the primary reason for being misgendered by others (i.e., incorrectly assumed to have a masculine gender identity). She was not concerned about her use of language; she felt it was sufficiently feminine. Z has presented with increasing feminine gender expression, full-time, for approximately 12 months including clothing, hair, and make-up. Her vocal load was moderate. She is a hair stylist and frequents loud bars and restaurants three to four times per week. She reported temporary hoarseness after going out and occasional difficulty being heard in loud environments. She was taking no medications, but she planned to start hormone replacement therapy in the coming month. She had no plans for surgery related to gender expression and was otherwise healthy. She weighed 125 pounds at 5 feet, 5 inches tall.

42.3 Clinical Testing

Perceptual observations were made on a variety of voice and speech parameters. Glottal fry, which resulted from mildly reduced breath control, was observed primarily at the end of approximately 25% of utterances. Vocal strain was also observed at pitches above 200 Hz. Intonation patterns were primarily downward and staccato-like. Resonance was focused more in the chest than in the face and head. Speech rate was unremarkable. Z successfully followed multiple cues and employed feedback modalities during diagnostic training tasks.

Acoustic measurement and analysis of sustained phonation and connected speech were conducted using commercially available speech analysis software, a stopwatch, a sound level meter, and manual calculations. Fundamental frequency (F_0) was 134 Hz and mean conversational frequency range was 15 semitones (86–213 Hz). Maximum phonation frequency range was 35 ST (103–770 Hz). Jitter and shimmer were 0.6 and 2.6%, respectively, at 133 Hz. Mean intensity during connected speech was 69 dB. Maximum phonation time was 21 seconds at 137 Hz. Spectral analysis indicated no vocal dysfunction. Last, videostroboscopy was performed, and laryngeal pathology was ruled out.

42.4 Questions and Answers for the Reader

1. The role of the speech-language pathologist (SLP) for training Z in feminine voice techniques includes:
   a) Using one's personal view of how a woman should act.
   b) Addressing Z's technical voice skills only, and referring to a psychotherapist for all related counseling.
   c) Specifying various services she should receive for transitioning.
   d) Guiding Z with techniques that are based on known gender norms in accordance with Z's needs.
   e) Confirming that Z has gender dysphoria.

Answer: d is correct. The SLP should use what is known about gender markers in voice and speech, based on biological differences and social expectations, to help Z feel more natural in her communication style and that will more likely be interpreted as feminine by others.

a is incorrect. The kind of woman Z should be is determined by Z, not the SLP. The clinician should use tools to assist Z achieve her own style of expression that allows her to reflect her individuality.

b is incorrect. As with any voice client, the clinician should not shy away from providing counseling that links feelings with communication skills so that understanding and overall satisfaction can be maximized. This may include discussions about (1) the connection between the client's changing voice and her gender identity, (2) acceptance of her best possible voice, and (3) managing situations when she is misgendered because of her voice. Psychotherapy referral is recommended only if distress or confusion regarding gender identity beyond voice is observed, or any related or unrelated mental health issues such as depression or anxiety become evident.

c is incorrect. Transgender needs are diverse. No predetermined set of transition services are required for transgender people. Transgender health providers, including SLPs, are resources for educating clients on what services exist.

e is incorrect. The SLP should assist Z change her gender expression regardless of whether she has gender dysphoria. The diagnosis of gender dysphoria is made by a mental health provider, not an SLP.

2. Z's glottal fry, vocal strain, hoarseness, and loudness level problems should:
   a) Not be addressed, since there was no vocal pathology shown on videostroboscopy.
   b) Be addressed and completely resolved before starting feminine voice training.
   c) Be addressed concurrently with feminine voice training.
   d) Be addressed by a laryngologist.
   e) Be addressed primarily by vocal hygiene instructions.

Answer: c is correct. In Z's case, exercises that increase feminine voice features can be integrated concurrently with vocal warm-up and rehabilitative tasks that address and resolve dysphonia.

a is incorrect. Dysphonia should be addressed even though no vocal pathology was observed on videostroboscopy. The goal of intervention is to alter her voice. The lack of findings on videostroboscopy does not preclude the need for intervention to address her vocal symptoms. Furthermore, her current dysphonia could worsen and/or lead to vocal fold pathology without appropriate guidance.

b is incorrect. Because Z's dysphonia was intermittent and vocal pathology was ruled out by videostroboscopy, there is no need to delay addressing Z's main complaint of feminine expression, which has a more negative impact on her life as long as the dysphonia is mild and can be addressed during treatment.

d is incorrect. Z's dysphonia appears to be behavioral, without any necessary medical or surgical intervention, and is thus treated by an SLP rather than a laryngologist.

e is incorrect. Though vocal hygiene instructions are important to include in treating Z's dysphonia, vocal warm-up and rehabilitative exercises should be primary.

3. More feminine resonance should be targeted through exercises that:
   a) Elicit more forward placement.
   b) Increase the size of the oral cavity.
   c) Lower the larynx.
   d) Change the length of the vocal folds.
   e) Lower the base of tongue.

Answer: a is correct. Forward placement of resonant energy in the mask of the face can result in a "smaller" or "brighter" tone that is considered to be more feminine.

b is incorrect. When the size of the oral cavity is increased, the resonance can sound "bigger" or more masculine.

c is incorrect. Lowering the larynx can lower pitch by reducing vocal fold tension. It can also create more masculine resonance, rather than feminine, by creating more space in the neck.

d is incorrect. Modifying the length of the vocal folds can affect pitch but not resonance.

e is incorrect. Lowering the base of tongue increases the size of the oral cavity, which results in more masculine resonance.

4. Z's prognosis for increasing feminine voice patterns to improve communication is:
   a) Excellent, because she is highly motivated.
   b) Very good, because of her current skills and current life situation.
   c) Good, because she will start hormone replacement therapy soon.
   d) Fair, because she has not opted for pitch-raising phonosurgery.
   e) Fair-to-poor, because, as a transgender person, Z faces physical limitations and uncontrollable reactions from others.

Answer: b is correct. Z has potential to sound feminine enough to meet her needs to feel more congruent and be gendered

correctly in most situations. This determination is based on (1) baseline F_0 that is on the higher end of normal for males, (2) relatively small body size, (3) the ability to practice and use her skills in daily life immediately, and (4) responsiveness to diagnostic therapy tasks during testing.

a is incorrect. Although motivation is an important factor for progress, it is not the only factor that determines eventual success in therapy.

c is incorrect. Hormone replacement therapy for transfeminine individuals has no known effect on voice. In contrast, testosterone therapy for transmasculine individuals has been shown to lower pitch.

d is incorrect. Behavioral training for transgender women is typically sufficient to elicit increasingly feminine communication. Pitch-raising surgery addresses one aspect of feminine speaking and is associated with widely varying client satisfaction.

e is incorrect. Physical limitations and uncontrollable reactions from others may limit Z's potential success in communicating with others. However, the positive factors far outweigh these negative factors. First, Z's current skills and life situation indicate that she will be able to modify her voice significantly and utilize these changes in her daily activities. Second, the task of increasing more feminine voice patterns is not as daunting as it could be, since there is significant overlap between feminine and masculine patterns as well as a variety of techniques that can be employed. Third, even small changes could make a positive impact on Z's life. Even though the possibility of being misgendered will not be eliminated, the chances of it happening could be reduced to a fraction of what it was before training.

42.5 Description of Problem and Recommended Treatment

Z presented with a masculine voice characterized by decreased pitch (134 Hz F_0), decreased conversational pitch range (86–213 Hz), primarily downward and staccato-like intonation, and chest resonance. In addition, her voice was characterized by glottal fry and strain. Z also reported episodes of worsening hoarseness and increased difficulty being heard in loud environments.

Z was seen for six skill-building sessions over 9 weeks followed by three maintenance sessions over 11 months. Her dysphonia was addressed concurrently with feminine voice training through vocal hygiene directives, vocal warm-up, rehabilitative breath control tasks, and semi-occluded vocal tract exercises. Because pitch is considered the most important factor for gender determination, it was the primary target for intervention. G3 (196 Hz) was used as a target average F_0 which is two semitones below the average female F_0 (224 Hz at 20–29 years of age) and four semitones above the lowest perceptual threshold for feminine pitch (155 Hz). Intonation was addressed through more overall expressiveness, including wider pitch movement and more legato-like or stretched vowels on stressed words. Resonance was addressed through more forward placement in the mask of the face to develop a "smaller" or "brighter" tone. As Z progressed to higher linguistic levels,

Numbering	Audio 1	Audio 2	Audio 3
Title	Before training	Session 4, week 7	Session 9, week 53
Description	Rainbow passage, 134 Hz	Rainbow passage, 180 Hz	Rainbow passage, 190 Hz
Duration	18 seconds	19 seconds	18 seconds

phrasing was introduced to allow her to reset pitch consistently over longer periods. Loudness was subsequently addressed with breath control and diaphragmatic breathing techniques to maintain feminine voice in loud environments and prevent voice deterioration.

Audio and visual feedback tools and recordings were employed to facilitate consistency of techniques, increase vocal awareness, and monitor therapeutic progress. Z was assigned daily homework as well as mindfulness strategies for carryover to daily life. Throughout therapy, Z was counseled extensively regarding voice and mind–body connection, such as identity development, risk-taking, empowerment, and acceptance of her best possible voice.

42.6 Outcome

Z improved on all targets within 9 weeks and maintained that improvement out to 13 months with continued morning vocal warm-up and mindfulness of voice techniques during daily interactions. Her F_0 increased to 180 Hz by the fourth session (week 7) and to 190 Hz at the end of training (ninth session, week 53). Her resonance shifted to a more forward placement and her intonation was more legato with a wider range. Glottal fry was eliminated almost completely and Z reported having no more difficulty speaking over noise. At the last session, Z reported that she was very happy with her progress, which has allowed her to lead a more fulfilling life, with less risk for negative reaction from others: "I hear my voice, and I think 'oh, what a sigh of relief!'"

42.7 Key Points

- Transgender voice training involves teaching multiple technical skills as well as extensive counseling related to the mind–body connection.
- Lead by the client's needs and interests for gender expression, the SLP uses known gender norms to guide the client in formulating an individualized skill set that she/he identifies with.
- It is possible to make a significant impact in the daily life of a transgender client, even with small voice changes, and this change can be done relatively quickly if the client is presenting full-time and has good responsiveness to training tasks.
- Dysphonia should be addressed either before or concurrently with feminine voice training, depending on the severity of the dysphonia.
- Transgender voice training requires advanced skills in voice and voice disorders as well as a deep understanding of transgender health, experience, and diversity.

Suggested Readings

[1] Adler RK, Hirsch S, Mordaunt M, eds. Voice and Communication Therapy for the Transgender/Transsexual Client: A Comprehensive Clinical Guide. 2nd ed. San Diego, CA: Plural Publishing; 2012

[2] Block C. Finding our voices, literally. In: Erickson-Schroth L, Ed. Trans Bodies Trans Selves. New York, NY: Oxford University Press; 2014:128

[3] Coleman E, Bockting W, Botzer M, et al. Standards of care for the health of transsexual, transgender, and gender nonconforming people, version 7. Int J Transgenderism. 2011; 13:165–232

[4] Davies S, Papp V, Antoni C. Voice and communication for gender non-conforming individuals: Giving voice to the person inside. Int J Transgenderism. 2015; 16(3):117–159

43 Cognitive Rehabilitation following Severe Traumatic Brain Injury

Joanna Close

43.1 Introduction

Along with physical, sensory, and behavior difficulties, traumatic brain injury (TBI) can impair cognitive function and communication, all of which can impair an individual's ability to function independently. Changes in cognition may occur in the areas of attention, memory/learning, and executive function such as planning, organizing, initiating, goal setting, problem solving, and self-awareness. Communication deficits can be characterized by difficulties in understanding or expressing both spoken and written language, or in the areas of pragmatics.

43.2 Clinical History and Description

PY was a 53-year-old man found unconscious for an unknown duration outside his home and taken by ambulance to the hospital. Imaging revealed left subdural hematoma (SDH), extensive subarachnoid hemorrhage, and right temporal bone fracture. He underwent emergency craniotomy for SDH evacuation in the context of a decreasing Glasgow Coma Scale score, reflecting a decline in his level of consciousness based on objective evaluation of eye, verbal, and motor responses. He remained in the acute hospital setting for 2 weeks, followed by 2 weeks in acute inpatient rehabilitation. His posttraumatic amnesia was estimated at more than 4 weeks.

43.3 Clinical Testing

The initial outpatient speech/language assessment took place more than 1.5 years following the acute brain trauma. Comprehensive evaluation included an extensive interview with PY and his daughter regarding his injury and course of recovery, ongoing cognitive-communication limitations, current routine and day-to-day activities, use of compensatory strategies, additional mitigating factors (e.g., poor sleep, symptoms of depression), and patient/family goals for rehabilitation.

Table 43.1 Pretreatment performance on the Repeatable Battery for Neuropsychological Status (RBANS); initial evaluation in the outpatient clinic nearly 1.5 years following PY's injury

	Index score	Percentile rank
Immediate memory	65	1st
Visuospatial/constructional	109	73rd
Language	75	5th
Attention	75	5th
Delayed memory	60	0.4th
Total scale	70	2nd

Prior to the injury, PY lived independently and was employed full time as a microchip-processing technician. Following the injury and subsequent recovery and rehabilitation, PY returned home to live with his wife and adult daughter. At the time of speech-language pathology (SLP) assessment, PY had not yet returned to work, but reported that employment was his primary goal. Although both he and his daughter reported significant improvement since his injury, he continued to require family assistance with many instrumental activities of daily living (IADLs) such as financial management, driving, shopping, meal preparation, and chores around the house. He primarily spent his time alone watching television, with weekly outings with family members.

PY initially denied cognitive-communication challenges, but ultimately reported having a difficult time "remembering stuff" including the television channels he preferred and the name of his dog. He also frequently forgot to eat at regular intervals. His daughter noted that she consistently observed PY having difficulty both initiating and completing tasks as well as decreased memory and word retrieval.

The Wechsler Test of Adult Reading (WTAR) and the Repeatable Battery for the Assessment of Neuropsychological Status (RBANS) were administered. His performance on the WTAR suggested premorbid intellectual functioning in the high average range (raw score = 44, standard score = 116). PY and his daughter each completed the Mayo-Portland Adaptability Inventory-4, Participation Index (M2PI) questionnaire to evaluate ability, activity, and social participation in patients following acquired brain injury. The results of the RBANS and M2PI are shown in ▶ Table 43.1 and ▶ Table 43.2, respectively.

43.4 Questions and Answers for the Reader

1. What additional standardized SLP assessment tools might be useful to guide treatment?
   a) Boston Naming Test (BNT).
   b) Montreal Cognitive Assessment (MoCA).
   c) Subjective rating scale.
   d) Formal driver's assessment.
   e) All of the above.

Table 43.2 Pretreatment patient and family member ratings (lower scores correlate to a higher level of independence) on a measure of social participation/overall level of disability, the Mayo-Portland Adaptability Inventory-4, Participation Index (M2PI); initial evaluation nearly 1.5 years following PY's injury

	Raw score	T score
PY	22	52
Daughter	21	50

Answer: a is correct. The BNT would likely provide more information about PY's difficulty with word retrieval, which was both reported by the patient and also noted by others.

b is incorrect. The MoCA is a cognitive *screening* tool, not a standardized assessment, and the RBANS provides more comprehensive information about cognitive function than the MoCA.

c is incorrect. Although a subjective rating scale might be useful to set treatment goals, it is not a standardized assessment.

d is incorrect. PY would likely benefit from driver rehabilitation, but this is typically addressed via occupational therapy (OT).

e is incorrect.

2. Given the results from the initial assessment, how would you characterize PY's deficits?
    a) Attention impairment.
    b) Language impairment.
    c) Memory impairment.
    d) Executive function impairment.
    e) All of the above.

Answer: c is correct. Based on initial formal and informal assessment, the most significant deficits are in the areas of memory and learning.

a, b, d, and e are incorrect. Although he did demonstrate difficulties with attention and language on standardized measures (performing in the fifth percentile rank in each domain), his performance on measures of immediate and delayed verbal recall reflected significant impairment (first and 0.4th percentile rank). Additionally, PY reported difficulty "remembering stuff."

3. What additional referrals to health care providers might you consider?
    a) Neuropsychology.
    b) Rehabilitation psychology.
    c) Sleep clinic.
    d) Vocational rehabilitation.
    e) All of the above.

Answer: e is correct. PY would benefit from referrals to neuropsychology, rehabilitation psychology, the sleep clinic, and vocational rehabilitation. Given the time since injury and PY's desire to return to employment, he would likely benefit from a more comprehensive neuropsychological assessment, which would also be useful to guide support from vocational rehabilitation. Given that cognitive-communication function and performance on standard assessment is sensitive to many factors, he might benefit from an intervention to address chronic insomnia and evaluation for possible depression; this would support a referral for formal sleep assessment and to a rehabilitation psychologist.

4. What cognitive rehabilitation approaches would you recommend initially?
    a) Environmental modifications.
    b) Direct attention training.
    c) Rote memory workbooks.

d) Assistive technology for cognition (ATC).
e) All of the above.

Answer: d is correct. Assistive technology for cognition has increasing evidence to support its effectiveness to improve independence and life participation for individuals with cognitive deficits. Given PY's memory impairment and dependence on his family for most of his IADLs, he would benefit from evaluation for a cognitive prosthesis.

a is incorrect. PY did not demonstrate significant need for environmental modifications to his physical space, such as labeling kitchen cupboards and drawers or establishing a filing system for paying bills.

b is incorrect. Given that PY's most severe deficits were in the memory domain, direct attention training such as Attention Process Training II (APT-II) would not be appropriate for mitigating his difficulties with immediate and delayed recall.

c is incorrect. Participation in rote memory tasks is not an evidence-based approach to cognitive remediation.

e is incorrect.

43.5 Description of Disorder and Recommended Treatment

PY performed below expectations on tests of processing speed, working memory, and semantic and phonemic verbal fluency, as well as immediate and delayed learning. PY demonstrated word-retrieval difficulties in conversation, poor initiation and planning, and reduced awareness and insight into his disabilities. His deficits were consistent with his injury and significantly impacted his general function and independence and life participation/quality of life. Treatment recommendations included both restorative and compensatory approaches. Initial treatment goals included evaluation for and training of ATC, development of a regular daily/weekly routine, increased activity, socialization and participation in ADLs, engagement in regular cognitive-linguistic stimulation, training word-retrieval strategies and semantic processing treatment activities, and components of goal management training.

43.6 Outcome

PY was seen a total of 36 times over the course of 14 months and demonstrated both objective and subjective gains in cognitive function and overall independence and life participation. During cognitive-communication therapy, PY learned to use and rely on an assistive device for technology to support memory (e.g., using an iPod/iPad to adhere to a regular routine, including home-related tasks and responsibilities, independent management of medical appointments, and regular participation in cognitively stimulating exercises) and wayfinding (e.g., smartphone GPS to support driving directions and geocaching). He independently employed word-retrieval strategies during conversation and reported subjective improvement in language output. He continued to struggle with cognitive inflexibility, goal setting, and problem solving. His daughter, however, reported improved

Table 43.3 PY's performance on the Repeatable Battery for Neuropsychological Status (RBANS) after 11 months of regular cognitive-communication therapy

	Index score	Percentile rank
Immediate memory	76	5th
Visuospatial/constructional	105	63rd
Language	79	8th
Attention	82	12th
Delayed memory	71	3rd
Total scale	78	7th

function initiating and completing more difficult home-related tasks (e.g., weekly meal planning and regular dinner preparation, installing new curtains). Overall, PY reported increased confidence in his cognitive functioning and reduced anxiety about his "new normal."

PY's gains following treatment were most significant with respect to his increased independence with ADLs, as reflected in pre- and posttreatment scores on the M2PI in ▶ Table 43.3 and ▶ Table 43.4. At discharge, PY was independently driving, shopping, and preparing meals, completing many home-related tasks, and managing his health and medical appointments, as well as becoming increasingly involved in social activities (e.g., brain injury support group, reengagement with geocaching club, weekly outings with friends and family). Although one of his initial goals was to return to his same employment, at discharge he had no plans to return to the workforce.

43.7 Key Points

- Comprehensive evaluation of patients with TBI should include extensive clinical interview with patient and family members in addition to standardized assessment instruments to collaboratively develop an individualized treatment plan and method for measuring progress.

Table 43.4 Following 7 months of regular cognitive-communication therapy, PY and his daughter noted functional improvements, as seen via ratings on a measure of social participation/overall level of disability, the Mayo-Portland Adaptability Inventory-4, Participation Index (M2PI); of note, a lower score correlates to a higher level of independence

	Raw score	T score
PY	8	37
Daughter	10	39

- Cognitive-communication therapy may incorporate both direct and indirect treatment approaches simultaneously, and draw on many other fields including aphasiology, counseling, OT, and neuropsychology.
- Therapy focused on training use of ATC must not only include the initial acquisition phase, but also emphasize generalization and maintenance to ensure continued use of the device to support optimal cognitive function.
- The success of cognitive-communication therapy may be measured via pre- and poststandardized assessment results, but should emphasize functional and patient-centered measures such as subjective reports, participation indices, or goal-attainment scaling to better reflect functional gains.

Suggested Readings

[1] Coelho C, Ylvisaker M, Turkstra LS. Nonstandardized assessment approaches for individuals with traumatic brain injuries. Semin Speech Lang. 2005; 26 (4):223–241

[2] Kennedy MR, Coelho C. Self-regulation after traumatic brain injury: a framework for intervention of memory and problem solving. Semin Speech Lang. 2005; 26(4):242–255

[3] Lewis VJ, Dell L, Matthews LR. Evaluating the feasibility of goal attainment scaling as a rehabilitation outcome measure for veterans. J Rehabil Med. 2013; 45(4):403–409

[4] Powell LE, Glang A, Ettel D, Todis B, Sohlberg MM, Albin R. Systematic instruction for individuals with acquired brain injury: results of a randomised controlled trial. Neuropsychol Rehabil. 2012; 22(1):85–112

[5] Sohlberg M, Turkstra L. Optimizing Cognitive Rehabilitation: Effective Instructional Methods. New York, NY: Guilford Press; 2011

44 Multiple Unmanaged Concussions in a Collegiate Rugby Athlete

Michael R. Fraas

44.1 Introduction

This case report discusses the management of an athlete with significant cognitive and emotional concerns following multiple concussions sustained playing collegiate rugby.

44.2 Clinical History and Description

A 21-year-old man, PP, studying physics at university reported to the Speech-Language and Hearing Clinic as a participant in a research study investigating sport-related concussions. PP arrived with his rugby teammates who were scheduled for pre-season baseline testing using a standard concussion assessment protocol that included concussion history, neurocognitive and balance testing, and symptom checklist. Following data collection, PP informed the lead investigator that, "I may be an outlier in your study," because he had received five concussions over the past 6 months playing rugby (▶ Table 44.1).

PP was diagnosed with depression at age 7 following the death of his father from cancer. In high school, he played football and wrestled. PP indicated that, "there were a lot of times where everything would go fuzzy, but I would just shake it off and keep playing." PP was a good student and graduated high school with a 3.7 GPA. He excelled in the sciences, but struggled with reading and writing. He acknowledged that he is close to his mother and friends, who provide him with strong emotional and social support. PP reported increased depression, anxiety, and cognitive difficulties as well as "emotional breakdowns" since his injuries.

Table 44.1 Concussion history over the course of a single season

Date of injury	Injury	Patient account
April 13, 2013	Kicked in the head	"Everything went black … but, I continued to play the rest of the game."
April 27, 2013	Knee to the head	"I got up slow and kept playing, until my head was hurting too much …. Then I came out."
April 28, 2013	"Bell rung"	"I didn't start this game, but a teammate broke his clavicle and I was put in the game … I got my bell rung a few times, but nothing too serious that I considered a concussion."
May 11, 2013	Head to head	"I instantly lost the feeling in the back left part of my skull, and blacked out for a brief moment."
September 23, 2013	Head to head	"We hit with less force than a typical hit, the next thing I remember, I was curled up face down on the turf. I opened my eyes but couldn't see anything."

With the fall quarter nearing completion, PP was instructed to maintain a schedule of mild cognitive and physical rest over the break and to report back to the clinic for a detailed clinical intake and cognitive evaluation at the start of the winter quarter. In January 2014, several days prior to the start of the quarter, PP was involved in an automobile accident resulting in his sixth concussion. PP denied hitting his head in the collision.

44.3 Clinical Testing

PP was evaluated by a neuropsychologist. It is important to note that these scores were obtained at the end of 2013, prior to his sixth concussion in January 2014. The following tests were administered and a summary of the results by cognitive domain is provided below: (1) Wechsler Adult Intelligence Scale-IV (WAIS-IV); (2) Wide Range Achievement Test-4; (3) Woodcock–Johnson III (WCJ-III) Tests of Cognitive Abilities (Concept Formation, Visual Matching, Numbers Reversed, and Decision Speed subtests); (4) California Verbal Learning Test-II; (5) Trail Making Test Parts A and B; (6) Wisconsin Card Sorting Test-64 (WCST-64); (7) Boston Naming Test (BNT); Controlled Oral Word Association Test (COWAT); (8) Beck Depression Inventory-2; and (9) the Oregon Concussion Awareness and Management Program (OCAMP) Post-Concussion Symptom Checklist.

44.3.1 Learning and Memory

Immediate recall of auditory information presented in a story was in the low average (25th percentile) range. His ability to recall this information after a 30-minute delay was in the average (50th percentile) range. Immediate recall of visual information related to day-to-day social activities was in the average (50th percentile) range. His ability to recall this information after a 30-minute delay was also in the average (63rd percentile) range.

44.3.2 Verbal and Nonverbal Reasoning, Concept Formation

On tests of perceptual reasoning (WAIS-IV) and concept formation (WCJ-III), PP's performance was average to above average.

44.3.3 Academic Functioning

On the Wide Range Achievement Test-4, PP obtained a word recognition score at the 37th percentile and a spelling score at the 23rd percentile.

44.3.4 Attention/Concentration

PP's working memory index from the WAIS-IV was in the average range (37th percentile). On the Digit Span subtest, he was able to repeat up to six digits forward fashion and up to four digits reverse, which is in the low average (25th percentile) range. His performances on a mental arithmetic task and on a task assessing visual working memory and attention (Spatial Span) were in the average (50th percentile) range.

44.3.5 Processing Speed, Executive Functioning, and Mental Flexibility

Processing speed was noted to be in the lower average (34th percentile) range on the WAIS-IV and below average on the WCJ-III. His ability to manipulate language symbols in a timed fashion was in the average (37th percentile) range. On a task assessing simple visual scanning and processing speed, performance was in the high average range. On a more complex version of this task, which also assesses mental flexibility, performance was in the average range. On a task of executive functioning, where individuals are required to complete test items in an unstructured environment (WCST-64), performance was in the low average range. The total number of errors was in the low average (18th percentile) range and the numbers of perseverative responses and perseverative errors were in the mildly impaired to low average (14th and 12th percentile) ranges, respectively.

44.3.6 Language Functioning

On tasks assessing verbal fluency (e.g., COWAT), performance was in the mildly impaired range. On a picture-naming task (BNT), performance was in the average range.

44.3.7 Emotional Functioning

PP was administered the Beck Depression Inventory-2 and obtained a score suggestive of moderate depression. He indicated areas related to feelings of sadness, discouragement, feelings of failure, anhedonia, loss of confidence, self-criticism, restlessness, difficulty making decisions, reduced energy, irritability, poor focus, and fatigue.

44.3.8 Concussion Symptoms

On the OCAMP Post-Concussion Symptom Checklist, participants indicate how much each of 23 symptoms has bothered them during the past 2 days. The symptoms are grouped into four categories, namely, Physical, Thinking, Sleep, and Emotional. In the Physical category, PP scored headache, fatigue, and numbness/tingling as severe. Within the same category, he scored dizziness, visual problems, and sensitivity to light and noise as moderately severe. In the Thinking category, PP scored all four symptoms (feeling mentally foggy, feeling slowed down, difficulty concentrating, and difficulty remembering) as severe. In the Sleep category, severe symptoms included drowsiness and sleeping more than usual. All four symptoms comprising the Emotional category (irritability, sadness, nervousness, and feeling more emotional) were scored as severe.

44.4 Questions and Answers for the Reader

1. A high school football player stumbles off the field in the first half of the game after receiving a "big hit." He did not lose consciousness but he fails the Sideline Concussion Assessment Tool administered by the athletic trainer (AT). At half time, he reports to the AT that he feels fine and is ready to go back into the game. Which of the following is the most appropriate decision for managing this athlete?
   a) The player knows best how he feels and should be allowed to make his own decision about when he is ready to return to the game.
   b) The player never lost consciousness; therefore, he never sustained a concussion. He should be cleared to return to play.
   c) The player should remain out for the remainder of the game. He should follow return-to-play guidelines and should only return to play following clearance from a medical practitioner trained in concussion management.
   d) He should sit out for the remainder of the game. If he is asymptomatic within 24 to 48 hours, he can return to full-contact practice.
   e) The athlete should report to the emergency department for an X-ray of his head. If the findings are negative for a concussion, he should be cleared to return to play.

Answer: c is correct. Guidelines have been established by the Concussion in Sport Group, which consists of medical and research specialists in the field of sport concussion. The guidelines outline safe and effective concussion management practices and include the following recommendations: (1) an athlete suspected of a concussion should be immediately removed from play and not allowed to return to play that day; (2) a graded return-to-play protocol should be implemented; (3) the athlete should not be allowed to return to play until a health practitioner trained in the management of concussions clears him or her. All 50 states have passed legislation that mandates similar recommendations.

a is incorrect. As many as 50% to 60% of concussions go unreported by athletes. The primary reasons for failing to report a concussion is that the athlete wanted to keep playing, he or she did not want to let their teammates down, or they did not realize they had a concussion.

b is incorrect. Loss of consciousness is not an indicator of concussion. Less than 10% of all concussions result in a loss of consciousness.

d is incorrect. It can take 7 to 10 days for the brain of a high-school-aged athlete to return to its normal level of functioning. The graded return-to-play protocol ensures that an athlete sits out a minimum of 7 days prior to clearance by a trained medical practitioner to return to play.

e is incorrect. The majority of concussions result in changes at the cellular level of the brain. Static imaging methods such as X-ray, computed tomography, or magnetic resonance imaging can only detect changes at the structural level. As a result, they are only capable of detecting the more severe concussions (e.g., those resulting in contusions or intercranial hemorrhages).

2. Which of the following statements about concussion is correct?
   a) Protective equipment (e.g., helmets and mouth guards) is effective in preventing concussion.
   b) Women are less likely to sustain a concussion than men.
   c) Sustaining one concussion does not elevate your risk of having another.
   d) There is no difference in concussion risk between athletes with a history of learning disabilities (LDs) or attention deficit hyperactivity disorder (ADHD) and those without a history of developmental disorders.
   e) None of these are correct.

Answer: e is correct. All of the previous choices were incorrect statements.

a is incorrect. There is no clinical evidence that currently available protective equipment will prevent concussion.[1] Biomechanical studies have shown a reduction in impact forces to the brain with the use of headgear and helmets, but these findings have not been translated to show a reduction in concussion incidence. Helmets have been found to reduce head (e.g., skull fracture) and facial injury in sports such as skiing, snowboarding, cycling, motor, and equestrian. Mouth guards have been found to protect against dental and orofacial injury. However, no studies have found a definitive reduction in concussions.

b is incorrect. There is evidence to indicate that females are more susceptible to concussions than males. In sports such as soccer, basketball, and softball/baseball, females have demonstrated higher rates of concussion compared to males. In addition, females perform worse on neuropsychological testing and report more symptoms following concussion than males. Females have also demonstrated protracted recovery times as compared to males.[2]

c is incorrect. There is an exponential increase in a person's risk for concussion following each subsequent injury. For an individual who has sustained one injury, their risk for a second concussion is one to two times greater. If a person has sustained two concussions, they are two to four times more likely to have a third, and if they have had three concussions, they are three to nine times more likely to have a fourth concussion.

d is incorrect. Recent findings have begun to demonstrate that individuals with a history of developmental disabilities such as ADHD and LD are more likely to sustain a concussion. They are also two to three times more likely of sustaining multiple concussions.[3] Individuals with a history of ADHD or LD also report more concussion symptoms and they perform worse on tests of neurocognitive function.

3. A 22-year-old female collegiate soccer player reports to a Speech-Language Pathology clinic with complaints of headache, memory problems, difficulty concentrating, and anxiety following two concussions sustained within 1 week of each other. Formal standardized cognitive testing determined the following: (1) she was within normal limits for problem solving, immediate and delayed auditory and verbal memory, visual-spatial awareness, and focused and sustained attention; (2) she demonstrated impaired selective, alternating, and divided attention, processing speed, and working memory. Which of the following would be a recommended treatment approach for addressing her deficits?

   a) Attention process training (APT).
   b) Errorless learning memory training.
   c) Scanning training to help increase focus.
   d) Time pressure management.
   e) a and d.

Answer: e is correct. Both APT and time pressure management are effective treatments for managing the deficits seen in this athlete.

a is correct. APT is a structured program that follows a hierarchically organized clinical theory of attention.[4] Tasks address all levels of attention processing, including focused, sustained, selective, alternating, and divided. APT focuses on generalization of skills throughout training and gradually progresses to novel contexts outside the clinic setting.

d is correct. Time pressure management utilizes a structured problem-solving strategy to compensate for mental slowness and deficits in higher levels of attention processing.[5]

b is incorrect. Errorless learning is a form of memory training that has been shown to be an effective method of learning for individuals with significant memory deficits following moderate-to-severe brain injury. Immediate and delayed memory performance was presumed to be within normal limits for the client.

c is incorrect. Scanning training can be an effective method for addressing focused and sustained attention, and for improving visual-spatial processing deficits. Neither of these was noted as problematic for the client.

44.5 Additional Testing

PP returned to the Speech-Language and Hearing clinic in January 2014 for a follow-up evaluation. Since he had been administered the Concussion Vital Signs computerized neuropsychological examination prior to his sixth concussion (i.e., the automobile accident), it was of interest to determine whether his performance changed. ▶ Table 44.2 displays PP's raw scores and subsequent converted percentile scores from October 2013, prior to the car accident, and from January 2014, 1 week following the accident.

Table 44.2 Computerized neuropsychological findings from two time periods

Cognitive domain	Time 1: October 2013		Time 2: January 2014	
	Score	%	Score	%
Verbal memory	41	1	39	1
Visual memory	47	47	37	37
Psychomotor speed	175	34	150	3
Executive function	49	42	28	6
Cognitive flexibility	46	34	25	1
Reaction time	735	5	942	1

As compared to normative data, PP's scores in October 2013 were in the average range for visual memory, psychomotor speed, executive functioning, and cognitive flexibility. His scores on reaction time were in the moderately impaired range, and verbal memory was severely impaired. Following the automobile accident, PP scored in the average range for visual memory, but his performance for psychomotor speed and executive function fell to the moderately impaired range, and verbal memory, cognitive flexibility, and reaction time fell within the severely impaired range.

44.6 Description of Disorder and Recommended Treatment

PP likely sustained multiple concussions throughout his high school and collegiate athletics career. Evidence from the sports literature indicates that each concussion sustained results in an elevated risk for a subsequent injury.[6,7] PP reported that his last rugby-related concussion resulted in hitting his head against that of a teammate, "with less force than a typical hit." In addition, PP denied hitting his head during his last concussion involving a motor vehicle accident. Concerns for PP's recovery center on the fact that multiple concussions have been linked to long-term deficits in neuropsychological function.[8,9]

Based on the evaluation findings from Neuropsychology and Speech-Language Pathology, and subjective reports from PP about his classroom performance concerns, several domains were targeted for cognitive rehabilitation. These targets include processing speed, executive function, higher levels of attention and working memory, and verbal memory. PP's reports of difficulty concentrating in the classroom, becoming easily distracted, overwhelmed, and frustrated, and word-finding difficulties lend support to the decision to target these domains.

Treatment was initiated two times per week for 50 minutes and followed a standard model for cognitive rehabilitation[4] consisting of three stages: Acquisition, Application, and Adaptation. During the Acquisition stage, PP was educated about concussions and how his injuries were contributing to his emotional and cognitive challenges. The clinician collaborated with PP to develop relevant and measureable goals to address his needs. During this initial stage, the clinician also explained to PP the cognitive strategies that would be used to address his deficits. These strategies included APT[4] to address sustained, selective, and alternating attention and deficits in working memory, time pressure management[5] to address issues related to processing speed, executive function, and attention, a memory strategy (PQRST) for recalling complex verbal and written information[10] was initiated as a means for generalizing his skills to the classroom, method of loci, a memory strategy for enhancing his verbal memory, and accommodations were set up through the university disability resource center to provide PP with additional support.

During the Application stage, PP began to apply the cognitive strategies in the clinic setting under the guidance and support of the clinician. The complexity of the treatment tasks gradually increased and the level of cueing began to fade as PP's performance progressed from session to session. The following provides a brief description of the treatments that were initiated.

44.6.1 Attention Process Training

This structured program follows a hierarchically organized clinical theory of attention. Following thorough assessment, treatment initiates with activities that match the areas of attention where the client functions suboptimally. APT focuses on generalization of skills throughout training and gradually progresses to novel contexts outside the clinic setting. In the case of PP, the goal was to transition from sustained, selective, and alternating attention drills in the clinic to activities such as reading textbooks or following a lecture without distraction.

44.6.2 Time Pressure Management

This strategy was chosen to address PP's challenges with slowed processing, which were leading to his sense of being overloaded. PP was taught to follow a problem-solving strategy to help him control and regulate information input. The strategy taught him how to develop a long-term plan to minimize his sense of being overloaded and short-term, moment-to-moment adjustments during the execution of a task. PP was particularly concerned with his difficulty reading, comprehending, and recalling large amounts of information. Therefore, the organizational memory strategy PQRST was implemented. The steps of PQRST include: preview the information to be recalled; ask key questions about the text; read the material carefully to answer the questions; state the answers; and test regularly for retention of the information. The strategy is self-instructional, promotes active learning, and engages elaboration and review of learned and remembered information.

PP learned to implement the method of loci strategy, which makes use of visual imagery to improve verbal memory skills. Target words are transformed into visual representations that are mentally linked with a different location in a well-known place, in this case, the rooms in PP's apartment.

Several classroom accommodations were set up for PP through the university disability resources center. These included a reduced course load, a note-taker during lectures, extended testing time, and extended due dates for assignments.

In the Adaptation stage, strategies learned in the application stage are applied to more functional and everyday tasks. The primary focus during this stage was to promote PP's success with comprehension and retention of reading assignments and with increasing his ability to sustain attention during lectures.

44.7 Outcome

Following two quarters of cognitive rehabilitation, PP reported that he was more attentive in the classroom, he was able to read and retain textbook content, his emotional outbursts were less frequent, he no longer experienced headaches, and he was able to manage a full-time (12-credit) course load. ▶ Table 44.3 displays PP's raw scores and subsequent converted percentile scores on computerized neuropsychological testing conducted at the end of treatment. PP demonstrated increased performance in all cognitive domains compared to testing conducted following his automobile accident. His scores in verbal memory, visual memory, and reaction time met or surpassed scores from initial baseline testing prior to the automobile accident. PP was able to graduate with a BS in physics 1 year after his originally scheduled graduation date.

Table 44.3 Computerized neuropsychological findings following cognitive rehabilitation

Cognitive domain	Time 3: June 2014	
	Score	%
Verbal memory	60	96
Visual memory	47	47
Psychomotor speed	158	12
Executive function	44	25
Cognitive flexibility	41	18
Reaction time	645	27

Throughout treatment, PP was educated and counseled about the seriousness of sustaining multiple concussions and the risk he faced if he returned to rugby. PP indicated that only one of his concussions was officially diagnosed, but it was clear from his description of the injuries that most were not well managed. The recommended course of management when an athlete is suspected of a concussion is to be removed from play immediately and not be allowed to return to play until cleared by a medical specialist trained in diagnosing and treating concussions.[11] It was recommended that PP not participate in rugby or any contact sport due to his elevated risk for further injury. Thankfully, PP had already come to the same conclusion and retired himself from further participation in high-risk sport.

PP's past medical history was significant for depression at age 7 when his father passed away from cancer. His current diagnosis of depression, anxiety, and difficulty with emotional regulation was cause for concern. Throughout the course of treatment, PP seemed to indicate increasing concern about his ability to control his emotions. PP was referred to a psychologist specializing in adolescent trauma. The clinician quickly identified issues related to the death of PP's father that were never fully addressed. Weekly psychotherapy sessions are ongoing and PP's ability to effectively regulate his emotions appears improved.

44.8 Key Points

- Sustaining a concussion can elevate the risk for subsequent brain injury, especially when the injury is poorly managed or the athlete is prematurely cleared to return to competition.
- Multiple concussions can result in a complex pattern of cognitive and emotional sequelae.

- Cognitive rehabilitation should follow an evidence-based approach, where goals are developed through a collaborative process between clinicians and their clients.
- Strategies learned in the clinic should be relevant to the client and treatment should focus on promoting generalization to functional activities in the client's natural environment.

Suggested Readings

[1] Cicerone KD, Langenbahn DM, Braden C, et al. Evidence-based cognitive rehabilitation: updated review of the literature from 2003 through 2008. Arch Phys Med Rehabil. 2011; 92(4):519–530

[2] Haskins EC, Cicerone K, Dams-O'Connor K, et al. Cognitive Rehabilitation Manual: Translating Evidence-Based Recommendations into Practice. Reston, VA: American Congress of Rehabilitation Medicine; 2012

References

[1] McCrory P, Meeuwisse WH, Aubry M, et al. Consensus statement on concussion in sport: the 4th International Conference on Concussion in Sport held in Zurich, November 2012. Br J Sports Med. 2013; 47(5):250–258

[2] Covassin T, Elbin RJ. The female athlete: the role of gender in the assessment and management of sport-related concussion. Clin Sports Med. 2011; 30(1): 125–131, x

[3] Nelson LD, Guskiewicz KM, Marshall SW, et al. Multiple self-reported concussions are more prevalent in athletes with ADHD and learning disability. Clin J Sport Med. 2016; 26(2):120–127

[4] Sohlberg MM, Mateer CA. Cognitive Rehabilitation: An Integrative Neuropsychological Approach. New York, NY: Guilford; 2001

[5] Winkens I, Van Heugten CM, Wade DT, Habets EJ, Fasotti L. Efficacy of time pressure management in stroke patients with slowed information processing: a randomized controlled trial. Arch Phys Med Rehabil. 2009; 90(10): 1672–1679

[6] Guskiewicz KM, McCrea M, Marshall SW, et al. Cumulative effects associated with recurrent concussion in collegiate football players: the NCAA Concussion Study. JAMA. 2003; 290(19):2549–2555

[7] Zemper ED. Two-year prospective study of relative risk of a second cerebral concussion. Am J Phys Med Rehabil. 2003; 82(9):653–659

[8] Covassin T, Elbin R, Kontos A, Larson E. Investigating baseline neurocognitive performance between male and female athletes with a history of multiple concussion. J Neurol Neurosurg Psychiatry. 2010; 81(6):597–601

[9] McCrory P, Meeuwisse W, Johnston K, et al. Consensus Statement on Concussion in Sport: the 3rd International Conference on Concussion in Sport held in Zurich, November 2008. Br J Sports Med. 2009; 43 Suppl 1:i76–i90

[10] Wilson B. Single-case experimental designs in neuropsychological rehabilitation. J Clin Exp Neuropsychol. 1987; 9(5):527–544

[11] McCrory P, Meeuwisse WH, Aubry M, et al. Consensus statement on concussion in sport: the 4th International Conference on Concussion in Sport held in Zurich, November 2012. Br J Sports Med. 2013; 47(5):250–258

45 Management of Swallow Function in a Patient with an Orocutaneous Fistula

Amy Fullerton

45.1 Introduction

Speech and swallowing outcomes following treatment of large-volume oral cavity tumors can have varying effects on speech and swallow function. Anticipation of these deficits and appropriate treatment planning can minimize loss of function due to disuse atrophy and facilitate safe resumption of oral diet. The literature also supports the role of preoperative counseling to reduce overall cost and length of stay as well as improve functional outcomes. Rehabilitative plans may need to be adjusted depending on the presence and duration of postoperative edema, flap dehiscence, and/or fistula formation and acute radiation toxicities, all of which contribute to complex rehabilitation.

45.2 Clinical History and Description

TL was a 65-year-old woman with pT4aN0M0 squamous cell carcinoma of the right alveolar ridge for which she underwent prophylactic gastrostomy tube placement and dental extractions in anticipation of adjuvant radiotherapy following composite mandibulectomy with fibular free flap and bilateral modified radical neck dissections. Five weeks following surgical resection, she received a total of 60 Gy at 2 Gy/fraction to the oral cavity and neck. Intensity-modulated radiotherapy (IMRT) was used instead of conventional radiotherapy to decrease the dose to normal tissues and, specifically, to decrease radiation exposure to the spinal cord, salivary glands, and brachial plexus.

45.3 Clinical Testing

Baseline evaluation of swallow function prior to oncologic therapy included the Functional Oral Intake Scale (FOIS), which is a 7-point ordinal scale that provides a measure of a patient's diet. Scores less than 6 indicate varying levels of oral intake dysfunction. TL's baseline score was 7, indicating she was on a total oral diet without restrictions. Measurements of oral aperture and tongue strength were obtained with the Iowa Oral Performance Instrument. Interdental oral aperture was 55 mm and lingua-palatal pressure (an indirect measure of tongue strength) was 56 kPa. These measures were within the normal range for her age. The Performance Status Scale for Head and Neck (PSS-HN) cancer is a 0 to 100 scale with 10-point ordinal increments correlating to the ability to eat an oral diet. A score of 0 indicates nothing by mouth and a score of 100 indicates no diet restrictions. Videofluoroscopic evaluation of swallow function followed the protocol for the Dynamic Imaging Grade of Swallowing Toxicity (DIGEST) tool, which is a reliable and valid scale incorporating pharyngeal residue and penetration/aspiration scores that give an indication of level of swallowing impairment. DIGEST scores include both safety and efficiency sub-scores (both of which were 0 at this time) as well as an overall score (which was also 0 at baseline). Preoperative scores were all within functional limits and no appreciable swallow deficits were identified. As expected, TL reported consuming a normal oral diet without restriction, denied appetite loss or dysgeusia, and reported her weight had been stable over the past several months. Preoperative evaluation of speech function included complete oral motor evaluation of cranial nerve integrity, diadochokinetics, and inventory of phonemes in isolated and connected speech. Baseline speech was also within functional limits without dysarthria or articulatory imprecision. TL denied changes to her speech and reported satisfaction with her current, baseline speech function.

45.4 Questions and Answers for the Reader

1. What is an appropriate time frame to schedule videofluoroscopic swallow study following free flap surgical reconstruction to an oropharyngeal structure(s) involved in speech production or deglutition?
   a) Postoperative day (POD) 1.
   b) POD 5 to 14.
   c) POD 30.
   d) No swallow study is indicated.

Answer: b is correct. Orocutaneous fistula may present at this point and postoperative swallow function can be reliably assessed.

a is incorrect. Acute postoperative edema will preclude a reliable result and surgical drains and/or tracheostomy, both of which are typically left in place 3 to 5 days postoperatively, will obscure views, and confound function.

c is incorrect. Thirty days is too long for a patient to remain without an oral diet unnecessarily and will delay functional rehabilitation.

d is incorrect. A swallow study is necessary to guide appropriate return to oral diet and rehabilitation as well as assess postoperative anatomical and physiological changes to structures involved in speech/deglutition.

2. What is an appropriate contrast material for initial postoperative swallow study when a leak or fistula may be present?
   a) Gastrografin.
   b) Cystografin.
   c) Omnipaque.
   d) Barium sulfate, $BaSo_4$.

Answer: c is correct. Omnipaque is appropriate for oral administration and, with a very low osmolarity of 520 mOsm/L, is nearly iso-osmolar. Although aspiration of this contrast is discouraged in copious quantities, it is better tolerated than hyperosmolar contrast materials.

a is incorrect. Gastrografin, a lemon-flavor Food and Drug Administration (FDA)-approved contrast material for oral ingestion has an incredibly high osmolarity of 1,900 mOsm/L or approximately six times that of extracellular fluid. If aspiration occurs, serious pulmonary complications including pulmonary edema, pneumonitis, or death through copious osmotic effusion may occur. Gastrografin may also have iodine-mediated thyrotropic effects, which would be contraindicated in a large proportion of head and neck cancer patients.

b is incorrect. Cystografin contrast material is not meant for oral ingestion.

d is incorrect. Although $BaSo_4$ is appropriate for oral consumption and routinely used for videofluoroscopic swallow studies due to water insolubility, it is inappropriate for patients with free flap reconstructions or where fistula is suspected as it will maintain patency of any postoperative fistula.

3. What speech deficits are anticipated following composite mandibulectomy?
   a) Labiodentals, bilabials, and interdentals: /m/, /f/, /v/, /b/, /p/, /ʃ/, /ʒ/.
   b) Alveolars and alveopalatals: /l/, /t/, /d/, /θ/.
   c) Palatals and velars: /k/, /g/, /ð/, /ŋ/, /j/.
   d) Glottals: /h/.

Answer: a is correct. Due to the dental extractions in anticipation of radiotherapy, these sounds will be affected.

b is incorrect. Lingual range of motion is preserved.

c is incorrect. Velar structure and lingual range of motion is preserved.

d is incorrect. Glottal movement is preserved.

4. How is adjuvant radiotherapy anticipated to affect speech outcomes?
   a) It will improve speech outcomes.
   b) It will not affect speech outcomes.
   c) It will hurt speech outcomes.

Answer: a is correct. Radiotherapy will further reduce flap bulk and improve conformity to native oral structures.

b is incorrect. See the above reasons.

c is incorrect. Development of mucositis may impede speech rehabilitation and slow progress temporarily however.

5. How is adjuvant radiotherapy anticipated to affect swallow outcomes?
   a) It will improve swallow outcomes.
   b) It will not affect swallow outcomes.
   c) It will hurt swallow outcomes.

Answer: c is correct. It is well known that radiotherapy has deleterious immediate and long-term effects on swallow function, including late-onset, radiation-associated dysphagia.

a is incorrect. Radiotherapy and its concomitant sequelae such as mucositis, erythema, and possibly thrush may promote disuse atrophy through periods of reliance exclusively on enteral nutrition.

b is incorrect. Radiotherapy generally has a deleterious effect on swallowing outcomes.

45.5 Description of Disorder and Recommended Treatment

Repeat swallow study on postoperative day 7 revealed oral stage deficits characterized by significant anterior loss of secretions as well as bolus materials. Floor of mouth (oral) bolus retention was also observed with poor anteroposterior propulsion. The pharyngeal phase was intact with functional airway protection. However, several submental lucencies were noted without an overt fistula (▶ Fig. 45.1) and it was recommended TL consume nothing by mouth. Three days later, TL developed a right orocutaneous fistula warranting packing (▶ Fig. 45.2). The packing was removed after 2 weeks and following two courses of antibiotics.

Postoperative oral motor evaluation revealed a nicely seated anterolateral thigh flap in the floor of mouth and right mandible. Neck incisions were slightly erythematous, but dry. Packing was observed per right neck incision, presumably where Penrose drain was removed. The patient was edentulous with malocclusion and open-mouth posture, resulting in the inability to achieve labial approximation, right less than left, due to flap edema. Lingual strength/range of motion was preserved. Anterior loss of secretions was resolved with adequate secretion management observed during speech/swallow tasks.

Postoperative speech evaluation revealed intact diadochokinesis, and remarkably preserved intelligibility despite an inability to approximate the lips with anticipated deficits in production of labiodentals, bilabials, and interdentals. These deficits were attributed to acute postoperative edema and anticipated to resolve in the following few days; thus, rehabilitation of these sounds was not indicated. Overall intelligibility was 95% in known contexts and 85% in unknown contexts.

	Pre-op	POD 7	POD 25	1month post-IMRT	3months post-IMRT
PSS-HN	100	0	0	60	80
FOIS	7	1	1	5	6
DIGEST	0	1	2	1	0
Safety	0	0	1	1	0
Efficiency	0	2	2	1	0
Deficit phonemes	None	/m/, /f/, /v/, /b/, /p/, /ʃ/, /ʒ/	/f/, /v/, /ʃ/, /ʒ/	/ʃ/, /ʒ/	/ʃ/, /ʒ/

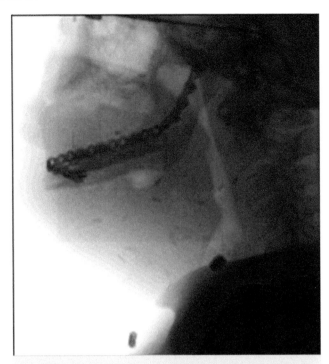

Fig. 45.1 Lateral postoperative radiographic view of composite mandibulectomy with several submental opacities; no overt leak.

Postoperative fistula is an unanticipated and uncommon complication following surgical resection that warrants vigilance from the speech-language pathologist (SLP) for identification and management of speech/swallowing functions during the healing process. Although not easily predictable, several risk factors warrant monitoring, including anemia, cachexia, history of radiation, large tumor volume warranting free-flap reconstruction, and glottal primary tumors that require total laryngectomy. The presence of one or more of these risk factors is associated with a 13% to 35% chance of postoperative fistula development.

Management of orocutaneous fistula is the responsibility of the surgical team and a conservative approach is generally taken that includes wound packing, administration of antibiotics, and delayed return to oral diet. SLPs play an important role in early identification or verification of fistula, guide return to oral diet, and provide interval rehabilitation during wound healing. Therapeutic exercises are not contraindicated with an active fistula. However, an oral diet is contraindicated because it may prolong wound healing and yield complications such as flap dehiscence, loss of flap viability, and persistent infection.

45.6 Outcome

Although TL remained nil per os for several weeks postoperatively and experienced delayed initiation of radiation therapy, she ultimately resumed a liberal oral diet without restriction and achieved intelligible speech, both of which she was pleased with. Speaking with her several months following completion of IMRT, TL and her daughter stated that routine contact with SLP and education regarding reliable time frames for expected

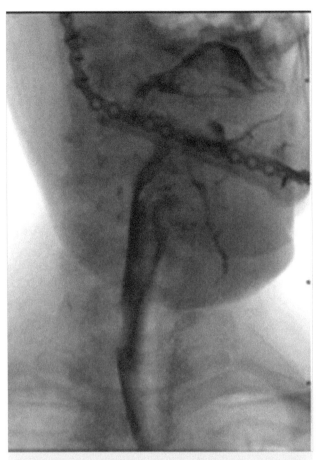

Fig. 45.2 anterolateral postoperative radiographic view of composite mandibulectomy with barium contrast per pharyngoesophageal lumen with visible left-sided anterior orocutaneous extravasation of contrast material concerning the leak.

return to oral diet and return of speech function made recovery manageable even during times of unanticipated complication. She was adherent with dysphagia therapy throughout her cancer treatment. Despite the absence of penetration/aspiration during instrumental swallow evaluation, super-supraglottic swallow, Mendelsohn's maneuver, and hard swallow were recommended 20 times a day to preserve function. Prophylactic intervention continued during IMRT, but her approach was altered to incorporate the Pharyngocise protocol, which consists of four sets of 10 of the following exercises:

- Sustained falsetto phonation for 5 seconds.
- Continuation of Mendelsohn's maneuver with 5-second hold.
- Tongue press with 5-second hold (instructions to patient: "Press your entire tongue against the roof of your mouth and hold it").
- Five-second manual jaw stretch (instructions to patient: "Open wide and pull down on your chin to increase the stretch").

She continued these exercises for 1 month following completion of IMRT and maintained an oral diet, which she modified to soft solids and thin liquids only during peak radiation toxicity. She was followed by the SLP with evaluations 1 and 3 months after IMRT, at which point she reported satisfaction with her swallow and speech and was deemed to have achieved maximal rehabilitative potential.

45.7 Key Points

- Identification of risk factors and early identification of fistula results in slightly prolonged return to oral diet.
- The SLP plays an integral role in educating the patient preoperatively, regarding likelihood of surgical and radiotherapy risks, delineating timeline for return to oral diet, as well as informing patients of anticipated speech and swallow deficits with guided postoperative rehabilitation.

- Guided SLP intervention is important in not only the postoperative period, but also pre-, peri-, and postradiation therapy.

Suggested Readings

[1] Clarke P, Radford K, Coffey M, Stewart M. Speech and swallow rehabilitation in head and neck cancer: United Kingdom National Multidisciplinary Guidelines. J Laryngol Otol. 2016; 130 S2:S176–S180

[2] Hutcheson KA, Barrow MP, Barringer DA, et al. Dynamic Imaging Grade of Swallowing Toxicity (DIGEST): scale development and validation. Cancer. 2017; 123(1):62–70

[3] van la Parra RF, Kon M, Schellekens PP, Braunius WW, Pameijer FA. The prognostic value of abnormal findings on radiographic swallowing studies after total laryngectomy. Cancer Imagi. 2007; 7:119–125

46 Evidence-Based Intervention for Dysarthria in a Patient with Amyotrophic Lateral Sclerosis

Amy Lustig

46.1 Introduction

Nearly all individuals diagnosed with amyotrophic lateral sclerosis (ALS) will experience a decline in speech communication at some point during their illness. Management of dysarthria to maximize communicative competence is a key target for speech-language pathologists and must employ evidence-based practices to optimize efficacy.

46.2 Clinical History and Description

DS was a 71-year-old, community-dwelling Caucasian man who was seen for speech pathology evaluation approximately 6 months after being diagnosed with ALS, following a long career as a civil engineer. His medical history included high blood pressure that was well controlled with diuretics, gastroesophageal reflux disease (GERD), including frequent heartburn symptoms (poorly managed with chewable antacids), and mild, untreated depression and anxiety. During the evaluation, DS reported increased difficulty speaking and swallowing. He also reported difficulty typing, which was particularly problematic as he was in the process of completing a book and also interfered with simple email communications. In addition, he reported difficulty ambulating and with self-care. He described his speech as "softer and quieter," as well as requiring increased effort to "get the words out." These issues were particularly noticeable later in the day, on the telephone, and in group settings. He also regularly coughed and occasionally drooled while speaking. DS's wife confirmed that his speech intelligibility was progressively worsening, and she occasionally had to ask him to repeat himself several times to increase intelligibility. They agreed that these speech changes had worsened over the past 9 to 12 months prior to receiving the ALS diagnosis (See Appendix).

46.3 Clinical Testing

Structured testing of DS's speech, language, and cognitive status was conducted. Each test has been standardized for diagnostic purposes except for the Montreal Cognitive Assessment (MoCA), which provides a cognitive screening score, and is not a comprehensive test of cognitive status. On the Frenchay Dysarthria Assessment (FDA-2),[1] DS was classified as having a moderately severe and mixed upper- and lower-motor neuron dysarthria. Lip function was better than laryngeal and tongue function, with a severely impaired cough reflex, visible lingual fasciculations, and variable palatal function, which were somewhat better during swallowing than speech. A mildly slumped posture and slow speech rate were identified as factors potentially influencing testing results, and the constant presence of oral secretions interfered with speech production and intelligi-

bility. On a perceptual dysarthria profile utilizing items from the Robertson Dysarthria Profile (Revised),[2] DS obtained a classification of moderately severe mixed spastic–flaccid dysarthria characterized by slow speech rate, equal and excess/reduced stress and pitch, hypernasality, strained-strangled vocal quality, and distorted consonant and vowel production, particularly for voiced/voiceless cognates, fricatives, and complex consonant blends. Overall speech intelligibility was 75% in conversation and 85% for single words and short phrases. Vocal intensity ranged between 59 and 64 dB during conversation (typical conversational range = 72–77 dB).

On the MoCA,[3] DS obtained a score of 27/30 within the normal range for his age; however, deficits in visuoconstruction skills, delayed word recall, and language fluency were observed. On the Boston Naming Test (BNT),[4] DS scored 14/15, within the normal range for his age. DS and his wife denied difficulties with word finding, language comprehension, reading, or writing, other than those associated with the physical mechanics of these activities (e.g., holding a pen, etc.).

46.4 Questions and Answers for the Reader

1. Are effortful exercises targeting articulatory or respiratory strength and range of motion appropriate for DS?
   a) Yes, because they will help increase muscle strength and control.
   b) No, because they will not improve muscle strength or control and will fatigue DS.
   c) Yes, because that is traditionally how speech pathologists treat dysarthria of speech.
   d) No, because respiratory strength does not affect the clarity of speech articulation.

Answer: b is correct. Because the pathophysiology of ALS is characterized by progressive and permanent decline in the numbers of functional motor neurons, the benefit of effortful exercise in ALS is controversial. No randomized trials of effortful exercise targeting speech articulation in ALS have been published, and a small handful of case studies report detrimental effects of intensive exercise on speech intelligibility and vocal quality.[5,6]

a is incorrect. A 2013 Cochrane review of randomized and quasi-randomized studies involving resistance and/or aerobic exercise training for individuals with ALS or other motor neuron disease found no studies regarding aerobic exercise in this population and little evidence of the benefits of resistance training.[7]

c is incorrect. Intervention goals and targets should be tailored to specific needs and circumstances, account for the nature of the underlying impairment, and be based on the best available clinical evidence for predicted treatment choices and effects. Dysarthria interventions targeting muscle strength are appropriate when the underlying impairment can accommodate the core target of the intervention (i.e., when motor neurons are available to facilitate increased muscle contractile strength). When the underlying condition is inconsistent with traditional interventions, such as in ALS, which is associated with progressive decline in the number of available motor neurons, alternative approaches to maximizing muscle strength for dysarthria management must be utilized.

d is incorrect. Strong and positive correspondences between respiratory muscle strength and intelligible speech are well recognized.

2. Would it be appropriate at this point in DS's illness trajectory to introduce the use of augmentative and alternative communication (AAC) strategies?
   a) No, because his speech is still understandable to others who know him well.
   b) No, because he would prefer to speak rather than employ a compensatory strategy.
   c) Yes, because he should stop speaking now to spare his strength.
   d) Yes, because it can provide him with communication options in the future.

Answer: d is correct. Individuals with ALS should be encouraged to maximize intelligibility through managing fatigue, conserving speech and voice output, and the use of augmentative/compensatory communication strategies.

a is incorrect. Even though DS may be reasonably well understood by familiar individuals, his speech intelligibility will continue to decline. Additionally, it would be useful for some of his closest relatives and friends to become familiar with the alternative communication strategies he may choose to employ, to improve his comfort with using them, and provide assistance.

b is incorrect. Virtually everyone would prefer to speak rather than utilize an alternative approach to communication with the critical caveat that if DS were to assert that he would rather rely solely on verbal communication for the duration of his illness, and was fully disinterested in exploring alternatives, it would be necessary to respect his wishes, assuming that he was fully aware of the consequences of this choice.

c is incorrect. Although alternative communication strategies can spare effort and conserve energy, DS would likely have little motivation to stop speaking if his speech was still reasonably intelligible. There is insufficient evidence to support substantially avoiding motor speech production in the interest of preserving energy while speech is still reasonably intelligible. However, it would be appropriate at this point to introduce the advantages of incorporating adjuncts to speech communication that DS might consider implementing for even short periods of time. For example, using a voice amplifier during telephone calls or in other challenging communication situations could increase intelligibility and communicative effectiveness.

3. What would you expect to happen with DS's speech intelligibility over the course of his illness?
   a) It will get progressively worse.
   b) It will remain at the current level indefinitely.
   c) There is a reasonable chance for improvement in speech intelligibility.
   d) It will change from day to day, from very intelligible to poor intelligibility.

Answer: a is correct. It is well recognized that speech intelligibility progressively worsens for the vast majority of ALS patients, with more rapid decline in bulbar cases.

b is incorrect. Different individuals decline at different rates, but over time, virtually all will show a decrement in speech articulation and clarity.

c is incorrect. No cases of improved speech intelligibility in patients with ALS have been reported.

d is incorrect. Although speech intelligibility can change to some extent from day to day due to factors including fatigue, stress, and medication effects, overall speech intelligibility is recognized to progressively worsen over time.

4. In addition to DS's articulatory distortions, what other factors could influence his intelligibility?
   a) Background noise, such as music, television, or conversation.
   b) A reluctance to speak in public due to feeling self-conscious about poor speech.
   c) Pressure to keep up with a rapidly paced discussion.
   d) All of the above.

Answer: d is correct. Many factors contribute to intelligibility. Background noise or other distractions can draw our attention away from the speaker or pose an auditory challenge that makes decoding spoken language more difficult. Many individuals with ALS with dysarthria and other morbidity associated with the disease struggle with these changes and suffer from negative effects on self-confidence and personal identity. Even with close friends or family, communication and cognitive issues co-occurring with ALS can result in difficulty participating in group conversations that are fast paced, have complex or frequent topic changes, or are competitive.

46.5 Description of Disorder and Recommended Treatment

ALS is a fatal, neurodegenerative disorder affecting upper and lower motor neurons of the spinal cord, motor cortex, and brainstem yielding progressive weakness and wasting of limb, bulbar, and respiratory musculature. Most individuals diagnosed with ALS experience progressive impairment of speech and swallowing function, typically associated with bulbar decline. Speech dysarthria in ALS is most often of the mixed flaccid/spastic type, given both upper and lower motor neuron involvement. Decreased speech intelligibility is due mainly to reduced movement of oral musculature and phonation changes resulting in slowed, slurred, and imprecise speech with harsh, hypointense, hypernasal, and monotonic vocal resonance.

DS was seen regularly for speech therapy visits for 8 months; therapy was scheduled weekly for 1 month, then biweekly for 2 months, once every 3 weeks for 2 months, and then again biweekly. DS was acutely aware of the decline in his speech intelligibility and voice quality. He initially requested exercises to maximize articulatory and vocal competence, but reluctantly acquiesced when provided with the rationale for avoiding them. A compromise was reached whereby he was provided with lists of challenging words and phrases on the condition that he agreed to practice them with another person for intelligibility feedback only, and not in a repetitive or fatiguing manner. Four lists were provided over the course of 10 weeks, and these were periodically reviewed during speech therapy visits. DS was provided a portable voice amplifier and lightweight headset microphone to increase loudness and phonemic contrasts while with minimal effort. DS employed this device in communication situations he considered particularly challenging, such as during mealtimes, automobile trips, and telephone conversations.

DS also participated in two trials (one during the first month of therapy and one at the end of the third month) of an AAC device capable of generating digital speech and a variety of interface modalities, including direct keyboard selection, head mouse, scan/switch interface, and eye-gaze technology. DS's speech intelligibility declined substantially over 8 months of therapy, from 75% to 45% in conversation. Though he was initially reluctant to consider using a speech-generating communication device, DS eventually recognized that he might eventually lose intelligible speech and use of his upper extremities. AAC approaches are typically successful with individuals with ALS often up to within a few weeks of death and are acknowledged as a central component of speech pathology intervention for this population.[8] AAC solutions range from "low-tech" approaches such as voice amplifiers, letter boards accessed via laser pointer, head mouse, scan/switch interface, or caregiver assistance with pointing or shared eye-gaze strategies to "high-tech" approaches such as speech-generating computerized systems accessed via sophisticated eye-tracking technology. The likelihood of upper and lower extremity impairment must be considered.

Additionally, it was suggested that DS contact his medical provider to discuss his reflux symptoms and the possibility of pharmacological management. Reducing oral secretions during speech as well as coughing/choking events during swallowing may be reduced by improved reflux management.

46.6 Outcome

A summary of treatment targets and outcomes is provided in ▶ Table 46.1. DS was generally willing to utilize the voice amplifier in a private setting, such as in his apartment, which his wife (who had mild hearing loss) found very helpful to improve his speech intelligibility, nearly eliminating her requests for him to repeat himself. He initiated use of the device himself only infrequently, but was generally receptive when it was suggested that he utilize it, and eventually self-initiated use of the voice amplifier on approximately 85% of appropriate opportunities. Initially, DS was particularly reluctant to utilize the device in public settings such as the dining room at the residential community where he lived. He had the device for approximately 2 months before he used it in public, at a meal with friends, about which he reported a benefit of having much better success at maintaining his presence during conversation, though he found the microphone interfered with the mechanics of eating when it was too close to his mouth. At the end of 8 months, DS and his wife both confirmed that he utilized the voice amplifier in public settings in approximately 65% of opportunities, with 75% success for conversation participation; limitations were associated with keeping up with the speed of group conversations, fatigue, and some distraction when the device was placed on the table rather than worn around the waist.

Table 46.1 Dysarthria intervention targets and outcomes

Intervention	Target	% Compliance	% Success
Voice amplifier (private setting)	Speech intelligibility	80	90
Voice amplifier (public setting)	Speech intelligibility	65	75
PPI use	Secretion management	100	100
AAC use (eye gaze)	Generated speech for communication; rapid assistance; manuscript writing/editing; book reading	90	70
AAC use (head mouse)	Generated speech for communication; rapid assistance; manuscript writing/editing; book reading	90	85

AAC, augmentative and alternative communication; PPI, proton pump inhibitor.

DS was prescribed a proton pump inhibitor (PPI) to manage his GERD symptoms and possibly reduce oral secretions. Within 2 weeks of starting the medication, DS reported he stopped coughing and choking while eating and that his GERD symptoms resolved. Coughing and drooling during speech was also eliminated.

Two therapy sessions consisted of trials of various AAC options; DS selected a dedicated speech-generating device that offered a variety of interface modalities, including eye-gaze, head mouse, and scan/switch approaches. This device was delivered during the fourth month of therapy. DS preferred the eye-gaze technology, which he used with approximately 70% success in approximately 90% of opportunities, and considered to be only a moderately successful outcome. Challenges in device use were associated with several factors, including fatigue, seating and positional issues, and eye-gaze calibration for accessing targets at the edges and corners of the display screen versus those in the more central screen. Modifications were made to the visual presentation of preferred programs to minimize the need to access targets at display edges and corners. DS's wife and children were also trained in device use, simple programming, and troubleshooting.

During the seventh month of therapy, DS's eyelids began to droop slightly and his ocular secretions became more viscous, two developments that further interfered with successful use of the eye-gaze interface. At that point, DS transitioned from eye-gaze to head mouse use, which he accomplished with somewhat better success (85%), again in approximately 90% of relevant opportunities. Difficulties with head mouse use were primarily associated with maintaining a comfortable upright head position and coordinating the timing of head movement to the desired target as well as persistent and rapid fatigue. For both eye-gaze and head mouse interface modalities, training was provided to generate spontaneous spoken words and phrases, to create a database of organized words and phrases that could be quickly accessed to communicate daily needs, and to ensure access to applications such as digitized books and quick select help options to meet DS's expressed needs and interests. DS also utilized the keyboard to continue work on his book; he completed the manuscript. DS's wife and children were essential partners to keep the device readily available to him through reminders, direct assistance, and solving problems as well as positive reinforcement.

46.7 Key Points

- ALS is a fatal disease, with progressive decline throughout disease trajectory, though the rate and magnitude of functional decline varies across individuals.
- AAC in patients with ALS is preferred over effortful exercise for maximizing speech communication and minimizing fatigue.
- People with ALS may be receptive to different types of AAC interventions at different points in time (e.g., voice amplifier vs. speech-generating device) and may require modifications to AAC strategies over time. It is critical to maintain contact over the course of the disease to ascertain shifting needs and priorities and to link the goals of device use with personally meaningful activities.
- Engaging family members to assist and encourage AAC use can make a substantial difference in patient access and success.
- It is important to identify and address symptoms, such as drooling or acid reflux, through medical management to maximize the benefit of functional speech therapy goals and objectives.

Suggested Reading

[1] Hanson EK, Yorkston KM, Britton D. Dysarthria in amyotrophic lateral sclerosis: a systematic review of characteristics, speech treatment and augmentative and alternative communication options. J Med Speech-Lang Pathol. 2011; 19(3):12–30

References

[1] Enderby PM, Palmer R. Frenchay Dysarthria Assessment. 2nd ed. Austin, TX: Pro-Ed; 2008
[2] Robertson SJ. Dysarthria Profile (Revised). Chesterfield, UK: Winslow Press; 1982
[3] Nasreddine ZS, Phillips NA, Bédirian V, et al. The Montreal Cognitive Assessment, MoCA: a brief screening tool for mild cognitive impairment. J Am Geriatr Soc. 2005; 53(4):695–699
[4] Kaplan E, Goodglass H, Weintraub S. The Boston Naming Test. 2nd ed. Philadelphia, PA: Lea & Febiger; 1983
[5] Dworkin JP, Hartman DE. Progressive speech deterioration and dysphagia in amyotrophic lateral sclerosis: case report. Arch Phys Med Rehabil. 1979; 60 (9):423–425
[6] Watts CR, Vanryckeghem M. Laryngeal dysfunction in amyotrophic lateral sclerosis: a review and case report. BMC Ear Nose Throat Disord. 2001; 1(1):1
[7] Dal Bello-Haas V, Florence JM. Therapeutic exercise for people with amyotrophic lateral sclerosis or motor neuron disease. Cochrane Database Syst Rev. 2008:CD005229
[8] Beukelman D, Fager S, Nordness A. Communication support for people with ALS. Neurol Res Int. 2011:714693

Appendix: Sound Clips Collected Approximately 10 Months following DS Acquiring the Diagnosis of Amyotrophic Lateral Sclerosis[1]

1. SMR (sequential motion rate) – pa-pa-pa.
2. SMR (sequential motion rate) – ta-ta-ta.
3. SMR (sequential motion rate) – ka-ka-ka.
4. AMR (alternate motion rate) – pa-ta-ka.
5. Counting 1 to 5.
6. Counting backward 5 to 1.
7. Pitch glide up.
8. Pitch glide down.
9. Prolonged /ah/.
10. One-syllable words: pet – thumb – dish – neck – safe – zero – juice.
11. Two-syllable words: behind – weather – rubbish – message – kitchen – power – finger.
12. Three-syllable words: yesterday – passenger – beautiful – visitor – tobacco – direction – charity.
13. Four-syllable words: population – development – majority – fundamental – generation – humanity – liberation.
14. Short phrases: You have to pay. – Go to bed. – She looks sad. – Where's my coat? – Do what you like. – Is that a joke? – I need my hat.
15. Longer phrases: My daughter is a nurse. – What do you think? – She gave me a coin. – Can you go to the shop? – Put it in a dish.
16. Spontaneous speech sample: Byberly has … has a greenhouse that my wife is very much involved with. Uh … she mainly has orchids there. And sometimes she has to repot them and she shows other ladies how to repot them. Uh … A couple days ago, a man put a plant in there that they think has a disease and would spread to the other plants. And she got an expert in there and they are attempting what disease they may have. Um … there is a great interest in orchids around here because several of the ladies have got them.

---

[1] Structured word and phrase targets were obtained from the Frenchay Dysarthria Assessment evaluation materials.

47 Rehabilitation of Right Hemisphere Disorder in the Chronic Phase of Recovery

Jamila Minga

47.1 Introduction

High-quality studies to direct treatment for cognitive-communication deficits associated with right hemisphere deficits are limited, likely related to the broad heterogeneity of this patient population. Theories and treatment approaches from other neurogenic populations can be employed, however, to guide rehabilitation.

47.2 Clinical History and Description

CP was a 48-year-old woman with a history of diabetes mellitus and hypertension who presented with left-sided weakness and facial droop after decreased responsiveness at the dinner table. Computed tomography (CT) of the brain revealed an infarct of the right middle cerebral artery (MCA) distribution. CP reported that she "lost her filter" and the ability to "organize her life." Close relatives and friends reported that CP frequently made inappropriate comments and did not allow them to participate in conversations. CP lived independently with her two daughters, aged 13 and 9 years. She had a graduate degree and worked as an administrator for a health care insurance company where she supervised eight employees. CP sought treatment for residual executive functioning deficits, and expressed a desire to reengage in community and occupational activities.

47.3 Clinical Testing

An initial cognitive profile was conducted approximately 10 months following CP's stroke. The Cognitive-Linguistic Quick Test was administered.[1] Cognitive domain severity ratings were mild for attention and visuospatial skills and moderate for executive functions (EF). Memory and language were within normal limits (WNL; ▶ Table 47.1). Empathy was measured as below average; she scored a 45 on the Toronto Empathy Questionnaire.[2]

Table 47.1 Pretreatment cognitive domain severity scores

Cognitive domain	Score	Ranges of severity		
		Within normal limits	Mild	Moderate
Attention	149	215–180	179–125	124–50
Memory	177	185–155	154–141	140–110
Executive functions	17	40–24	23–20	19–16
Language	33	37–29	28–25	24–21
Visuospatial skills	60	105–82	81–52	51–42

Visuospatial neglect was also observed; CP eliminated numbers 6, 7, and 8 from her clock drawing and eliminated the leftmost aspect of the page during maze and design generation tasks. Neglect was assessed further using the Apples Cancellation Test.[3] Both egocentric and allocentric left neglects were observed. The total number of complete apples selected was 40/50 and the total number of false positives, selection of apples open on the left side, was 6/50. False positives were isolated to the lower left quadrant of the page.

47.4 Questions and Answers for the Reader

1. Knowledge of brain–behavior relationships can guide assessment and treatment approaches. CP had damage to the right MCA distribution. What cerebral lobes are most likely involved when EF and visuospatial skills are impaired?
   a) Right frontal lobe and temporal lobe.
   b) Right frontal lobe and parietal lobe.
   c) Left frontal lobe and temporal lobe.
   d) Left temporal lobe and right occipital lobe.

Answer: b is correct. The MCA supplies most of the lateral surface of the cerebral hemispheres, the thalamus, and basal ganglia. Since the right MCA was involved, damage to the right frontal lobe (EF) and the right parietal lobe (visuospatial skills) is likely.

a is incorrect. The temporal lobe is not associated with impaired EF or visuospatial skills.

c is incorrect. The cerebrovascular accident (CVA) occurred in the right MCA, which does not supply the left hemisphere.

d is incorrect. The CVA occurred in the right MCA, which does not supply the left hemisphere. The occipital lobe is associated with visual perception.

2. CP scored below average on the Toronto Empathy Questionnaire. If she plans to return to the workforce in her previous position, which of the following areas may be impacted by diminished empathy?
   a) Communication.
   b) Organization.
   c) Supervision.
   d) Both a and c.

Answer: d is correct. Empathy can be thought of as the ability to take another's point of view with respect to desires, needs, and emotional state. Empathy plays a role in communication in that the manner in which a person decides how and when to communicate includes the perspective of communication partners. Supervision requires the ability to communicate effectively and to demonstrate empathy for employees.

b is incorrect. Empathy does not influence organizational capabilities. Organization can be subsumed under EF.

3. If a clinician seeks to employ the client's concerns as the basis for prioritizing treatment, which area should be prioritized?
   a) EF.
   b) Left neglect.
   c) Pragmatic communication.

Answer: a is correct. Most of CP's limitations can be captured under EF. She reported difficulty organizing her life and filtering communication. Furthermore, her prior occupation necessitated intact executive functioning. Since evidence-based treatment exists for deficits of executive functioning in the literature of acquired disorders (e.g., traumatic brain injury), therapy should target executive functioning first.

b is incorrect. Neglect was not identified by CP as one of the primary motives for seeking treatment. In addition, her neglect was isolated to one visual field quadrant and she seems to be functioning with the neglect. Additional testing may be warranted to further assess visual capabilities, and specifically to determining whether the observed deficit is truly neglect or an anopsia.

c is incorrect. Cognitive processes are thought to contribute to deficits in pragmatic communication, with respect to language production, in adults with right hemisphere brain damage (RHD). Pragmatic communication may be observed concurrently with improvement in cognitive domains, especially if the cognitive treatment includes the use of communicative tasks.

47.5 Description of Disorder and Recommended Treatment

RHD can result in cognitive-linguistic deficits that impact quality of life. The representation of these deficits can vary greatly. Adults with RHD typically express themselves with appropriate grammar, morphology, and syntax (i.e., preserved basic language abilities). However, as noted in the current case, pragmatic aspects of language may be impaired. Underlying cognitive deficits have been postulated to contribute to abnormal pragmatic communication.[2,4] Although pragmatic communication is not widely examined in the RHD literature, literature can direct the treatment of cognitive deficits.[5] Targeting cognitive deficits may result in improved communication.

CP had deficits of attention, executive functioning, and pragmatic communication in the chronic phase of recovery. A functional approach to rehabilitation utilizes patient motivation; considering CP's goal to return to work and her perceived inability to organize, skilled treatment for EF and visuospatial neglect was recommended. EF therapy was consistent with the EF/frontal lobe dysfunction model. Deficits of EF can impact all aspects of communication; impaired social interactions may be related to an inability to organize thoughts, shift attention, and plan. Within this model, treatment foci included organization, planning, and problem solving. Moreover, it was recommended that communicative activities and tasks be embedded in EF treatment. CP was motivated to return to work and desired improved organization at home.

An approach to the treatment of chronic neglect is prism adaptation intervention. Growing evidence supports this approach in the chronic phase of recovery. This approach, however, requires close interaction with a neuro-ophthalmologist. In the absence of such collaboration, standard therapy for neglect is visual scanning training. Career counseling was also recommended. CP supervised eight employees, and at the onset of therapy, it was unclear whether she could return to work in this capacity.

47.6 Outcomes

CP participated in individual treatment once per week for 10 weeks and then transitioned to ongoing group treatment. Individual treatment focused on executive functioning with embedded communicative activities and visuospatial skills. Group treatment continued with a frequency of once a month. Group treatment focused on EF skills, planning, problem solving, and organization.

A cognitive profile was gathered after 12 weeks of treatment. Improvement was noted for the domains of attention, visuospatial skills, and EF (▶ Table 47.2). Anecdotally, CP reported that communication with close friends and loved ones improved. She reported that she was more conscious of what and how she communicates and that she asked more questions in conversation. CP returned to work part time as an administrative assistant.

Given that CP was in the chronic stage of recovery, it was likely that the gains were related to treatment and not spontaneous recovery. This concept, however, was not formally assessed. An inability to determine whether such improvements would have occurred simply with time precludes such a conclusion.

47.7 Key Points

- RHD can result in a number of cognitive-linguistic deficits that can negatively impact quality of life. There is an increasing need to understand the utility of improved cognitive process on pragmatic communication.
- EF is one cognitive deficit that may contribute to aberrant communication behaviors in RHD.
- EF can be targeted in structured context using evidence-based treatments. Targeting EF may result in improvements in pragmatic communication, particularly if communicative activities are used in treatment (e.g., organizing a speech or problem solving what goes wrong in a conversation).

Table 47.2 Posttreatment cognitive domain severity scores

Cognitive domain	Score	Ranges of severity		
		Within normal limits	Mild	Moderate
Attention	189	215–180	179–125	124–50
Memory	172	185–155	154–141	140–110
Executive functions	22	40–24	23–20	19–16
Language	34	37–29	28–25	24–21
Visuospatial skills	62	105–82	81–52	51–42

47.8 Acknowledgments

The author acknowledges Dr. Robert Mayo and Dr. Margaret Blake for their ongoing mentorship and contribution to her professional development.

Suggested Readings

[1] Lehman Blake M, Frymark T, Venedictov R. An evidence-based systematic review on communication treatments for individuals with right hemisphere brain damage. Am J Speech Lang Pathol. 2013; 22(1):146–160

[2] Minga J. Discourse production and right hemisphere disorder. Perspect ASHA Spec Interest Groups.. 2016; 1(2):96–106

[3] Spreng RN, McKinnon MC, Mar RA, Levine B. The Toronto Empathy Questionnaire: scale development and initial validation of a factor-analytic solution to multiple empathy measures. J Pers Assess. 2009; 91(1):62–71

References

[1] Bickerton WL, Samson D, Williamson J, Humphreys GW. Separating forms of neglect using the Apples Test: validation and functional prediction in chronic and acute stroke. Neuropsychology. 2011; 25(5):567–580

[2] Helm-Estabrooks N. Cognitive-Linguistic Quick Test. San Antonio, TX: Psychological Corporation; 2001

[3] Martin I, McDonald S. Weak coherence, no theory of mind, or executive dysfunction? Solving the puzzle of pragmatic language disorders. Brain Lang. 2003; 85(3):451–466

[4] Tompkins CA. Right Hemisphere Communication Disorders: Theory and Management. San Diego, CA: Singular Publishing Group; 1994

[5] Cicerone KD, Langenbahn DM, Braden C, et al. Evidence-based cognitive rehabilitation: updated review of the literature from 2003 through 2008. Arch Phys Med Rehabil. 2011; 92(4):519–530

48 Reading as Intervention for a Skilled Nursing Facility Resident with Dementia

Susan Ostrowski

48.1 Introduction

Reading impairment may evolve early in the progression of dementia. However, the true incidence of reading impairment is unknown. Accessible reading material can be of significant benefit to people living with dementia in numerous functional and therapeutic ways.

48.2 Clinical History and Description

EB was an 87-year-old former homemaker and community volunteer. Her husband was deceased, her daughter lived nearby, and her son lived out of state. She was diagnosed with Alzheimer's disease (AD), chronic heart failure, and diabetes. For the last 10 years, EB lived independently near her daughter. Three months ago, EB was admitted to a skilled nursing facility (SNF) due to increased difficulty with self-care and failure to thrive. EB was subsequently referred for speech pathology evaluation as a component of the multidisciplinary team by the nursing staff primarily related to decreased cognitive functioning as well as anxious wandering, occasional agitation, and possible depression.

48.3 Clinical Testing

To determine whether speech pathology services were clinically justifiable for EB and to identify EB's needs and strengths, formal and informal cognitive and language assessment was performed. The evaluation was initiated by spending quiet, one-on-one time with EB in relaxed conversation to acquire a sense of what is important and meaningful. Referring to her new living environment, EB stated: "I'm not sure how it all works here" and "I would like to know where I'm supposed to be." EB discussed meaningful activities in her past including a sewing circle, reading, and volunteer work. She also added that she "missed being with friends."

EB's family and the SNF staff were also interviewed. EB's children said they were happy with their mother's care, but would like to "be able to communicate better" with her. In the past, EB followed a schedule, she liked being with people, and enjoyed reading, although "she hasn't read in a long time." EB's daughter reported that her mother "has pretty much lost her ability to read." She added that EB "always wears her eye glasses" and "has never worn hearing aids." The date of EB's last vision or hearing evaluation was unknown.

The nursing staff reported that every day, for about an hour prior to dinner, EB wandered anxiously and asked the same questions repeatedly. She also occasionally raised her voice in agitation when the staff attempted to direct her away from the exit or to an activity. The recreation staff reported that EB was invited to three recreation activities a day, but she only attended about two activities a week. The staff added that "EB is afraid that if she goes to an activity, she will miss her children's visits," and when they encourage EB to socialize and converse with other residents "it's never successful."

Interactions between EB and staff were observed. Multiple miscommunications and incidences of confusion were noted. EB's memory as well as problem-solving ability and language were formally evaluated via the Cognitive Linguistic Quick Test (CLQT) and a spaced retrieval (SR) screen. Cumulatively, these tools suggested significant working memory and problem-solving deficits. She retained and recalled new information (maximum 2–3 elements) with appropriate visual scaffolding, SR practice, and vanishing cues.

In addition, informal cognitive/language assessments were conducted in low- and high-stimulation environments. EB demonstrated functional verbal expression in both environments. However, in high-stimulation environments, decreased language comprehension and increased requests for repetition were observed.

Hearing screening included an outer ear exam, as well as spoken word/sentence identification tasks, with speechreading and without, in noisy and in quiet settings. This screening revealed bilateral, moderate cerumen impaction and difficulty perceiving speech in noise without visual cues. Under ideal listening conditions during social conversation, EB displayed rudimentary, functional speech perception, but poor auditory processing of lengthy speech input.

Vision and reading screenings were performed with and without eyeglasses and included the Arizona Battery for Communication Disorders of Dementia (ABCD) visual field screen, color identification screen, reading signs in the environment, and an oral reading screen. Although no apparent difference in visual perception was noted with and without glasses, EB chose to wear her glasses throughout the evaluation. No visual field neglect or deficit in color perception was noted. EB's ability to notice and read signage was inconsistent. EB showed limited comprehension of common schedule aids in her current environment (e.g., calendars, recreation schedules, weekly menus, etc.), but she could read and comprehend an analog clock.

EB was unable to fluently read and comprehend typical book and newspaper material. However, when presented with print adaptations such as high-contrast, extra white space, large font, nonserif, evenly weighted typeface, EB showed intact letter identification and good decoding skills. With adapted, accessible print, EB read aloud slowly but fluently with functional comprehension. EB's written language comprehension proved to be functional and commensurate with her oral language comprehension. EB reported that adult books for leisure reading would be enjoyable to her.

48.4 Questions and Answers for the Reader

1. What information was obtained from EB and her personal history that would influence the focus of therapy?
   a) EB's wandering and agitation is most likely due to her need for physical exercise.
   b) In the past, EB has derived security and comfort from scheduling her day. Reading, working in groups, and helping others have provided fulfilment and purpose in her life.
   c) EB has not had to adapt to many new situations in her life and, therefore, may be struggling to adjust to her long-term care residence.
   d) EB enjoyed living independently and exercising control over her life. Reliance upon others for care may be the source of her distress and depression.

Answer: b is correct. Personality traits present before the disease process often persist, even in the presence of cognitive decline. In the past, EB enjoyed significant organization to her days. Presently, she may feel unsettled without that sense of structure. EB was sociable and community oriented. At this time, without conversation and personal contact with others, she may feel lost and anxious.

a is incorrect. Although exercise may benefit EB, neither EB nor her family mentioned physical exercise as important to EB in her past.

c is incorrect. This statement is too broad and universal to be helpful in determining the focus of an individualized plan for EB.

d is incorrect. Similar to c, this statement is too broad and universal to be helpful in constructing an individualized therapy plan with meaningful, practical goals unique to EB's needs and strengths.

2. What goals would be clinically justifiable and functional for EB?
   a) Use of a typical workbook to improve language skills and participation in cognitive games (e.g., concentration, trivia) would be effective therapy goals to improve EB's memory and word finding and to enable her to better communicate her wants and needs.
   b) No goals are appropriate for EB at this time due to the progressive nature of her disease.
   c) Engineering situations in which EB may engage in the types of activities that she enjoyed in the past (socializing, participating in groups, reading) to lessen EB's probable feelings of social isolation, disorientation, and restlessness.
   d) Given EB's signs of anxiety and depression, completion of the Cohen–Mansfield Agitation Inventory and the Geriatric Depression Scale is warranted to provide objective information in support of pharmacological treatment of EB's anxiety and distress.

Answer: c is correct. A justifiable, functional therapy approach for EB should focus on making modifications to foster EB's participation in the types of activities she enjoyed in her past.

a is incorrect. Although language exercises and memory games are common in traditional speech therapy, no scientific evidence exists that isolated language or memory activities improve recall or communication skills in people with dementia. A plan of care must use evidence-based interventions aimed at improved safety, communication, independence, and quality of life (e.g., a communication book to recall family visits, comprehending the dinner menu, speaking on the phone, using the nurse's call button, remembering to use a walker, remembering the steps for safe transfers, comprehending the activity calendar, using the TV remote, managing mealtime items, using a life storybook to increase socialization, using simulated presence therapy to decrease agitation, actively participating in activities of daily living, accepting medication, etc.).

b is incorrect. Therapy for memory-challenged seniors need not be restorative. Therapy is justified when the goal is to improve function, often via memory aids, environmental modifications, care partner training, and use of adapted materials.

d is incorrect. Although standardized assessments can provide helpful information in some cases, these scales are not of primary importance for EB's plan of care at this time. Given that EB is of no danger to herself or to others, the first priority is to determine EB's response to evidence-based therapy techniques and strategies to increase her comfort and engagement with the people, materials, and activities in her current environment.

3. How can SR and errorless learning (EL) be used to benefit EB in a functional way?
   a) To assist with recall and retrieval of a daily schedule.
   b) To assist with recall and retrieval of her eyeglasses.
   c) To assist her to remember the day of the week.
   d) To assist her to remember the name of the facility.

Answer: a is correct. For EB, a daily schedule is an excellent visual orientation aid that could reduce confusion and anxiety. However, its efficacy is affected by her independent use of the aid. SR and EL will enhance EB's cued recall, and possibly free recall, of this visual aid throughout the day.

b is incorrect. Although remembering to wear her eyeglasses is a functional goal, EB has shown no forgetfulness in this area. Wearing her glasses is in her procedural memory and does not need to be addressed in therapy.

c is incorrect. Recalling the day of the week is not a functional goal because it will not affect EB's behavior, activity level, engagement, or emotions.

d is incorrect. Although recall of the name of the facility is often a goal of therapy, EB's recall of the name of the facility will not likely affect her behavior, activity level, engagement, or emotions.

48.5 Description of Disorder and Recommended Treatment

Formal and informal assessment results confirmed that EB was functioning with vision and hearing limitations, moderate deficits in working memory and short-term memory, and a severe deficit in executive functioning. With regard to language, reading, and sustained attention, EB demonstrated functional skills for her age and environment. A significant component of EB's anxiety and agitation was not inherent to her AD diagnosis. As with many people living with dementia, much of EB's frustration and restlessness was due to the limitations of her environment and inadequate communication by her care partners. Hearing loss and decreased vision may also contribute to EB's social isolation, disassociation, loss of control, and disorientation.

Broadly, the goals of intervention for people living with dementia are to decrease disability, maximize functional abilities, and contribute to the design of a system of care to allow the individual to live symptom free as much as possible in the least restrictive environment. The justification for speech therapy (three times per week for 4 weeks) for EB was as follows:

There is reasonable expectation that therapeutic intervention in the form of environmental modifications, communication-partner training, visual memory aids, and meaningful activities with adapted materials will result in attainment of measurable, functional objectives for EB.

The objectives for EB are as follows:

- Increased attendance in recreation activities.
- More positive social interactions with peers.
- Less anxious wandering.
- Less agitated verbal exchanges.

A plan of care was designed to work collaboratively with EB, family members, and care professionals. The plan of care included the recommendations and treatment strategies below.

- Audition recommendations: Treatment for bilateral cerumen impaction and audiological evaluation was recommended. The impact of background noise on speech perception, confusion, and frustration level was discussed with family and staff. A quiet environment was created, with EB's consent, during care and during visits and involved turning TV/radio off, shutting the door, silencing pagers/phones, and refraining from side conversations with other individuals when with EB.
- Vision-related recommendations: Complete optometric evaluation was recommended. In addition, increased task lighting and ambient lighting was recommended in EB's room.
- Communication compensatory strategies: To minimize the frustration of miscommunication, the following communication recommendations for EB's conversational partner were suggested:
  ○ Maintain eye contact during discourse.
  ○ Introduce a topic before asking about it or elaborating on it.
  ○ Do not shift topics frequently.
  ○ Ask yes/no questions and offer binary choices rather than open-ended questions.
  ○ Do not ask direct questions about recent events.
  ○ Use one-idea sentences.
  ○ Do not speak quickly.
  ○ Give EB quiet time to process what was said and to formulate her response.
  ○ Be comfortable with silence.
- Daily schedule cue card (▶ Fig. 48.1, blank and ▶ Fig. 48.2, completed).
- Given EB's past reliance on a daily schedule, EB collaboratively designed a highly readable daily schedule form with place of residence and date printed on the top. EB communicated where she would like the schedule to be kept for easy access (i.e., in the bag on her walker). The importance of filling in the schedule every day with such items as meals, therapy, recreation activities, favorite TV programs, doctor appointments,

and especially family/friend visits was emphasized. Necessary print considerations were implemented to make the schedule readable for EB (i.e., using black ink, print letter formation not cursive, not block letters, large size font, and no print distractions). By observing staff's use of the form, the efficacy of the written daily schedule to decrease EB's feelings of disorientation and her anxiety about missing family visits was assessed as well as increased attendance at recreation activities. The nursing staff reviewed the schedule with EB in the morning and after her afternoon nap. Evidence-based memory interventions (e.g., SR and EL) were implemented to increase EB's recall of the daily schedule and its location.

- Independent, solo reading of adapted material: Given EB's past interest in reading and present ability to read, evidence-based, dementia-care Montessori principles (use of meaningful activities, preserved abilities, adapted materials, and prepared environment) were implemented to facilitate independent reading with the goal of reduced boredom, restlessness, and anxiety. Books with print adaptations (such as wide margins, nonserif, evenly weighted typeface, bold print, large font, short sentences with simple syntax, and supportive images) were identified; EB discussed her preference of books with nursing and recreation staff.

Environmental factors were also optimized to enhance EB's independent reading experience including the following:

- Bright lighting above and behind.
- Quiet environment.
- Use of a tabletop book stand.
- Optimal back, shoulder, arm, neck and head positioning and support.
- Reading to enhance family communication: Family members were introduced to interactive reading with adapted books as a means of enhanced communication with EB. These recommendations included the following:
  ○ Allow EB to explore the book at her own pace, in her own way, which may not be sequential.
  ○ Follow her lead.
  ○ Avoid a teacher–student dynamic.
  ○ Accept periods of silence as she reads and formulates her ideas.
  ○ Use gentle comments more than direct questions.
- Accessible reading material created by the family: EB's family was educated regarding the creation of personalized, accessible reading material for their mother (e.g., adapted online articles, high interest books, life storybooks).
- Reading with a friend (▶ Fig. 48.3): Typically, conversations with peer residents were unsuccessful for EB due to auditory, speech, and memory issues. Adapted books were implemented as an effective means of fostering EB's communication with peers. EB and a peer partner remained engaged with the book and with each other for a prolonged period of time without relying on staff intervention. The burden of understanding each other's speech and remembering what was said was lifted by the tangible, visual support provided by accessible reading material. To reduce EB's frequent late afternoon agitation, the staff encouraged EB to read an adapted book with another resident (i.e., reading with a friend). The environmental and interaction recommendations (treatments Nos. 5 and 6) to optimize the reading experience

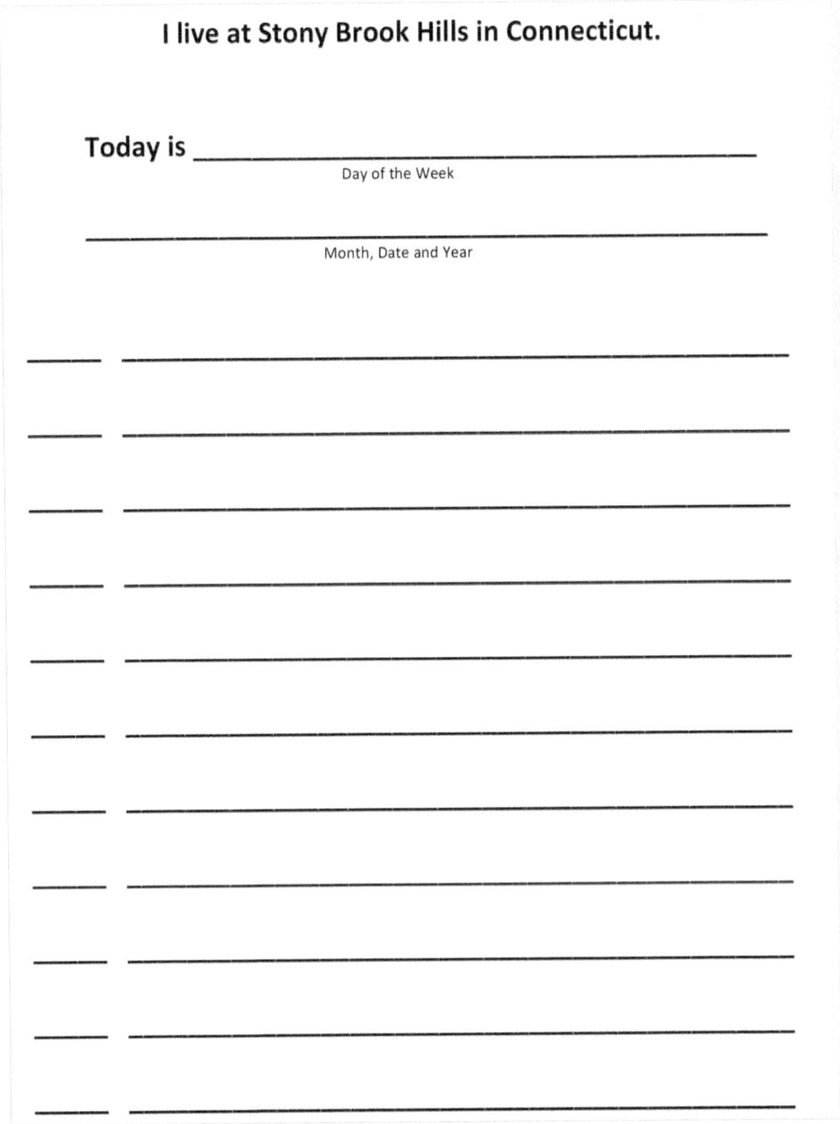

I live at Stony Brook Hills in Connecticut.

Fig. 48.1 Daily schedule cue card blank.

Today is _____
Day of the Week

_____
Month, Date and Year

___ _____

___ _____

___ _____

___ _____

___ _____

___ _____

___ _____

___ _____

___ _____

___ _____

were reinforced. "Reading with a friend" was added as an afternoon activity on EB's daily schedule form and added to EB's nursing care plan.

- Reading2Connect groups (▶ Fig. 48.4): Given EB's past experience with committees and social groups, EB, with the speech pathologist, attended one of the weekly recreation department Reading2Connect groups. The speech-language pathologist modeled and reviewed the optimal reading environmental and interaction recommendations (▶ Fig. 48.5 and ▶ Fig. 48.6) to foster EB's comfort level and engagement with the group. In addition, the weekly Reading2Connect group was also included in EB's daily schedule.

48.6 Outcome

By the end of therapy, visual memory aids, environmental adaptions, and communication strategies were implemented. Recreation staff reported that EB's activity attendance had increased from twice a week before therapy to twice a day.

According to recreation staff, EB "seemed to respect the authority of print" and most of the time willingly attended activities that were written on her daily schedule. EB also reported enjoying reading. However, staff observed that EB rarely read independently. Family and staff concluded that EB read and enjoyed books most when reading interactively with a family member or another resident. One staff member reported, "She lights right up when we invite her to read with another resident."

Nursing reported that EB consented to and enjoyed the scheduled reading with a friend four to five afternoons a week. Staff also reported that periods of afternoon wandering and agitated verbal exchanges decreased from about approximately 1 hour a day, 7 days a week, to approximately 15 minutes, about three times a week. Companionship reading appeared to be an effective nonpharmacological strategy to address EB's agitation, repeated questions, high confusion, and restlessness. In addition, EB's family reported that their awareness of environmental factors, use of communication strategies, and the adapted reading material made conversations with their mother more successful, substantial, and relaxed.

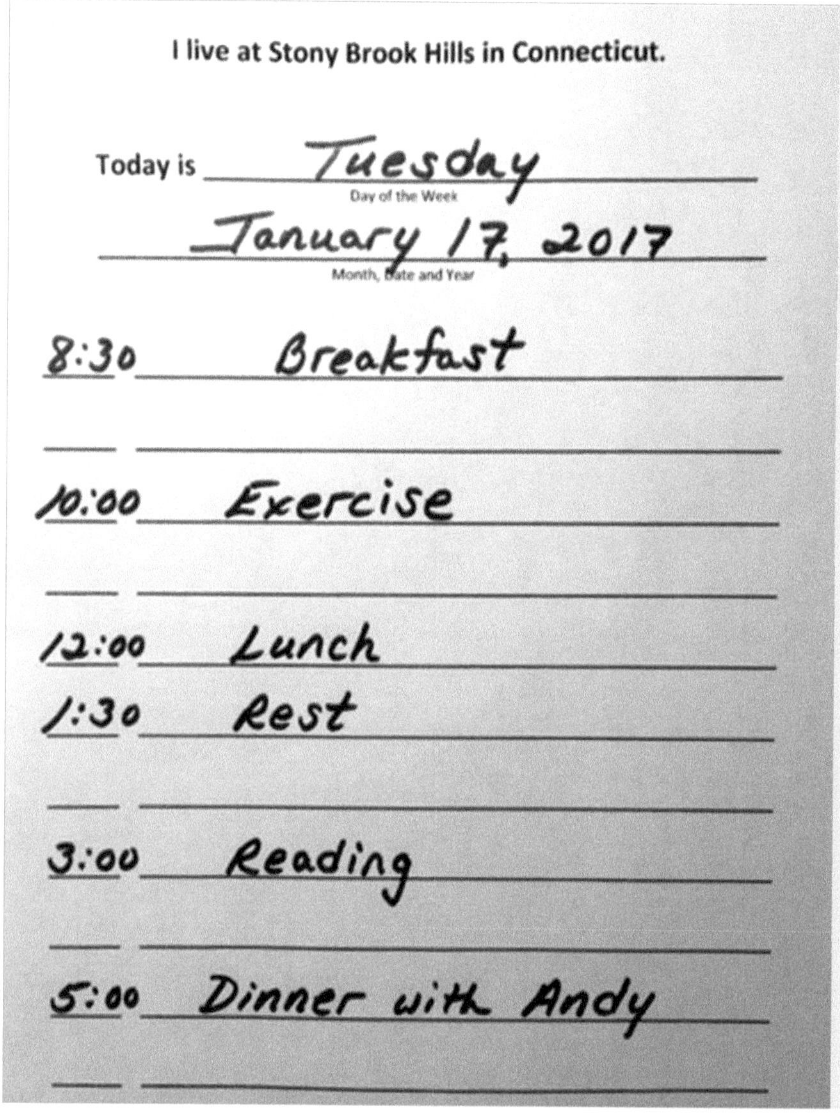

I live at Stony Brook Hills in Connecticut.

Today is _____ *Tuesday* _____
Day of the Week

_____ *January 17, 2017* _____
Month, Date and Year

8:30 _____ *Breakfast* _____

_____ _____

10:00 _____ *Exercise* _____

_____ _____

12:00 _____ *Lunch* _____

1:30 _____ *Rest* _____

_____ _____

3:00 _____ *Reading* _____

_____ _____

5:00 _____ *Dinner with Andy* _____

_____ _____

Fig. 48.2 Daily schedule cue card completed.

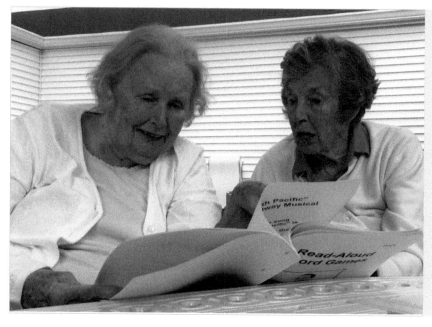

Fig. 48.3 Reading with a friend.

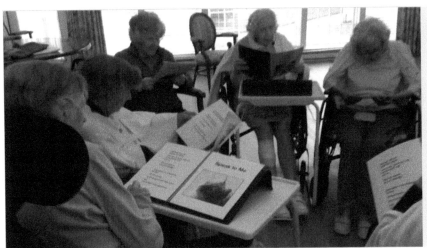

Fig. 48.4 Reading2Connect group.

reading2connect

Fig. 48.5 Environmental recommendations.

TO FACILITATE READING FOR MEMORY-CHALLENGED ADULTS

ENVIRONMENTAL RECOMMENDATIONS

Decrease Environmental Stimuli
Decrease background noise (TV, music, voices).
With their consent, position them where they can't see people moving around them.

Lighting
Maximize lighting above and behind.

Not Facing a Window
Bright light in front of them darkens the page.
Also, seniors have difficulty with glare.

Postural Support
Close to table.
Table height at or above elbows.
Pillow/cushion behind back – no hunching over.
Elbows resting on a surface (chair arm rests or table).

Book Placement
Book should be raised and at an angle; not lying flat on the table.
Slant board, document holder, edge of table.

Eyeglasses
Always find out if the resident wears glasses.
However, don't assume the reader can see more clearly with glasses (could be outdated prescription, for distance, or another person's glasses).
Using our vision screens, informally assess adult's reading comfort with and without glasses.
If glasses are needed, clean them.

www.reading2connect.org   860.235.4348   reading2connect@gmail.com reading**2**connect

...rediscovering the joy of reading

What does our *Invitation to Read*™ entail?

1. Social connection first and foremost.
   When approaching a resident,
   - approach from the front slowly
   - use eye contact
   - smile
   - use a gentle voice
   - engage in social, pleasant, introductory discourse
   - use judicial, calming touch

2. Presenting the book.
   When the individual appears to be at ease,
   - gently bring the book into her line of vision.
   - comment or ask an indirect, nonthreatening question about the cover.
   - look for signs of interest or withdrawal.
   - help her take the book and explore it if that is what she wants.

3. Preparing for reading.
   If the individual is showing interest in the book,
   - gently assist her in optimal body positioning (back support, close to the table, table at elbow height).
   - support and positioned the book properly.
   - adjust lighting as needed.
   - minimize extraneous environmental stimulation.
   - clean and adjust eye glasses as needed.
   - assess functional vision.

4. Interacting with the book.
   Each person will need different kinds and different degrees of support with the reading process. Some ways to support the reader are as follows.
   - preview the book
   - follow the reader's lead
   - honor her choices and independence
   - quietly assist without disrupting the person's exploration of the book
   - determine if conversation facilitates the reading process or hinders it
   - be comfortable with the quiet time needed for the reading process
   - no need to insist on sequential reading
   - avoid teacher-student dynamic

www.reading2connect.org   860-235-4348   reading2connect@gmail.com

Fig. 48.6 Interaction recommendations.

48.7 Key Points

- Cognitive/language therapy for people living with dementia should be functional, focusing on optimizing visual and auditory reception, educating communication partners, and modifying the environment to circumvent deficits and capitalize on the individual's spared abilities.
- Difficult behaviors exhibited by persons living with dementia are not random. They are a form of communication, and may more accurately be referred to as *responsive* behaviors. These behaviors are generally related to physical discomfort or pain, inadequate communication by care partners, and/or suboptimal environmental factors.
- Cognitive/language assessment of people with dementia is a dynamic and highly individualized process, occurring throughout the duration of therapy and involves the examination of the efficacy of interventions.

Suggested Readings

[1] Bourgeois M. Memory Books and Other Graphic Cuing Systems. Baltimore, MD: Health Professions Press; 2007

[2] Dixon PS, Ostrowski S. Making reading easier for people with dementia. vertical bar Advance Senior Care. 2016. Available at: http://www.iadvanceseniorcare.com/article/memory-care/making-reading-easier-people-dementia

[3] Kitwood T. Dementia Reconsidered: The Person Comes First. Philadelphia, PA: Open University Press; 1999

[4] Basting AD. Forget Memory. Baltimore, MD: The Johns Hopkins University Press; 2009

49 Speech-Language and Dysphagia Assessment in a Bilingual Female Post Cerebrovascular Accident

Luis F. Riquelme

49.1 Introduction

This case describes the speech-language/dysphagia assessment and intervention following a left hemisphere cerebrovascular accident (CVA) in an 81-year-old bilingual (Spanish/English) woman. This patient initially presented equal language impairment in both her native, Spanish, and second language, English. Patients like these can benefit immensely from assessment and treatment by a bilingual speech-language pathologist (SLP), who is able to accept responses in either language, as well as provide stimuli in either language.

49.2 Clinical History and Description

AS, an 81-year-old woman, presented to the emergency room at a local acute care hospital with a past medical history of diabetes mellitus, hypertension, and hyperlipidemia. Initial computed tomography of the brain revealed no evidence of acute intracranial hemorrhage, mass effect, or midline shift. A focal area of diminished attenuation in the right basal ganglia compatible with lacunar infarct was noted. Given that AS arrived at the emergency room with signs/symptoms of stroke, she underwent and failed dysphagia screening (i.e., she coughed upon being given 3 ounces of water to drink without interruption) and was temporarily kept NPO (nil per os). According to AS's daughter, AS was fully bilingual (Spanish/English) prior to this incident, but her native/primary language was Spanish. AS was a retired seamstress. In addition, AS was also employed as a home health aide for a short period of time. AS was originally from Honduras and had lived in the United States for more than 20 years.

49.3 Clinical Testing

AS was admitted to the Acute Stroke Unit and seen by speech-language pathology early the next morning. The available clinician was a monolingual/English speaker. The initial evaluation focused on AS's most immediate need: her ability to eat by mouth. Use of an interpreter was explored, but due to the complexity of linguistic symptomatology, the clinician chose to await full speech-language evaluation by a Spanish-speaking clinician. Results of this evaluation revealed a mild oropharyngeal dysphagia, characterized by mild bolus management delays noted clinically. Further, the initial monolingual evaluation left queries regarding possible aphasia versus apraxia of speech for further exploration by a bilingual clinician. This evaluation resulted in the following recommendations: chopped diet with neutral liquids and further speech-language assessment by a Spanish-speaking examiner. Neutral liquids are a classification used at the local institution to describe a set of liquids that do not include acidic or fatty substances. All other liquids are allowed. This classification is thought to reduce risk for development of aspiration pneumonia given that acidic/fatty substances are thought to be more invasive for the lungs than other "neutral" substances.

A second SLP evaluation was conducted by a Spanish-speaking clinician. AS presented with poor comprehension skills (< 10%) for simple yes/no questions, following commands, and object identification in a field of two. These findings were consistent when stimuli were presented in Spanish and in English. Verbal output was unintelligible with prosodic features of both Spanish and English. Approximately 10% real words were produced within jargon; these words were judged to be low content. Again, some productions were in English and some in Spanish. Overall, AS was well related and cooperative. Results of this evaluation revealed a moderate-to-severe fluent aphasia and speech-language treatment provided by a bilingual Spanish/English clinician was recommended.

Subsequent magnetic resonance imaging of the brain without contrast, conducted 4 days postadmission, revealed acute infarct in the left temporoparietal region, with foci of diminished gradient within the infarcted region compatible with hemorrhagic components. In addition, mild chronic microvascular changes and mild cortical atrophy were noted. AS was discharged home after a 2-week admission. She was then referred for outpatient rehabilitation, including speech-language reassessment and treatment. Approximately 8 weeks post onset, AS was seen in the outpatient center and reassessed for speech-language treatment services by a bilingual Spanish-/English-speaking clinician. Results revealed continued moderate-to-severe fluent aphasia, with improvements observed in comprehension and slightly for expression. Data from testing in Spanish revealed the following: simple yes/no questions—62% correct; common object identification in a field of two—66% correct. Verbal output continued to comprise mostly jargon with increasing use of concrete words. Jargon now included simple phrases, which increased intelligible productions to 30%. In this context, some confabulation was noted. More direct testing for output was conducted via adapted subtests of the Boston Diagnostic Aphasia Examination (BDAE; available informally in Spanish version from Spain or from Argentina). Confrontation naming: 20% correct; picture description via the cookie theft picture was similar to conversational output described. Reading was at 60% for matching labels to common objects, while writing was limited to producing AS's name. Similar results were noted in English.

49.4 Questions and Answers for the Reader

1. What was the significance of having a speaker of the patient's native language conduct an assessment? (In view of the fact that patient was bilingual Spanish/English prior to the CVA.)

a) Testing in dominant language would have sufficed.
b) Need to compare proficiency and breakdown in both languages concurrently.
c) Important for patient to feel comfortable.
d) No real need to have a bilingual examiner see patient.

Answer: b is correct. Differences in comprehension, processing, and selection for expression are significant factors in determining choice of language for treatment and overall prognosis. It is known that bilinguals possess an intermixed lexical and morphosyntactic neural organization; however, inconsistent evidence exists for cross-language transfer post CVA. Kohnert[1] questions whether L1 and L2 are equipotent for language/communication gains.

a is incorrect. AS was bilingual prior to CVA; therefore, the interaction of both languages needs to be addressed post neurological event.

c is incorrect. The patient's language proficiency is likely insufficient for feelings of comfort. Overall communicative effectiveness needs to be taken into account.

d is incorrect. The argument for testing in both languages of proficiency prior to CVA has been made.

2. Would results be different if the assessment had been conducted using an interpreter?
   a) Yes, using an official interpreter always yields more accurate data.
   b) Yes, using a bilingual SLP always yields more accurate data.
   c) There is minimal evidence to support large diagnostic differences when using an interpreter.

Answer: c is correct. Clinical intuition suggests that the use of an interpreter is the "second" best alternative; however, no empirical evidence exists to support this. The SLP team at this local institution conducted a small performance-improvement project in 2012 using interpreters and native-speaking SLPs for patients of Spanish or Russian background who were referred for a speech-language evaluation post CVA. The hypothesis was that results from evaluations conducted at bedside would differ when conducted by a native speaker of the patient's native language versus when conducted with the use of an interpreter. All testing was conducted on the same day and examiners were blinded to results from the previous evaluation. Nine patients participated in the project, four Russian and five Spanish speakers. We found that the resulting impressions did not differ when the assessment was conducted by an SLP in the native language of the patient versus when conducted with a native-speaking interpreter. These results should be interpreted cautiously given the small number of participants.

a is incorrect. There is insufficient research evidence available to make this statement.

b is incorrect. There is insufficient evidence on this issue.

3. Knowledge of the neuroimaging results assist in reaching a communication diagnosis. True or false?
   a) True.
   b) False.

Answer: a is correct. The fact that damage was multifocal helped explain some language-processing behaviors. Simply stated, focal damage may result in one-dimensional language breakdown, whereas in the presence of diffuse damage, cognitive factors play a stronger role in neural relations with language processing.

If only considering behavioral communication factors during assessment, many clinical judgments may be questioned. While neuroimaging data are not always available, location and circumstances of the brain damage help the examiner form a stronger hypothesis for impressions and recommendations.

49.5 Description of Disorder and Recommended Treatment

AS presented with significant moderate-to-severe fluent aphasia. Her comprehension was limited, ranging 60% to 70% for simple auditory input, yet she appeared socially appropriate, as expected with this clinical population. While her language output was mostly jargon, prosodic features from both Spanish and English were observed. An increase in concrete productions and simple phrases, mostly in Spanish, was also of note. The mild oropharyngeal dysphagia noted acutely when first examined 1 day post admission had resolved by the time of discharge from the hospital. As there were no complaints of any swallowing deficits, a dysphagia evaluation was not included in the outpatient assessment protocol.

AS's family support, mostly from her only daughter, was excellent. Her daughter was present for approximately 80% of the sessions, supporting carryover of the treatment goals to the home. Language proficiency in one language versus the other was difficult to ascertain in the context of fluent aphasia. Given that both L1 and L2 are processed in the dominant hemisphere, in overlapping areas, it was anticipated that both languages were affected by her CVA.

During outpatient language therapy, an important decision had to be made regarding the choice of language to employ in treatment. Several hypotheses exist regarding language recovery post focal cerebral lesion in bilingual speakers. The most known are parallel and nonparallel recovery (where proficiency in L1 and L2 are similar or dissimilar to levels prior to the brain injury), Ribot's rule (proposed in 1881: L1 will be the stronger language post injury), and Pitre's rule (proposed in 1895: the dominant language at the time of injury will be the first to recover). The following three components should be considered when making decisions regarding language of treatment decisions in bilingual patients:[2]

- Premorbid language history, including educational/occupational history and estimated extent of premorbid bilingualism.
- Strengths and weaknesses in each language.
- Environmental factors: the language that the patient selects for rehabilitation, the language of family choice, and the sociocultural language needs upon discharge.[3]

Given that AS presented stronger skills in Spanish, with some emerging English output, treatment was conducted in Spanish with allowances for English productions. This ideal clinical scenario was possible given the availability of a bilingual SLP for treatment. Encouragingly, evidence suggests that regardless of language of treatment, the other language will also benefit. A recent systematic review of 14 studies examining the effect of treatment for bilingual individuals with aphasia revealed evidence for cross-linguistic transfer in over half of the studies included. This review also showed that treatment in L2 resulted in receptive and expressive language changes in L1, even in chronic bilingual aphasia.[4]

49.6 Outcome

As treatment progressed, comprehension and content of verbal output increased in both Spanish and English. Comprehension for structured and nonstructured tasks increased to 95% with no notable difference by language of presentation (Spanish vs. English). Expressive language increased from simple phrases to high-content narratives, 80% for accuracy. While output was often in Spanish, the emergence of greater support from English was evident. Literacy skills were also targeted and facilitated presentation of in-home activities (i.e., homework). Improved reading comprehension increased to 90% (BDAE Reading Sentences and Paragraphs subtest) in English. While not tested formally, the patient was able to read stories in newspapers and discuss with daughter as well as clinician. AS was eventually able to conduct her own banking business and manage her real estate properties in the United States and abroad. Her communication disorder evolved into a mild nonfluent aphasia with mild comprehension deficits. Her bilingualism was supported, as she often retrieved lexical items in one or the other, with intermittent ability to translate as needed.

49.7 Key Points

- Patients can greatly benefit from working with a bilingual SLP, who is able to accept responses in either language, as well as provide stimuli in either language.

- Treatment goals need to target language processing for input or output, regardless of language used to provide the context.
- Neuroimaging data can be of benefit when attempting to understand the pathophysiology of the language breakdown in the context of bilingualism.
- The choice of which language to target in treatment in language-impaired bilingual adults has received some attention; however, important unanswered questions remain. Future research should focus on whether comprehension networks continue to improve for the language not being used in treatment and whether the rate of treatment progress is delayed when the nondominant language is used for treatment.

Suggested Reading

[1] Riquelme LF. Working with limited-English speaking adults with neurological impairment. Perspect ASHA Spec Interest Groups (SIG 15). 2006; 11(2):3–8

References

[1] Kohnert K. Language Disorders in Bilingual Children and Adults. San Diego, CA: Plural Publishing; 2008
[2] Riquelme LF. Clinical issues with Hispanic and Asian populations: Part 1: Choice of language for intervention with adult populations. Maui, Hawaii: ASHA Teleseminar; 1994
[3] Wallace G. Multicultural Neurogenics: A Clinical Resource for Speech-Language Pathologists Providing Services to Neurologically Impaired Adults from Culturally and Linguistically Diverse Backgrounds. Tucson, AZ: Communication Skills Builders; 1997
[4] Faroqui-Shah Y, Frymark T, Mullen R, Wang B. Effect of treatment for bilingual individuals with aphasia: A systematic review of the evidence. Neurolinguistics. 2010; 23(4):319–341

50 Accent Modification in a 30-Year-Old L1 Ukrainian Speaker

Darlene M. Monda

50.1 Introduction

This case involves the evaluation and management of a female English speaker with a moderate Ukrainian accent. Accent modification is often sought by professionals hoping to enhance their career trajectory. NS specifically desired to improve her communicative effectiveness and confidence in the use of Standard American English (SAE) in daily contexts at home with her children, in social contexts with friends, and in her professional life. As a future speech-language pathologist (SLP), she was particularly concerned regarding her ability to deliver services effectively.

50.2 Clinical History and Description

NS, a 29-year-old woman, was self-referred for accent modification. NS is a native speaker of Ukrainian, but she currently speaks English in almost all settings including with her two young children. She moved to the United States from Ukraine in 2001 at the age of 15 following intensive English language studies. She continues to speak Ukrainian with her husband and parents. At the time of the evaluation, she was enrolled in her first year of a Master's program in Communicative Sciences and Disorders. NS referred to herself as a "perfectionist," and expressed an acute awareness of specific components of her accent, an academic and personal interest in treatment methodologies, and a strong desire to improve her speech and language skills to sound "as close to native as possible."

50.3 Clinical Testing

Expressive and receptive language, assessed informally during conversational speech, were functional for academic purposes. However, frequent omission of articles was observed in statements such as: "I like restaurant Spotted Pig." Cognition, voice, and fluency were informally determined to be within normal limits. An oral-sensorimotor exam revealed unremarkable strength, steadiness, symmetry, rate, range of motion, and coordination of the orofacial mechanism. Speech production was formally assessed using the Compton Phonological Assessment of Foreign Accent Test (▶ Table 50.1), as well as via informal observations throughout the session. NS read single words, self-corrected productions without cueing, produced each word in a sentence, and orally read the passage provided in the Compton.

NS presented with a moderate Ukrainian accent, characterized by vowel distortion, incorrect syllable stress, and sound substitutions in English consistent with those of a native Ukrainian speaker. An informal speech/language sample was obtained to evaluate language use, syllable stress, prosody, rate, intensity, fluency, and resonance during conversational speech.

Phonemic errors occurred in the conversational context with increased frequency; syllable stress, fluency, and prosody were negatively impacted by both increased rate of speech and decreased self-monitoring. Additionally, resonance was perceived as mildly nasal during conversational speech. Speech rate was increased during conversational discourse, matching perceptually with that of a typical New York City–based speaker, with mildly reduced fluency, prosody, and oral resonance. Vocal loudness was considered below normal limits, but attributed to self-consciousness about her accent. NS exhibited functional hearing and reported that a hearing evaluation "two semesters ago" revealed intact hearing acuity.

50.4 Questions and Answers for the Reader

1. What further formal and/or informal testing would assist in the formation of a treatment plan?
   a) A test of phonological processes to acquire more information on production.
   b) Use an acoustic analysis program (such as Praat) to measure vocal intensity, pitch, and resonance for comparative baseline data.
   c) Analyze a recorded speech/language sample to evaluate language use, syllable stress, prosody, rate, intensity, fluency, and resonance in conversational contexts.
   d) Employ word lists to determine coarticulatory variability for target sounds.

Answer: c is correct. Each of these elements influences the perception of accent. To employ SAE across all communicative contexts, it is essential to address all aspects of output, which calls for a comprehensive overview of speech patterns. Analysis of these speech parameters at the conversation level will complement information gathered from isolated words, sentences, and oral reading.

a is incorrect. Phonological processes may be present in nonnative speech, but they are not the cause for the presenting accent. The client does not have a disorder of speech, rather habits influenced by the client's first language (L1) patterns.

b is incorrect. Instrumental analysis of voice is not necessary to determine the presence of, or indicate solutions to, accent-related production differences. Informal assessment did not indicate the need for more comprehensive voice evaluation.

d is incorrect. Coarticulatory influences on phoneme production are useful in treatment, but will be best assessed via a connected speech sample rather than words in isolation.

2. How would you formulate a prognosis for this client's therapeutic success?
   a) Contrast the number of error versus correct sounds produced in SAE.
   b) Consider interests, motivation, educational level, language mastery, and daily use.

Table 50.1 Results of the Compton stimulus word responses subtest, February 1, 2014

Intended vowel	Spoken vowel: single words	Examples in SW	Spoken vowel: sentences	Examples in sentences	English words
/e/	/ɛ/	/snɛk/	–	–	Snake
/ɪ/	/i/	/witʃ/	/i/		Witch
/ɪ/	/ɛ/	/kɹɛb/, /twɛnz/	–	–	Crib, twins
/i/	/ɛ/	/ʃtʃin/	/ɛ/	ʃtʃiŋ	
/ɛ/	/æ/	/θɹæd/	/æ/		Thread
/ɪ/	/ɛ/	/pɛg/, /pɹɛnt/	/ɛ/ x 1	/pɹɛnt/	Pig, print
/ʌ/	/æ/	/gæm/, /glæv/	/ æ /	/glæv/	Gum, glove
/a/	/o/	/bol/	/o/	/bol/	Ball
/ʊ/	/ʌ/	/pʌt/	/u/	/luk/	Put, look
Intended consonant	**Spoken consonant: single words**	**Examples in SW**	**Spoken consonant: sentences**	**Examples in sentences**	**English words**
/ŋ/ final	/ŋg/	/ɹɪŋg/			Ring
/θ/ initial	Distorted /θ/	/θɝd/	–	–	Third
/θ/ final	/t/	/tit/	–		Teeth
/k/ final	–	–	/g/	/tʃɹæg/	Truck
/z/ final	–	–	/s/	/nois/	Noise

c) Compare the inventory of phonemes absent in L1 to the number of SAE phonemes mastered.

d) None of the above.

Answer: b is correct. Prognosis is based on several factors. Most significantly, NS is highly motivated to improve intelligibility to ensure career success. Furthermore, she self-corrected during the assessment. Adequate intellect and executive functioning were observed as evidenced by her academic and professional achievements to date; both are favorable prognostic indicators for accent modification. Finally, her choice of profession and her current use of L2 in most settings offer substantial opportunities to attain her desired outcome. Challenges to progress, however, may include the lack of excellent SAE models at home and significant time constraints secondary to the demands of graduate school as well as parenting and other obligations. In addition, prolonged poor use of L2 resulting in habituation of error patterns and her perfectionism may also limit motivation over time if expectations are not met.

a is incorrect. Assessing severity by contrasting number of error sounds versus number of correct sounds produced in SAE narrows the evaluation by yielding a quantitative assessment of a predominantly qualitative parameter. Although number of error phonemes is a factor in considering the length of treatment, it is not a sufficient prognostic indicator without consideration of the complex of factors considered in answer b.

c is incorrect. Comparative inventories of phonemes between languages are of interest academically, but not a practical measure of potential for change. Numerous unknown but influencing extralinguistic features not evidenced in a phonological inventory make this impractical.

d is incorrect?

3. Which taxonomies would guide your treatment plan and what treatment modalities would best enhance the adoption of appropriate and natural SAE use?
   a) Frequency of occurrence of error phonemes in SAE and correction via education, and treatment via practice at the word, sentence, and conversational levels.

b) Severity of impact on intelligibility and correction via self-monitoring and opportunities for self-correction, as well as training in the use of environmental cues.

c) Hierarchy of stimulability for errors with drill and practice in various contexts.

d) All of the above.

Answer: d is correct. Identification of productions negatively impacting intelligibility is a primary indicator for the selection of production targets. The most efficient path to change is via learned self-monitoring and self-correction. The use of environmental cues to note, assess, and accommodate listener comprehension is also critical to functional communicative change. The frequency of occurrence of error phonemes in SAE is also a main determinant in treatment planning. Correct production of frequently occurring phonemes will strongly impact the perception of accent improvement. Practice at the conversational level starting at the onset of education regarding sound production creates early awareness of the need for change. In some cases, stimulability may be the most critical factor for the selection of early targets for those who respond to success by increased dedication to practice. In all cases, drill and naturalistic practice are essential.

4. What are the best discharge criteria to use with accent modification clients?
   a) Client satisfaction with status or clinician determination of lack of measurable benefit from treatment.
   b) Decreased frequency of occurrence of error phonemes and inappropriate syllable stress, and correct production of frequently occurring phonemes and language use at the conversational level.
   c) Accurate production of all target sounds, consistently appropriate intonation patterns, with mastery determined through a phonemically balanced oral reading sample, produced at a moderate rate of speech.
   d) Accurate self-monitoring and self-correction of target sounds, emerging intonation patterns, and correct language usage at a moderate speech rate at the conversation level.

Answer: a is correct. Each person with a desire to modify a naturally occurring speech pattern, as in the case of a foreign or regional accent, has a personal rationale and outcome criteria for treatment. If the individual attains satisfaction with progress, conviction that continued progress can be made outside of treatment, or a balancing point between desire for change and willingness to work at it, a logical end point has been reached. An equally powerful rationale for discharge exists when no progress can be observed or measured by the clinician or the client. When this occurs, there is no longer a "reasonable prognosis" for improvement, and reevaluation at a later time may be suggested as the American Speech-Hearing-Language Association's Preferred Practice Patterns indicate.

b is incorrect. Decreased frequency of occurrence of error phonemes and inappropriate syllable stress, and correct production of frequently occurring phonemes and language use at the conversational level are desirable and measurable outcomes, but they do not indicate client readiness to end therapy. If a particular person has not demonstrated mastery for skills of self-monitoring and correction, or simply wishes to continue to work toward further mastery, discharge is not indicated.

c is incorrect. Accurate production of target sounds and consistently correct intonation patterns are positive treatment outcomes, but mastery cannot be determined at the reading level. Even if the client has no familiarity with the text, both positive and negative conditions exist when producing speech from text. These include influences through visual representation, the words of others, and the lack of connectivity to conversational speech. While selected reading passages provide a means of practice and exposure to various forms of production, conversational speech remains a greater indicator of mastery.

d is incorrect. Although accurate self-monitoring and self-correction of target sounds, emerging intonation patterns, and correct language usage at a moderate speech rate at the conversation level are the keys to success, client goals must also be met when possible. For example, in professional situations where being recognized as a native speaker is crucial, it is important to progress beyond the level of self-correction to be perceived as such. For this reason, client satisfaction, along with continued demonstration of benefit from treatment, is the preferred discharge criteria for accent modification clients.

50.5 Diagnosis, Therapy Recommendation, Goals

NS presented with moderately accented English, characterized by phoneme errors, inappropriate syllable stress and intonation, and article misuse and deletion. A rapid speech rate and mildly decreased speaking volume further compromised intelligibility. Language errors were primarily article misplacement and deletion. Fluency was within normal limits for an English speaker, but prosody was marked by inconsistent stress patterns. It was recommended that NS undergo weekly, 50-minute sessions focused primarily on discrimination and production of SAE vowels and consonants, correct use of articles, and appropriate intonation. These therapeutic goals were addressed during the course of treatment in naturalistic contexts such as conversation, presentation practice, test administration, and interview role-playing as well as dialogue readings. Early goals included appropriate production of tense and lax vowels in both words and phrases, accurate production of final word voicing of consonants, demonstration of self-awareness of incorrect productions of specific targeted sounds, self-correction, the use of appropriate English grammatical elements, and vowel substitutions and distortions in words and phrases across all communicative contexts. Goals were added as mastery of phonemes was achieved. An emphasis was placed on self-monitoring and correction, which aided in the reduction of rate and improved syllable stress, prosody, and use of articles. Correction of SAE vowels also aided in increased oral resonance. NS participated in 41 fifty-minute sessions of accent modification services over a 15-month period, and was discharged in May 2015.

50.6 Outcome

In follow-up testing, again using the Compton (▶ Table 50.2), NS demonstrated reduced frequency of errors of target phonemes, improved syllable stress, improved overall prosody, and the elimination of article deletion and misplacement. By her own report, NS speaks with increased awareness, particularly with regard to "overarticulation" and reduced speech rate. NS states that although she feels "more free and fluent" in her expression, she still catches errors and then "I go home and practice." Most significantly, NS described adequate self-confidence to enter her clinical placements as an SLP intern. Follow-up testing confirmed these improvements while providing goals for continued progress. Supplied with the tools of self-awareness, self-monitoring, and self-correction, NS was discharged from treatment.

50.7 Key Points

- Prognosis for successful accent modification is complex, demanding high-level motivation and independence with overarching skills such as rate control.

Table 50.2 Results of the Compton stimulus word responses subtest, April 29, 2015

Intended vowel	Spoken vowel: single words	Examples in SW	Spoken vowel: sentences	Examples in sentences	English words
/ɛ/	/æ/	/θɹæd/	/æ/		Thread
/ɪ/	/ɛ/	/pɛg/, /ʃtʃɛŋ/	/ɛ/	ʃtʃɛŋ	Pig
/ʌ/	/o/	/glov/	/ o /	/glov/	Glove
Intended consonant	**Spoken consonant: single words**	**Examples in SW**	**Spoken consonant: sentences**	**Examples in sentences**	**English words**
/ŋ/ final	/ŋg/	/ɹɪŋg/			Ring
/z/ final	–	–	/s/	/nois/	Noise

- Training of self-monitoring and self-correction skills is essential for continued progress even after the course of treatment ends.
- Client-centered materials and naturalistic practice are most generalizable to daily life.

Suggested Readings

[1] Menon MS. Foreign Accent Management. San Diego, CA: Plural Publishing; 2007

[2] ASHA Preferred Practice Patterns. Guidelines on admission and discharge criteria. http://www.asha.org/policy/GL2004–00046.htm#sec1.4

51 Influence of Cognitive Status on AAC Intervention in a Case of Amyotrophic Lateral Sclerosis

Michelle Gutmann

51.1 Introduction

Amyotrophic lateral sclerosis (ALS) can yield substantial speech, language, and cognitive deficits. Both low- and high-tech alternative and augmentative communication (AAC) options should be considered for this challenging population.

51.2 Clinical History and Description

RL, a 62-year-old woman, was seen for an initial speech pathology consultation at a multidisciplinary ALS clinic, having been diagnosed with bulbar-onset ALS 1 month prior. RL was accompanied by her husband who expressed concern about his wife's speech. When questioned, RL reported that she noted changes in her voice and speech for approximately 8 or 9 months. She visited her family doctor when her "raspy voice" would not clear. The doctor was unable to identify the etiology of this voice change and referred RL to a local otolaryngologist (ENT). According to RL, the ENT was unable to diagnose any organic pathology underlying the voice change. RL continued to engage regularly in social and community activities and was an avid exerciser as well. Speech changes began to compound over time, and RL revisited her family doctor who referred her to a local neurologist. The neurologist suspected ALS and referred RL for further workup. RL was then seen by a neurologist affiliated with a multidisciplinary clinic at a large teaching hospital. RL underwent a series of testing including electroencephalogra-

phy, nerve conduction studies, and magnetic resonance imaging to confirm the diagnosis of ALS. Both RL and her husband were significantly distressed by this diagnosis. Of note, RL's husband traveled regularly for work and was not home much of the week.

51.3 Clinical Testing

At the time of initial visit, the clinician explained the role of speech-language pathologist (SLP) as part of the multidisciplinary team, provided both verbal and written information regarding speech, language, and swallowing deficits in ALS, and discussed the need to schedule a full evaluation. RL and husband agreed to an outpatient visit approximately 3 weeks from the time of the first ALS clinic visit. Speech, language, and cognitive screening were conducted at that time. Results are summarized in ▶ Table 51.1.

RL was independently ambulatory at the time of evaluation and was independent in all ADLs (activities of daily living). Bulbar functions such as speech, swallowing, and, to a lesser extent, respiration were most affected. Notably, RL could generally follow conversation, although verbal perseverations were noted as was poor performance on cognitive tasks such as executive function and overall language comprehension elicited by the MoCA (Montreal Cognitive Assessment).

Given the severity of RL's dysarthria at the time of the outpatient evaluation, AAC options were discussed and demonstrated. To meet RL's current communication needs and provide

Table 51.1 Summary of clinical speech, language, and cognitive assessment

Test	Description	Results
Sentence Intelligibility Test (SIT)	Set of 11 decontextualized sentences of increasing length are presented onscreen. Patient reads each sentence while they are being taped. Unfamiliar listener transcribes the sentences. Comparison between the actual sentences presented vs. what listener transcribed provides basis for calculations.	• 64% intelligible • Communication efficiency ratio of 0.59
Word Intelligibility Test (WIT)	57 individual words presented onscreen. Patient reads each one while being taped. Comparison between the actual words presented vs. what listener transcribed provides basis for calculations. Options for coding and for presentation of stimuli (i.e., in a phrase or as a single word) exist.	• 52% intelligible
Montreal Cognitive Assessment (MoCA)	Cognitive screening tool that taps executive function, memory, attention, language, and abstraction.	• 21/30 (≥ 26 is WNL for people with 12th-grade education) • Range for MCI: 19–25.2/30
ALS Functional Rating Scale-Revised (ALSFRS-R)	Standard rating scale widely used to characterize function across domains such as motor skills, ability to dress, speech, and respiration. Scores range from 0 (maximum disability) to 48 (no disability) points.	• 35/48: Score taken from RL's electronic medical record reflecting patient's recent clinic visit
Dysarthria staging	Speech staging system widely used in ALS.	• Stage 4:speech + nonvocal communication (writing)

ALS, amyotrophic lateral sclerosis; WNL, within normal limits; MCI, mild cognitive impairment.

Table 51.2 AAC options presented

Device	Features supported	Skills needed to operate
Lightwriter SL-40	• Text-to-speech • QWERTY or ABCD layout • Attention-getting bell • Word prediction • Memory for phrases • Memory for longer, prepared texts	• Direct selection • Single finger sufficient for operation • Typing (single finger or more)
iPad with Verbally app (free version)	• Text-to-speech • Various onscreen text layouts • Attention-getting bell • Word prediction • Some preprogrammed phrases • Premium version supported additional features such as better voice, categorization of phrases to be stored in memory, etc.	• Direct selection • Swipe, tap, and push home button • Typing (single finger or more)
iPad with AssistiveChat app	• Text-to-speech • Word prediction • Memory for phrases	• Direct selection • Swipe, tap, and push home button • Typing (single finger or more)

ABCD, alphabetic layout of keyboard; app, application; QWERTY, layout of typical keyboard.

an option for an ambulatory patient, several AAC options were selected for demonstration. The Lightwriter, a dedicated device that supports text-to-speech synthesized speech output with a proprietary dual-sided screen and a keyboard that could support either QWERTY or ABCD layouts, was attempted. A mobile tablet with a variety of commercially available text-to-speech apps was also demonstrated. ▶ Table 51.2 summarizes the features of each AAC option.

51.4 Additional Assessment

The majority of the outpatient assessment was devoted to trials of AAC options. Each AAC option was introduced and demonstrated for both RL and her husband. RL then had the opportunity to try each option. The clinician asked RL questions and had her answer using the AAC option she was trialing at the time. In this way, RL was put in communicative situations that required use of similar phrasing while trialing each device. Performance across options could be more readily compared than when each option was trialed with a unique and dissimilar task. Considerations at this point included personal preference as well as objective data from device trials. ▶ Table 51.3 summarizes RL's performance with each AAC option trialed.

At the end of the assessment, RL indicated that she would like to try a Lightwriter at home. The clinician agreed that this was a viable option and indicated that she would locate a loaner unit for the patient. Despite RL's significant speech challenges and likely imminent total loss of speech, cognitive involvement had the greatest influence on selection of an AAC option. Use of a tablet was contraindicated by RL's inability to perform basic functions such as "swipe," "tap," and "touch the home button" during trials. Although RL was capable of executing motor tasks such as "tap the icon" with hand-over-hand assistance, she was unable to reliably understand and independently perform the required movements. Use of a basic dedicated device with customizable

features was the device of choice, given her ability to use it functionally during the assessment. She could type single words and short phrases and locate keys on the keyboard. She could also use the erase function and the bell to get attention. Interestingly, RL's husband advocated strongly for use of a mobile tablet. His rationale for such was that many of his wife's friends had tablets and that it would not be socially stigmatizing for her to use one when with them. He underplayed the significance of RL's inability to perform basic tasks (e.g., "tap the icon to open the app," or "press the 'home' button") with the tablet.

51.5 Questions and Answers for the Reader

1. A patient with ALS, having a moderately severe mixed (spastic-flaccid) dysarthria, agrees to participate in an assessment for AAC. What domains should be evaluated so that you have a solid overview of your patient's basic skills prior to exploring AAC options?
   a) Fine, gross, and oral motor skills.
   b) Speech, language, and cognition.
   c) Fine motor, auditory comprehension.
   d) Higher-level language skills.

Answer: **b is correct.** Without a basic overview of your patient's speech, language, and cognitive skills, you may over- or underestimate patient's abilities given their ease and familiarity with conversational communication in context. Given how effortful speech is for a patient with dysarthria, you need to assess judiciously, not overtaxing any one system but sampling across domains of function.

Once thought of as purely a motor disorder, it is now known that cognition is often affected in ALS. It is important to assess this function as it has clear implications for both assessment and implementation of AAC.

Table 51.3 Performance with various AAC options trialed

Device	Skills needed to operate	Performance
Lightwriter SL-40	• Direct selection • Single finger sufficient for operation • Typing (single finger or more)	• Preferred ABCD layout • Able to spell single words and short phrases • Hunt and peck typist still able to use right index finger of dominant right hand • Liked double-sided screen
iPad with Verbally app (free version)	• Direct selection • Swipe, tap, and push home button • Typing (single finger or more)	• Extreme difficulty following commands to swipe and tap • Could perform under imitation but only fleetingly • Liked the bell function • Word prediction options were potentially confusing
iPad with AssistiveChat app	• Direct selection • Swipe, tap, and push home button • Typing (single finger or more)	• Same as above for swipe and tap commands • Liked large "speak" icon • Liked idea of saving phrases in categories

ABCD, alphabetic layout of keyboard; app, application.

a is incorrect. Although a thorough assessment of all functional domains is important, SLPs are not trained to provide a detailed assessment of fine and/or gross motor skills. Since fine motor skills have implications for AAC with respect to access, and gross motor skills have implications for AAC with respect to portability and the potential need for mounting, this information is important but outside the SLP's purview. Assessment of oral motor skills is within the SLPs purview and should be a critical component of the assessment for AAC.

c is incorrect. Although it is important to know about a patient's fine motor ability and his/her auditory comprehension, assessing only these functions does not provide enough information with respect to the potential use of AAC to meet the requirement of a thorough assessment.

d is incorrect. Information regarding higher-level language skills is important and may be relevant to the type of vocabulary/language a patient may use with an AAC system. However, these skills alone are insufficient to provide the breadth of information necessary for hypothesis testing with AAC options.

2. Given the RL's current status, what features of AAC systems should you consider?
   a) A dedicated eye-tracking system that needs to be mounted to a wheelchair.
   b) A picture-based communication app that runs on a mobile tablet.
   c) A large, picture-based commercially available communication display.
   d) A lightweight, portable option that supports text-to-speech output.

Answer: **d is correct.** Since the patient is still independently ambulatory and literate, it is important to meet patient's needs with an AAC option that is portable and supports direct selection as a method of input (i.e., the ability to activate the desired cell by direct touch), and exploits the patient's existing spelling skills. Patient also has to talk on the phone with her husband who often travels for work, so the AAC option should support that need as much as possible.

a is incorrect. An eye-tracking system that needs to be mounted to a wheelchair is not a portable option; it is likely too heavy to carry around for someone who is independently ambulatory. As technology improves, it is quite possible that tablets that support eye gaze as a method of input for communication will become accessible. At this time, however, dedicated eye gaze systems tend to be bigger and heavier than mobile tablets.

b is incorrect. A picture-based communication app that runs on a mobile tablet would not support patient's use of her literacy skills and would require additional learning. Use of a tablet is unlikely to be practical for her, given her difficulty using the clinic's tablet during the assessment.

c is incorrect. A large, picture-based commercially available communication display would not meet patient's need for speech output, and it would likely be limited in terms of options that she could express given that it would only have room for a finite number of pictures.

3. Knowing the typical clinical trajectory of speech and motor deterioration in ALS, which AAC options should you consider for later on in your patient's disease progression?
   a) AAC options that support direct selection via touch because that is what your patient uses now.
   b) AAC options that support a variety of access methods to accommodate motor deterioration.
   c) A picture-based commercially available communication display with a head pointer for access.
   d) An electronic magic slate that the patient can print/write messages on and erase with the press of a button.

Answer: **b is correct.** The typical clinical trajectory of deterioration in speech and motor functions in ALS means that patients' needs often change as the disease progresses. In terms of AAC, this means that patients may require alternate means of access (i.e., they may no longer be able to type on a keyboard or tap an icon/letter on a tablet) to use an AAC system. Likewise, as speech deteriorates, they may become more reliant on AAC. Clinicians need to plan ahead for these changes and aim to have a variety of equipment options available to meet the patient's changing needs.

a is incorrect. Direct selection means that the person using the AAC system selects the desired item directly from among the available options (e.g., typing on a keyboard, or touching a picture of desired item/phrase). Direct selection via touch may not be viable as an access method as motor function continues to deteriorate as the disease progresses.

c is incorrect. Although use of a picture-based commercially available communication display may become part of the communication system for a person with ALS, use of a head pointer (i.e., a stylus or stick that is attached to a headband worn around the head and situated at the forehead) may be precluded by decline in motor function. Often, muscles of the neck weaken significantly, so the ability to move one's head may be lost.

d is incorrect. Writing may not be viable as motor function declines. Likewise, not having speech output would be extremely limiting, especially as speech function may deteriorate or be lost as the disease progresses.

4. The spouse of a patient with ALS purchases a mobile tablet after the AAC assessment. From what you know about the patient's inability to use a tablet during the assessment, you counsel the husband about:
   a) The nature of cognitive and physical decline in ALS as they relate to communication.
   b) How he may need to stop working and become his wife's full-time caregiver.
   c) How his wife's cognition is more than likely to stay as it is at the present time.
   d) How his wife will learn to use the tablet if he forces her to use it every day.

Answer: **a is correct.** Informational counseling—the nature of cognitive and physical decline in ALS, as they relate to communication, in general, and to use of AAC, in particular—should be provided judiciously. The amount of information provided should dovetail with husband's readiness to receive and integrate it. Affective counseling would likely be quite appropriate at this juncture as well.

b is incorrect. Although this may be one course of action, this option is not related to purchase of a mobile tablet and patient's inability to use it.

c is incorrect. Cognitive decline in ALS is not static and it is more than likely that patient's cognitive status will continue to deteriorate over the course of her disease.

d is incorrect. In addition to being unethical, forcing someone to use an AAC option, or any equipment, is not a guarantee that the system will be used functionally. Given the wife's inability to use independently a mobile tablet during the assessment, it is unlikely that she will acquire this skill under duress.

51.6 Description of Disorder and Recommended Treatment

ALS may be accompanied, or preceded, by cognitive impairment, which influences both the type and extent of AAC intervention. Cognitive impairment in ALS is not the same as in a disease such as Alzheimer's, and it tends to be associated with a more rapid course of the disease. In terms of AAC intervention, when cognitive decline is suspected and/or documented, introduction of devices should be initiated as soon as possible so that procedural memory, which is usually preserved, can be exploited when learning device operation. Had RL been diagnosed with ALS closer in time to symptom onset, and had she been willing to consider AAC options instead of relying on speech beyond the point when it was viable as a primary means of communication, intervention for AAC may have been more successful.

Although a portable AAC option that supported text-to-speech may not have continued to meet her needs for the duration of the disease, at the time of assessment, it was a reasonable therapeutic option. Once the use of AAC is integrated into a patient routine,

transfer of those skills to another device and/or means of access, if needed, may be predicated on this earlier success. Since the natural trajectory of ALS involves increasing physical and motor deterioration, it is likely that RL would later require different AAC options. For this reason, access to a pool of loaner AAC equipment is critical to supporting the needs of patients with ALS. Since needs change, and may do so many times over the course of the disease, it is vital to have access to all sorts of options so that people are able to use them while needed and then return the item to the pool when it is no longer useful to them.

51.7 Outcome

In subsequent phone follow-up with RL's husband, he told the clinician that on their way back to their hometown, they had stopped at a local retailer to look at tablets. The sales clerk demonstrated a few options to RL and her husband, and when the clerk asked RL whether she thought she would use it and a variety of other innocuous questions, RL repeatedly responded "yes." To obviate the need for another trip, the tablet was purchased at that time.

The clinician verbally reviewed all the results from the assessment and highlighted the difficulty that RL demonstrated in following the steps to use the basic functions of the tablet. RL's husband remained hopeful that she could learn how to use a tablet for communication. Similarly, RL's husband reiterated that RL answered "yes" to all the clerk's questions. The clinician explained about verbal perseveration and how it fulfilled a pragmatic function even if the answer did not reflect the speaker's true intent.

The clinician located a loaner Lightwriter and arranged to send it to the family who had identified a clinician in their community who would provide support in its implementation. RL's husband suggested that it would be too overwhelming to have both the Lightwriter and the tablet, and he preferred that she learn to use the tablet.

Subsequently, a clinician more local to the family contacted this clinician to strategize and optimize intervention. We sourced an app that supported communication of "yes" and "no," but did not require typing of actual words. We also discussed use of an option such as a MessageMate with recorded messages for common requests, comments, and social interaction. The local clinician thought this might be a consideration since, despite repeated instruction in how to use basic functions of the tablet, RL was unable to use it functionally. Lower tech AAC options such as a picture-based communication display accompanied by text were implemented by the local clinician.

Although viable AAC options were identified and a loaner unit sourced for RL, AAC intervention took another route. RL's husband's desire for her to have her own mobile tablet to use as a communication device superseded RL's inability to use the tablet. RL's husband spent significant time attempting to convince RL to use the mobile tablet rather than learning to use other AAC devices. A precipitous decline in RL's physical condition resulted in only limited progress with the low-tech communication option (e.g., display). Both cognition and communication continued to decline, with the deterioration in cognition further compounding communication deficits. At the time of her death, RL was anarthric and had not mastered functional use of AAC.

51.8 Key Points

- Despite the proliferation of mobile tablets and apps in the marketplace, no randomized controlled trials have been performed with mobile tablets as AAC devices for people with ALS.
- The decision regarding AAC options should be made on a case-by-case basis, based on current and projected needs.
- When at all possible, access to a pool of AAC equipment that can be loaned to patients is well suited to the needs of the person with ALS. This applies to AAC as well as all other equipment they may need (e.g., wheelchair, shower chair, Hoyer lift).
- Cognitive impairment in ALS is well documented and may both shorten life span and diminish cognitive resources available for the implementation of AAC.

Suggested Readings

[1] Elamin M, Phukan J, Bede P, et al. Executive dysfunction is a negative prognostic indicator in patients with ALS without dementia. Neurology. 2011; 76 (14):1263–1269

[2] Hanson EK, Yorkston KM, Britton D. Dysarthria in amyotrophic lateral sclerosis: a systematic review of characteristics, speech treatment, and augmentative and alternative communication options. J Med Speech Lang Pathol. 2011; 19(3):12–30

[3] Körner S, Sieniawski M, Kollewe K, et al. Speech therapy and communication device: impact on quality of life and mood in patients with amyotrophic lateral sclerosis. Amyotroph Lateral Scler Frontotemporal Degener. 2013; 14(1): 20–25

52 Dysarthria Associated with Parkinson's Disease

Jessica E. Huber

52.1 Introduction

People with Parkinson's disease (PD) often present with significant speech and voice changes, called hypokinetic dysarthria.[1,2] Speech characteristics most commonly associated with PD include reduced loudness, weak voice, breathiness, hoarseness, fast rate of speech, and imprecise articulation.[3] PD also impacts self-monitoring[4] and cognitive resources,[5] reducing their ability to perceive changes in their speech and alter their production in everyday communication environments. This is a case of an individual with fairly advanced PD and significant dysarthria as a result. Lack of previous treatment response was a complicating factor in devising a treatment plan.

52.2 Clinical History and Description

DG was a 73-year-old woman diagnosed with idiopathic PD approximately 12 to 14 years ago. She lived at home with her husband. Her primary concern was decreased vocal intensity, which varied with dopaminergic medication. Although she did not complain of voice fatigue, she frequently lost her voice by the time her husband returned from work in the evening. DG was a retired nurse and her husband was often the only communication partner that she had all day. She had occasional visitors, but was otherwise mostly homebound. DG stated that she generally avoided communicative situations due to her difficulty speaking. Her voice was typically better when she had some vocal use during the day; she reported that her voice improved in the evening on days she had visitors. Three years ago, an evaluation by an otolaryngologist revealed unremarkable vocal folds. She underwent the Lee Silverman Voice Treatment program (LSVT LOUD)[6] at two facilities in the past 2 years. LSVT LOUD is an intensive behavioral treatment program to increase loudness, clarity, and self-monitoring. She and her husband reported no significant improvement after the program. She scored in the normal range on the Montreal Assessment of Cognition (MoCA).[7]

52.3 Clinical Testing

Perceptual characteristics: Perceptually, her speech consisted of moderate-to-severe hypophonia, slightly decreased speech rate, and occasional articulation errors. Her vocal quality was moderately severely breathy and moderately hoarse. She was mostly intelligible (75%) in conversation with careful listening. Her husband assisted with communication repair.

Oral mechanism examination: DG demonstrated a slight right lip droop, but adequate protrusion, retraction, and labial seal. Eye and mandibular dystonia were observed. Tongue lateralization and strength were moderately reduced, and tongue tremor was observed as well as a weak volitional cough. Alternating and sequential motion rates were slow but rhythmic.

Respiratory function: Inspiratory and expiratory muscle strength were assessed by measuring maximal inspiratory and expiratory pressures. Pressures were much lower than expected (see ▶ Table 52.1).

Voice evaluation: DG's sound pressure level was 66.3 dB on average during conversation (using a 6-cm mouth-to-microphone distance), significantly lower than published norms (about 80 dB).[8] The SpeechVive device[9] was implemented to determine whether she was stimulable for increased vocal intensity in noise. The SpeechVive device is a small wearable device that elicits increased sound pressure level by playing noise in one ear, eliciting the Lombard effect. DG increased sound pressure level to 69.3 dB on average with the SpeechVive device in place during conversation. However, increased intensity varied across conversation. Intensity tended to be lower at the ends of sentences and for short (one- to two-word) utterances. The Communication Participation Item Bank (CPIB)[10] was administered; she scored 3/30 and reported her condition interfered very much with communication. Her husband scored 2/30, indicating agreement with significant difficulties in communication participation.

Swallowing evaluation: DG and her husband indicated some coughing during most meals, particularly when ingesting thin liquids. DG reported that occasionally she has difficulty starting to swallow chewed solids, but that pureed foods did not cause any difficulty. DG was referred for a Videofluoroscopic Swallow Study (VFSS) at a local medical facility.

52.4 Questions and Answers for the Reader

1. What muscle(s) is/are likely weak, as reflected by reduced maximum expiratory pressure?
   a) Diaphragm.
   b) Scalene muscles.
   c) External intercostals.
   d) Abdominal muscles including the rectus abdominis, internal and external oblique muscles, and transverse abdominis muscle.
   e) Posterior and lateral cricoarytenoid muscles.

Table 52.1 Maximum inspiratory and expiratory pressure results

Measurement	Client's pressures: evaluation (cm H$_2$O)	Client's pressures: after 6 weeks of therapy (cm H$_2$O)	Expected pressures[13] (cm H$_2$O)
Maximum expiratory pressure	52	102	121
Maximum inspiratory pressure	24	44	56

Answer: d is correct. The abdominal muscles act to increase alveolar pressure and cause expiration.

a is incorrect. The diaphragm is the main muscle of inspiration.

b is incorrect. The scalene muscles are small, relatively weak muscles that elevate the first rib.

c is incorrect. The external intercostals are mostly muscles associated with inspiration.

e is incorrect. The posterior and lateral cricoarytenoid muscles are associated with arytenoid movement, resulting in true vocal fold movement.

2. Given her physiological presentation, which of the following issues are you most concerned with assessing, in addition to her speech production?
   a) Walking.
   b) Balance.
   c) Feeding and swallowing.
   d) Cognitive function.
   e) Language skills.

Answer: c is correct. Given her voice quality and oral mechanism exam results, it is likely that she experiences both oral and pharyngeal swallowing issues and is at risk for aspiration.

a and b are incorrect. They are not in the scope of practice for speech-language pathologists.

d is incorrect. She and her husband report no change in cognition. Her primary complaint is speech-related. She scored normally on the MoCA screening. She seems able to adequately judge her communication and report her condition.

e is incorrect. Generally, language changes in PD are related to cognitive change. Given that any changes in cognition are subtle, language is likely acceptable.

3. Which treatment might you try with DG to improve her communication?
   a) LSVT LOUD.
   b) SpeechVive alone.
   c) SpeechVive with vocal warm-ups and behavioral therapy to improve voicing and communication repair strategies.
   d) Pacing therapy to increase speech rate.
   e) Oral motor exercises to increase lip and tongue strength.

Answer: c is correct. The SpeechVive was effective in cueing increased vocal intensity. However, the effects were variable, suggesting the need for behavioral therapy in addition to daily use of the SpeechVive device.

a is incorrect. She has had two courses of LSVT LOUD in the last 2 years without improvement. However, effortful voice production training may assist her.

b is incorrect. Due to the variable effects of the SpeechVive device, additional behavioral therapy is indicated to improve speech and communication. Her reports of better voice with use suggest that vocal warm-ups would be of benefit to her.

d is incorrect. We would not want to increase her speech rate, even though it is slow. Her slower speech rate likely contributes to intelligibility.

e is incorrect. Oral motor exercises have not been shown to have clinical efficacy for speech.

4. If you were to attempt treatment to increase respiratory muscle strength, which would you choose?
   a) Inspiratory muscle strength training with the PowerBreathe.
   b) Expiratory muscle strength training with the EMST 150.
   c) Both inspiratory and expiratory muscle strength training with the breather.
   d) Both inspiratory and expiratory muscle strength training with an incentive spirometer.
   e) Both inspiratory and expiratory muscle strength training with the PowerBreathe and EMST 150.

Answer: b is correct. Since she is experiencing significant issues with vocal intensity, strengthening the respiratory system is critically important. There are excellent data demonstrating that expiratory strength can be improved in people with PD as a result of expiratory training.[11] Additionally, treatment with the EMST 150 has been shown to improve hyolaryngeal elevation, which may mitigate issues with aspiration, depending on the findings of a swallowing evaluation.[11] Finally, it is possible for treatment of expiratory muscle strength to increase maximum inspiratory pressure by improving abdominal support for the diaphragm and rib cage during breathing.

a and e are incorrect. There are less efficacy data regarding the use of inspiratory strength in people with PD. Also, it is often difficult for patients to keep up with both treatments at once. This would require 60 minutes per day of respiratory exercise, at least 5 days per week.

c and d are incorrect. Neither of those devices provide enough overload to result in increased strength.

52.5 Description of Disorder and Recommended Treatment

DG presented with moderate-to-severe dysarthria as a result of PD. Major impairments were associated with respiratory weakness and laryngeal valving. Treatment was recommended twice a week for 6 weeks. Treatment focused on improving vocal quality, speech breathing patterns, and clear speech,[12] along with communication repair strategies including augmentative low-tech systems. Expiratory muscle strength training using the EMST 150 was initiated, five sets of five breaths five times per day for at least 5 days. Vocal warm-up exercises were taught and she was asked to perform them twice daily, once in the morning and again in the afternoon before her husband comes home. Treatment with the SpeechVive device was also initiated. She wore the device daily for at least 3 to 8 hours and read aloud with the device for 30 minutes per day. She was also encouraged to engage in more social communicative situations during the week. Safety and efficiency of swallow was also assessed via VFSS. The evaluation indicated that DG had (1) intermittently reduced oral transit with chewed solids, (2) delayed initiation of the swallow, (3) moderately reduced laryngeal elevation, (4) moderate aspiration of thin liquids during the swallow, and (5) moderate pharyngeal residue for solids leading to inconsistent aspiration after the swallow.

52.6 Outcome

DG improved her voice quality and vocal intensity within 6 weeks of therapy. Her speech was clearer and she used a text-to-speech system well for communication repair. However, she was unable to maintain increased vocal intensity without the

SpeechVive device. It was recommended she continue to use the device daily during communicative situations. Her inspiratory and expiratory muscle strength increased, but she remained below norms (see ▸ Table 52.1). It was recommended that she continue expiratory muscle strength training. Treatment for swallowing was conducted during speech therapy sessions since much of the speech work could be practiced outside of the therapy room with the SpeechVive.

52.7 Key Points

- It is important to consider respiratory muscle strength, particularly expiratory strength, in individuals with PD.
- The lack of success with LSVT LOUD suggests the need for modified or alternative therapies.
- Oral motor exercises are not acceptable approaches to improve speech, even in the context of oral motor weakness.
- Technological treatments such as the SpeechVive can be used in combination with other speech and swallowing treatment approaches.

Suggested Readings

[1] Sapienza CM. Respiratory muscle strength training applications. Curr Opin Otolaryngol Head Neck Surg. 2008; 16(3):216–220
[2] Fox CM, Morrison CE, Ramig LO, Sapir S. Current perspectives on the Lee Silverman Voice Treatment (LSVT) for individuals with idiopathic Parkinson disease. Am J Speech Lang Pathol. 2002; 11:111–123
[3] Stathopoulos ET, Huber JE, Richardson K, et al. Increased vocal intensity due to the Lombard effect in speakers with Parkinson's disease: simultaneous laryngeal and respiratory strategies. J Commun Disord. 2014; 48:1–17

References

[1] Logemann JA, Fisher HB, Boshes B, Blonsky ER. Frequency and cooccurrence of vocal tract dysfunctions in the speech of a large sample of Parkinson patients. J Speech Hear Disord. 1978; 43(1):47–57
[2] Ho AK, Iansek R, Marigliani C, Bradshaw JL, Gates S. Speech impairment in a large sample of patients with Parkinson's disease. Behav Neurol. 1999; 11(3):131–137
[3] Darley FL, Aronson AE, Brown JR. Differential diagnostic patterns of dysarthria. J Speech Hear Res. 1969; 12(2):246–269
[4] Ho AK, Bradshaw JL, Iansek T. Volume perception in parkinsonian speech. Mov Disord. 2000; 15(6):1125–1131
[5] Zgaljardic DJ, Borod JC, Foldi NS, et al. An examination of executive dysfunction associated with frontostriatal circuitry in Parkinson's disease. J Clin Exp Neuropsychol. 2006; 28(7):1127–1144
[6] Fox CM, Morrison CE, Ramig LO, Sapir S. Current perspectives on the Lee Silverman Voice Treatment (LSVT) for individuals with idiopathic Parkinson disease. Am J Speech Lang Pathol. 2002; 11:111–123
[7] Armstrong MJ, Duff-Canning S, Psych C, Kowgier M, Marras C. Independent application of montreal cognitive assessment/mini-mental state examination conversion. Mov Disord. 2015; 30(12):1710–1711
[8] Huber JE. Effects of utterance length and vocal loudness on speech breathing in older adults. Respir Physiol Neurobiol. 2008; 164(3):323–330
[9] Stathopoulos ET, Huber JE, Richardson K, et al. Increased vocal intensity due to the Lombard effect in speakers with Parkinson's disease: simultaneous laryngeal and respiratory strategies. J Commun Disord. 2014; 48:1–17
[10] Baylor C, Yorkston K, Eadie T, Kim J, Chung H, Amtmann D. The Communicative Participation Item Bank (CPIB): item bank calibration and development of a disorder-generic short form. J Speech Lang Hear Res. 2013; 56(4):1190–1208
[11] Troche MS, Okun MS, Rosenbek JC, et al. Aspiration and swallowing in Parkinson disease and rehabilitation with EMST: a randomized trial. Neurology. 2010; 75(21):1912–1919
[12] Lam J, Tjaden K. Clear speech variants: an acoustic study in Parkinson's disease. J Speech Lang Hear Res. 2016; 59(4):631–646
[13] Enright PL, Kronmal RA, Manolio TA, Schenker MB, Hyatt RE, Cardiovascular Health Study Research Group. Respiratory muscle strength in the elderly. Correlates and reference values. Am J Respir Crit Care Med. 1994; 149(2, Pt 1):430–438

53 Stroke-Induced, Moderate, Acquired Apraxia of Speech and Nonfluent Aphasia

Lisa D. Bunker and Julie L. Wambaugh

53.1 Introduction

Apraxia of speech (AOS) is an acquired neurogenic communication disorder resulting from disrupted planning/programming of motor speech production. Although, historically, there has been some disagreement regarding the characteristic features of AOS, most experts in the field agree that the following features are characteristic of AOS: sound errors (i.e., distortions, often perceived as sound substitutions), increased segment and/or intersegment durations, and slowed speech rate with a tendency to segregate syllables and equalize stress across syllables.[1,2] Other common features that may be present, but are not unique to AOS include articulatory groping (silent or audible), increased errors with increased length and/or complexity of utterances, motor perseveration, difficulty initiating speech, self-awareness of errors, improved automatic speech production, and periods of errorless speech (e.g., social conventions). Differentiating AOS from other neurogenic speech and language disorders (e.g., aphasia with phonemic paraphasia) has also been an area of concern for researchers and clinicians alike. This case will present the history and assessment tasks necessary to adequately differentiate and diagnose AOS with subsequent intervention as indicated.

53.2 Clinical History and Description

BB was a 64-year-old Caucasian man who was referred for a speech and language evaluation and subsequent treatment due to complaints of difficulty "[saying] the right words, but [knowing] what [he wants] to say," and poor intelligibility. BB's wife reported that his speech/language symptoms began 6 months ago following a stroke. A review of the neurologist's computed tomography scan report confirmed an ischemic cerebrovascular accident in the left middle cerebral artery. Residual symptoms included a mild-negligible right lower extremity weakness, a mild-to-moderate right upper extremity weakness, and speech/language impairment.

53.3 Clinical Testing

After collecting BB's case history, an oral-mechanism examination was administered to identify possible characteristics associated with dysarthria and nonverbal oral apraxia.[3] Additional tasks were requested to determine the presence of limb apraxia (e.g., making a "thumbs up," clapping, or snapping fingers).

BB was then given a series of AOS screening tasks,[3] which included repetition of sounds, syllables, monosyllabic words, and polysyllabic words incorporating a thorough inventory of consonants in various word positions. He was also asked to repeat words with similar phonemic structure, but with increasing length (e.g., "car," "carpet," "carpenter," and "carpetbagger"), and repeated productions of polysyllabic words (e.g., "octopus" repeated three times). Sentence repetition was completed as well (approximately five to seven words in length; "The boy is raking leaves"). Diadochokinetic tasks, including alternating and sequential motion rates, were elicited and audiorecorded to verify the calculation of syllables per second. Several automatic language tasks were given, including counting, reciting days of the week, and singing a familiar tune (i.e., "Mary had a little lamb"). Lastly, BB was engaged in brief conversational, narrative, and reading tasks to determine the impact of any deficits on connected speech. The preceding speech samples were audiorecorded.

After completing these screening tasks, the presence of apraxic symptoms was rated using the Apraxia of Speech Rating Scale (ASRS),[4] which rates the presence/severity of 16 features associated with AOS (both differential and nondifferential, such as sound distortions or articulatory groping) on a 5-point scale. Single-word speech intelligibility was assessed using the computerized Chapel Hill Multilingual Intelligibility Test (CHMIT),[5] which involved BB repeating 50 monosyllabic words. Responses were recorded and then scored by three unfamiliar listeners.

The Western Aphasia Battery-Revised (WAB-R)[6] was administered to assess presence, type, and severity of aphasia. Tasks include spontaneous speech (conversation and picture description), auditory verbal comprehension (question comprehension, word recognition, and following directions), repetition, and naming/word-finding (object naming, fluency, sentence completion, and short-answer questions). To assess functional communication, BB completed the general short form (10 questions) of the Communicative Participation Item Bank (CPIB),[7] which included questions such as "Does your condition interfere with giving someone *detailed* information?" All assessment results are reported in ▶ Table 53.1.

53.4 Questions and Answers for the Reader

1. Which of the following characteristics must be present for a diagnosis of AOS?
   a) Articulatory groping.
   b) Sound distortions.
   c) Increased errors with increased utterance length.
   d) Islands of error-free speech.

Table 53.1 Speech and language assessment results for BB

Assessment task	BB's performance/response
Oral mechanism exam (and limb apraxia)	• No characteristics of dysarthria (e.g., weakness, hypo-/hypertonicity, unilateral deviations) • Symptoms of nonverbal oral apraxia were absent • No apparent limb apraxia; some difficulty with bilateral tasks due to his right upper extremity paresis
Sound, syllable, and monosyllabic word repetition	• Slight slowed rate on some monosyllabic words • Occasional consonant errors on monosyllabic words (about 10%)
Repetition of words of increasing length	• Slow rate, slower on longer words • Consonant errors = 40%; voicing, fronting/backing, and other distortion errors; errors were predominantly on stops, affricates, and clusters • Vowel errors = 10%; errors were generally on diphthongs
Polysyllabic word repetition	• Slow rate on most productions (prolonged and segmented syllables) • 60% consonant errors, 15%–20% vowel errors, on words 3 + syllables in length • Errors predominantly on stops, affricates, clusters, and diphthongs • Moderate difficulty initiating, particularly words beginning with affricates/clusters • Articulatory groping, increased on longer utterances
Repeated productions (3 ×)	• Slow rate, false starts/self-corrections • 56% consonant errors; 10% vowel errors • Error type/place was generally consistent • Stop errors in medial and final syllable positions • Affricates/cluster errors in all positions • Vowel errors in longer utterances
Sentence repetition	• Slow rate on most productions (prolonged and segmented syllables)
Conversation, narrative, and reading tasks	• Overall slow rate (prolonged and segmented syllables) • Similar frequency and pattern of consonant and vowel errors as word and sentence repetition tasks
DDK rates	
• AMRs	• 5.2, 4.8, and 4.3 syllables/second for /p/, /t/, and /k/, respectively • Mild difficulty after several repetitions
• SMRs	• Unable without integral stimulation (i.e., "watch me, listen to me, say it with me")
Automatic language tasks	• Slightly slow, but within functional limits
Prosody	• Overall monotone quality with occasional inappropriately stressed syllables
CHMIT	• Intelligibility was rated, on average, at 63%
Other	• Perseveration (during speech repetition tasks) and periods of fluent speech were infrequent
ASRS score	• Scored 2 or 3 on *most* items (i.e., frequent or pervasive but not significantly impacting intelligibility) • Overall score of 38/64 (cutoff of 8 for diagnosis of AOS)
WAB-R	• BB's aphasia quotient (AQ) was 65, and was categorized as Broca's aphasia • Language production characterized as moderately agrammatic, anomic, and perseverative, but with relatively good comprehension
CPIB	• BB scored 18/30 (higher scores indicate less participation interference).

AMRs, alternating motion rates; ASRS, Apraxia of Speech Rating Scale; CHMIT, Chapel Hill Multilingual Intelligibility Test; CPIB, Communicative Participation Item Bank; DDK, diadochokinetic; SMRs, sequential motion rates; WAB-R, Western Aphasia Battery-Revised.

Answer: b is correct. A diagnosis of AOS can be made if key features, including sound distortions, are present.

a is incorrect. Although persons with AOS often demonstrate articulatory groping, this symptom is also present in some individuals with aphasia without AOS. Thus, it cannot be reliably attributed to only AOS.

c is incorrect. Increased errors with increased syllable length is a common feature of apraxic speech production, but it is also associated with aphasia. Thus, its presence—in the absence of the compulsory features of AOS—should not be used to make a diagnosis.

d is incorrect. Brief periods of error-free speech may be noted for an individual with AOS, especially for very automated or stereotypic responses. However, this characteristic may be observed for some types of aphasia and cannot be used to differentiate AOS from aphasia.

2. AOS usually co-occurs with aphasia. AOS symptoms overlap somewhat with symptoms often considered diagnostic of nonfluent aphasia. Which symptoms are characteristic of both Broca's aphasia and AOS?
   a) Word-retrieval difficulties.
   b) Significantly reduced comprehension of spoken language in comparison to production of verbal language.
   c) Difficulty with reading comprehension.
   d) Effortful speech and language production.

Answer: d is correct. Effortful speech production is considered characteristic of both Broca's aphasia and AOS.

a is incorrect. Impaired word retrieval is a symptom of aphasia (i.e., it is a language disorder and not a motor speech disorder).

b is incorrect. Language comprehension problems may be evident in Broca's aphasia, but tend to be less severe than language production problems. Impairment of language is not a symptom of AOS, which is a motor speech disorder.

c is incorrect. As with a and b, language problems, such as difficulty with reading, are not symptoms of motor speech disorders, but may be found with many types of aphasia.

3. In seeking reimbursement, which of the following assessment results would be *most* important to include in any report given to insurance justifying a need for skilled speech-language pathologist (SLP) services (i.e., documenting a risk that warrants treatment by an SLP)?
   a) Communicative Participation Item Bank (CPIB).
   b) Apraxia of Speech Rating Scale (ASRS).
   c) Western Aphasia Battery-Revised (WAB-R).
   d) Apraxia screening tasks.

Answer: a is correct. Any inability to communicate wants/needs or participate in functional communication settings presents a risk to the individual/patient. The CPIB is the best choice to provide an assessment of *functional* communication, as it reports on the individual's ability to participate in various, and often critical, contexts.

b is incorrect. The ASRS assists a clinician in making a differential diagnosis of AOS (vs. dysarthria or aphasia with phonemic paraphasia) and quantify the severity of symptoms. This rating can be useful in description, treatment planning, and measuring progress/outcomes, but it does not specifically report any medical risks associated with decreased communication skills. This assessment would not be necessary for justifying the need for treatment.

c is incorrect. Just as with the ASRS, the WAB-R quantifies the type and severity of a communication disorder—aphasia—but in and of itself does not directly describe the impact of aphasia on various communication contexts. It may be used for descriptive purposes, treatment planning, and measuring progress/outcomes, but would not be necessary for justifying the need for treatment.

d is incorrect. Apraxia screening tasks are used for assessment and diagnosis and provide no quantifiable score related to safety risks secondary to decreased functional communication skills.

53.5 Description of Disorder and Recommended Treatment

BB presented with moderately severe AOS and Broca's-type aphasia. An accurate diagnosis of AOS may be difficult to make, particularly with co-occurring aphasia, but BB demonstrated all required characteristics for an AOS diagnosis (i.e., sound distortions, slow rate, and prosodic abnormalities) as well as several commonly associated characteristics (e.g., articulatory groping). A "moderate" severity rating was based on his ASRS score, speech intelligibility, and type and percentage of sound errors. BB's language and speech impairments negatively impacted his communicative abilities and participation in desired activities.

Due to the need to improve both verbal language and speech skills, BB's clinician felt that he would be an excellent candidate for Combined Aphasia and Apraxia of Speech Treatment (CAAST).[8,9] CAAST combines Sound Production Treatment (SPT)[10] for AOS with Modified-Response Elaboration Training for aphasia (M-RET),[11] which allowed the clinician to target both impairments in the same session. SPT is the most extensively researched treatment for AOS, and has been shown to be effective in improving targeted sounds for both trained and untrained stimuli.[12] SPT consists of a repeated practice of a target sound—typically embedded in a one- to two-word context—after clinician model, with a response-contingent hierarchy. That is, that subsequent steps—which include practicing minimal contrasts, graphemic cues, integral stimulation, and isolated practice with placement cues—are completed depending on the response of the previous step. M-RET involves presenting a picture of an action/scene and eliciting a descriptive response. The clinician then prompts an elaboration by asking a question and modeling, if needed, to encourage the client to add additional content (e.g., BB said "She drive" to describe a picture of a woman driving. The clinician asked, "What is she driving?" BB responded "car," and was encouraged to repeat the new, longer response, "She drive car"). CAAST combines both treatments by applying SPT to any sound errors produced during the M-RET portion of treatment (i.e., in response to a picture stimulus).

BB was scheduled for three 1-hour sessions per week for 8 weeks. Using the Life Interests and Values (LIV) cards,[13] BB's clinician was able to select 16 personally relevant pictures of actions/activities (e.g., hobbies, interests, occupation, etc.) to use during treatment. The 16 pictures were divided into two sets of eight with 3 to 4 weeks of treatment for each set (targeting too many pictures at a time would have lengthened the session unnecessarily and restricted the amount of time spent on SPT). SPT typically targets preselected sounds, but with CAAST, it was applied as needed for each picture stimulus. An example of the protocol and BB's response (for a single stimulus item) is shown in ▶ Table 53.2.

53.6 Outcome

BB enjoyed and participated well in treatment. After 8 weeks, he was administered the CHMIT, WAB-R, and CPIB again. Clinically significant increases in speech intelligibility were observed, and modest improvements were noted in his WAB-R AQ and CPIB scores. Both BB and his wife report improved intelligibility, particularly for face-to-face conversations, although telephone conversations remain difficult. They also reported an increase in sentence length and use (i.e., using a sentence where he had typically used single words or short phrases before), with a greater variety of words. BB's clinician documented that although his speaking rate and prosody did not improve perceptually, he was able to produce a greater amount of content, with improved grammatical productions, as well as increased articulatory accuracy. These changes, combined, contributed to a "significant" improvement in functional communication. BB and his wife were educated regarding resources and home exercises

Table 53.2 Example of CAAST treatment for a single picture stimulus for BB

Clinician instruction/feedback	BB's response
(After explaining the sentence frame and components of a sentence, the clinician presented a picture of a man talking on the phone.) "BB, can you tell me what is happening in this picture, or anything it reminds you of?"	"A woman, no … a man … talk (pronounced /dak/) on … um … te- te- … um … phone."
Great! "A man talks on the phone." *(Response was written onto the sentence frame.)* Who might he be talking to?	"Um … um … a fff- … ff- (Oh! That is hard for me) … friend (pronounced /f: ɛn/). Not right … close (/kos/)."
"'Friend' works well." "A man talks on the phone with a friend." *(Clinician added the new content to sentence frame.)* Let's practice that longer sentence now. Can you say the whole thing for me? "A man talks on the phone with a friend." *(Clinician pointed to each word as BB repeated the sentence.)*	"A man … talks (/dakʃ/) on … a- … the (/θə/) phone … uh … with a f- ff- … (Oh man!) a … friend (/f: ɛn/)."
"Nice job! There were a few sounds that weren't quite right—these sounds here" *(Clinician underlined /t, s, ð, fr, and nd/.)* Think about those sounds and try it again. "A man talks on the phone with a friend."	"A man talks (/dakʃ/) … on … the phone … with a f-…a…friend (/f: ɛn/)."
"Good try! A couple of those were still a little off. Let's practice each of those words and then we will do the whole sentence again. Let's start with 'talks,' you had trouble with both the first sound 't' and the last sound 's.' Can you try that word for me, 'talks'."	"/dakʃ/."
"That 't' was closer, but it still sounds a little like a 'd.' The 's' on the end sounds almost like an 'sh.' Let's try it together, watch me, listen to me, and then say it with me. 'Talks, talks, talks …'" *(integral stimulation up to 3 ×.)*	*(Joined in with clinician)* "… /takʃ/, /taks/, /taks/."
"Excellent! Let's try the next word and work on this (pointed to /ð/) sound." *(Clinician proceeded in a similar manner to apply SPT to each errored consonant in a single word context … BB's responses are not all reported here, but were similar to his response on "talks".)* "Okay, now that we've practiced each of those sounds, let's try the whole sentence together again. 'A man talks on the phone with a friend'." *(Clinician pointed to each word on the sentence frame as BB responded.)*	"A man talks (/daks/) on the te- … phone … with his f- ff- … friend (/frɛnd/ with slight distortion on /r/)."
"Very nice! You hung on to most of those sounds! I'm going to move the picture and sentence; let's wait just a sec." *(Clinician waited 5 seconds and then replaced the picture.)* "Okay, can you describe this picture for me again?"	"A…a man talks…on the…f- phone phone…with his…with his f-… friend (/frɛnd/ with slight distortion on /r/)."
"Great job BB! Okay, let's move on to our next picture." *(Clinician presented the next item and the treatment protocol was repeated. Cueing and feedback were gradually faded as treatment progressed across sessions. After all pictures were presented, if time permitted, additional SPT was applied to any previously produced responses.)*	

53.7 Key Points

- BB received a diagnosis of AOS because he demonstrated slowed rate, prosodic abnormalities, and a predominance of sound distortion errors. Additional features were present, but not necessary for his diagnosis.
- BB's AOS and aphasia were relatively equal in severity and it was difficult to determine which disorder had a greater impact on his communication. Thus, BB's clinician selected a treatment (i.e., CAAST), which effectively addresses both disorders in the same protocol.

Suggested Readings

[1] McNeil MR, Duffy JR, Ballard KJ, Wambaugh J. Apraxia of speech, theory, assessment, differential diagnosis, and treatment: past, present, and future. In: van Lieshout P, Massan B, Terband H, Eds. Speech Motor Control in Normal and Disordered Speech: Future Developments in Theory and Methodology. Rockville, MD: ASHA; 2016:195–221

[2] Miller N, Wambaugh JL. Apraxia of speech. In: Papathanasiou I, Coppens P, Eds. Aphasia and Related Neurogenic Communication Disorders. 2nd ed. Burlington, MA: Jones & Bartlett Learning; 2016:493–526

References

[1] Ballard KJ, Wambaugh JL, Duffy JR, et al. Treatment for Acquired Apraxia of Speech: A Systematic Review of Intervention Research Between 2004 and 2012. Am J Speech Lang Pathol. 2015; 24:316–337

[2] McNeil MR, Robin DA, Schmidt RA. Apraxia of speech: definition and differential diagnosis. In: McNeil MR, Ed. Clinical Management of Sensorimotor Speech Disorders. New York, NY: Thieme; 2009:249–268

[3] Duffy JR. Motor Speech Disorders: Substrates, Differential Diagnosis, and Management. 3rd ed. St. Louis, MO: Elsevier; 2013

[4] Strand EA, Duffy JR, Clark HM, Josephs K. The Apraxia of Speech Rating Scale: a tool for diagnosis and description of apraxia of speech. J Commun Disord. 2014; 51:43–50

[5] Haley KL, Roth H, Grindstaff E, Jacks A. Computer-mediated assessment of intelligibility in aphasia and apraxia of speech. Aphasiology. 2011; 25(12): 1600–1620

[6] Kertesz A. The Western Aphasia Battery-Revised. San Antonio, TX: Pearson; 2007

[7] Baylor C, Yorkston K, Eadie T, Kim J, Chung H, Amtmann D. The Communicative Participation Item Bank (CPIB): item bank calibration and development of a disorder-generic short form. J Speech Lang Hear Res. 2013; 56(4):1190–1208

[8] Wambaugh JL, Wright S, Nessler C, Mauszycki SC. Combined Aphasia and Apraxia of Speech Treatment (CAAST): effects of a novel therapy. J Speech Lang Hear Res. 2014; 57(6):2191–2207

[9] Wambaugh JL, Wright S, Mauszycki SC, Nessler C, Bailey D. Combined Aphasia and Apraxia of Speech Treatment (CAAST): Systematic replications in the development of a novel treatment. Intern J Speech Lang Pathol. 2018; 20(2): 247–261

[10] Wambaugh JL, Kalinyak-Fliszar MM, West JE, Doyle PJ. Effects of treatment for sound errors in apraxia of speech and aphasia. J Speech Lang Hear Res. 1998; 41(4):725–743

[11] Wambaugh JL, Martinez AL. Effects of modified response elaboration training with apraxic and aphasic speakers. Aphasiology. 2000; 14(5-6):603–617

[12] Bailey DJ, Eatchel K, Wambaugh J. Sound production treatment: synthesis and quantification of outcomes. Am J Speech Lang Pathol. 2015; 24(4):S798–S814

[13] Haley KL, Womack J, Helm-Estabrooks N, Caignon D, McCulloch K. Life Interests and Values Cards. Chapel Hill, NC: Department of Allied Health Sciences, University of North Carolina at Chapel Hill; 2010. Available at: https://www.med.unc.edu/ahs/sphs/card/resources/livcards

54 Compensatory and Restorative Application of AAC in Chronic, Severe Aphasia

Kimberly A. Eichhorn

54.1 Introduction

Alternative and augmentative communication (AAC) strategies in persons with aphasia (PWA) require careful consideration. Cognitive and linguistic strengths and limitations directly influence device and field complexity as well as language content and layout. Without a general understanding of the PWA's phonological, semantic, syntactic, and input/output span abilities, the effectiveness of AAC for PWA can be significantly limited.

54.2 Clinical History and Description

GA was a 68-year-old left-handed man status post multiple, remote, cerebrovascular accidents (CVAs), the most recent of which was 10 years ago. His medical history and the course surrounding the CVAs were limited as his care was at a different facility. However, a head computed tomography was available for review, which showed a large wedge-shaped area of infarction in the left hemisphere in the area of the middle cerebral artery (MCA) distribution extending from the frontal to the parietal lobe. Per report, he received speech-language therapy immediately following one of his strokes, but he had not received services within the past 5 years.

GA earned an associate's degree, served in the army for 2 years, and worked for a local gas company for 20 years. His brothers and sisters were his primary caregivers; he never married. At the time of evaluation, GA was completely dependent for care, including all activities of daily living. Verbal output was limited to several automatic, overlearned phrases (such as "I don't know" or "here we go") with islands of appropriate single word content. Additional past medical history was significant for chronic myeloid leukemia, peripheral vascular disease, diabetes mellitus, visual field deficit, prostate cancer, chronic obstructive pulmonary disease, benign hypertension, deep vein thrombosis, and right above the knee amputation.

54.3 Clinical Testing

54.3.1 Clinical Interview

Some key information obtained during interviews of GA's family included the following: GA received "some speech therapy" following a CVA 16 years ago, GA typically used gestures to communicate at home and was relatively effective expressing his needs, and GA's family expressed a desire for him to have more input in his daily activities, such as meal selection.

54.3.2 Oral Motor Examination/Motor Speech Evaluation

Completion of a full oral motor examination was limited by GA's inability to complete many of the tasks requested, even with a model. Of note, mild right-sided weakness of the upper and lower face was observed. Facial sensation was intact bilaterally. Jaw strength was intact bilaterally. Significantly reduced range of motion was observed during labial retraction. GA was unable to complete alternating nonspeech motion tasks. Speech tasks were slow, but articulatory precision was grossly intact for bilabial plosives and lingual-alveolar stops. Vocal quality was mildly harsh and wet at baseline. Maximum phonation time was not assessed due to poor coordination of respiration/phonation. GA presented with lower dentition only.

54.3.3 Cognitive Linguistic Quick Test

The Cognitive Linguistic Quick Test (CLQT) is a brief measure of five cognitive domains in adults with known or suspected cognitive dysfunction. Criterion-referenced severity ratings for the five cognitive domains and overall severity rating and a clock drawing severity rating are provided for two age range categories. GA presented with severely impaired attention, memory, executive functions, language, and visuospatial skills. These results were interpreted with caution given his known aphasia and observed low frustration tolerance with testing.

54.3.4 Comprehensive Aphasia Test

The Comprehensive Aphasia Test (CAT) contains both a cognitive screening and complete language battery. The design of this assessment tool permits the clinician to determine patterns of errors, such as complexity and phonological versus semantic errors. Consistent with previous evaluations, low frustration tolerance and task abandonment were occasionally observed. Behavioral observations led to concern for mild right neglect.

In addition, GA was unable to gesture object use or complete word fluency tasks. On a semantic memory task, he recalled items previously seen, but the errors he made were consistently related to semantic distractions. Comprehension of spoken simple sentences was a relative strength, with significant impairment noted with comprehension of single words and complex language structures. Comprehension of written language was consistent with spoken language; a relative strength was seen with simple written sentences. Again, errors in comprehension were most consistently related to semantic relationships. Relative strengths were seen in the ability to repeat simple/short words with notable breakdown in polysyllabic structures. Repetition of digit strings was also impaired, with maximum repetition of two information units following multiple practice trials.

No items were named to confrontation. First syllable cueing paired with visual model increased appropriate verbal productions in naming tasks. GA was unable to read any words aloud. He did, however, write his name and copy letters. He was unable to write picture names or write to dictation. He was unable to provide any information for a picture description task, verbally or in writing.

54.4 Informal Assessment

As part of the evaluation, several communication pages were trialed in a grid layout of both four and six options. Given observations regarding GA's semantic deficits, content was organized with icons and text of semantically distinct targets as well as semantically similar targets (▶ Fig. 54.1). Performance for identification of targets (auditory comprehension) was accurate for fields of four semantically different items. Breakdown occurred in larger fields and with semantically related items. Additionally, for semantically distinct items, he was able to choose correct items from a field of four when presented with more abstract questioning (i.e., which one would you pick if you were hungry?).

54.5 Questions and Answers for the Reader

1. A 55-year-old woman post left temporoparietal CVA presents to your clinic with her tablet device requesting applications to assist with her communication deficits. What is your first course of action?
   a) Complete a thorough case history, interview, and evaluation of cognitive-language skills.
   b) Recommend applications as requested by the patient.

Answer: a is correct. The first course of action in this case would be to evaluate the patient. Discuss previous therapies and goals. Determine the type of device she has and which applications might be appropriate based on your impressions from the evaluation.

b is incorrect. Unless you already have testing results from another source, it is important to establish a baseline that should drive your recommendations. Input from the patient regarding goals and expectations will also direct your treatment/recommendations.

2. An 80-year-old PWA presents with his family who are requesting a "communication device." Family reports that since the stroke, their father has been able to communicate in a very limited fashion. Although they have developed a form of gesture communication, they are convinced that some form of technology will increase the effectiveness of their interactions with their father. Throughout the course of the interview and evaluation, the patient rarely makes eye contact with you, does not engage in any type of device trial you attempt, and only periodically uses gesture or a single word to communicate with you. What are your primary concerns regarding the use of technology for this patient?
   a) Family/caregiver support.
   b) Visual acuity/perception.

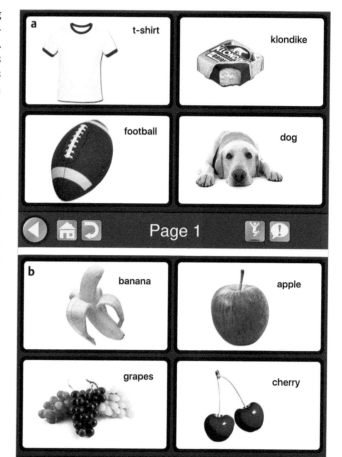

Fig. 54.1 Sample pages from GoTalkNow designed with semantically distinct and similar nouns.

   c) Fine motor skills.
   d) Motivation to use technology.

Answer: d is correct. This patient's seemingly limited interest in device trials within the session should raise a concern. Although the family is very motivated for use of a device, the patient must also be on board. It is possible that given his age, he has limited exposure to technology. It would be wise to spend some time alone with the patient to ascertain his personal goals regarding communication. A thorough evaluation of his language/communication skills should be undertaken as well as his candidacy/desire for traditional, restorative therapy based on his language deficits. Consideration of low/no technology supports (such as boards or picture books) as well as family education may be the appropriate place to start.

a is incorrect. This patient clearly has a supportive family who are attempting to advocate for him. This is paramount for successful use of AAC. However, without patient "buy-in," AAC will not be an effective tool.

b is incorrect. Although a thoughtful consideration, visual acuity/perception should not be the immediate concern in this case.

c is incorrect. Again, fine motor skills as they relate to access to device (touch, mouse, eye gaze, as examples) are considerations that should be made in all cases, but this should not be the primary focus at this time.

3. A 67-year-old man post MCA distribution CVA is referred to you for AAC. Results of his testing show severe expressive (verbal and written) language deficits, moderate receptive (spoken and written) language deficits, and a working memory span of 3 units. Additional testing revealed impairment in semantic access. Which of the following will most likely be the greatest barrier to success with dynamic display AAC?
   a) Amount of information they can "hold onto" at one time (i.e., input and output span).
   b) Comprehension/distinction of semantic relationships.
   c) Comprehension of written words.

Answer: b is correct. Inability to understand and determine accurate semantic relationships will likely inhibit the patient's ability to make correct/desired selections within categorical fields (even small numbers)—he/she will not be able to accurately specify a want/need with choices from closely related items.

a is incorrect. Whereas input/outspan should be a careful consideration when choosing/using AAC, a span of 3 in this case *might* suggest that the patient can accurately complete some navigation and chain some information together *if* organized appropriately.

c is incorrect. For some PWA, written words in combination with icons/photos can enhance comprehension. In this case, however, the ability to determine specific semantic characteristics (as above) would likely not be overcome with the addition of a written word.

54.6 Description of Disorder and Recommended Treatment

GA was diagnosed with chronic, severe aphasia, severe apraxia of speech, and moderate-to-severe nonverbal oral apraxia. Additionally, he was diagnosed with moderate-to-severe attentional impairment and mild memory deficits. Relative strengths appeared in word repetition, copying, and verbal/written simple sentence level comprehension. It was postulated that context enhanced comprehension.

Restorative as well as compensatory treatment was initiated. Following training and in-home trials with "low tech" paper communication boards, several assistive communication applications (GoTalkNow, SnapScene) were procured to translate items into accessible verbal output with hopes of priming GA's repetition and overall verbal output. For restorative treatment, a modified version of Beeson and Egnor's[1] Copy and Recall Treatment with Repetition (CART + R) was attempted with a flashcard app to allow visual (static and video of production) and auditory input from treatment targets (▶ Fig. 54.2). Functional vocabulary was provided by the family and divided into trained and untrained stimuli. Trained treatment targets were practiced in sessions with companion application as well as home practice between sessions. Functional and concrete visual scenes were initiated to enhance functional communication regarding preferences in daily life (▶ Fig. 54.3). Device navigational support was recommended and GA's family was trained and included in this process.

54.7 Outcome

Following 6 weeks of modified CART + R treatment, GA demonstrated learning and retention of trained nouns less than five letters in length. However, no generalization to untrained nouns was observed, and his verbal perseveration limited the consistency of his accurate productions. Although he consistently generated one or two letters of the treatment targets, he was unable to use these fragments functionally for written communication or to prime verbal productions. Given these factors, the treatment plan was adjusted to trial modified script training,[2] again using flashcard applications with audio/video models for home practice. Consistent with other restorative treatment attempts, gains were limited by verbal perseveration and short input/output span.

Treatment and training transitioned to solely focus on compensation, employing AAC with a visual scene display to enhance participation in daily activities. Using photographic images and recorded hot spots (a selectable area on the screen embedded with text and/or audio), with navigational support from family, GA could play a larger role in selection of activities and meals. The content of the scenes was driven by GA's motivation (▶ Fig. 54.4). The concrete photograph with some context appeared to assist with semantic impairment where a grid display was less effective. Given his strength in single word repetition, he was afforded the opportunity, when able, to repeat the message himself. Ongoing training and work in this regard continued with the goal of increased participation in everyday interactions.

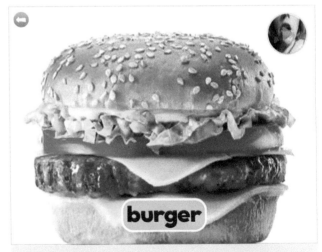

Fig. 54.2 Screenshot of INKids Kids Flashcard Maker adapted as tool for copy and repetition practice. (Note option for embedded video of verbal production in upper right corner.)

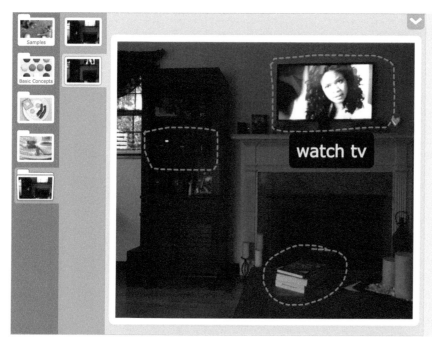

Fig. 54.3 Screenshot of Tobii Dynavox's SnapScene with recorded "hot spots." Optional text support.

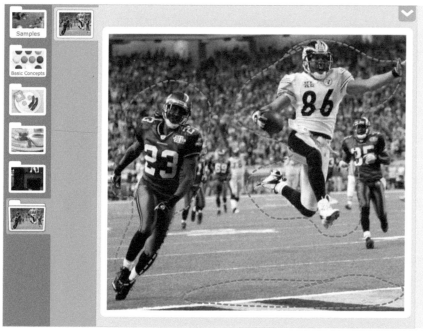

Fig. 54.4 Screenshot of Tobii Dynavox's SnapScene with recorded "hot spots" to discuss this GA's interests.

Anecdotally, despite marginal gains toward restorative treatment goals and limited observation of carryover of skills by clinicians, GA's family and other health care providers reported increased meaningful and appropriate verbal output to request wants/needs, such as asking for a "cup of coffee" or "socks" as opposed to tapping the table and pointing.

54.8 Key Points

- Use of AAC in PWA should not be considered until a thorough evaluation of language and cognitive function has been completed.

- Functional communication page set layouts must be designed to maximize a PWA's residual language strengths and modified throughout the treatment process.
- AAC can be a successful tool in restorative treatment approaches if careful device selection and treatment planning occurs from the outset.
- Family/caregiver support and engagement is paramount for successful outcomes when using AAC with PWA.

Suggested Readings

[1] Beukelman DR, Hux K, Dietz A, McKelvey M, Weissling K. Using visual scene displays as communication support options for people with chronic, severe

aphasia: a summary of AAC research and future research directions. Augment Altern Commun. 2015; 31(3):234–245

[2] Beukelman DR, Fager S, Ball L, Dietz A. AAC for adults with acquired neurological conditions: a review. Augment Altern Commun. 2007; 23(3):230–242

[3] Wilkinson KM, Jagaroo V. Contributions of principles of visual cognitive science to AAC system display design. Augment Altern Commun. 2004; 20(3): 123–136

[4] Vigneau M, Beaucousin V, Hervé PY, et al. Meta-analyzing left hemisphere language areas: phonology, semantics, and sentence processing. Neuroimage. 2006; 30(4):1414–1432

[5] Helm-Estabrooks N. Cognitive Linguistic Quick Test: CLQT. Toronto, Canada: PsychCorp; 2001

[6] Swinburn K, Porter G, Howard D. Comprehensive aphasia test. East Sussex: Psychology Press; 2004

References

[1] Beeson PM, Egnor H. Combining treatment for written and spoken naming. J Int Neuropsychol Soc. 2006; 12(6):816–827

[2] Youmans G, Holland A, Muñoz M, Bourgeois M. Script training and automaticity in two individuals with aphasia. Aphasiology. 2005; 19(3–5):435–450

55 Functional Language Rehabilitation in Nonfluent Aphasia

Lisa McQueen

55.1 Introduction

This case describes a patient presenting in an acute rehabilitation facility for assessment and treatment of language post-stroke. Of particular interest, this report outlines the patient's language presentation, concomitant mental health considerations, and lack of social support at discharge.

55.2 Clinical History and Description

FG was a 65-year-old man who presented to an acute rehabilitation facility 6 days following cerebral vascular accident. Computed tomography scan confirmed an acute stroke in the left middle cerebral artery region with specific areas of foci noted in the left frontal operculum, left insular cortex, and left parietal lobe. Prior to the insult, FG lived alone and had no immediate family. A neighbor and family doctor were listed as next of kin. FG was a retired ultrasound technician and had been receiving government support for an unknown disability prior to the stroke. His friend described him as "reclusive." Previous medical history included high blood pressure, diabetes, high cholesterol, and depression. He had been treated pharmacologically for these conditions, but medication compliance was often poor, according to his friend.

55.3 Clinical Testing

FG presented with low frustration tolerance, which limited testing. FG was also given a very short length of stay, further limiting assessment. FG was admitted on a regular texture diet. No dysphagia was identified. A formal oral-motor exam was not completed as there was no evidence of change to vocal function or motor speech.

Portions of the Boston Diagnostic Aphasia Exam (BDAE, 3rd edition) Short Form were administered. Results are summarized in ▶ Table 55.1 and ▶ Fig. 55.1, ▶ Fig. 55.2, ▶ Fig. 55.3. ▶ Table 55.1 summarizes the BDAE test results; ▶ Fig. 55.1: depicts the BDAE rating scale profile; ▶ Fig. 55.2: cookie theft transcription pretreatment (admission); and ▶ Fig. 55.3: cookie theft transcription posttreatment (discharge).

55.4 Questions and Answers for the Reader

1. Based on the assessment findings, suggest a possible aphasia type for FG:
   a) Broca's aphasia.
   b) Conduction aphasia.
   c) Transcortical motor aphasia.
   d) Anomic aphasia.

Table 55.1 BDAE assessment results

Subtest	Score	Comments
Aphasia severity rating scale	1	"All communication through fragmentary expression; great need for inference, listener carries burden of communication"
Word comprehension	12/16	Impulsivity in responses
Commands	6/10	Perseveration noted
Complex ideational material	3/6	Written cues increased accuracy when trialed informally
Automatized sequences	3/4	Perseveration
Repetition of words	5/5	
Repetition of sentences	1/2	Difficulty with longer sentences
Responsive naming	1/10	No response or "I can't" for most trials
Boston Naming Test (short)	4/15	Phonemic paraphasias = 4 Semantic = 5 Multiword = 2 Phonemic cues helpful approximately 50% of the time
Reading: words	4/4	
Oral word reading	15/15	
Oral reading sentences	5/5	Fluent, no hesitations, no pausing
Comprehension of orally read sentences	2/3	
Reading comprehension sentences and paragraphs	3/4	Impulsive responding
Writing	Not formally completed due to frustration	Wrote single words to dictation (three to four letters) with 70% accuracy, unable/unwilling to do narrative writing task. Able to write name and address accurately

Answer: c is correct. Many patients with aphasia do not fall definitively into one category; given the assessment findings for this case, this category would be the best choice. Transcortical motor aphasia is a nonfluent aphasia and as such one would expect short phrases, lack of content words, and difficulty with grammatical structures. FG exhibited this presentation. In addition, he had strong repetition and oral reading, which are often hallmarks of transcortical motor aphasia.

a is incorrect. Most individuals with Broca's aphasia have much less verbal output and dramatically reduced prosody. Additionally, these patients generally present with poor repetition and poor oral reading. Comprehension may be relatively preserved despite severe verbal expression deficits.

SEVERITY AND SPEECH OUTPUT CHARACTERISTICS PROFILE
(BASED ON FREE CONVERSATION, PICTURE DESCRIPTION, AND AESOP'S FABLES)

APHASIA SEVERITY RATING SCALE

0. No usable speech or auditory comprehension

1. All communication is through fragmentary expression; great need for inference, questioning, and guessing by the listener. The range of information that can be exchanged is limited, and the listener carries the burden of communication.

2. Conversation about familiar subjects is possible with help from the listener. There are frequent failures to convey the idea, but the patient shares the burden of communication.

3. The patient can discuss almost all everyday problems with little or no assistance. Reduction of speech and/or comprehension, however, makes conversation about certain material difficult or impossible.

4. Some obvious loss of fluency in speech or facility of comprehension, without significant limitation on ideas expressed or form of expression.

5. Minimal discernible speech handicap; the patient may have subjective difficulties that are not obvious to the listener.

RATING SCALE PROFILE OF SPEECH CHARACTERISTICS

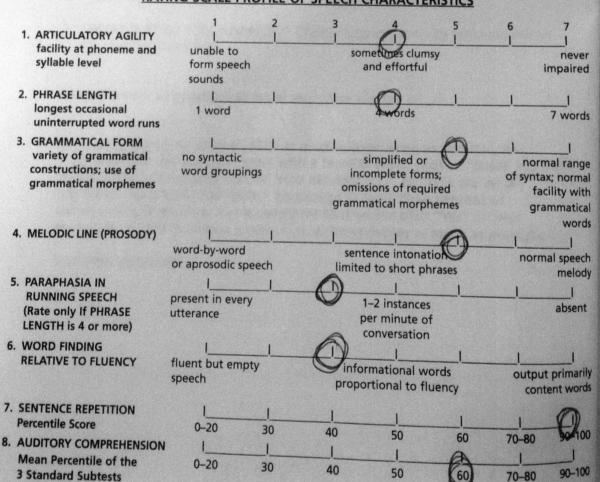

Fig. 55.1 BDAE rating scale profile.

Cookie Theft: Mr. F.G. - March 21, 2016 (total time = 3.5 minutes)

"it's ty-typ-typical and then it's um uh, it's sp – sp – splashing on the floor ... two open" (patient gestured to taps of sink; needed cues to look at whole page because ignored left side while focusing on right)

"they – they ... uh um th- they Kaplunk! ... well, he was was, he was – uh he (pointing to boy) ... um uh ... th- the – that was kaplunk.."

Content units = 1

Phrase length = 2–3 (average = 2)

Fig. 55.2 Cookie theft admission.

Cookie Theft: Mr. F.G. - April 7, 2016 (total time = 2 minutes)

"He is falling off the chair getting a cookie from the cookie jar...and the – the –the – her...she was helping him off the chair and he um – he enlisted her help and she was basically looking at him" (patient covered mouth in gesture of little girl)

"and the – ok, yeah – the fi- fi- just the midding. She's talking to something over there and she wasn't talking anything about it (referring to mother in picture) – it's falling – she's doing the outside of the dish and the inside is facing her ..."

Content units = 14

Phrase length = 3–13 (average = 6.1)

Fig. 55.3 Cookie theft discharge.

---

b is incorrect. A defining feature of conduction aphasia is poor repetition. Additionally, patients may produce more sound and word repetitions in speech. This presentation is often referred to as "conduit d'approche."

d is incorrect. This type of aphasia has a more fluent presentation with longer phrases and stronger melodic lines. Production of nouns and verbs is impaired. Grammar is frequently intact.

2. When considering a starting point for treatment for this patient, which technique may yield greatest success given the assessment profile?
   a) "PROMPT" type therapy.
   b) Script training.
   c) Semantic feature analysis–based therapy.
   d) Picture–word matching tasks.

Answer: b is correct. Based on assessment findings, treatment tasks that capitalize on FG's intact oral reading may provide a feasible therapeutic starting point. Script training may be beneficial because the patient could practice various grammatical structures and functional vocabulary in practical contexts that may generalize well to other environments.

a is incorrect. This technique is very useful for patients with motor planning deficits and difficulties sequencing sounds in words. It is often useful for patients who have an apraxia of speech in addition to a nonfluent aphasia.

c is incorrect. Results from the Boston Naming Test suggest that phonemic cueing might enhance therapeutic progress and a phonological approach may be more useful. However, given that this patient demonstrated both semantic and phonemic paraphasias, it is unclear whether semantic-based therapy may yield benefits with FG.

d is incorrect. This technique is often used to treat reading comprehension impairments. FG did not identify reading comprehension as a goal for therapy. In fact, reading comprehension was relatively preserved based on assessment results.

3. What are some factors to consider when planning specific treatment tasks aside from the patient's language presentation?

Answer: This patient was provided a very short length of stay in rehab. Treatment activities that allow for greatest generalization with significant functional impacts in terms of a safe discharge must be prioritized. Given FG's limited familial support, soliciting the help of friends/neighbors may be useful to learn about his baseline conversation partners and language requirements and contexts. Maximizing rehabilitation intensity would also be an important factor in treatment planning. Ideally, patients with aphasia poststroke should receive at least 1 hour of therapy daily for optimal outcomes. Providing homework and utilizing assistants/students or volunteers can potentially increase therapy exposure each day. Another important factor is this patient's mental health status. Depression may impede overall recovery. Patient mood and engagement should be observed and discussed with the treatment team. Finally, given FG's limited social support, the clinician should work closely with other team members to provide the communication skills for the safest discharge possible. Treatment may involve spending more time on targeting functional language tasks such as calling a pharmacy or phoning the police in an emergency.

4. Completing formal assessment of speech and language in the acute rehabilitation setting poststroke can be challenging due to issues with patient fatigue, tolerance of testing, and impaired insight. What are some informal tasks that could be used to gather useful baseline data and guide with treatment planning?

Answer: Routine conversational interaction is useful for gaining information about functional verbal expression and can often yield a more robust language sample than formalized testing. Engaging the patient in discussion about hobbies or asking them to describe a typical day provides themes for conversations. Asking the patient to share what they know and understand about stroke can provide insight into their level of awareness and education needs. Spending your first session explaining what to expect during the rehabilitation process can provide information about verbal expression and auditory comprehension as well as increase patient comfort. Yes/no or multiple choice questions should be employed to determine patient comprehension. A food menu choice card or a bedside brochure such as "falls prevention" can yield basic information about reading ability. Additionally, the speech-language pathologist (SLP) plays a fundamental role in overall patient education related to safety. When informally assessing written expression, ensure that the assessment targets tasks that are functional for the patient's baseline status. For example, many patients will indicate that their common writing tasks prior to stroke included simple tasks such as checks, grocery lists, and to-do lists.

55.5 Description of Disorder and Recommended Treatment

Based on the initial assessment (formal and informal), FG presented with a moderate-to-severe communication impairment with characteristics most consistent with a nonfluent aphasia, quite possibly transcortical motor in nature. Deficits were identified across all modalities, but verbal expression was most severely impaired and was determined to be the most important goal for treatment. FG's communication impairment was expected to have a significant impact on his ability to function independently at home. Given his short length of stay and lack of familial/social support, it was critical to select and develop treatment targets that would provide maximal functional outcomes to help him achieve his goal of returning home safely.

FG was physically quite well and consequently could tolerate intensive speech and language therapy. He agreed to participate in daily 45-to-60 minute speech therapy sessions five times per week. Additionally, he had 30-minute sessions with a therapy assistant, which provided further practice. Recommended treatment included training of scripts using an oral reading

technique.[1] Topics for scripts were generated together with patient using facilitative language techniques (picture support, yes/no questions, written choices) and practiced in a variety of contexts (face-to-face, over the phone, small groups) and with multiple communication partners in the hospital. The focus of therapy was twofold. First, the scripts provided sentence production practice using intact skills that enhanced grammatical formulation as well as word finding for functional vocabulary. The material was motivating given that it was generated by the patient with multiple opportunities for repetition. Second, the patient saved all the scripts in a binder and was able to use them as a low-tech communication aid in various scenarios (e.g., when he had to request medication from nursing staff during training in self-medication). This secondary benefit was very important in terms of increasing independence at discharge.

55.6 Outcome

FG was discharged home on his target discharge date. His communication improved such that he was able to use the telephone for simple conversations, request assistance as needed, ask for directions, make appointments, and participate in simple interactions with friends. On admission, his verbal expression was assessed with the hospital-based outcome tool FIM (Functional Independence Measure) and he scored a 1/7 (able to communicate basic information less than 25% of the time). At discharge, his FIM verbal expression score increased to a 4/7 (able to express basic information 75% of the time). On admission, he spoke in one-to three-word utterances with limited content. On discharge, he produced utterances over 10 words in length and his content improved significantly, both in spontaneous speech and on reassessment (▶ Fig. 55.3).

Functionally, at time of discharge, FG managed his medications and was able to take public transit and use the phone. He agreed to further therapy as an outpatient. Given his ongoing difficulties with sentence formulation and grammatical usage, treatment using techniques such as "Verb Network Strengthening Treatment (VNeST)" were suggested.[2]

55.7 Key Points

- Therapy techniques should be chosen based on assessment findings, patient strengths, and patient interests/goals. A patient will be most engaged by tasks he/she finds valuable and motivating, which will yield increased generalization and improved outcomes. The clinician may be the "expert" in his/her field, but it is the patient who is the expert in his/her impairment. Patient partnership in the rehabilitation process is paramount.

- For patients in the acute phase of rehabilitation, in-depth assessment may be deferred. Patient presentation may change rapidly in the first 2 weeks poststroke. Choosing to spend too much time in the early phase on assessment may not be the best use of time. Consider collecting initial baseline assessment information and then moving into diagnostic therapy. Allowing time for education and counseling in these early days poststroke is also critical.

- Depression is common poststroke, particularly in the context of aphasia, and can impact rehabilitation outcomes. An SLP can help screen for depression and should engage team/family doctor as required.

Suggested Reading

[1] Graven C, Brock K, Hill K, Ames D, Cotton S, Joubert L. From rehabilitation to recovery: protocol for a randomised controlled trial evaluating a goal-based intervention to reduce depression and facilitate participation post-stroke. BMC Neurol. 2011; 11(1):73

References

[1] Cherney LR. Oral reading for language in aphasia (ORLA): evaluating the efficacy of computer-delivered therapy in chronic nonfluent aphasia. Top Stroke Rehabil. 2010; 17(6):423–431

[2] Edmonds LA, Mammino K, Ojeda J. Effect of Verb Network Strengthening Treatment (VNeST) in persons with aphasia: extension and replication of previous findings. Am J Speech Lang Pathol. 2014; 23(2):S312–S329

56 Differential Diagnostics in Spasmodic Dysphonia versus Muscle-Tension Dysphonia

Shirley Gherson

56.1 Introduction

Referrals for diagnostic evaluation and treatment for a patient with possible spasmodic dysphonia (SD) can be challenging given that symptoms are not always categorical. In addition, symptoms related to muscle-tension dysphonia (MTD), a much more common dysregulation of muscle coordination, can mimic those of SD, making accurate diagnosis even more difficult. This case represents an example of a clinical pathway for the differential diagnosis of SD and MTD.

56.2 Clinical History and Description

C is a 29-year-old female marketing professional referred for evaluation and diagnostic therapy to define whether her symptoms were related to MTD or SD. C summarized her problem with the following statements: "I sound nervous even when I'm not. It feels like my voice just sort of seizes up, but it feels shaky." She reported a functional voice until late 2012 when she noticed a subtle and intermittent tremor in her voice, especially while on the telephone; her tremor often occurred in the absence of anxiety or stress. In October 2012, C developed an upper respiratory infection with several days of hoarseness. Upon recovery, her vocal symptoms became much more frequent and exacerbated in severity to the point where her friends began commenting on the quality of her voice. Her voice was characterized by worsening voice quality while on the telephone, primarily during conference calls, and when initially arriving somewhere and initiating voice. Her voice progressively improved with increased use. She denied significant improvement in voice with alcohol. She stated, "It's hard for me to know since it seems to be better, but then once I start to notice it, the voice breaks start to happen." She also reported some voice symptoms during singing.

C's work required substantial voice use. At the time of referral, her symptoms were increasingly evident and she found them to be limiting both social and occupational activities. C was otherwise in good health and denied any past voice problems. With respect to family history, she reported a possibility of a cousin with the same type of voice symptoms, although she was unsure.

C was evaluated by an otolaryngologist who performed laryngostroboscopy, which revealed some signs of a possible neurological voice issue. In this case, behavioral therapy was indicated to attempt to differentiate between SD and a more functional presentation.

56.3 Clinical Testing

C underwent extensive acoustic and functional testing. Stimuli included sentences loaded with unvoiced and voiced consonants. In addition, she was instructed to perform the following tasks: sustain a comfortable /a/ at modal pitch, whisper voiced-consonant stimuli, sing "happy birthday," yell "taxi!," and count in her normal voice and count again in her falsetto voice (▶ Table 56.1).

56.4 Questions and Answers for the Reader

1. A 55-year-old man presents to your clinic with a strained-strangled voice quality that has developed gradually over the course of 2 years. The patient was diagnosed with MTD and referred for eight sessions of speech therapy. Speech therapy was ineffective despite the patient compliance with exercises. During the evaluation, you notice that the patient's strained-strangled voice quality improves with sustained vowels, whispering, and falsetto voicing. Voice quality worsens when reading "We rode along rainy island avenue" and improves slightly when reading "The puppy bit the tape." Laryngeal palpation reveals moderate-to-severe muscle tone in the neck muscles and tongue base during speech. Muscle tone normalizes at rest. What is the most likely diagnosis given the findings of your evaluation?
   a) Adductor SD (ADSD) without compensatory MTD.
   b) Abductor SD (ABSD) with compensatory MTD.

Table 56.1 Diagnostic tasks for differentiating spasmodic dysphonia from muscle-tension dysphonia

Task	Result
Falsetto voice/singing/yelling	Significantly improved vocal quality
Mid-vowel, mid-word voice breaks	Present
Sustained vowel vs. speech	Significant difference in quality with greater vocal stability noted on sustained tones
Unvoiced consonant-heavy phrases vs. voiced consonant-heavy phrases	Increased frequency of spasms noted during voiced consonant-heavy phrases
Laugh/cry/coughing/throat clearing	Voice improved during laugh. No other activities noted
Digital manipulation and laryngeal massage	Palpation revealed mild tongue base tension with excellent range of motion of the larynx
Change in voice with masking	N/A

c) ADSD with compensatory MTD.

d) Mixed ADSD with a tremor component.

e) MTD.

Answer: c is correct. The most likely diagnosis for the patient's evaluative findings is ADSD with a component of compensatory MTD. Clues to this diagnosis include failure to respond to speech therapy treatment, strained-strangled voice quality that worsened with a vowel initial, voiced consonant-heavy sentence and improved with an unvoiced consonant-heavy sentence and improved quality with non-speech-related tasks such as falsetto voicing, whispering, and sustained vowels. MTD can develop in compensation to the primary SD diagnosis.

a is incorrect. Although the patient does present with ADSD, he is also presenting with signs and symptoms of MTD with positive finds of laryngeal palpation.

b is incorrect. ABSD is characterized by breathy voice breaks and typically triggered by unvoiced consonant-heavy phrases.

d is incorrect. The patient did not present with a tremorous voice during sustained voice tasks.

e is incorrect. MTD is characterized by positive findings on laryngeal palpation, improved voice quality with ongoing voice therapy (given a lack of secondary gain), and improved voicing with masking and diversion tasks (e.g., lip trills). Voice quality would not typically improve with non-speech-related tasks such as falsetto voicing, whispering, or sustained vowels.

2. What might account for the abrupt improvement in vocal quality with non-speech-related tasks (e.g., singing, laughing, crying, falsetto voicing) for a person with SD?

a) A relaxation of their laryngeal musculature.

b) These tasks trigger an alternate motor pathway that is not speech related.

c) Nonspeech tasks are less psychologically stressful.

d) Emotional voicing is cathartic and releases pent-up tension.

Answer: b is correct. The defining characteristic of SD is that it is a task-specific condition that presents itself mainly in speech tasks. Therefore, when triggering alternate pathways of phonation such as those used in singing, SD symptoms can be seen to drop significantly.

a is incorrect. Although laryngeal musculature may relax by way of using a non-speech-related motor pathway and having reduced triggers of spasms, release of muscle tension is a symptom and not a cause of the improved voice quality.

c is incorrect. SD has historically been misdiagnosed as a psychological condition because of this phenomenon. It is now understood to be related to the use of an alternate motor pathway rather than a psychological release.

d is incorrect. This observation is related to C in that the task specificity of improved voicing with emotive speech is more related to the brain using an alternate motor pathway.

3. A reading task during perceptual testing finds that voice quality is worse with frequent breathy voice breaks during sentences such as "He is hiding behind the house" and "The puppy bit the tape," and better with "We rode along rainy island avenue" and "We eat eels every day." All things considered, what diagnosis would you start to consider?

a) ADSD.

b) Mixed SD.

c) Vocal tremor.

d) ABSD.

e) MTD.

Answer: d is correct. ABSD is characterized by breathy voice breaks that are triggered by unvoiced consonants. An increase in symptom frequency can be observed with sentences that use a significant number of unvoiced consonants as compared to those that use primarily voiced consonants.

a is incorrect. ADSD is characterized by vocal spasms that are triggered by voiced consonants and vowel-initial heavy sentences.

b is incorrect. Mixed SD has components of both ABSD and ADSD and possibly a component of tremor. Therefore, symptoms can be appreciated in both voiceless-consonant and voiced-consonant/vowel-heavy sentences.

c is incorrect. Vocal tremor is characterized by a rhythmic wavering of the voice. Although severe tremor may also present as ADSD, symptoms are not triggered by speech-specific tasks.

e is incorrect. MTD is characterized by tension of the peripheral nervous system and would not present with abrupt changes based on speech-specific tasks.

56.5 Description of Disorder and Recommended Treatment

SD is a task-specific focal dystonia characterized by involuntary, action-induced muscle spasms of the larynx during speech.[1] The two most common subtypes of SD are ADSD, where the vocal folds abruptly adduct causing voice breaks and a strained-strangled quality, and ABSD, where the vocal folds abduct inappropriately causing breathy voice breaks. The subtypes can be identified by their phonetic patterns: ADSD is triggered by voiced consonants and ABSD by unvoiced consonants. In mixed SD, characteristics of both types are present.[2]

Approximately one-third of patients with SD have concurrent tremor. "Islands" of normal speech may be present and voicing may also be normal during emotional vocal expression (e.g., laughing, crying), singing, sustained vocalizations, or with non-typical speech patterns (e.g., speaking in falsetto, shouting). The disorder is chronic, can be progressive, and is thought to be a central motor-processing disorder of the basal ganglia and its connections.[3] Recent studies suggest reduced brain activation between the sensory and motor regions, which could theoretically result in the disruption of sensory processing and subsequent processing by the motor cortex.[4] A brain imaging study using magnetic resonance imaging (MRI) and functional MRI, by Simonyan and Ludlow,[2] found abnormal structure–function relationships in key areas of the speech control system, including the laryngeal sensorimotor cortex, inferior frontal gyrus, superior/middle temporal and supramarginal gyri, and in the cerebellum. The pathophysiology of SD may involve a multilevel disruption of speech-controlling networks involving both sensorimotor output and auditory monitoring.

Current standard treatment for SD is type A botulinum toxin or BT.[5] BT has been traditionally combined with voice therapy; however, evidenced-based research has not been conclusive as to whether this combined modality treatment increases efficacy. Murry and Woodson[6] suggest that the combination of BT treatment and voice therapy functions to prolong the effects of BT by reducing compensatory muscle strain. To date, however, no additional studies have been published on this combined effect. When BT is not effective or a patient refuses BT treatment, voice therapy may reduce the overall handicapping effects of the condition. It is important to note that there are no curative effects of behavioral therapy. Other surgical treatments for SD include lateralization thyroplasty[7] and selective laryngeal adductor denervation–renervation.[8]

MTD, by contrast, is not related to any structural or neurological dysfunction of the larynx. MTD is thought to be caused by excessive or poorly regulated muscle tension of the laryngeal and extralaryngeal musculature.[9] Although the specific mechanism related to the causation and persistence of the problem has not been clearly identified, anecdotal evidence reveals an association with compensatory strain during or following an upper respiratory infection. Excessive stress and psychological conflict has also been related to an exacerbation of symptoms.[10] Symptoms can appear gradually or suddenly and are exacerbated by stress and vocal usage. Although singing and non-speech-related vocalizations may result in improved voice quality, this effect is typically brief as dysphonia sets in once the muscles return to their default patterns of tension. The gold standard treatment is speech therapy. Techniques are primarily used to target muscle relaxation and may include laryngeal massage, semi-occluded vocal tract postures, and exercises to re-coordinate breath flow and resonance. At times vocal improvement can be immediate. Other times gains are made over a longer period of time with ongoing speech therapy.

56.6 Outcome

In the case of C, several diagnostic indicators pointed toward the diagnosis of SD over MTD. Most significantly, C's voice quality improved during laughing, singing, speaking in falsetto voice, and yelling. In addition, a noticeable decrease in the overall frequency of C's tremor and voice breaks was observed during sustained voicing compared to connect speech. Roy[11] purported that although patients with ADSD may have voice breaks during non-speech-related tasks, improved vocal quality with these tasks during diagnostic testing significantly increased the likelihood of a positive SD diagnosis. Although C did not appear to present with a clear phonetic pattern of spasms during spontaneous speech, an appreciable increase in spasm frequency was observed during voiced consonant-loaded phrases. Minimal muscle strain with digital manipulation of extrinsic musculature (typically present with MTD) and a clear absence of secondary gain were also contributory to the final diagnosis. MTD can co-occur; however, it is compensatory in nature. Spectrographic analysis clearly showed abrupt voice breaks and irregular vertical striations. Diagnostic indicators in the patient's medical history included her reports that her voice is involuntarily "shaky," intervals of normal voice quality, and the potential for a positive family history. By contrast, MTD would likely present as a more consistent disruption in vocal quality across all tasks, and can also be associated with vocal dose, levels of stress, and secondary gain. In addition, MTD is associated with persistent and significant muscle tenderness and strain that can be identified during laryngeal palpation.

Following a brief period of counseling with a focus on defining the diagnosis of SD, which C already suspected by way of independent research, and discussing treatment options, she agreed to medical treatment with BT. She was asked to call in at 3-week intervals for the first several months following the injection to touch base with the therapist and discuss any ill effects or concerns. C expressed concern and sadness over the diagnosis itself; however, she was relieved to have a clear plan of treatment. She also requested several sessions of voice therapy following her first BT treatment. However, this treatment was advised against given the lack of significant secondary muscle tension noted on evaluation. C was provided several links to the National Spasmodic Dysphonia Association for further social support groups and general information about the condition.

56.7 Key Points

- SD is task specific and voice quality is often (but not always) improved during non-speech-related tasks such as laughing, singing, falsetto voicing, and yelling.
- Speech-specific items that trigger spasms may be vowel-initial phrases (e.g., "We eat eggs every Easter") for ADSD and voiceless consonants (e.g., "He is hiding behind the house") for ABSD. Mixed SD will have a tremor component (a regular wavering in pitch) that can be appreciated on sustained voicing.
- There is a much greater likelihood of SD if voice quality improves with sustained phonation.
- MTD without a significant psychogenic component will respond to speech therapy techniques focused on release of extrinsic laryngeal musculature.
- Most confusing is that SD is characterized by "islands" of normal speech and an exacerbation of voice quality with stress, both of which may appear to be more functional in nature.
- Although SD can co-occur with MTD, vocal function will only improve temporarily with even the best of relaxation techniques.

Suggested Readings

[1] Rees CJ, Blalock PD, Kemp SE, Halum SL, Koufman JA. Differentiation of adductor-type spasmodic dysphonia from muscle tension dysphonia by spectral analysis. Otolaryngol Head Neck Surg. 2007; 137(4):576–581

[2] Tanner K, Roy N, Merrill RM, Sauder C, Houtz DR, Smith ME. Spasmodic dysphonia: onset, course, socioemotional effects, and treatment response. Ann Otol Rhinol Laryngol. 2011; 120(7):465–473

References

[1] Ludlow CL, Adler CH, Berke GS, et al. Research priorities in spasmodic dysphonia. Otolaryngol Head Neck Surg. 2008; 139(4):495–505

[2] Simonyan K, Ludlow CL. Abnormal structure-function relationship in spasmodic dysphonia. Cereb Cortex. 2012; 22(2):417–425

[3] Blitzer A, Brin MF, Stewart CF. Botulinum toxin management of spasmodic dysphonia (laryngeal dystonia): a 12-year experience in more than 900 patients. Laryngoscope. 2015; 125(8):1751–1757

[4] Ali SO, Thomassen M, Schulz GM, et al. Alterations in CNS activity induced by botulinum toxin treatment in spasmodic dysphonia: an H215O PET study. J Speech Lang Hear Res. 2006; 49(5):1127–1146

[5] Blitzer A, Sulica L. Botulinum toxin: basic science and clinical uses in otolaryngology. Laryngoscope. 2001; 111(2):218–226

[6] Murry T, Woodson GE. Combined-modality treatment of adductor spasmodic dysphonia with botulinum toxin and voice therapy. J Voice. 1995; 9(4):460–465

[7] Isshiki N, Tsuji DH, Yamamoto Y, Iizuka Y. Midline lateralization thyroplasty for adductor spasmodic dysphonia. Ann Otol Rhinol Laryngol. 2000; 109(2): 187–193

[8] Berke GS, Blackwell KE, Gerratt BR, Verneil A, Jackson KS, Sercarz JA. Selective laryngeal adductor denervation-reinnervation: a new surgical treatment for adductor spasmodic dysphonia. Ann Otol Rhinol Laryngol. 1999; 108(3):227–231

[9] Roy N, Gouse M, Mauszycki SC, Merrill RM, Smith ME. Task specificity in adductor spasmodic dysphonia versus muscle tension dysphonia. Laryngoscope. 2005; 115(2):311–316

[10] Roy N, Bless DM, Heisey D, Ford CN. Manual circumlaryngeal therapy for functional dysphonia: an evaluation of short- and long-term treatment outcomes. J Voice. 1997; 11(3):321–331

[11] Roy N. Differential diagnosis of muscle tension dysphonia and spasmodic dysphonia. Curr Opin Otolaryngol Head Neck Surg. 2010; 18(3):165–170

57 Aphasia and Dysphagia in a Resident of a Skilled Nursing Facility

Kelly A. Bridges

57.1 Introduction

Each practice setting comes with a unique set of challenges and limitations. It is critical for speech-language pathologists (SLPs) to provide in-service education to staff when faced with complex cases in the skilled nursing, subacute, and/or long-term care rehabilitation settings.

57.2 Clinical History and Description

MM, a 75-year-old man, was admitted to an acute care hospital following reports from his long-time girlfriend that "after breakfast, he couldn't speak" and "couldn't move his right arm." A computed tomography of the brain at admission (~4 hours after symptoms began) revealed a left middle cerebral artery ischemic cardiovascular accident (CVA) in the posterior distribution. MM was not a candidate for tissue plasminogen activator, as his symptoms began more than 3 hours prior to admission and he presented with other contraindications. Following admission, MM was transferred to a specialized inpatient rehabilitation institute (IRI) for 4 weeks to receive intensive physical, occupational, and speech therapy. MM was then transferred to a subacute rehabilitation center/skilled nursing facility (SNF), approximately 6 weeks after his CVA.

According to the transfer records, MM's prior medical history was significant for uncontrolled hypertension, high cholesterol, diabetes mellitus type 2, benign prostatic hyperplasia, and four prior "mini strokes" with no known lasting symptoms (~11 years prior, 5 years prior, and two last year). Additionally, the discharge documents stated that MM was a fall risk, required 2:1 assistance with transfers and 1:1 supervision at all times, was on aspiration precautions, and was discharged on a mechanical soft solid consistency diet with thin liquids. Reportedly, he was making slow but steady progress in physical, occupational, and speech therapy, but frequently refused to participate and was increasingly agitated. MM was recently upgraded from a pureed solid consistency diet with nectar-thickened liquids to a mechanical soft solid consistency diet with thin liquids after significant improvement with dysphagia therapy. MM had also received intensive language therapy, targeting expressive and receptive language. No details were provided in the transfer records regarding language goals or progress.

The SNF's nursing admission notes stated that he was "agitated and had trouble speaking," that he "ate 100% of lunch and dinner," and was consuming a "regular solid and thin liquid diet." It is also stated that he planned to discharge home with his girlfriend and continued assistance/care as needed.

57.3 Clinical Testing

MM was seen for dysphagia and speech-language evaluation 1 day following admission. Dysphagia evaluation was performed to assess safety and tolerance of swallowing of the least restrictive diet and possible return to prior level of function (reportedly, a regular solid and thin liquid consistency diet). An oral motor examination revealed natural dentition with attrition of only one right posterior molar. Facial symmetry at rest and during movements, labial retraction, protrusion, and strength were within functional limits (WFL). Lingual elevation, depression, protrusion, right and left lateralization, and strength were WFL. Velar elevation was symmetrical and functional during phonation. Vocal quality was clear and loudness was adequate. MM produced a strong cough and functional throat clear on command. He adequately managed secretions and exhibited functional hyolaryngeal elevation/excursion to digital palpation during a dry swallow. He was trialed with mechanical soft solids, regular solids, and thin liquids during evaluation. MM self-fed large, unsafe bites of all solid consistencies trialed, and did so at a very rapid pace. He required frequent reminders to slow pace and to take small bites during the assessment. With all solid consistencies, he exhibited functional labial seal/containment, timely rotary-pattern mastication, relatively cohesive bolus formation, timely oral transport, and timely initiation of pharyngeal swallow with functional hyolaryngeal elevation/excursion to digital palpation. Minimal bilateral lingual residue was noted postswallow on regular solid consistency trials only; this residue was cleared with liquid wash (after first bite, the patient performed liquid wash with verbal cue from the clinician; MM utilized liquid wash strategy without cueing on remainder of trials). No overt signs or symptoms of penetration/aspiration were observed with solid consistencies. Two 4-ounce cups of thin liquids were attempted via continuous cup and straw sips; MM demonstrated gross functional tolerance, with clear voice postswallow and no overt signs or symptoms of penetration/aspiration during or following oral intake.

MM's motor speech function was judged to be WFL based on informal conversation before and during his swallowing evaluation. Expressive and receptive language were assessed informally due to increased agitation, reduced attention, and increased distractibility. He required consistent encouragement, redirection, and positive reinforcement to engage in language tasks. MM was alert and oriented to person and partially to place (stated he was "in the hospital") and situation ("I had a stroke"), but not to time (he did not provide the correct day/date/month/year). Receptive language was characterized by 9/10 correct in response to simple yes/no questions pertaining to himself and his immediate environment (he verbalized "yes" and "no"), 1/10 correct in response to complex yes/no questions (e.g., Do you eat dinner at night? Do you peel a banana before you eat it?), 5/10 correct in following one-step commands (e.g., touch your head, stick out your tongue), and increased to 9/10 correct when provided with additional visual cues and repetition of the command, 4/5 identifying body parts (error on "elbow," where he pointed to his wrist), 5/5 identifying objects in his immediate environment in a field of two and 1/5 objects correctly identified in a field of four, and 3/5 identifying color photos in a field of two and 0/5 in a field of four.

Regarding MM's expressive language, informal evaluation revealed functional production of formulaic language/conversational greetings/nonpropositional speech (e.g., stated "Hi, how are ya?" upon SLP entering the room, "damn" when frustrated during lexical retrieval tasks, frequent production of pause-fillers and "you know"), fluent speech (produced approximately five to six words per utterance) with appropriate use of function words, 5/5 repeating single words (e.g., cup, pizza, money), 4/5 repetition of short phrases/sentences (e.g., I love you, babies cry, I'm hungry), 0/5 repeating complex sentences (e.g., before you eat dinner, take the trash out), 3/10 naming objects around the room, 3/5 naming body parts, and 3/10 naming common objects in color photographs. Across naming tasks, errors were often in the form of semantic paraphasias (e.g., produced "spoon" for fork, and "bed" for chair) and perseveration on prior target words (e.g., perseverated on "bed" across several stimuli while naming objects, body parts, and photographs). MM appeared to be inconsistently aware of these errors; he expressed frustration (e.g., "damn") and increasing agitation as the evaluation progressed (e.g., he stated "are we done yet?" and "I don't have time for this" toward the end of the session).

57.4 Questions and Answers for the Reader

1. What should the SLP do after observing conflicting information regarding MM's diet between the IRI discharge documents and the SNF nurse's admission notes?
   a) Recommend continue with the nurses' orders for a regular solid diet consistency. A swallowing evaluation is not necessary.
   b) Recommend continue with the IRI discharge orders for a mechanical soft solid diet consistency. A swallowing evaluation is not necessary.
   c) Recommend continue with the nurses' orders for a regular solid diet consistency and perform a swallowing evaluation to determine whether this is the safest consistency diet.
   d) Recommend continue with the IRI discharge orders for a mechanical soft solid diet consistency and perform a swallowing evaluation to determine the least restrictive diet.
   e) Recommend diet downgrade to pureed solid consistency pending results of a swallowing evaluation.

Answer: d is correct. It is critical that facilities have clear communication during the transfer process; however, it is not always the case that recommendations are implemented correctly from facility to facility. The SLP, upon noting this discrepancy, should inform nursing of the diet recommendation at discharge, notify the dietary staff of the diet recommendation, and immediately request a diet change from the erroneous "regular solid" diet consistency to the "mechanical soft" consistency as recommended by the discharging facility and pending results from the dysphagia evaluation. It is also advisable to conduct in-service education to nursing and/or administrative staff on the importance of obtaining and adhering to diet consistency recommendations from the discharging facility and the risks associated with not doing so. Above all else, the safety of the patient must be maintained, and if one is unsure of the appropriate diet consistency prior to an evaluation by the SLP, it is necessary to err on the side of caution and adhere to the downgraded diet. Following this downgraded diet back to the discharge recommendation, the SLP should conduct a thorough dysphagia evaluation to further evaluate the appropriateness of the current diet consistency and goals for therapy.

a is incorrect. While nurses have some knowledge of dysphagia, they do not receive the same level of training as the SLP and, as such, we should always follow recommendations of the SLP at discharge from the IRI. As IRI discharge documents note a downgraded diet of mechanical soft solid consistency, a swallowing evaluation would be necessary to determine the least restrictive and safest diet as well as to inform the therapy plan.

b is incorrect. As MM was admitted on a downgraded diet and reportedly was consuming regular solids with thin liquids prior to his stroke, it is appropriate for the SLP to conduct a dysphagia evaluation to determine the safest and least restrictive diet and to inform the plan for therapy with the goal of MM returning to his prior level of function.

c is incorrect. The IRI discharge orders of mechanical soft solid diet consistency should be adhered to, as the discharging SLP is more highly trained in swallowing physiology and is considered the expert opinion. A swallow evaluation should also be conducted to assess the safety and efficiency of MM's swallow for the least restrictive diet consistency.

e is incorrect. The IRI discharge documents note that MM was upgraded from pureed solids to mechanical soft solids by the IRI SLP. As such, one should be confident in these recommendations to continue with mechanical soft solid diet consistency prior to the SLP's evaluation. If during a subsequent dysphagia assessment, the SLP finds that MM is unsafe with mechanical soft solids, it could be appropriate for a diet downgrade to pureed solids.

2. Why did the SLP choose not to assess MM's tolerance of nectar-thickened liquids during the evaluation?
   a) Because it is more important to assess thin liquids, since everyone is given regular (thin) water in a facility regardless of their recommended diet/liquid consistency.
   b) Because MM was upgraded to thin liquids during his time in therapy in the IRI and has been safely tolerating them according to hospital discharge records.
   c) Because MM demonstrated safety and gross functional tolerance of thin liquids during his skilled dysphagia evaluation.
   d) Because MM would have been too fatigued to complete additional testing after drinking 8 ounces of thin liquids.
   e) b and c.

Answer: e is correct (both b and c are correct). According to the IRI discharge documents, after participating in swallowing therapy, MM was successfully upgraded to a thin liquid consistency diet. Additionally, the SLP assessed MM's tolerance of 8 ounces of thin liquids via continuous cup and straw sips, at which time he demonstrated functional tolerance and did not exhibit any overt signs or symptoms of penetration or aspiration. As such, it was unnecessary to evaluate tolerance of thickened liquids during this evaluation.

a is incorrect. Unless explicitly stated in a diet order, individuals with orders for thickened liquids should never be given thin liquids (including water). It is possible for patients to aspirate when drinking water, which may lead to complications including respiratory distress and/or pneumonia.

d is incorrect. Fatigue was not reported during the dysphagia evaluation. In fact, he completed a speech-language evaluation following his swallowing assessment.

3. What should be the main focus of dysphagia therapy?
   a) Improving the timeliness of triggering his pharyngeal swallow.
   b) Increasing hyolaryngeal elevation and excursion.
   c) Increasing strength of labial seal during mastication to reduce oral spillage.
   d) Improving safety at meals with reduced pace and bite size when consuming solids.
   e) Improving base of tongue retraction for pharyngeal clearance.

Answer: d is correct. As MM did not demonstrate impairments in the pharyngeal phase of swallowing and only minimal postswallow residue, characteristic of mild oral phase dysphagia, the main concern is MM's unsafe and impulsive self-feeding behaviors (rapid rate of self-feeding and large bite sizes). The focus of dysphagia therapy should center on increasing safety during meals, increasing awareness of his self-feeding behaviors, educating on potential risks associated with unsafe eating, and educating on the continued use of compensatory strategies to clear postswallow oral residue. The goal of the patient is to return to eating regular solid consistency foods, and the goal of the SLP is for the patient to do so *safely*. Due to MM's desire to return home with increased independence (and additional assistance as needed), it is also important to provide education on safe feeding strategies to his long-time girlfriend and any other family members/caregivers that will be present and assisting in his daily activities after discharge.

a is incorrect. Per the dysphagia evaluation, MM exhibited a timely trigger of the pharyngeal swallow.

b is incorrect. According to the assessment, hyolaryngeal elevation and excursion was WFL for all consistencies trialed.

c is incorrect. There was no anterior oral spillage observed during intake and his labial seal was WFL during the assessment.

e is incorrect. MM's pharyngeal phase of swallowing was WFL during all consistencies trialed at bedside. The SLP did not suspect pharyngeal residue and he exhibited no overt signs or symptoms of penetration/aspiration during the assessment.

4. Of the following, which is not an appropriate short-term language goal early on in his treatment plan?
   a) MM will express orientation to person, place, time, and situation with 100% accuracy with visual calendar aid and minimal verbal cues.
   b) MM will provide two alternative solutions to complex problem scenarios 5/5 × with minimal to no cues.
   c) MM will follow one-step directions with 80% accuracy (8/10 ×) with minimal verbal cues.

d) MM will name 7/10 objects in his immediate environment in a field of four with moderate verbal (semantic, phonemic) and visual cues.
e) MM will answer complex yes/no questions with 90% accuracy (9/10 ×) with minimal verbal cues.

Answer: b is correct. When prioritizing goals, we can consider several factors, including improving safety, promoting independence, and facilitating the patient's engagement in activities of enjoyment. For MM, he is currently residing in a subacute rehabilitation center and frequently expresses frustration and occasionally agitation when there are communication breakdowns between him and staff. To reduce frustration and improve interactions with staff, it would be beneficial to MM to initially focus on increasing accuracy in following commands, in answering complex yes/no questions about himself, preferences, and care, and in improving lexical retrieval for common objects and items in his daily environment (the SNF). Additionally, to further reduce frustration and confusion, targeting improved orientation is desirable. Later goals may target more complex areas, including higher-level cognition (e.g., problem-solving goals), auditory comprehension (e.g., reading comprehension), and improving lexical retrieval for objects and photographs that are not found in the SNF setting but that represent items present in and applicable to his home-life and leisure activities.

a is incorrect. An individual's knowledge and awareness of person, place, time, and situation are very beneficial in the recovery process. Orientation is often one of the first goals that clinicians establish for people with neural injury.

c is incorrect. MM would benefit greatly from making improvements in following simple one-step commands, as he and the nursing staff have expressed frustration in their daily care interactions due to receptive limitations.

d is incorrect. Due to his increasing frustration with lexical retrieval and communication breakdowns with staff, MM would also benefit from improved naming of objects in his immediate environment (his room, the bathroom, the dining room, etc.), which would facilitate his communication of basic wants and needs.

e is incorrect. Again, the communicative breakdowns with staff negatively affect MMs quality of life. By initially targeting improved comprehension of complex yes/no questions, staff would be better equipped to meet MMs needs and MM would exhibit less frustration and improved integration into this present environment.

57.5 Description of Disorder and Recommended Treatment

MM presented with mild oral phase dysphagia characterized by mild postswallow residue for regular solids and impulsive and unsafe rate and bite sizes during self-feeding. Dysphagia therapy was recommended with a focus on compensatory strategy training and increased safety during oral intake with the goal of MM returning to his prior level of function (safely tolerating regular solid consistency with thin liquids). Prior to MM's evaluation, nursing and dietary staff were informed of a necessary diet downgrade to mechanical soft solid consistency with thin liquids. Following dysphagia evaluation, nursing was informed that MM should remain on the downgraded diet due to safety concerns with advanced consistencies at this time.

MM also presented with moderate receptive and mild expressive aphasia with reduced attention and frequent agitation, which impacted his participation in tasks. Language therapy was recommended to increase MM's functional communication of wants, needs, thoughts, and medical decisions to facilitate reintegration into his social/living environment. Family education was an important component of therapy, as MM and his girlfriend expressed that the goal was for him to return home with additional support as needed.

57.6 Outcome

MM participated in dysphagia therapy for 2 weeks and was seen 3 days per week for 30-minute sessions to target swallowing goals. MM was pleasant; participation and engagement in tasks were generally good across dysphagia therapy sessions. While trialing regular consistency solids initially with small quantities and then at full lunch meals, MM was trained to increase swallow safety via verbal and visual cueing to reduce his bite sizes, take his time while eating, and alternate liquids and solids (to promote clearance of postswallow residue and to facilitate reduced pace during meals). Initially, MM required verbal cues on 70% of bites (to reduce rate, take small bites, and alternate liquids and solids) with occasional visual cues to slow pace. However, MM gradually increased independence in reducing pace, bite size, and utilizing liquid wash, and, at discharge, he required minimal to no cueing. After completing three sessions with small-quantity trials of regular solid consistency and one session at a full meal, MM demonstrated improved tolerance with minimal to no oral residue postswallow with and without use of liquid wash and no overt signs or symptoms of aspiration. His diet was upgraded to regular solid consistency with thin liquids and he participated in two final sessions with the SLP at lunch to assure safety with upgraded diet consistency and continued use of safe-swallow and compensatory strategies. He was discharged from swallowing therapy at his prior level of function, safely consuming regular solid and thin liquid consistencies. At discharge, nursing and certified nursing assistant staff were educated on safe swallow strategies and recommendations to provide verbal cues to slow pace and reduce bite size as needed. Due to MM's other safety concerns and physical therapy/occupational therapy recommendations for constant supervision (due to fall risk and patient's impulsivity in attempting to self-transfer), MM continued to eat with supervision at all times. MM's girlfriend was present during the final session and two prior sessions. She verbalized and demonstrated knowledge of safe swallow and compensatory strategies.

MM also participated in language therapy for the 4 weeks he resided in the SNF. He was seen for 30- to 45-minute sessions 3 to 4 days per week for aphasia therapy, with a focus on improving receptive language (specifically increasing accuracy of answering complex yes/no questions about self and medical care and activities of daily living, and following one- and two-step commands with minimal cueing) and expressive language

(increasing lexical retrieval of concrete objects in his immediate environment via semantic features analysis with variable levels of cueing). These skills were targeted first, as they were expected to improve MM's quality of life in the SNF by reducing communicative breakdowns between MM and staff, and increasing his accurate expression of wants and needs to improve overall functional communication. During therapy, MM exhibited inconsistent participation and engagement, as some days he was pleasant and put forth optimal effort, and other days he was easily frustrated and agitated. Often, he benefited from positive reinforcement, occasional breaks from therapy (with the therapist reapproaching later to finish the session), and encouragement from his girlfriend to continue. MM exhibited increased distractibility during aphasia therapy as compared with his dysphagia therapy, but he benefited from gentle redirection to tasks and a quiet therapy environment. Receptive language skills slowly improved over 4 weeks of therapy. At discharge, MM exhibited 70% accuracy when answering complex yes/no questions, 100% accuracy in following one-step commands without visual cues, and 80% accuracy in following two-step commands with minimal visual cues. Using a modified form of semantic feature analysis treatment, lexical retrieval also improved for the naming of common objects in his immediate environment (90% correct with minimum semantic and phonemic cueing). MM continued to exhibit occasional semantic paraphasias and perseveration, but they were more common when he was tired or frustrated. He was occasionally resistant to using compensatory strategies (e.g., circumlocution) when lexical retrieval proved difficult and required consistent encouragement to do so. The SLP recommended continued aphasia therapy services as an outpatient or via home health care upon discharge from the facility.

57.7 Key Points

- Different rehabilitation settings present different challenges. One must understand that issues arise and errors may occur in documentation and adherence to clinical recommendations. It is the responsibility of the SLP to provide education to other health professionals when this happens in an effort to reduce these potentially harmful situations and improve patient safety and quality of life.
- In SNFs (subacute rehabilitation units, short- and long-term care units), each patient will be different and may progress at different rates. Some may demonstrate great strides in their recovery and others may not. It is important to initially prioritize goals that will help to meet that individual's needs in their current environment (e.g., functional communication of basic wants and needs, improving patient–staff–family communicative interactions, and increasing safety) in an effort to improve quality of life.
- People with brain injuries (stroke, disease, or trauma-related) may have co-occurring impairments that can impede progress in swallowing, language, or cognitive-linguistic therapy. The clinician–patient dynamic benefits from finding optimal methods to encourage participation and increase motivation during therapy, which may include incorporation of family and/or caregivers into the treatment program.

Suggested Readings

[1] Kristensson J, Behrns I, Saldert C. Effects on communication from intensive treatment with semantic feature analysis in aphasia. Aphasiology. 2015; 29 (4):466–487

[2] Ownsworth T, Clare L. The association between awareness deficits and rehabilitation outcome following acquired brain injury. Clin Psychol Rev. 2006; 26 (6):783–795

[3] Winstein CJ, Stein J, Arena R, et al. American Heart Association Stroke Council, Council on Cardiovascular and Stroke Nursing, Council on Clinical Cardiology, and Council on Quality of Care and Outcomes Research. Guidelines for adult stroke rehabilitation and recovery: A guideline for healthcare professionals from the American Heart Association/American Stroke Association. Stroke. 2016; 47(6):e98–e169

58 Multiple Cranial Neuropathies and Posterior–Inferior Cerebellar Artery Aneurysm following a Traumatic Brain Injury

Gemma Bailey

58.1 Introduction

Acquired brain injuries are complex and require thorough assessment to determine the most suitable rehabilitation plan for each patient.

58.2 Clinical History and Description

TD was a 20-year-old helmeted, male driver involved in a motorcycle accident. A computed tomography scan of the head revealed occipito-cervical dissociation and subarachnoid hemorrhage (SAH). Magnetic resonance imaging revealed an incidental finding of a left posterior-inferior cerebellar artery (PICA) aneurysm, which was subsequently stented and coiled, as well as evidence of diffuse axonal injury. TD presented with multiple cranial neuropathies, including bilateral glossopharyngeal nerve palsy (CN IX) and bilateral vagal nerve palsy (CN X). Otolaryngology assessment revealed bilateral vocal fold immobility with the vocal folds in a lateralized position (▶ Fig. 58.1).

58.3 Clinical Testing

TD was evaluated approximately 2 months following the injury. At that time, he reported difficulty swallowing and was only receiving nutrition via percutaneous endoscopic gastrostomy (PEG) tube feeds. Oral-motor evaluation (OME) revealed symmetrical facial appearance; moist oral cavity; natural dentition; and adequate strength, range, and speed of movements relevant to the musculature of the tongue, lips, and mandible. TD's vocal quality was breathy and he demonstrated difficulty altering pitch and volume. Palatal elevation was observed during phonation tasks. TD presented with a volitional cough and throat clear. Laryngeal movement was detected during a saliva swallow. However, a saliva swallow was immediately followed by a cough and expectoration of secretions. Given the severity and complexity of TD's presentation, clinical swallowing trials were limited to ice chips. Oral management was adequate; however, TD demonstrated difficulty triggering a pharyngeal swallow. Repeated laryngeal movements (i.e., "bobbing") were observed, followed by a coughing episode and expectoration of pharyngeal secretions (i.e., water and frothy saliva). Inspiratory stridor

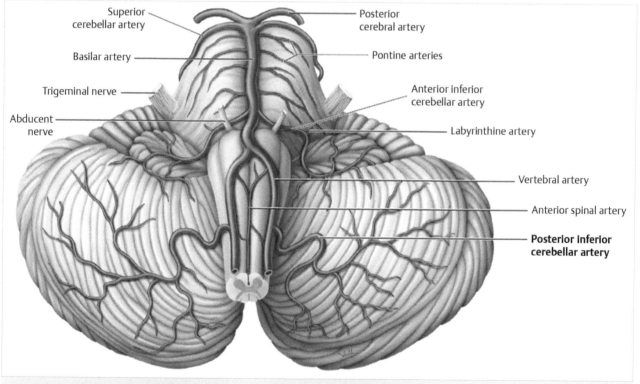

Fig. 58.1 Circle of Willis: posterior-inferior cerebellar artery (PICA).

was observed during coughing episodes. The clinical swallowing evaluation was discontinued (▶ Table 58.1).

Follow-up laryngoscopy revealed improved left vocal fold movement, but no movement of the right vocal fold. Pooling of secretions in the pharyngeal recesses was observed. Videofluoroscopic swallow study (VFSS) was performed; honey-thick liquids were attempted initially. TD's oral phase was unremarkable. TD's pharyngeal phase was profoundly impaired. Hyoid elevation was absent anteriorly and notably reduced superiorly. Epiglottic deflection was marginal. Laryngeal elevation was noted. Incomplete supraglottic closure resulted in high penetration. The bolus did not pass through the upper esophageal sphincter (UES) and remained in the pyriform sinuses. After the initial swallow attempt, further penetration to the level of the vocal folds was observed. No cough was noted. The bolus was expectorated after 7 to 10 unsuccessful swallow attempts. A small volume of material passed through the UES on one of three bolus trials when TD spontaneously moved his chin forward during the swallow.

58.4 Questions and Answers for the Reader

1. A 67-year-old woman was found at home with her eyes open, unable to verbalize or move any of her extremities. She now has a tracheostomy and difficulty managing oral secretions. An OME reveals movement of the upper face and eyebrows, no movement of lower face, wet oral cavity, and tongue paralysis. She is nonverbal, but can subtly nod her head "yes" in response to questions. She is oriented to person, place, and time. She can roll her eyes upward on command. She is most likely presenting with:
   a) Guillain–Barré syndrome.
   b) Myasthenia gravis.

Table 58.1 TD's oral-motor evaluation

Structure	Function
Face	• Symmetrical appearance
Oral cavity	• Moist
Mandible	• Adequate range of motion • Adequate speed of movement • Adequate strength against resistance
Dentition	• Natural dentition—no missing teeth
Lips	• Adequate retraction and pucker • Adequate strength of lip seal • Adequate speed and coordination during alternating movements
Tongue	• Adequate range of movements • Adequate strength against resistance • Adequate speed and coordination of movements
Palate	• Elevation noted during sustained and intermittent phonation • No obvious asymmetry
Larynx	• Breathy vocal quality and difficulty altering pitch and volume • Adequate volitional cough and throat clear • Laryngeal movement observed during dry swallow attempt

   c) Unresponsive wakefulness syndrome.
   d) Locked-in syndrome.
   e) Amyotrophic lateral sclerosis.

Answer: d is correct. Locked-in syndrome is a neuromuscular disorder, resulting from damage to the pons. Damage is typically caused by a lack of blood flow (infarct) or bleeding (hemorrhage). Individuals cannot consciously swallow, breathe, speak, or produce any other voluntary movements. Cognitive function is unaffected.

a is incorrect. Guillain–Barré syndrome is an autoimmune disease, which attacks the peripheral nervous system. It results in a gradual onset of symptoms.

b is incorrect. Myasthenia gravis is a chronic autoimmune neuromuscular disease. It often presents as increased muscle weakness during activity. It often affects muscles controlling eye and eyelid movement.

c is incorrect. In unresponsive wakefulness syndrome, the patient is awake but lacks cognitive function.

e is incorrect. Amyotrophic lateral sclerosis is a progressive neurodegenerative disease where the nerve cells that control muscles die.

2. A 21-year-old man presents with dysphonia. He was involved in a serious motor vehicle accident (MVA) and intubated for a period of 2 weeks. When asked to speak, the patient is hesitant and presents with a soft whisper. An otolaryngology assessment reveals adequate bilateral vocal fold movement and a hemorrhage on the left true vocal fold. The patient is eager to start treatment. As his clinician, you:
   a) Note that treatment is not necessary and promote talking loudly throughout the day.
   b) Encourage 1 to 2 weeks of complete vocal rest, followed by a reassessment.
   c) Recommend hard glottal attacks to improve volume.
   d) Liaise with the otolaryngologist to discuss a left thyroplasty.
   e) Liaise with the otolaryngologist to discuss a Botox injection to the left vocal fold.

Answer: b is correct. Vocal fold hemorrhages result from a rupture of a blood vessel. A sudden change in vocal quality is the most common symptom. Treatment is vocal rest.

a is incorrect. This may result in worsening of symptoms and permanent voice changes.

c is incorrect. This may result in worsening of symptoms and permanent voice changes.

d is incorrect. A thyroplasty utilizes a surgical implant to "push" a paralyzed vocal fold toward the glottal midline to improve glottic closure.

e is incorrect. Botox injections are used to treat spasms of the vocal folds.

3. You complete an OME on a stroke patient, presenting with notable dysarthria and reported swallowing difficulties. You observe a right-sided lower facial droop and reduced lip retraction on the right. You further note tongue deviation to the right on protrusion. The patient's volitional cough is strong and vocal quality is unremarkable. The oral cavity is dry, and the patient reports impaired taste. You might expect to see the following physiological impairments during a VFSS:

a) Absent pharyngeal swallow.

b) Premature spillage, impaired bolus preparation, and slow posterior transfer with solids.

c) Reduced UES relaxation, resulting in pyriform sinus residue and aspiration post swallow.

d) Premature spillage, reduced base of tongue contact with the posterior pharyngeal wall, and impaired velopharyngeal closure.

e) Reduced airway protection resulting in aspiration and pharyngeal stasis.

Answer: b is correct. The OME suggests right lower motor neuron involvement of the facial nerve (CN VII) and the hypoglossal nerve (CN XII).

a is incorrect. This impairment involves the brainstem (medulla).

c is incorrect. This impairment is likely to involve the trigeminal nerve (CN V), the glossopharyngeal nerve (CN IX), and the vagus nerve (CN X). You would likely note impairments specific to the jaw and volitional cough.

d is incorrect. This impairment is likely to involve the hypoglossal nerve (CN XII) and the pharyngeal plexus (CN IX and X). You would note impairments specific to the tongue and possibly an absent gag reflex.

e is incorrect. This impairment involves the vagus nerve (CN X). You would likely note difficulty initiating a volitional cough and impaired vocal quality.

58.5 Description of Disorder and Recommended Treatment

TD presented with multiple cranial neuropathies likely caused by severe head trauma, and Wallenberg's syndrome, likely related to the PICA aneurysm and SAH. Bilateral involvement of CN XI and X resulted in vocal fold paralysis. Improved left vocal fold movement was observed within 2 months of the MVA. TD presented with a breathy vocal quality and difficulty changing pitch. Wallenberg's syndrome is often the result of a unilateral lateral medullary infarction, which negatively impacts the pharyngeal phase of swallowing. An acute unilateral event is capable of causing bilateral dysfunction. The pharyngeal swallowing impairment is severe and often necessitates nonoral feeding. Recovery is slow compared with hemispheric stroke patients, and symptoms may persist years after the event.

Improved swallowing function was TD's main goal. Based on clinical and instrumental testing, a personalized swallowing rehabilitation program was created. TD participated in therapy sessions two to three times per week, 12 sessions prior to discharge. Sessions were 45 to 60 minutes in length and consisted of regular-effort saliva swallows, effortful swallows, supraglottic swallows, and Mendelsohn's maneuvers. A total of 60 saliva swallows per session were completed. Once TD was familiar with the prescribed swallowing exercises, bolus trials with yogurt were introduced. By the time of discharge, TD was completing 10 to 15 bolus trials per session. The number of expectorations during a session was also tracked. Improvement was suggested by an overall reduction in the number of expectorations within a session.

58.6 Outcome

Upon discharge, TD continued to require all nutrition and hydration via PEG. He was transferred to a private speech-language pathology clinic specializing in the provision of neurorehabilitation services. The staff at this facility was updated on TD's therapy program and progress. Prior to discharge, TD was referred for a follow-up VFSS. It was also recommended that TD participate in therapy directed at improved vocal efficiency. The receiving clinic had an experienced voice clinician and was equipped (i.e., videostroboscopy) to complete the evaluation and initiate intervention.

58.7 Key Points

- Acquired brain injuries are complex and require a detailed review and understanding of the patient's clinical history.
- Dysphagia is often multifaceted. The completion of a thorough oral motor exam and a clinical swallowing evaluation is necessary and provides critical information regarding the nature and potential severity of swallowing impairments, and determines the need for further instrumental evaluation.
- Dysphagia often coincides with dysarthria and/or voice disorders. A multidisciplinary approach to assessment and rehabilitation is essential.
- Patient and/or family should be included in the prioritization of treatment goals.
- Treatment should be planned and evidence based. A comprehensive plan promotes the likelihood of success.

Suggested Readings

[1] Aydogdu I, Ertekin C, Tarlaci S, Turman B, Kiylioglu N, Secil Y. Dysphagia in lateral medullary infarction (Wallenberg's syndrome): an acute disconnection syndrome in premotor neurons related to swallowing activity? Stroke. 2001; 32(9):2081–2087

[2] Daniels SK, Huckabee ML, eds. Dysphagia Following Stroke. San Diego, CA: Plural Publishing; 2008

59 Script Training in Nonfluent/Agrammatic-Primary Progressive Aphasia

Michael de Riesthal and Sarah Diehl

59.1 Introduction

An evidence-based approach to managing communication deficits is critical to therapeutic success. In the current case, we describe an approach to therapy for an individual with nonfluent/agrammatic-primary progressive aphasia (nf-PPA) based on patient history, as well as his social, community, and vocational environment, and best clinical evidence.

59.2 Clinical History and Description

BH, a 64-year-old, right-handed man, was actively employed as a pharmacist. He presented with a 4-year history of decline in communicative function. Early in this decline, he was incorrectly diagnosed with Alzheimer's disease. He then received a thorough neurological assessment. On examination, BH was alert and oriented to person, place, and time. He named all of the pictures on the NIH Stroke Scale and followed a three-step command. His speech was hesitant and groping, and he made inconsistent errors when producing multisyllabic words. He repeated "no ifs, ands, or buts" and was able to spell WORLD forward and backward. When presented with words to remember, he was able to register 3/3 words and recalled all three words after a 10-minute delay. He was able to copy the intersecting pentagon figure and drew a clock with properly placed numbers and hands. BH's pupils were equal and reactive to light, his visual fields were full, and his extraocular movements were full without nystagmus. His facial movements and palatal elevation were symmetric, and his tongue protruded at midline. BH did not demonstrate arm drift, focal weakness, or dysmetria. He was able to walk on a narrow base and perform a tandem walk without difficulty. Magnetic resonance imaging indicated minimal ischemic white matter changes in the left periventricular regions. Based on this assessment, with the primary findings being issues with motor speech production, the neurologist diagnosed BH with a primary progressive apraxia of speech (AOS). He was referred for a speech and language evaluation and treatment.

59.3 Clinical Testing

During speech and language evaluation, BH and his wife reported that, at first, he had difficulty "getting his words out," followed by progressive difficulty communicating in conversational interactions at home, in the community, and at work. At the time of this assessment, BH was having more difficulty initiating speech. He denied difficulty comprehending language or with memory function. According to BH and his wife, he was still able to perform most aspects of his job, although he reported increased difficulty communicating with customers and pharmacy technicians.

BH participated in a motor speech evaluation and the Revised Token Test,[1] Story Retell subtest from the Arizona Battery for Communication Disorders of Dementia (ABCD),[2] a picture description task including the "cookie theft" picture from the Boston Diagnostic Aphasia Examination,[3] the Pyramid and Palm Trees Test (PPT),[4] Boston Naming Test (BNT),[5] and a word fluency measure. His word fluency was examined for both spoken and written generation of words beginning with "f," "a," and "s" to determine the influence of a potential motor speech disorder (e.g., AOS) on the efficiency of performance during a timed generative naming task.

On the motor speech evaluation, BH presented with slow rate, inconsistent articulatory errors, distorted substitutions, sound repetitions, voicing errors, and excess and equal stress. His performance was consistent with a moderately severe AOS.

On language testing, his overall score on the Revised Token Test was 13.35, which placed BH in the 80th percentile compared to individuals with left hemisphere lesions. He made a few frank errors (e.g., selecting the wrong color or shape); however, primarily, he demonstrated "self-corrections" and "immediacy" responses (i.e., he initiated the gestural response to a command before the command was completed). During the picture description, BH's number of correct information units (CIUs) and percent CIUs were consistent with nonaphasic performance as described by Nicholas and Brookshire[6]; however, his CIUs per minute and percent CIUs per minute were consistent with the performance of individuals with aphasia. He was able to recall 15 of 17 elements on the Story Retell subtest from the ABCD immediately after presentation and following a 10-minute delay, which was consistent with his report of little difficulty with memory. BH named 13 of 15 pictures on the BNT and correctly answered all 52 items on the PPT, suggesting naming and the ability to identify semantic associations were relative strengths. Performance on the word fluency measure, for both spoken and written naming, was impaired—17 and 19 total words, respectively—across the three letter categories. BH spoke in complete sentences, with rare omission of function words. He was able to write in complete sentences. The most striking aspect of BH's communication was the delay in initiating utterances, inconsistent articulatory errors (groping for articulatory position, self-correction), and halting speech during motor speech and language testing. Based on this assessment and his history of a progressive decline in communication function, he was diagnosed with nf-PPA.[7]

59.4 Questions and Answers for the Reader

1. The results of BH's testing suggest that memory is not impaired. This finding is important because it potentially rules out the presence of
   a) Stroke.
   b) Traumatic brain injury.

c) Dementia of the Alzheimer's type.

d) Tumor

Answer: c is correct. Memory must be impaired to have a diagnosis of dementia of the Alzheimer's type.

a is incorrect. One can have a stroke and not have an impairment in memory.

b is incorrect. One can have a traumatic brain injury.

d is incorrect. One can have a tumor and not have an impairment in memory.

2. Given BH's primary deficit appears to be AOS, how would you justify a diagnosis of nf-PPA?

a) The classification of the nonfluent/agrammatic variant of PPA includes the presence of agrammatism and/or effortful halting speech with inconsistent speech sound errors and distortions.

b) AOS is a phonological deficit that is reflected in the agrammatism that is associated with the nonfluent/agrammatic variant of PPA.

c) The diagnosis is not the nonfluent/agrammatic variant of PPA.

d) The classification of the nonfluent/agrammatic variant excludes the presence of AOS as a significant sign or symptom.

Answer: a is correct. AOS is considered one of two primary characteristics of the nonfluent/agrammatic variant of PPA.

b is incorrect. AOS is a disorder of motor programming and not a disorder of language or phonological encoding.

c is incorrect. The diagnosis of nonfluent/agrammatic variant of PPA is accurate.

d is incorrect. The classification of nonfluent/agrammatic variant includes the potential presence of AOS as a significant sign or symptom.

3. A 63-year-old patient presents with a 2-year history of progressive decline in communication. Upon exam, you observe impaired confrontation naming and single-word comprehension and dyslexia. His repetition is intact and speech production is normal. What type of progressive speech and/or language disorder would you diagnose the patient with?

a) Logopenic variant of PPA.

b) Semantic variant of PPA.

c) Primary progressive AOS.

d) Nonfluent/agrammatic variant of PPA.

Answer: b is correct. The semantic variant of PPA may result in surface dyslexia, as well as preserved speech production.

a is incorrect. A primary feature of the logopenic variant of PPA is impaired repetition, and surface dyslexia is *not* an expected feature.

c is incorrect. Primary progressive AOS would result in impaired repetition and speech production.

d is incorrect. The nonfluent/agrammatic variant is characterized by impaired repetition and possible speech production deficits.

4. A 58-year-old patient presents with a 3-year history of progressive decline in communication. Upon exam, you observe impaired word retrieval in conversation and on naming tasks and impaired repetition of sentences and phrases. Phonemic paraphasic errors are noted in spontaneous speech. Single-

word comprehension and motor speech production are spared. What type of progressive speech and/or language disorder would you diagnose the patient with?

a) Nonfluent/agrammatic variant of PPA.

b) Semantic variant of PPA.

c) Primary progressive AOS.

d) Logopenic variant of PPA.

Answer: d is correct. A hallmark of the logopenic variant of PPA is impaired repetition and the presence of phonemic paraphasias in conversational speech.

a is incorrect. Nonfluent/agrammatic variant of PPA is not characterized by phonemic paraphasias and motor speech production is impaired.

b is incorrect. The semantic variant of PPA is not characterized by phonemic paraphasias and repetition is typically spared.

c is incorrect. Primary progressive AOS, by definition, must include impaired motor speech production.

59.5 Description of Disorder and Recommended Treatment

Treatment planning focused on educating BH and his family, exploring potential alternative and augmentative communication options for the future, and implementing treatment targeting his speech and language impairments and functional communication needs. A particular limitation for BH was that, due to transportation issues and his work schedule, he could only attend therapy every other week. Script training was selected as one intervention because it permitted targeting BH's relatively scripted daily work interactions and he could practice with his wife at home. The purpose of script training is to improve automatic natural language. Functional scripts are developed by the individual with aphasia, his or her family, and the clinician. The training protocol utilizes the principles of motor learning, including the use of massed practice through repetitive, cue-based drill of the individual utterances within a script and the script in its entirety, and the distributed practice of whole scripts in natural conversational contexts. The therapeutic effect of script training on speech and language production in individuals with aphasia has been reported in published studies.[8,9]

BH's primary concern was difficulty communicating at work. Seven scripts were developed: five related to workplace interactions and two related to social interactions. One or two scripts were trained at a time using a multiple baseline design. A modified script training protocol based on work by Youmans and colleagues[9] was employed. Initially, the sentences of a script were trained individually. Training included the use of reading, repetition, choral reading, and immediate and delayed spontaneous productions to practice accurate productions of each sentence. The script was then practiced in its entirety. BH was expected to practice the scripts with his wife daily. In addition, he had opportunities to use the scripts in the targeted home and workplace interactions on a daily basis. An example of a script for interacting with pharmacy customers is provided ▶ Fig. 59.1. For the three scripts that dealt with this type of interaction, training included practice "cutting and pasting" parts of the three scripts. That is, the clinician would merge elements from different scripts to build flexibility to use the scripts functionally.

59.6 Outcome

During baseline and treatment probes, BH's performance on the scripts was scored online at the beginning of a session. The percentage of lines produced accurately within a script was measured. A response was considered accurate if it was initiated in a timely manner, contained all words within the script, and all words were produced accurately with the exception of mild distortions.

BH was seen for a total of 15 one-hour treatment sessions over an 8-month period. His baseline performance on the first three scripts (▶ Fig. 59.2), which targeted interactions with cus-

tomers, ranged from 20% to 40% accuracy. By the seventh session for each script, he reached 100% accuracy. Some variability was noted during the maintenance phase of the first three scripts. This variability was determined to be related to a decrease in BH's level of home practice during one period of treatment. Scripts 4 and 5 targeted two specific social interactions with two visitors to his home during the summer. Scripts 6 and 7 targeted interactions with his pharmacy technicians (▶ Fig. 59.3). Baseline performance ranged from 0% to 33% accuracy. He reached 100% accuracy on scripts 4 to 7 by the first session. Throughout treatment, BH and his wife reported that he was communicating more effectively at work, both with customers and staff members, and in the targeted social interactions. The first three scripts targeting interactions with customers were monitored for a longer period as they were deemed to be the most important interactions.

59.7 Key Points

- Treatments designed for individuals with nonprogressive communication disorders may be applied successfully to individuals with progressive speech and language disorders.
- The data from this case report suggest that script training may be successful in improving the communication of an individual with nf-PPA.
- When practiced in functional contexts, a patient's ability to utilize scripts in everyday communication will improve in these contexts.
- A combined treatment approach, including education, direct language training, and augmentative and alternative communication is necessary for individuals with PPA.

Suggested Readings

[1] Carthery, Goulart MT, da Costa da Silveira A, Machado TH, et al. Nonpharmacological interventions for cognitive impairments following primary progressive aphasia: a systematic review of the literature. Dement Neuropsychol. 2013; 7(1):122–131

P:	Hi, have you been waited on?
C:	No, I haven't.
P:	How can I help you?
C:	I have a prescription to fill.
P:	Do you have the `script number?
C:	Yes, here it is.
P:	This medication is out of refills. I'll fax your doctor.
C:	How long will that take?
P:	It depends on when the doctor gets it.

Fig. 59.1 Example of script for interacting with pharmacy customers.

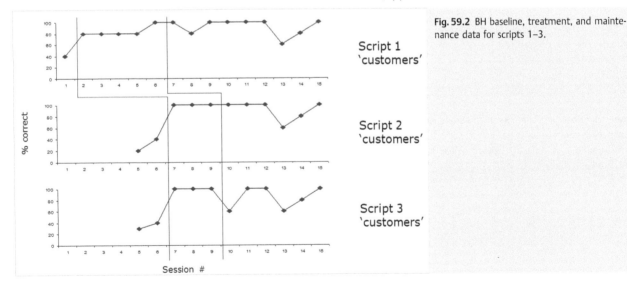

Fig. 59.2 BH baseline, treatment, and maintenance data for scripts 1–3.

Script 1 'customers'

Script 2 'customers'

Script 3 'customers'

% correct

Session #

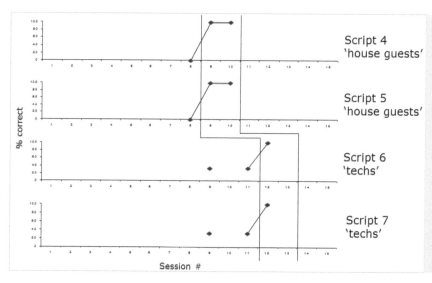

Fig. 59.3 BH baseline, treatment, and maintenance data for scripts 4–7.

References

[1] McNeil MR, Prescott TE. Revised Token Test. Austin, TX: Pro-Ed; 1978

[2] Bayles KA, Tomoeda CK. Arizona Battery for Communication Disorders of Dementia. Tucson, AZ: Canyonlands Publishing; 1993

[3] Goodglass H, Kaplan E, Barresi B. Boston Diagnostic Aphasia Examination. 3rd ed. Philadelphia, PA: Lippincott Williams & Wilkins; 2001

[4] Howard D, Patterson KE. The Pyramids and Palm Trees Test: A Test of Semantic Access from Words and Pictures. Bury St. Edmunds, UK: Thames Valley Test Company; 1992

[5] Kaplan E, Goodglass H, Weintraub S. Boston Naming Test. Pro-Ed; 2001

[6] Nicholas LE, Brookshire RH. A system for quantifying the informativeness and efficiency of the connected speech of adults with aphasia. J Speech Lang Hear Res. 1993; 36(2):338–350

[7] Gorno-Tempini ML, Hillis AE, Weintraub S, et al. Classification of primary progressive aphasia and its variants. Neurology. 2011; 76(11):1006–1014

[8] Cherney LR, Kaye RC, van Vuuren S. Acquisition and maintenance of scripts in aphasia: a comparison of two cuing conditions. Am J Speech Lang Pathol. 2014; 23(2):S343–S360

[9] Youmans G, Holland A, Muñoz M, Bourgeois M. Script training and automaticity in two individuals with aphasia. Aphasiology. 2005; 19(3–5):435–450

60 Hyperkinetic Dysarthria: Dystonic Features in a Patient with a History of Brainstem Encephalitis

Heather M. Clark

60.1 Introduction

One role of the speech-language pathologist (SLP) is to differentially diagnose motor speech disorders to aid physicians, typically neurologists, in establishing a medical diagnosis.[1] This case highlights several aspects of clinical decision-making: (1) selection of assessment procedures commensurate with clinical goals; (2) differential diagnosis based on patterns of speech features; and (3) exploration of behavioral interventions to inform recommendations to the treating clinician. The case further highlights the similarities and differences in clinical features arising from underlying spasticity and dystonia.

60.2 Clinical History and Description

RM was a 29-year-old right-handed man who, 8 months prior to presentation, developed brainstem encephalitis treated with antibiotics followed by speech and physical rehabilitation (▶ Fig. 60.1). His symptoms had been stable for several months when he developed new-onset dysphagia, jerking of the right arm and face, blurred vision, and left temporomandibular joint pain during speech. Prior to his evaluation at a tertiary medical center, RM had 6 months of speech therapy, twice per day, 5 days per week, focusing on breath control and oral motor exercises. He did not feel his speech improved as a result of therapy.

A summary of RM's assessment is provided in ▶ Table 60.1. RM was evaluated by three neurology subspecialties over the course of 3 days. The first neurologic examination was remarkable for dysarthria, described by the neurologist as spastic with nasality, as well as several other subcortical features consistent with the previous diagnosis of brainstem encephalitis. Imaging revealed symmetric bilateral hypertrophic olivary degeneration. The movement disorder neurology specialist documented pursing mouth movements, intermittent thrusting of the jaw down and to the left, and intermittent jaw clenching. These symptoms, along with other clinical findings, yielded a diagnosis of oromandibular and upper limb dystonia and palatal tremor, consistent with hypertrophic olivary degeneration. Multichannel electromyogram with multiple electrodes over the face, jaw, and palatal region revealed intermittent 8-Hz tremor in the upper orbicularis oris muscle bilaterally and speech-induced high-amplitude tonic contractions of palatal muscles. These findings were determined to be consistent with palatal dystonia. The final diagnoses were brainstem encephalitis without active infection or inflammation and dystonia.

60.3 Clinical Testing

RM underwent motor speech examination that included observation of orofacial structure and function during nonspeech tasks, and speech during picture description, word and sentence repetition, and diadochokinetic tasks.[1] RM's face was symmetric at rest. Volitional lip retraction and rounding were normal. Intermittent lip pursing, which appeared unintentional, was noted at rest. The tongue protruded at midline and moved laterally with full range, strength, and speed. No lingual atrophy or fasciculations were noted. The velum was immobile during phonation but moved with full range with elicitation of gag reflex and cough. Cough was normal with respect to sharpness. Suck, snout, and palmomental reflexes were negative.

Alternate and sequential motion rate (AMR/SMR) movements were produced at a rate of approximately five repetitions per second and with good regularity, but were imprecise and associated with reduced pressure of articulatory contacts. RM sustained phonation for 14 seconds with mild strain, but subsequent attempts were more normal with regard to vocal quality, without evidence of strain or tremor.

RM's connected speech was characterized by severe hypernasality with intermittent audible nasal emissions, mild intermittent phonatory strain, and moderately imprecise articulation. Speaking rate was equivocally reduced, associated with pauses between words and phrases rather than prolonged segments. Overall loudness and pitch variation were within normal limits. Intelligibility was fair in conversation, but repetition and/or clarification were required for most utterances without contextual cues.

Videofluorographic evaluation, conducted separately by another SLP, revealed oropharyngeal swallowing within functional limits. Palatal elevation was mildly and inconsistently reduced, without evidence of nasal regurgitation.

60.4 Questions and Answers for the Reader

1. The presence of adventitious movements of lips raised the potential for dystonia. Several sensory tricks were introduced to assess the potential to reduce adventitious movements. Chewing gum had minor facilitative effects but did not completely normalize speech. A small stick placed between the lips or a finger resting on the lips resulted in equivocal reduction in lip pursing during speech. Involuntary (or adventitious) movements are most closely associated with what type of dysarthria?
   a) Ataxic.
   b) Spastic.
   c) Hypokinetic.
   d) Hyperkinetic.

Answer: d is correct. Hyperkinetic dysarthria is defined by the presence of involuntary movements. The features present in hyperkinetic speech reflect the underlying movement disorder and the speaker's efforts to suppress or compensate for the involuntary movements.

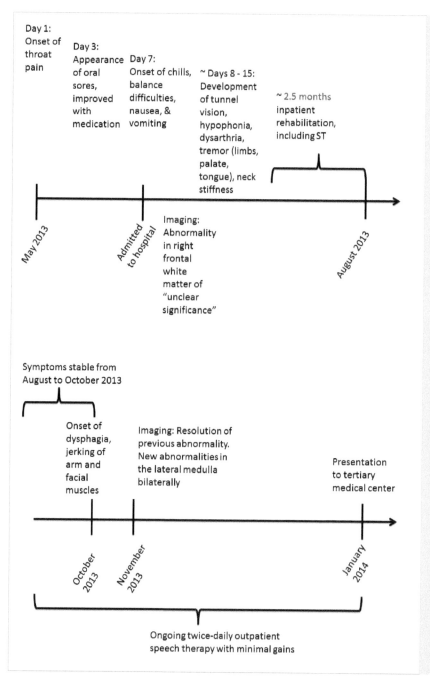

Fig. 60.1 Timeline of illness and care prior to presentation at tertiary medical center.

a is incorrect. Ataxic dysarthria is associated with uncoordinated movements.

b is incorrect. Spastic dysarthria is associated with slow movements.

c is incorrect. Hypokinetic dysarthria is associated with movements that are difficult to initiate and that are reduced in range. Some speakers with hypokinetic dysarthria exhibit tremors in the jaw or tongue, and these movements are, in fact, involuntary. However, the most prominent features of hypokinetic dysarthria arise from impairments other than involuntary movements.

2. Which aspects of RM's performance are consistent with spastic dysarthria?
   a) Breathy voice and slow rate.
   b) Strained voice and hypernasality.

   c) Oral weakness and absent pathologic reflexes.
   d) Involuntary movements and pathologic reflexes.

Answer: b is correct. The referring neurologist characterized RM's speech disorder as spastic dysarthria, which would indeed be expected in the context of brainstem encephalitis.[1] The classic presentation of spastic dysarthria is strained vocal quality (typically constant and consistent across speech tasks and sustained phonation), slow rate, monopitch and monoloudness, imprecise articulation, hypernasality, and slow and regular AMRs.[2,3] Nonspeech observations supporting the diagnosis of spastic dysarthria include orofacial weakness,[4] slow oral movements, reduced sharpness of glottal coup, pathologic oral reflexes, and pseudobulbar affect.[2] Of these features, RM demonstrated strained phonation (although this was mild, intermittent, and typically absent during sustained phonation) and hypernasality, which was disproportionate to all other speech features. Speaking rate was only equivocally slow, associated with intermittent interword pauses rather than lengthened segments. Articulatory precision was reduced in the absence of weakness or slowness of the lips or tongue. Defining features of spastic dysarthria absent from RM's speech were monopitch and monoloudness and slow AMRs. Moreover, none of the supporting nonspeech observations typical of spastic dysarthria were evident (▶ Fig. 60.2).

a is incorrect. Slow rate is a prominent feature of spastic dysarthria, but RM's speaking rate was only equivocally slow. RM exhibited mild and intermittent strained vocal quality, which may be observed in spastic dysarthria. Breathy vocal quality would be very unusual in spastic dysarthria.

c is incorrect. Although speakers with spastic dysarthria may demonstrate oral weakness, pathologic oral reflexes are more often present than absent. RM demonstrated a normal nonspeech exam—no oral weakness or pathologic oral reflexes were observed.

d is incorrect. RM demonstrated involuntary movements, but such movements are associated with hyperkinetic dysarthria, not spastic dysarthria. Speakers with spastic dysarthria often exhibit pathologic oral reflexes, but RM did not.

3. Which of the following statements about RM's previous therapy is false?
   a) The intensity (frequency and duration) of therapy RM received in the outpatient setting is typical of treatment schedules for adults receiving speech therapy in the United States.
   b) The intensity of therapy may have been warranted given the severity of RM's dysarthria.

c) RM's therapy included oral strengthening exercises even though oral weakness is not typical of hyperkinetic dysarthria.
d) RM's recollection of the goals and activities of therapy may have been inaccurate or incomplete.

Answer: a is correct. Treatment twice per day for several months would be highly unusual in the United States. A growing literature is informing the development of guidelines for treatment "dose." For now, many decisions about treatment dosage in the United States are dictated by third-party payer policies and availability of clinical and financial resources.

b is incorrect. As mentioned, the literature does not yet provide clear guidance about whether or how dysarthria severity might influence decisions about treatment intensity. However, in the absence of limitations in clinical or financial resources, it would be understandable for a speaker to seek intensive therapy for a communication disorder so disruptive to participation and quality of life.

c is incorrect. Hyperkinetic dysarthria is not typically associated with oral weakness, yet RM completed oral strengthening exercises as part of his speech therapy. It is tempting to judge negatively the decisions made by the treating clinician, but a number of factors may have influenced the goals and activities selected for RM. First, not all (and probably only a small percentage of) SLPs arrive at a differential speech diagnosis and those who do will likely make occasional mistakes. In RM's case, it is quite possible that the diagnosis of hyperkinetic dysarthria had not been made previously, so the logical conclusion that strengthening exercises were not needed may have not been obvious. Moreover, RM may have displayed different clinical signs at the time of the earlier therapy. It is possible that he

Table 60.1 Timeline of medical workup and speech pathology assessment/intervention

Date	Subspecialty/test	Key findings
1/13	General neurology	Spastic dysarthria with nasality, myoclonic jerks of right arm
1/13	Speech pathology (dysphagia)	Mildly and inconsistently reduced velar elevation without nasal regurgitation
1/14	Speech pathology (communication)	Normal language Hyperkinetic dysarthria (dystonia)
1/14	MRI	Symmetric bilateral hypertrophic olivary degeneration
1/15	Speech therapy	Improvement in hypernasality with gum chewing Initial progress in eliminating nasal flow during production of "sh" and /s,z/
1/16	Speech therapy	Extended and expanded RM's ability to sustain appropriate oral resonance to additional phonetic contexts and longer utterances; established normal intonation of short phrases
1/17	Speech therapy	Severe dystonia; sensory tricks less successful; reducing speaking rate exacerbates dystonic effects on hypernasality
1/17	Movement disorder consultation	History of brainstem encephalitis Dystonia, with oropharyngeal/palatal and upper extremity involvement, secondary to encephalitis Tremor versus dystonia, secondary to encephalitis Possible palatal tremor, secondary to encephalitis Vertical nystagmus, secondary to encephalitis
1/20	Speech pathology exit counseling	
1/20	Movement disorders laboratory	Palatal dystonia Mild facial tremor
1/21	EEG	No EEG correlate for tremor and shiver
1/21	Neurology exit counseling	Brainstem encephalitis Dystonia Anxiety

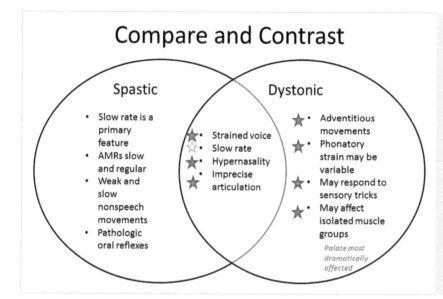

Fig. 60.2 Venn diagram illustrating similarities and differences in features associated with spastic dysarthria and hyperkinetic dysarthria associated with dystonia. Features displayed by RM are starred.

demonstrated oral weakness, perhaps from disuse or deconditioning associated with his illness; what was observed at the tertiary medical center may have been, in fact, evidence of effective treatment.

d is incorrect. Most people have at least slightly inaccurate or incomplete recollection of most life events. Moreover, it is possible that RM *never* fully understood the rationale for the activities he completed during therapy. Finally, it is common for two or more individuals involved in an interaction to have different perspectives about the nature, reason for, and success of any undertaking. For this reason, it is very helpful to have access to the written reports related to previous assessments or therapy. At the very least, differences in perspective can be identified, and in many cases the information in the reports provides insight into the current clinical picture.

60.5 Description of Disorder and Recommended Treatment

The diagnosis of hyperkinetic dysarthria associated with dystonia was informed by the following observations: (1) Hypernasality disproportionate to other deviant speech features, with preserved reflexive velar movements and effective velopharyngeal valving in select nonspeech movements (blowing bubbles through a straw). Hypernasality more severe than other speech features is most typically observed in flaccid dysarthria affecting the 10th cranial nerve; however, in that case, reflexive movements would also be affected. In the absence of evidence of lower motor neuron impairment, focal dystonia best accounts for disproportionate impairment of specific muscle groups. (2) Adventitious lip pursing at rest and during speech: focal dystonia may be speech-induced but can also be observed at rest and during vegetative movements.[1] (3) Modest improvement in speech with the use of sensory tricks. RM reported that chewing gum improved oral motor function (he attributed the benefit to "relaxing [of] the jaw"). Moreover, introduction of sensory tricks during the examination improved hypernasality and articulatory precision. (4) Mild and intermittent phonatory strain. Focal laryngeal dystonia most commonly presents in the form of spasmodic dysphonia,

but can be observed in the context of generalized dystonia as well.[1] It is not unusual for phonatory strain associated with laryngeal dystonia to vary across tasks or even across trials.[1] (5) Normal nonspeech oral motor function (with the exception of adventitious lip movements). Finally, the remaining speech features displayed by this patient (slow rate, articulatory imprecision) were not incompatible with dystonia. In summary, hyperkinetic dysarthria secondary to dystonia accounted for nearly all of the deviant speech features observed (▶ Fig. 60.2). Moreover, the subsequent identification of limb, oral, and palatal dystonia by the movement disorder specialist lent additional support to the communication diagnosis.

The following recommendations were offered during the postassessment counseling session:

- Botulinum toxin (Botox) injection is a first-line treatment for cervical,[5] laryngeal,[6] and oromandibular[7] dystonia and has been explored with mixed success for lingual dystonia.[8] Although no literature was identified describing the use of Botox for palatal dystonia, it has been used to treat palatal tremor and palatal myoclonus.[9,10] SLPs do not administer this treatment but can offer input regarding potential benefit and risks for speech and swallowing. Risks of palatal Botox injection to the palatoglossus include reduced posterior oral seal, placing RM at risk for aspiration before the swallow. Positive indicators include normal baseline swallowing assessment; postinjection assessment could identify potential compensatory strategies to mitigate effects of reduced posterior seal. Potential benefits include direct improvement from relaxation of injected muscles, as well as possible secondary benefits for noninjected muscles due to altered sensorimotor function acting as a sensory trick. These potential risks and benefits were reviewed with RM and family members.
- Fitting with a palatal lift to address hypernasality. A palatal lift could hypothetically improve speech via two mechanisms. First, the lift could facilitate velopharyngeal closure and thus improve oral resonance, as previously demonstrated for other types of dysarthria.[11] Second, the lift had the potential to serve as a sensory trick, alleviating the dystonia and allowing the palate to elevate more freely. RM indicated that his local SLP collaborated with an orthodontist who may have the

necessary expertise to fit a palatal lift/prosthesis. He was also provided with the name of a prosthodontist in his home city with experience with palatal lifts.

- Sensory tricks. Gum chewing and, to a lesser extent, placing the finger on the lips, had some benefit for improving speech production. RM was cautioned that the benefits of sensory tricks can decline with their use[12,13] and that he should therefore use gum chewing expeditiously and only when it is most important for his speech to be clear.[1]
- Speech therapy/oral motor exercises. No evidence of weakness was detected in the speech mechanism; therefore, it was no longer necessary for him to continue with exercises targeting breath support, vocal cord adduction, or movements of the speech articulators outside of speech movements. Instead, it was recommended that the emphasis shift to speech production.
- Speech therapy/speech production. A motor learning–based approach emphasizing RM's auditory, tactile, and kinesthetic awareness during relaxed phonation and oral airflow during speech was recommended.[14,15,16] It was further recommended that a speech subsystems approach be adopted, establishing integrity of the systems in the following order: velopharyngeal closure, phonation, articulation, and prosody.[17,18] The respiratory system was not impaired and was not recommended as a target for intervention. Although categorized as independent systems, the systems function interactively during speech production. The order of the targets is intended to reflect the area of "attention" that will guide the focus of feedback during speech tasks. Ideally, medical and/or prosthetic interventions would facilitate speech movements so that speech production-focused therapy would be more fruitful.

60.6 Outcome

As is often the case in tertiary medical centers, ongoing treatment was not sought as RM and his family returned to their home country. The author had the opportunity to use RM as a teaching case for neurology staff and trainees.

60.7 Key Points

- Differential diagnosis of dysarthria requires consideration of the pattern of speech features, and is supported by nonspeech and neurologic findings.
- Adventitious movements, as well as speech features that vary in severity across tasks, should raise suspicion of hyperkinetic dysarthria.
- Diagnostic therapy can help confirm or refute the differential diagnosis.

Suggested Readings

[1] Esper CD, Freeman A, Factor SA. Lingual protrusion dystonia: frequency, etiology and botulinum toxin therapy. Parkinsonism Relat Disord. 2010; 16(7): 438–441

[2] Sinclair CF, Simonyan K, Brin MF, Blitzer A. Negative dystonia of the palate: a novel entity and diagnostic consideration in hypernasal speech. Laryngoscope. 2015; 125(6):1426–1432

References

[1] Duffy J. Motor Speech Disorders: Substrates, Differential Diagnosis, and Management. 2nd ed. St. Louis, MO: Elsevier Mosby; 2013

[2] Clark HM, Duffy JR, Whitwell JL, Ahlskog JE, Sorenson EJ, Josephs KA. Clinical and imaging characterization of progressive spastic dysarthria. Eur J Neurol. 2014; 21(3):368–376

[3] Darley FL, Aronson AE, Brown JR. Differential diagnostic patterns of dysarthria. J Speech Hear Res. 1969; 12(2):246–269

[4] Clark H, Duffy J, Strand E, Hanley H, Solomon NP. Orofacial muscle tone & strength across the dysarthrias. In: Annual Convention of the American Speech-Language Hearing Association. Atlanta, GA; 2012

[5] Marsh WA, Monroe DM, Brin MF, Gallagher CJ. Systematic review and meta-analysis of the duration of clinical effect of onabotulinumtoxinA in cervical dystonia. BMC Neurol. 2014; 14(1):91

[6] Watts C, Nye C, Whurr R. Botulinum toxin for treating spasmodic dysphonia (laryngeal dystonia): a systematic Cochrane review. Clin Rehabil. 2006; 20(2): 112–122

[7] Persaud R, Garas G, Silva S, Stamatoglou C, Chatrath P, Patel K. An evidence-based review of botulinum toxin (Botox) applications in non-cosmetic head and neck conditions. JRSM Short Rep. 2013; 4(2):10

[8] Budak F, Aydın E, Koçkaya A, Ilbay G. Botulinum toxin in the treatment of lingual dystonia induced by speaking. Case Rep Neurol. 2013; 5(1):18–20

[9] Conill Tobías N, de Paula Vernetta C, García Callejo FJ, Marco Algarra J. Objective tinnitus from palatal myoclonus. Use of botulinum toxin: a case report. Acta Otorrinolaringol Esp. 2012; 63(5):391–392

[10] Penney SE, Bruce IA, Saeed SR. Botulinum toxin is effective and safe for palatal tremor: a report of five cases and a review of the literature. J Neurol. 2006; 253(7):857–860

[11] Yorkston KM, Spencer K, Duffy J, et al. Evidence-based practice guidelines for dysarthria: management of velopharyngeal function. J Med Speech Lang Pathol. 2001; 9(4):257–274

[12] Albanese A. The clinical expression of primary dystonia. J Neurol. 2003; 250 (10):1145–1151

[13] Loyola DP, Camargos S, Maia D, Cardoso F. Sensory tricks in focal dystonia and hemifacial spasm. Eur J Neurol. 2013; 20(4):704–707

[14] Clark HM. Neuromuscular treatments for speech and swallowing: a tutorial. Am J Speech Lang Pathol. 2003; 12(4):400–415

[15] Maas E, Robin DA, Austermann Hula SN, et al. Principles of motor learning in treatment of motor speech disorders. Am J Speech Lang Pathol. 2008; 17(3): 277–298

[16] Verdolini K. Principles of skill acquisition applied to voice training. NCVS Status Prog Rep. 1994; 6:155–163

[17] Dworkin JP. Motor Speech Disorders: A Treatment Guide. St. Louis, MO: Mosby; 1991

[18] Yorkston KM, Beukelman D, Strand E, Hakel M. Management of Motor Speech Disorders in Children and Adults. 3rd ed. Austin, TX: Pro-Ed; 2010

61 Exploring Clinician Readiness for Interstate Telepractice

Ellen R. Cohn and Jana Cason

61.1 Introduction

Telepractice (i.e., telespeech and teleaudiology) is a rapidly evolving service-delivery model. The American Speech-Language-Hearing Association (ASHA) defines telepractice as: "... the application of telecommunications technology to the delivery of speech-language pathology and audiology professional services at a distance by linking clinician to client/patient or clinician to clinician for assessment, intervention, and/or consultation."[1] Other rehabilitation and medical disciplines employ different terms, including telemedicine, telehealth, and telerehabilitation. This case describes the process for speech-language pathologists (SLPs) and audiologists to determine the appropriateness of this service-delivery model (▶ Fig. 61.1).

61.2 Clinical Description

RS, a school-based SLP with 15 years of experience, lives near Toledo, Ohio, close to the border of Michigan. RS works full time during the school year in a suburban public school district. Because she is very new to telepractice, she joined ASHA's Special Interest Group on Telepractice to learn more. She has no other experience or training in telepractice. To earn extra money, RS wishes to engage in private telepractice during the summer months, especially when she spends time at the ocean visiting relatives in New Jersey and Maryland. She decided to focus on a school-aged caseload located in a neighboring state (Michigan) that will not pose a conflict of interest with her full-time employment in Ohio.

61.3 Clinical Scenario

It is currently mid-June, and RS intends to begin telepractice in July. The following is in place for her to begin telepractice with patients in Michigan:

1. RS holds a state license to practice in the state of Ohio and is qualified to work in the public schools.
2. RS has access to a laptop computer equipped with a camera. This laptop belongs to her husband and he intends to keep using the computer when RS is not using it.
3. RS intends to use a free version of a popular videoconferencing software. She already employs this software to talk with friends and relatives. The address is posted on her public Facebook account. She uses the same password for all of her communication technologies so that she does not forget.
4. RS intends to use her personal, free e-mail account for scheduling, billing, and to send communications about therapy.
5. RS has password-protected Internet service in her home. She also intends to use free Wi-Fi provided at hotels or coffee shops to maintain her practice when she travels.
6. RS owns assessment instruments for both articulation and language. Because these are not yet adapted for use over the Internet, she plans to hold them up to the camera, as needed.

She will follow the same practice for commercially available therapy materials presented in kits or spiral notebooks.

61.4 Questions and Answers for the Reader

1. What aspects of RS's preparation and clinical readiness are positive indicators for safe and successful telepractice with a school-aged population?
   a) RS holds the ASHA Certificate of Clinical Competence and is a school-based clinician with 15 years of experience.
   b) RS has access to her husband's laptop computer that is equipped with a camera and she is experienced with a free version of a videoconferencing program.
   c) RS has a password-protected service to access the Internet in her home and will use free Internet access when she travels.
   d) RS owns assessment instruments for both articulation and language and has identified a strategy to adapt their use for telepractice.

Answer: a is correct: RS holds the ASHA Certificate of Clinical Competence, and is a school-based clinician with 15 years of experience. She is qualified to provide services to a school-aged population.

b is incorrect: RS must further evaluate the use of private and secure technology and software before delivering services via telepractice.

c is incorrect: Public Internet is not secure. RS must use password-protected Internet access when engaging in telepractice.

d is incorrect: RS must consult with the assessment publishers for their guidance on the use of the assessments when delivered through telepractice.

2. What aspects of RS's preparation and clinical readiness need to be bolstered?
   a) Selection and use of telepractice technology.
   b) Knowledge of assessment tools and materials sanctioned by their publishers for use with telepractice.
   c) Acquisition of appropriate state licenses to practice speech therapy.
   d) All of the above.

Answer: d is correct: RS is not yet demonstrating the preparation and clinical readiness to engage in telepractice in a manner that ensures privacy and security. She requires further training in both the selection and use of telepractice technology. She is not yet knowledgeable about what commercially available and copyrighted assessment tools and materials are sanctioned by their publishers for use with telepractice. She does not yet hold a license in the state where her prospective clients are located. The "location of practice" is identified as the location of the client; thus, in most cases, a practitioner must be licensed in the state where the client is located.

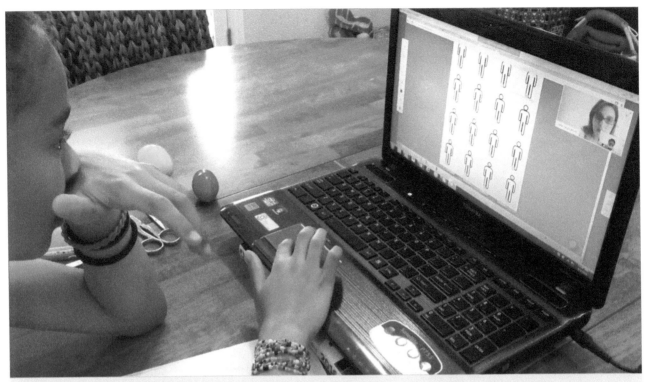

Fig. 61.1 Telepractice, a fast-developing service-delivery model that employs telecommunications, typically conducted via synchronous videoconferencing.

3. What aspects of RS's professional credentials including licensure will be supportive of her telepractice?
   a) RS is a member of ASHA's Special Interest Group on Telepractice and is an active member of the group.
   b) RS holds state licensure in Ohio, and is recognized as qualified to practice in schools.
   c) RS holds the requisite number of continuing education (CE) credits to satisfy her Ohio licensure requirements.
   d) RS intends to participate in CE opportunities specific to telepractice within the next 3 months.

Answer: b is correct. RS holds state licensure in Ohio, and is recognized as qualified to practice in schools, which facilitates her ability to gain licensure in other states where her potential clients are located.

a is incorrect. Though membership and participation in ASHA's Special Interest Group on Telepractice may be beneficial for gaining knowledge about telepractice and networking, it is not an aspect of professional credentialing.

c is incorrect. Although having the requisite CE credits to satisfy her Ohio licensure requirements is important, holding the Ohio license and her Certificate of Clinical Competence facilitates her ability to gain licensure in other states where her prospective clients are located.

d is incorrect. Although it is advantageous for RS to participate in CE opportunities specific to telepractice, gaining licensure where her prospective clients are located is most critical to support her telepractice.

4. What, if any, aspects of RS's professional credentials including licensure are not yet aligned with her intended telepractice?

a) All of RS's professional credentials are aligned with her intended telepractice.
b) RS must obtain a limited license for school-based SLPs in the state of Michigan.
c) RS must obtain state licensure in Michigan and adhere to the state's requirements for professional practice, inclusive of telepractice.
d) RS must engage in CE opportunities from state-approved CE providers in both Ohio and Michigan.

Answer: c is correct. RS does not yet hold state licensure in Michigan, and is unfamiliar with the state's requirements for professional practice, inclusive of telepractice. RS can utilize ASHA's state-by-state advocacy resource to gain preliminary information and then check the currency and accuracy of the information by contacting the appropriate licensure board or regulatory agency.

a is incorrect. RS will need to obtain a state license to practice speech therapy in Michigan, the state where her prospective clients are located and become familiar with the state's requirements for professional practice, inclusive of telepractice.

b is incorrect. RS's telepractice work will not be affiliated with a school district or school-based services, rather she will be providing private (solo) telepractice during the summer months.

d is incorrect. Although it is advantageous for RS to participate in CE opportunities specific to telepractice, gaining licensure where her prospective clients are located is most critical to support her telepractice. For license renewal purposes, RS should review CE requirements of each state where she holds a license, as activities that receive CE credit vary by state; also, some states require CE credits from state-approved CE providers.

5. What action should RS take first to be fully prepared to deliver telepractice during her upcoming vacations in New Jersey and Maryland?
   a) RS should become familiar with New Jersey and Maryland's requirements for telepractice, including vacation-related telepractice.
   b) RS should utilize a password-protected service to access the Internet while vacationing in New Jersey and Maryland.
   c) RS should travel with the requisite assessment tools and telepractice materials.
   d) RS should coordinate schedules with her husband to secure designated times to utilize the shared laptop computer.

Answer: a is correct. RS should become familiar with New Jersey and Maryland's requirements for telepractice, including vacation-related telepractice. She should determine whether the licensure boards claims jurisdiction if she is physically located in the state (even if the client is not located/residing in the state). Many state licensing boards do not claim jurisdiction in this case and defer to the licensing board in the state where the client is located. Some states have temporary practice provisions, which may allow RS to continue to work with her clients while she or they are temporarily vacationing in the state.

b is incorrect. Although it is true that RS should utilize password-protected services to access the Internet while vacationing in New Jersey and Maryland, it is not the first action she should take. The first action should be determination of New Jersey and Maryland's requirements for telepractice, including vacation-related telepractice.

c is incorrect. RS should have the necessary telepractice materials with her while vacationing; however, it is not the first action she should take.

d is incorrect. RS risks compromising protected health information (PHI) by sharing a computer with other family members (i.e., her husband). RS should utilize available resources to determine strategies to assure the privacy and security of PHI when utilizing a shared computer. However, becoming familiar with New Jersey and Maryland's requirements for telepractice, including vacation-related telepractice, is the first action she should take to fully prepare to deliver telepractice during her vacation.

61.5 Description of Readiness for Telepractice and Recommended Measures

RS has identified a clinical population with which to engage in telepractice and is beginning to consider what is required. Unfortunately, the time to prepare is very brief with less than a month before the projected start of therapy. RS is not yet licensed in Michigan and it is unlikely that she can successfully apply for and gain her new license within 2 to 3 weeks. The same constraints and expense could apply to practice in the states in which she, and/or her clients, will be vacationing in,

and will require preparatory contact with the state licensure boards of the vacation sites.

RS is similarly not prepared to begin telepractice via technologies and connectivity methods she intends to employ. Greater attention must be given to practices that will uphold the privacy and security of the clinical session, as well as other electronic communication between the client and the clinician. RS must also verify that any copyrighted diagnostic and therapeutic materials have been approved by their publishers for use with telepractice. Finally, RS has but a brief time to become more broadly trained in how to effectively engage in the conduct of telepractice sessions, as well as the research evidence for such practice.

61.6 Outcome

Telepractice (i.e., telespeech and teleaudiology) is rapidly evolving within a complex and dynamic environment. This new service-delivery model is simultaneously subject to transformation and constraint by numerous external influencers, including historical roots and current practices in telemedicine and telehealth; new and developing technologies; state licensure and federal regulations; reimbursement and healthcare economics; and professional association-based policies that dictate nomenclature, tele-ethics, and practice guidelines. RS read content provided on the ASHA website (http://www.asha.org/Practice-Portal/Professional-Issues/Telepractice/) and realized she was not yet prepared to begin telepractice in 2 to 3 weeks as an independent, sole provider with no identified mentor or prior training in telepractice.

RS further relied upon ASHA's Code of Ethics (http://www.asha.org/Code-of-Ethics/) to guide her decision. While the entirety of the Code applies to service delivery via telepractice, two Rules of Ethics (in Principles of Ethics I) were especially relevant to RS's decision making:

1. "Individuals who hold the Certificate of Clinical Competence shall not provide clinical services solely by correspondence, but may provide services via telepractice consistent with professional standards and state and federal regulations."
2. "Individuals shall protect the confidentiality of any professional or personal information about persons served professionally or participants involved in research and scholarly activities and may disclose confidential information only when doing so is necessary to protect the welfare of the person or of the community, is legally authorized, or is otherwise required by law."

61.7 Key Points

- Telepractice is a fast-developing service-delivery model that employs telecommunication that is typically conducted via synchronous videoconferencing. All technologies associated with telepractice must be deployed in a manner that upholds privacy and security.
- An SLP must hold a valid state professional license in both the state in which they are practicing and, if different, the state where the client is present. If the client and/or the clinician wishes to engage in telepractice from yet another state during vacation, the clinician must abide by that state's licensure

requirements. (The requirement for multiple state licenses does not apply to clinicians employed by the U.S. Department of Veterans Affairs or the U.S. Department of Defense.)

Suggested Readings

[1] American Speech-Language-Hearing Association. ASHA state-by-state requirements for state licensure. Available at: http://www.asha.org/advocacy/state/. Last accessed April 30, 2016

[2] American Speech-Language-Hearing Association. Telepractice overview. Available at: http://www.asha.org/Practice-Portal/Professional-Issues/Telepractice/. Last accessed April 30, 2016

[3] Cason J, Brannon J. Telehealth regulatory and legal considerations: frequently asked questions. Int J Telerehabil 2011; 3(20): 15–18. Available at: http://telerehab.pitt.edu/ojs/index.php/Telerehab/article/view/6077.

[4] Cohn ER, Brannon JA, Cason J. Resolving barriers to licensure portability for telerehabilitation professionals. Int J Telerehabil. 2011; 3(2):31–34

[5] Towey MP. Speech telepractice: installing a speech therapy upgrade for the 21st century. Int J Telerehabil. 2012; 4(2):73–78

[6] Watzlaf VJ, Moeini S, Firouzan P. VOIP for telerehabilitation: a risk analysis for privacy, security, and HIPAA compliance. Int J Telerehabil. 2010; 2(2):3–14

References

[1] Cohn ER (2012). Tele-ethics in telepractice for communication disorders. Perspect Telepract 2012; 2(1): 3-15. Available at: http://sig18perspectives.pubs.asha.org/article.aspx?articleid=1811135. Last accessed April 30, 2016

62 Paradoxical Vocal Fold Motion in a High-Level Athlete

Karen Drake

62.1 Introduction

Paradoxical vocal fold motion (PVFM), also known as vocal cord dysfunction or paradoxical vocal cord motion is a nonorganic episodic breathing condition often mistaken for asthma. It involves abnormal adduction of the true vocal folds during inspiration and/or exhalation resulting in narrowing of the upper airway with perceived shortness of breath and/or stridor. It is commonly seen in young, competitive athletes but can occur in adults or in young nonathletes.

62.2 Clinical History and Description

DR was in his early 20s and a very high-level runner, regularly competing in distance events at national and international meets. At presentation, he reported a 7-month history of breathing problems that began after a bad flu. He was initially diagnosed with asthma and was taking Advair as well as two puffs of Albuterol prior to exercise. This treatment protocol provided some relief of his dyspnea, but he still felt like his throat "constricted" when running. When symptomatic, he reported increased difficulty inspiring relative to expiring and he was occasionally stridorous on inhalation. His symptoms affected his ability to train as intensely as required and affected his running performance. He denied any limitations related to his voice, but reported increased difficulty with voicing when symptomatic.

62.3 Clinical Testing

Perceptual/observational assessment of voice and breathing was completed. DR's resting breathing was primarily thoracic. He was neither short of breath nor stridorous at rest. His voice was moderately tight and characterized by low pitch and nearly constant glottal fry. Flexible fiberoptic laryngoscopy was employed to visualize laryngeal anatomy and function during both speaking and breathing. Normal laryngeal anatomy was observed with normal vocal fold mobility. Significant supraglottic activity was observed during connected speech primarily characterized by severe anterior-posterior squeeze with the arytenoid cartilages postured toward the epiglottis, which limited visualization of the vocal folds during conversational speech. The vocal folds remained abducted during rest breathing.

In addition, an exercise challenge was completed by having DR run on a treadmill at a fast pace until he became symptomatic. Flexible fiberoptic laryngoscopy was then performed to visualize the larynx while symptomatic. Some paradoxical motion of the vocal folds toward midline during the breath cycle was observed. Excess vertical motion of the larynx was also observed during respiration with some "hooding" of the airway with the arytenoid cartilages pulling anteriorly and inward on inhalation. Stimulability was also determined during the evaluation; DR was very stimulable for more efficient breathing (▶ Fig. 62.1 and ▶ Fig. 62.2).

62.4 Questions and Answers for the Reader

1. In what ways can PVFM be differentiated from asthma?
   a) Asthma responds to a "rescue" inhaler and symptoms are fairly immediately relieved.
   b) Asthma typically causes more difficulty breathing out and PVFM typically causes more difficulty breathing in.
   c) Asthma may cause wheezing in the lungs and PVFM may cause stridor at the level of the vocal folds.
   d) All of the above.

Answer: d is correct. All of the above is the correct answer.

a is correct. Asthma typically responds to a rescue inhaler (Albuterol) and symptoms improve fairly quickly. PVFM does not respond to a rescue inhaler, though brief relief of symptoms may be related to the deep inhalation associated with the inhaler, which leads to increased vocal fold abduction.

b is correct. Both asthma and PVFM are associated with shortness of breath or dyspnea. However, asthma is typically associated with increased difficulty with exhalation. In contrast, PVFM is typically associated with increased difficulty inspiring. However, occasionally, patients may have difficulty with both inspiration and expiration.

c is correct. With an asthma attack, wheezing is common and can be heard via stethoscope to the lungs, or in severe cases, without a stethoscope. During a significant PVFM attack, stridor from the vocal folds is common and patients are typically aware of tightness in their throat.

2. It is not uncommon for patients with PVFM to also have laryngeal tension during phonation or laryngeal hyperfunction with voicing. Why do you think this might happen?
   a) PVFM is a focal neurological disorder, which can cause problems with breathing and voicing.
   b) PVFM is caused by vocal cord edema, which can affect breathing and voicing.
   c) Tightness in the intrinsic and/or extrinsic muscles during the breathing cycle contributes to PVFM. Tension in those same muscles can contribute to laryngeal hyperfunction while voicing.
   d) Voice disorders cause PVFM.

Answer: c is correct. Patients often present with co-occurring tension of the extrinsic and/or intrinsic laryngeal muscles during voicing. Many of those same muscles have increased tension when exercising or otherwise symptomatic.

a is incorrect. PVFM is not a focal neurological disorder. It is a functional or nonorganic episodic breathing disorder improved behaviorally, rather than with medication.

b is incorrect. Vocal cord edema does not cause PVFM. It can contribute to dysphonia. If a patient has severe edema such as

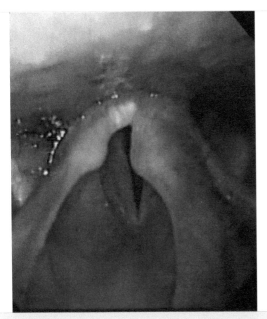

Fig. 62.1 The larynx elevating, the vocal folds moving toward midline, and the arytenoid cartilages partially hooding the airway on inhalation just after triggering symptoms during exercise.

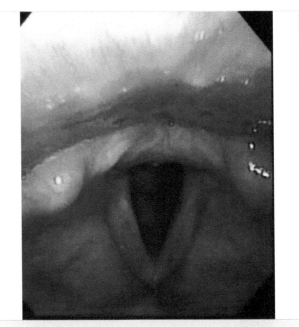

Fig. 62.2 Normal, abducted vocal cord position during inhalation and exhalation in the same patient.

with polypoid corditis, shortness of breath may be related to the vocal folds obstructing the airway, not PVFM .

d is incorrect. Voice disorders do not cause PVFM. The cause of PVFM is unknown and thought to be multifactorial.

3. Treatment for PVFM in young athletes should include:
   a) Botox injections to limit vocal fold adduction.
   b) Behavioral treatment to train more efficient breathing patterns at rest and during exercise.
   c) Medication such as valium prior to exercise.
   d) Discontinue athletics to avoid breathing problems.
   e) All of the above.

Answer: b is correct. Behavioral treatment aimed at more efficient breathing patterns at rest as well as specific breathing strategies to use during exercise has been shown to successfully reduce or eliminate symptoms. These strategies and their application may need to be modified to meet the demands of a specific sport.

a is incorrect. Botox injections are not typically indicated for the treatment of PVFM. Botox to the vocal folds can also have temporary negative side effects including difficulty swallowing and breathy voice.

c is incorrect. Although many patients with PVFM have anxiety associated with their symptoms, which is understandable given the degree of dyspnea, treating anxiety with a muscle relaxant is not indicated, as it may negatively affect athletic performance.

d is incorrect. Quitting sports may temporarily decrease episodes of PVFM, but is not an optimal long-term solution. The implications for limiting physical activity are significant.

e is incorrect. All of the above is not correct for reasons already stated.

4. Evaluation of a patient with suspected PVFM should include:
   a) Laryngoscopic evaluation to ensure that there is no vocal fold pathology and no conditions such as subglottic stenosis that could result in dyspnea.

b) Educating the patient regarding normal laryngeal appearance and physiology during both breathing and speech.
   c) Visualizing the larynx when symptomatic to see laryngeal motion/vocal fold motion when the patient is feeling short of breath.
   d) Initiating visual biofeedback. The laryngoscope can be employed to show the patient the larynx and visualize the vocal folds as they adduct. Strategies can be employed to decrease adduction with concurrent visual feedback.
   e) All of the above.

Answer: e is correct. All of the above is the correct answer.

a is correct. Laryngoscopy is a critical component of a PVFM evaluation to rule out any condition or pathology that could contribute to shortness of breath as well as to confirm paradoxical motion of the vocal folds. The larynx should be imaged before beginning treatment and patients must be seen in collaboration with an otolaryngologist to make a medical diagnosis. If the speech pathologist is not part of a voice/PVFM team, they should engage an otolaryngologist to obtain this information before initiating therapy. Occasionally, patients referred for the evaluation of PVFM present with subglottic stenosis or bilateral vocal fold paralysis. Treatment for these two conditions is quite different from PVFM treatment.

b is correct. The vast majority of patients and their families are unaware of PVFM. Allowing patients to view their laryngeal examination is extremely helpful to increase awareness of the issues underlying their shortness of breath.

c is correct. It can be extremely helpful to trigger symptoms of PVFM by an exercise or scent challenge (exposing them to whatever scent triggers their symptoms) and then visualize the larynx while symptomatic. This examination allows both the clinician and patient to see what is happening during an attack. PVFM can be "classic," with the vocal folds adducting on inhalation and opening on exhalation, but several variants of PVFM have been described. In some patients, the arytenoids pull forward, a condition referred to as "hooding" the larynx during inhalation. In contrast, the vocal folds can remain fairly abducted, but the larynx rises excessively in the neck. Some patients maintain significant vocal tension during inhalation and exhalation, while others maintain some vocal fold tension during the breathing cycle, even during rest breathing.

d is correct. Visual biofeedback can be critical for patient education and "buy in" for therapy as well as self-efficacy or the belief that he/she can control his/her symptoms. The clinician can instruct the patient to imitate an attack if they are not actually symptomatic and the patient can see abnormal vocal fold motion and how this affects the airway. Patients can then be instructed to release laryngeal tension by using a strategy such as breathing in through the nose and out through the lips and cheeks, which commonly allows the larynx to drop into a more natural position in the neck and facilitates vocal fold abduction.

62.5 Recommended Treatment

DR had fairly classic PVFM with movement of the vocal folds toward midline on inhalation during strenuous aerobic exercise. He had also had excess laryngeal elevation during the breathing cycle and his arytenoid cartilages pulled forward during inhalation. He demonstrated an inefficient breathing pattern at rest and tended to hold his breath frequently throughout the day as an unconscious habit. We recommended behavioral treatment to train preventative breathing strategies, including efficient breathing at rest and warm-up breathing exercises aimed at releasing laryngeal tension during the breathing cycle as well as rescue breathing strategies or tasks to prevent symptoms while running and to immediately interrupt symptoms when they occur. DR also demonstrated laryngeal hyperfunction during voicing and spoke with a low-pitch, throat-focused resonance and poor airflow likely related to significant anterior-to-posterior compression. Voice treatment was also initiated, as he was tightening his extrinsic laryngeal muscles with speaking as well as with breathing.

For athletes, it is critical to gain confidence with efficient breathing during sport. In this case, we recommended front-focused, open-throat breathing, which involved shifting the focus of the breath from the throat to the front of the mouth as if the air was going in and out through a large straw. Allowing the air to be gently exhaled through the lips and cheeks opened the vocal folds during exhalation, and focusing inhalation at the lips instead of the throat maintained vocal fold abduction. He began implementing this technique during a slow jog on the treadmill working up to a sprint. Success was emphasized to build self-efficacy and confidence that he could control his symptoms. DR was highly motivated throughout treatment as his running performance had suffered due to his PVFM.

DR was able to complete negative practice while running on a treadmill by returning to his baseline breathing and then switching to the new, more efficient breathing technique. He could feel the difference between running with his habitual throat-focused breathing and running with the more efficient,

front-focused breathing. As he became more aware of his throat/laryngeal muscles and his breathing, he also became more aware that he had constant tension in his throat likely related to increased laryngeal tension while speaking and breath holding. Although DR initially had no voice complaints, he began to understand and feel how he was also tightening his laryngeal muscles and stopping airflow while voicing. Optimal vocal technique was implemented to address this issue. He was given daily vocal warm-up exercises, and, during therapy sessions, improved breath support, coordination of breath and sound, and front vocal resonance in conversation were targets.

62.6 Treatment Outcome

DR completed the initial evaluation and three treatment sessions (once per week for 3 weeks). His track coach was involved and was motivated to assist with implementation of therapeutic techniques. Both DR and his coach were educated during the initial evaluation. It was helpful for them to see what was happening at the level of the vocal folds via laryngoscopy at baseline, and also when symptomatic after running on a treadmill. DR progressed rapidly through treatment as he was skilled at differentiating between his habitual respiratory pattern and more efficient front-focused breathing. By the end of the third session, he reported significant improvements in his workouts. Two weeks after the completion of treatment, he set a personal record in his event. In follow-up, he reported excellent control over his symptoms. His dyspnea index scale score[1] improved from 27 before treatment to 4 after treatment. He had no further symptoms, but occasionally had to think about controlling his symptoms during especially hard workouts and races. He also reported improved vocal function and decreased vocal fatigue. Furthermore, he reported that he felt much more confident with voicing when he had to do a running workshop or give interviews.

62.7 Key Points

- PVFM is a functional or nonorganic episodic breathing disorder that responds very well to behavioral treatment with a speech pathologist trained to work with this challenging population.
- PVFM differs from asthma in which tightness is usually felt in the upper chest and/or throat and the breathing limitation is typically most obvious on inhalation. Rescue inhalers are not associated with lasting relief of PVFM. Asthma is typically felt more on the exhalation, though further into an attack, patients can feel difficulty with both inhalation and exhalation. In addition, with asthma, tightness is typically reported in the mid-chest area and rescue inhalers typically relieve symptoms very quickly.
- In PVFM treatment, breathing strategies used during resting breathing will differ from breathing strategies used during aerobic exercise, as the oxygen demands are greater and the rate of breathing increases.
- Many patients with PVFM experience tightness or laryngeal tension during phonation as well laryngeal tension during the breathing cycle.

- All patients with PVFM must see a physician to rule out laryngeal and/or upper airway pathology before initiating PVFM treatment.
- Imaging the larynx at baseline and when symptomatic, often with an exercise challenge, is extremely beneficial to educate the patient on normal and aberrant vocal fold anatomy and physiology.

Suggested Readings

[1] Mathers-Schmidt D. Paradoxical vocal fold motion: a tutorial on a complex disorder and the speech pathologist's role. Am J Speech Lang Pathol. 2001; 10:111–125

Reference

[1] Gartner-Schmidt JL, Shembel AC, Zullo TG, Rosen CA. Development and validation of the Dyspnea Index (DI): a severity index for upper airway-related dyspnea. J Voice. 2014; 28(6):775–782

[2] Murry T, Sapienza C. The role of voice therapy in the management of paradoxical vocal fold motion, chronic cough, and laryngospasm. Otolaryngol Clin North Am. 2010; 43(1):73–83, viii–ix

[3] Newman KB, Mason UG, III, Schmaling KB. Clinical features of vocal cord dysfunction. Am J Respir Crit Care Med. 1995; 152(4, Pt 1):1382–1386

[4] Sullivan MD, Heywood BM, Beukelman DR. A treatment for vocal cord dysfunction in female athletes: an outcome study. Laryngoscope. 2001; 111(10): 1751–1755

63 Accent Modification in a Thai-Speaking Graduate Student

Dana Rissler Fritz

63.1 Introduction

Persons seeking to modify accents typically have strong English language skills in terms of comprehension and production, but have increasing difficulty with details of the English language that do not match with linguistic patterns of their first language, specifically with the use of phonemes, coarticulation, and intonation patterns.

63.2 Clinical History and Description

P was a 28-year-old woman originally from Thailand referred to a university accent modification program. P was pursuing a doctorate in chemical engineering and sought to improve her research-presentation skills as well as her ability to be understood by her fellow students, professors, and friends. She studied English for more than 10 years in Thailand with primary emphasis in reading and writing, but relatively limited practice in listening and speaking. She began using English for daily communication 2 years ago when she started her academic program. P presented as an outgoing person with a large international cohort of friends.

63.3 Clinical Testing

The Proficiency in Oral English Communication (POEC)[1] was administered to determine P's strengths and weaknesses related to American English pronunciation and intonation. The POEC provides information regarding word-level intonation, sentence-level intonation, use of contrastive stress, and articulation of consonants and vowels, as well as auditory discrimination abilities with common minimal pairs. Words with second-syllable stress (whether two or three syllables in length, such as "aCROSS" and "conSIStent") were particularly difficult for P; she had a tendency to stress the first syllable irrespective of appropriate stress placement. Pitch, volume, and duration changes to syllables within sentences were observed during conversation and within the question–answer intonation task of the POEC. However, these changes did not wholly conform to what would be expected of American speakers. She had a tendency to raise pitch or use a monotone pitch at the end of "WH" questions and statements; many utterances sounded as if she were asking a helping verb question ("Do you...?"; "Will we...?") rather than employing falling pitch with high points for important words, which is more typical of American speakers. Contrastive stress or the ability to highlight a particularly important word to improve listener comprehension of utterances was an area of relative strength for P. During a brief conversation sample, very little linking or coarticulation between words was observed.

With regard to phoneme production, P demonstrated commonly deleted word-final consonants and reduced consonant clusters in initial, medial, and final positions. Consonant substitutions noted during the assessment were /d/ for /θ, ð/ and /w/ for /v/. Consonant sounds used interchangeably included /s/ and /z/, /ʃ/ and /tʃ/, /ʒ/ and /dʒ/. Auditory discrimination tasks revealed difficulties distinguishing most voiced and voiceless English consonants. Regarding vowels, P had difficulty consistently producing /ɪ/, /ɛ/, /e/, /ə/, /œ/, and /o/; she tended to overuse canonical vowels when lip rounding was not needed. She also had a tendency to make errors related to orthography (e.g., always pronouncing words with the spelling pattern "ou" as /ɑ/). Schwa insertion was commonly noticed, particularly when three consonants were strung together (e.g., /str/).

The Sentence Intelligibility Test (SIT),[2] which consists of 11 semantically unpredictable, yet grammatically correct sentences of 5 to 15 words in length was administered. The testing protocol involves recording these productions and these recordings are then transcribed by three unfamiliar American listeners. P was 80% intelligible.

63.4 Questions and Answers for the Reader

1. What is a likely language difference in the area of phonology between English and Thai?
   a) Fewer pitch changes are expected and utilized to impact meaning in Thai.
   b) Consonant clusters are more common in Thai than in English.
   c) Linguadental phonemes are more often used in English than in Thai.
   d) All of the above.
   e) None of the above.
   Answer: c is correct. Linguadental phonemes (voiced and voiceless "th") are uncommon in most Asian languages, and not used in Thai.
   a is incorrect. Pitch change in the Thai language is common and expected by the listener.
   b is incorrect. Within-word consonant clusters are more common in English than in Thai.
   d is incorrect. Not all of the above answers are correct.
   e is incorrect. At least one of the above answers is correct.
2. P's accent modification and pronunciation should primarily focus on:
   a) Improving correct production of consonants and vowels.
   b) Word-level stress.
   c) Sentence intonation and appropriate pitch variation.
   d) All of the above.
   e) None of the above.
   Answer: d is correct. Although targets for pronunciation vary among participants, all of the above should be employed in

this case—consonants, word stress, and sentence intonation. Linking or coarticulation is also a common area of work in accent modification. Once these foundational aspects of pronunciation are addressed, therapy shifts toward applying these skills to real-world communication needs.

a is incorrect. Phoneme practice is only one component of therapy.

b is incorrect. Word-level stress is also only one part of intervention.

c is incorrect. Therapy should focus not only on sentence intonation and pitch variation but also on other areas.

e is incorrect. At least one of the above answers is correct.

3. P's difficulty in effectively producing syllable-stress differences was mostly related to:
   a) Volume.
   b) Pitch.
   c) Syllable duration.
   d) Coarticulation.
   e) Air support.

   Answer: b is correct. P could produce differences in syllable volume and duration—two of the three ways English speakers stress key syllables, but pitch was more difficult for her to change consistently. Overall, her pitch was more monotone in nature, as compared to her clinician's target model analyzed on PRAAT (to be discussed in the following section).

   a is incorrect. Although overall volume was sometimes aberrant, it was not an issue when P was using louder volume on stressed syllables.

   c is incorrect. P was able to increase the length of stressed syllables with relative ease.

   d is incorrect. Coarticulation does not directly relate to distinguishing stressed syllables at the word level.

   e is incorrect. Air support was not a relevant clinical issue related to syllable stress.

4. In terms of voiced and voiceless consonants, P had difficulty differentiating between many fricative and affricate consonants. It could be assumed that:
   a) P had a hearing and/or speech disorder.
   b) The use of fricatives and affricates in Thai is less common than in English.
   c) The importance of voicing distinctions in terms of listener perception and comprehension is less in Thai than in English.
   d) a and c are correct.
   e) b and c are correct.

   Answer: e is correct. In the Thai language, only three fricatives are used (/s/, /f/, and /h/) and no affricates are used. Voiced/voiceless correlates common and frequently used in the English language are infrequent in Thai, and only include p/b and d/t.

   a is incorrect. As an English-language learner, P's main concern was a difference in her ability to be understood by American listeners, not problems related to a disorder in speech or hearing.

   b alone is incorrect. It is not the only aspect of auditory discrimination that can be assumed.

   c alone is incorrect. It is not the only aspect of auditory discrimination that can be assumed.

   d is incorrect because a is incorrect; P's issues are related to a language difference, not disorder.

63.5 Description of Language Difference and Recommended Treatment

P's intelligibility to American listeners fell within tier III in the Missouri University Accent Modification and Pronunciation program's constructs (tier III describes listeners who are greater than 75% intelligible to unfamiliar listeners; see ▶ Table 63.1). This score likely indicated that she was asked to repeat herself regularly in situations where she was meeting new people, in noisy environments, or when the scientific jargon of engineering was challenging. Likely she was seldom misunderstood by close friends and fellow students. P was active and involved on campus, which involved significant communicative demands. Similarly, she had many opportunities to practice. Generalizability of newly learned pronunciation skills is key to effective accent modification work; her active social life was a favorable prognostic indicator.

Based on these issues, it was determined that P would likely benefit from an individualized "American phonetics" class with an intense focus on the specific phonemes and phonological rules that were challenging for her. An approach focusing on classes of sounds with significant direct practice and multimodal feedback (visual, auditory, and tactile) was determined to be ideal. Using information gained from the POEC, treatment focused on vowels and consonants in error, contrasting them with phonemes that were generally produced correctly and subsequent discussion regarding their similarities and differences. Explicitly teaching common word stress patterns would be helpful as well to ensure that increased volume and increased duration and increased pitch are required for syllable stress. Focusing on the language of origin of English words is helpful in predicting stress patterns (e.g., Latin words tend to have first syllable stress or penultimate syllable stress; Germanic words tend to have first syllable stress, etc.). In considering overall sentence-level intonation, the freeware program PRAAT[3] can be an effective tool for visual feedback of pitch lines and word-to-word linking (▶ Fig. 63.1 and ▶ Fig. 63.2). Determining P's fundamental frequency using a yawn-sigh technique or a piano keyboard would be helpful in determining what four notes she would most likely shift among in American English. In English, most speakers generally move among four notes as they speak,

Table 63.1 Intelligibility improvement as related to beginning performance levels

MU AMP tier	Average SIT baseline	Average SIT endline	Average improvement
Tier I: < 50% at baseline	43%	73.67%	30.67%[a]
Tier II: 50%–75% at baseline	65.85%	80.51%	14.66%[a]
Tier III: > 75% at baseline	86.37%	91.75%	5.38%[a]

Notes: To quantify progress and effectiveness of the Missouri University Accent Modification and Pronunciation program (MU AMP), baseline and endline data using the sentence intelligibility test (SIT) with unfamiliar American listener transcribers has been gathered since the program's inception in 2006. This table documents our results to date.

[a]$p < 0.001$.

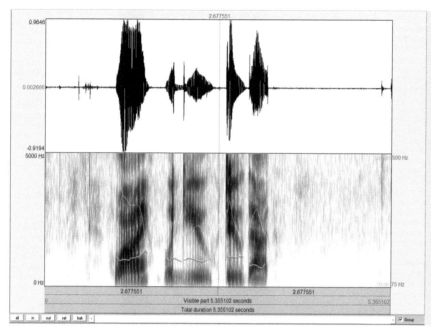

Fig. 63.1 In this PRAAT sound file, you can see changes in speaker volume on the intensity bar as well as on the spectrogram (yellow line). You can also observe pitch changes by examining the blue line on the spectrogram as P says, "Why would you do that?" Although she is changing volume of stressed syllables in a somewhat appropriate fashion, you can see very little pitch change in this question utterance, ranging from 137 to 187 Hz. You can also see very little coarticulation between the syllables, as if she is saying each word on its own. Coarticulation or linking improves intelligibility overall.

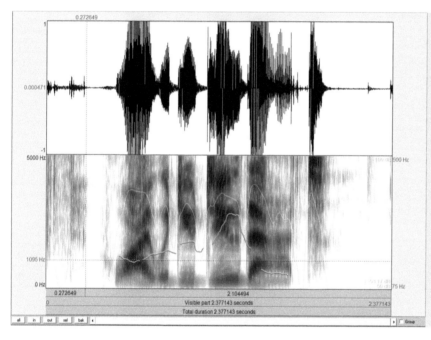

Fig. 63.2 In this PRAAT sound file, P's accent modification and pronunciation clinician is saying the same question as in ▶ Fig. 63.1: "Why would you do that?" In this example, you can observe a greater range in volume overall (intensity bar and yellow line on the spectrogram), but in terms of pitch (blue line on the spectrogram), the difference is dramatic. P's clinician shows the typical WH-question intonation, with peak pitch change near the end of the question and a steep drop in pitch after that. Her pitch range is from 124 to 314 Hz, which is more typical of American speakers and approximately 72% more pitch variation than in P's example. You can also see more coarticulation between syllables with the only real spaces in voicing because of stopgap consonants.

with their lowest note near their fundamental frequency and the three notes above serving as contrast points for stress variation and to show emotional differences (e.g., higher pitches used for excitement or to indicate a helping-verb question have been asked such as "Can we talk later?").

63.6 Outcome

P attended twenty-four, 50-minute sessions and was an active, involved participant. Initially, treatment was clinician directed with specific phoneme and intonation targets, and as improvements were observed at the syllable and word level, treatment shifted to pronunciation skills in phrases and sentences. Since accents are not disorders, rapid progression to more difficult targets is common; "real-world" communication activities typically accelerate this process. By mid-semester, a more client-led

approach was initiated where P brought in research presentations, stories from the radio related to her educational interests, and even a restaurant menu that she wanted to practice as she felt frequently misunderstood when ordering. All pronunciation skills directly targeted during the first part of the semester were then critiqued as the focus shifted to more relevant communication tasks. VoiceThread, a cloud-based educational application, was employed for P to record herself along with her presentation slides. Commentary and feedback were provided directly within the recorded presentation. This software was a motivating, yet asynchronous, homework tool employed to ensure generalization of clinic-based practice to everyday communication.

At discharge, the SIT was readministered and distributed again to three unfamiliar American listeners. P's overall sentence-level intelligibility improved to 91%. P reported that she was asked to repeat herself less often and she was more confident in her overall speaking skills. She stated that she understood continued and ongoing practice was critical to maintain and further improve her pronunciation skills. She was provided with many recommendations and online resources to support continued practice.

63.7 Key Points

- Multimodality cueing and feedback (visual, auditory, and tactile) is imperative for effective work in accent modification.
- Tailoring accent modification work to communication interests and demands of the participant is the best way to ensure transfer and generalization.
- Careful examination of L1 can be helpful in establishing targets for pronunciation and intonation work.
- Significant qualitative and quantitative improvements in overall intelligibility can be made in accent modification work.

Suggested Readings

[1] Avery P, Ehrlich S. Teaching American English Pronunciation. Oxford, UK: Oxford University Press; 1992

[2] Fritz DR, Sikorski LD. Efficacy in accent modification services. Quantitative and qualitative outcomes for Korean speakers of American English. Perspectives on Communication Disorders and Sciences in Culturally and Linguistically Diverse Populations. 2013; 20:118–126

[3] McLeod S. The International Guide to Speech Acquisition. Lexington, KY: Delmar Cengage Learning; 2007

References

[1] Sikorski L. Proficiency in Oral English Communication Manual. Santa Ana, CA: LDS and Associates; 2011

[2] Yorkston K, Beukelman DM, Hakel, M. Sentence Intelligibility Test for Windows. Lincoln, NE: Institute for Rehabilitation Science and Engineering at Madonna Rehabilitation Hospital; 1996

[3] Boersma P, Weenink D. PRAAT: Doing phonetics by computer (computer program, version 6.0.26). 2016. Available at: http://www.praat.org

64 Conversation Training Therapy for a Professional Voice User

Amanda I. Gillespie and Jackie Gartner-Schmidt

64.1 Introduction

This case demonstrates the use of conversation training therapy (CTT) in a professional voice user with phonotraumatic vocal fold lesions. CTT is a voice therapy approach based on motor learning theory that teaches patients with voice disorders the traditional therapeutic targets of phonotrauma reduction, resonance, negative practice, prosody, and breath control without the traditional therapeutic hierarchy of skill building from least to most complex. CTT exclusively relies on patient-driven conversation as the therapeutic stimulus upon which therapy skills are layered.

64.2 Clinical History and Description

JB was a 47-year-old man with gradual onset of hoarseness for 6 months with no inciting events. He reported a raspy and constricted speaking voice with difficulty projecting and decreased vocal endurance. He was a middle-school reading teacher and a semiprofessional rock singer. At the time of referral, he had been singing solo and in rock bands for over 20 years with at least one performance weekly. His singing voice also had a reduction in quality with frequent voice breaks, loss of high notes, and increased effort. He reported that his voice quality was so degraded by the end of a teaching week that he has stopped scheduling Friday singing events to rest his voice for Saturday performances. He had never taken singing lessons. He attended one session of voice therapy at another facility that consisted of diaphragmatic breathing exercises, which he stated were not helpful.

64.3 Clinical Testing

JB underwent a comprehensive multidisciplinary evaluation by a speech-language pathologist (SLP) and laryngologist. The voice evaluation included auditory-perceptual, acoustic, and aerodynamic testing, as well as stimulability assessment. The overall perceived severity of JB's voice was assessed by the SLP in accordance with the Consensus Auditory-Perceptual Evaluation of Voice (CAPE-V) parameters, and a score of 38/100 was obtained. For acoustic and auditory-perceptual analyses, JB read the six sentences of the CAPE-V and produced a sustained vowel.[1] Acoustic measures of cepstral peak prominence and cepstral-spectral index of dysphonia were taken from the all-voiced sentence, "we were away a year ago" and the sustained /a/.[2,3] See ▶ Table 64.1 and ▶ Table 64.2 for results of acoustic analyses.

The first four sentences of The Rainbow Passage[4] were analyzed for phonatory aerodynamics.[5] Following the initial reading, JB was instructed to use "clear speech" and increase intonational variety as he reread the passage to assess stimulability for immediate voice change in connected speech.[6] Clear speech requires the speaker to use crisp, clear consonants and precise articulation; it was used here with an added focus on pitch variation when speaking.[7–9] The use of clear speech is associated with immediate improvement in acoustic and aerodynamic voice outcomes in some patients with voice disorders.[6] ▶ Table 64.3 provides the aerodynamic result for both the original and stimulability productions.

Table 64.1 Acoustic analysis of sustained /a/ vowel pretreatment

ADSV measures	JB's score	Male norm	SD
CPP (dB)	8.02	13.03	1.68
CPP SD	2.97	0.63	0.24
CSID	36.22	3.58	10.37

ADSV, analysis of dysphonia in speech and voice; CPP, cepstral peak prominence; CSID, cepstral-spectral index of dysphonia; SD, standard deviation.

Table 64.2 Acoustic analysis of all-voiced sentence "we were away a year ago" pretreatment

ADSV measures	JB's score	Male norm	SD
CPP (dB)	6.11	8.04	1.33
CPP F0 (Hz)	130 Hz	127.65	19.79
CPP F0 SD	67 Hz	41.23	25.56
CSID	8.97	−4.48	7.94

ADSV, analysis of dysphonia in speech and voice; CPP, cepstral peak prominence; CSID, cepstral-spectral index of dysphonia; SD, standard deviation.

Table 64.3 Phonatory aerodynamics in connected speech (Rainbow Passage) pretreatment

	Number of breaths	Passage duration in seconds	Mean SPL in dB	Mean pitch (F0) in Hz	Mean phonatory airflow in mL/s
Original	8	25	74	93	340
Clear speech	12	33	74	111	350

SPL, sound pressure level.

Table 64.4 Patient-based questionnaires pretreatment

VHI-10 (out of 40)	25
RSI (out of 45)	6
DI (out of 40)	2
CSI (out of 40)	1
SVHI-10 (out of 40)	22

CSI, Cough Severity Index; DI, Dyspnea Index; RSI, Reflux Symptom Index; SVHI-10, Singing Voice Handicap Index-10; VHI-10, Voice Handicap Index-10.

Table 64.5 Posttreatment patient-based questionnaires

VHI-10 (out of 40)	3
RSI (out of 45)	1
DI (out of 40)	1
CSI (out of 40)	0
SVHI-10 (out of 40)	9

CSI, Cough Severity Index; DI, Dyspnea Index; RSI, Reflux Symptom Index; SVHI-10, Singing Voice Handicap Index-10; VHI-10, Voice Handicap Index-10.

JB reported that he heard and felt positive improvement in his voice following clear speech and intonation stimulability trials, and the SLP concurred. He then underwent stimulability testing using resonant voice, which has also demonstrated immediate voice improvement and utility as a stimulability tool,[10] and he reported an improvement in kinesthetic awareness ("the feel") of his voice with that strategy.

A number of self-perception questions were asked of JB about his voice. He stated that his voice bothered him a "moderate" amount (on a scale from *none* to *severe*), his complaint was in both the sound and the feel of his voice, and he rated his vocal effort as a 6/10 in severity. Furthermore, he completed a series of patient-symptom and voice handicap questionnaires, the Voice Handicap Index-10 (VHI-10),[11] Reflux Symptom Index (RSI),[12] Dyspnea Index (DI),[13] Cough Severity Index (CSI),[14] and the Singing Voice Handicap Index-10 (SVHI-10).[15] The results of these instruments are shown in ▶ Table 64.4. For all indices, a higher score is indicative of increased severity.

Following SLP assessment, JB underwent rigid stroboscopic laryngeal examination with the laryngologist. His exam revealed a right true vocal fold, mid-subepithelial lesion. Glottic closure was complete (normal), mild asymmetry of vibration was observed, and the mucosal wave was mildly decreased on the right true vocal fold and normal on the left true vocal fold.

64.4 Questions and Answers for the Reader

1. A patient with confirmed vocal fold paralysis is evaluated in the voice lab. Which tests are appropriate for this patient?
   a) Acoustic, aerodynamic, auditory-perceptual, and stimulability testing.
   b) Acoustic only.
   c) Aerodynamic only.
   d) Acoustic, aerodynamic, and auditory-perceptual testing.
   Answer: a is correct. Voice therapy and voice assessment is not a disorder-specific process. Regardless of the vocal fold anatomy, it is critical to assess all aspects of the voice as well as the individual's ability to achieve voice change following a cue or model (stimulability testing).
   b is incorrect. Acoustic testing provides only a part of the voice picture.
   c is incorrect. Aerodynamic testing provides only a part of the voice picture.
   d is incorrect. Omitting stimulability testing does not allow the SLP to assess a patient's ability to modify her/his voice and determine appropriateness for referral for voice therapy.

2. A professional speaker diagnosed with muscle tension dysphonia is referred for voice therapy. She had 23 voice therapy sessions already at another facility and is reluctant to commit to therapy again. Which approach do you suggest to treat her voice?
   a) Indirect vocal hygiene so that she will not have to practice exercises again.
   b) Do not treat her because she has already exhausted her therapy options.
   c) Treat her with CTT.
   Answer: c is correct. CTT immediately uses conversational stimuli; therefore, the patient can start to see gains in voice therapy during the first session and she will likely need to attend only three to four sessions.
   a is incorrect. Voice hygiene alone cannot rehabilitate a voice.
   b is incorrect. She clearly was not treated appropriately because she still has a voice problem.

3. True or False? During stimulability testing, a 17-year-old semi-professional volleyball player admits that she cannot hear a difference in her voice with any of the stimulability probes. You should not recommend therapy because she is not stimulable.
   Answer: False is correct. Often voice change can occur by focusing on the *feel* of the voice (kinesthetic awareness) by reducing strain, fatigue, and effort, even in the absence of awareness of a change in sound. Therefore, therapy should be recommended at least on a trial basis.

64.5 Description of Disorder and Recommended Treatment

JB was diagnosed with a unilateral benign vocal fold lesion. Based on the result of his multidisciplinary assessment, JB was referred for voice therapy. Voice therapy was completed with one 45-minute session weekly with the same therapist. The first session of voice therapy began with indirect voice therapy techniques,[16] which included an overview of relevant, personalized vocal hygiene strategies. JB revealed that he consumed an inadequate amount of daily water, cleared his throat, spoke loudly, and had frequent uncomfortable throat sensations associated with speaking. He had a history of laryngopharyngeal reflux disease, which was now controlled on medication. He exercised daily (a mixture of aerobic and strength) and did not report significant life stressors outside of his current voice problem. Following indirect voice therapy, the SLP introduced JB to CTT.[9] A full description of each skill and their scientific rationale is provided in publications regarding the conceptual development of CTT.[9] CTT begins by asking the patient to start a conversation with the SLP on any topic of his or her choice, and to use clear speech when speaking. The patient is asked to focus on the different sensations he feels with consonant production as he speaks. JB recalled using CTT during stimulability assessment in the voice lab and noted a positive change in his voice, using it during the first session of voice therapy. The SLP noted a distinct change in the patient's old and new voice, which was noted by the patient as well. The SLP then introduced negative practice by asking JB to alternate between his "old/problem voice" and the "clear voice."[17,18] To make the voices personal and distinct, the patient was also asked to name the two different voices. JB referred to his old voice as "stale" and the new voice as "fresh."

Sessions two and three remained focused in conversation. However, the SLP instructed JB on adding intonational variety when speaking, and the use of linguistically appropriate pauses for breath replenishment. Pauses also helped to slow down his rate of speech, so he was better able to focus on maintaining consistent airflow and avoiding dropping into reduced flow (e.g., "vocal fry") at the ends of his phrases. Ecologically valid classroom teaching scripts from JB's lesson plans were used to train safe and efficient vocal loudness. Intensity targets were achieved by focusing on increased consonant energy, reduced speech rate, and using a larger oral aperture when speaking. Of note, after the first session, JB reported that he did not like alternating between the "fresh" and "stale" voice, because the "stale" voice was so dysphonic and painful that he wanted to abandon its use. He also noted that his students and family had commented on his vocal improvement, and his wife said he no longer sounded in pain when speaking. By the start of session three, JB reported he had no difficulty in his speaking voice the prior week despite teaching a full 5-day week. At the completion of the third session, JB and the SLP determined that he had shown sufficient independent adjustment to the target speaking techniques, and that no further treatment was needed.

64.6 Outcome

Six weeks following the final (third) voice therapy session, JB returned to the clinic. The time between the final treatment session and follow-up was intentional to allow JB the time to integrate his new voice techniques into daily life and for learning to occur. At follow-up, he reported he was 90% better following voice therapy. His self-assessment scores all improved (▶ Table 64.5) as did his acoustic and aerodynamic outcomes (▶ Table 64.6, ▶ Table 64.7, and ▶ Table 64.8). His auditory-perceptual evaluation of overall voice severity also decreased from

38 to 7. His laryngeal examination revealed a reduction, but not complete resolution, of the vocal fold lesion. Based on the resolution of his symptoms, JB was discharged from further treatment and recommended to return to the clinic as needed.

CTT is appropriate for patients with ongoing professional voice demands because it targets voice therapy techniques in conversation immediately, instead of building hierarchically through skills, with conversational, spontaneous voice addressed last. Teachers, like other voice professionals, cannot professionally or financially afford to take weeks away from their voice demands while in voice treatment, or continue dysphonic speaking. It is essential that these professionals learn healthy, balanced speaking techniques that can immediately transfer to conversational voice, which is the goal of CTT. CTT was developed based on motor learning theory, which encourages learning through the practice of challenging tasks in real-life contexts. CTT emphasizes real-world narratives and is designed to efficiently teach phonatory techniques in ecologically valid patient-driven contexts, such as teaching, phone, and meeting scripts. Patients leave the first CTT session able to use their "new voice" in some contexts. Because of this focus on conversational voice from the first session, the number of sessions required for CTT is dramatically reduced compared to traditional therapies. Early data show that patients benefit from CTT in less than four sessions, as was the case for JB.

64.7 Key Points

- Stimulability assessment as a part of the SLP voice evaluation is critical to determining patient appropriateness for voice therapy and for guiding voice therapy approaches and goals.
- CTT eliminates the need for a therapeutic skill hierarchy and trains healthy, balanced phonatory techniques in the most difficult context—patient-driven conversation—at the start of therapy and in all subsequent sessions.
- CTT results in voice goals being achieved in a reduced number of sessions compared to traditional voice therapy approaches with measurable improvement in voice outcomes following treatment.

Table 64.6 Acoustic analyses of the sustained vowel /a/ posttreatment

ADSV measures	JB's score	Male norm	SD
CPP (dB)	10.94	13.03	1.68
CPP SD	1	0.63	0.24
CSID	9.6	3.58	10.37

ADSV, analysis of dysphonia in speech and voice; CPP, cepstral peak prominence; CSID, cepstral-spectral index of dysphonia; SD, standard deviation.

Table 64.7 Acoustic analyses of all-voiced sentence "we were away a year ago" posttreatment

ADSV measures	JB's score	Male norm	SD
CPP	9.07	8.04	1.33
CPP F0 (Hz)	124	127.65	19.79
CPP F0 SD	69	41.23	25.56
CSID	6.8	−4.48	7.94

ADSV, analysis of dysphonia in speech and voice; CPP, cepstral peak prominence; CSID, cepstral-spectral index of dysphonia; SD, standard deviation.

Table 64.8 Phonatory aerodynamics in connected speech (Rainbow Passage) posttreatment

	Number of breaths	Passage duration	Mean SPL in dB	Mean pitch	Mean phonatory airflow
Posttreatment	7	26	73	126	190

SPL, sound pressure level.

Suggested Readings

[1] Bonilha HS, Dawson AE. Creating a mastery experience during the voice evaluation. J Voice. 2012; 26(5):665.e661–665.e667

[2] Gartner-Schmidt J, Gherson S, Hapner ER, et al. The development of conversation training therapy: a concept paper. J Voice. 2016; 30(5):563–573

[3] Gillespie AI, Gartner-Schmidt J. Immediate effect of stimulability assessment on acoustic, aerodynamic, and patient-perceptual measures of voice. J Voice. 2016; 30(4):507.e9–507.e14

References

[1] Kempster GB, Gerratt BR, Verdolini Abbott K, Barkmeier-Kraemer J, Hillman RE. Consensus auditory-perceptual evaluation of voice: development of a standardized clinical protocol. Am J Speech Lang Pathol. 2009; 18(2):124–132

[2] Awan SN, Roy N, Zhang D, Cohen SM. Validation of the Cepstral Spectral Index of Dysphonia (CSID) as a screening tool for voice disorders: development of clinical cutoff scores. J Voice. 2016; 30(2):130–144

[3] Awan SN, Roy N, Jetté ME, Meltzner GS, Hillman RE. Quantifying dysphonia severity using a spectral/cepstral-based acoustic index: Comparisons with auditory-perceptual judgements from the CAPE-V. Clin Linguist Phon. 2010; 24(9):742–758

[4] Fairbanks G. Voice and Articulation Drill Book. 2nd ed. New York: Harper and Row; 1960

[5] Gartner-Schmidt JL, Hirai R, Dastolfo C, Rosen CA, Yu L, Gillespie AI. Phonatory aerodynamics in connected speech. Laryngoscope. 2015; 125(12):2764–2771

[6] Gillespie AI, Gartner-Schmidt J. Immediate effect of stimulability assessment on acoustic, aerodynamic, and patient-perceptual measures of voice. J Voice. 2016; 30(4):507.e9–507.e14

[7] Picheny MA, Durlach NI, Braida LD. Speaking clearly for the hard of hearing. II: Acoustic characteristics of clear and conversational speech. J Speech Hear Res. 1986; 29(4):434–446

[8] Picheny MA, Durlach NI, Braida LD. Speaking clearly for the hard of hearing. I: Intelligibility differences between clear and conversational speech. J Speech Hear Res. 1985; 28(1):96–103

[9] Gartner-Schmidt J, Gherson S, Hapner ER, et al. The development of conversation training therapy: a concept paper. J Voice. 2016; 30(5):563–573

[10] Bonilha HS, Dawson AE. Creating a mastery experience during the voice evaluation. J Voice. 2012; 26(5):665.e1–665.e7

[11] Rosen CA, Lee AS, Osborne J, Zullo T, Murry T. Development and validation of the voice handicap index-10. Laryngoscope. 2004; 114(9):1549–1556

[12] Belafsky PC, Postma GN, Koufman JA. Validity and reliability of the reflux symptom index (RSI). J Voice. 2002; 16(2):274–277

[13] Shembel A, Gartner-Schmidt J, Rosen CA, Zullo TG. Two Novel Instruments: Development and Validation of the Dyspnea Index (DI) and Cough Severity Index (CSI). The Voice Foundation Annual Symposium, June 5, 2011, Philadelphia, PA

[14] Shembel AC, Rosen CA, Zullo TG, Gartner-Schmidt JL. Development and validation of the cough severity index: a severity index for chronic cough related to the upper airway. Laryngoscope. 2013; 123(8):1931–1936

[15] Cohen SM, Jacobson BH, Garrett CG, et al. Creation and validation of the Singing Voice Handicap Index. Ann Otol Rhinol Laryngol. 2007; 116(6):402–406

[16] Ziegler A, Gillespie AI, Abbott KV. Behavioral treatment of voice disorders in teachers. Folia Phoniatr Logop. 2010; 62(1–2):9–23

[17] Verdolini K. Resonant voice therapy. In: Stemple J, Ed. Voice Therapy: Clinical Studies. 2nd ed. San Diego: Singular; 2000:46–61

[18] Grillo EU. Clinical investigation of the Global Voice Therapy Model. Int J Speech-Language Pathol. 2012; 14(2):156–164

65 Psychogenic Stuttering in an Adult

Suzanne Hungerford

65.1 Introduction

Individuals with conversion disorders have motor or sensory symptoms that resemble those associated with neurological conditions such as stroke, but no medical disorder fully explains the symptoms. Such "pseudoneurological" or psychogenic symptoms can mimic neurogenic communication disorders such as aphonia, dysarthria, or stuttering.

65.2 Clinical History and Description

WB was a 25-year-old veteran with a 1-year history of abnormal speech. He had a diagnosis of posttraumatic stress disorder (PTSD) and was taking several psychotropic medications to manage sleep difficulties, depression, and anxiety. WB had severe speech disfluency resembling stuttering, accompanied by quick hyperkinetic movements of the neck and face, facial grimacing, and clenching of the jaw and hands. He reported that his speech difficulties and accompanying hyperkinetic movements were context dependent. He did not have difficulty speaking at home except when speaking on the phone, and therefore WB avoided talking and traveling outside his home. He attributed his speech difficulties to "nervousness" and reported speech disfluency caused significant stress and frustration. He had no personal or family history of developmental stuttering, and medical records indicated a normal magnetic resonance imaging (MRI) and no neurologic diseases or disorders.

65.3 Clinical Testing

A conversational speech sample confirmed that WB's disfluencies were mostly sound, syllable, part-word, and whole-word repetitions with a few sound prolongations. Significant disruption of airflow during speech was observed and he could not prolong a vowel for more than 2 seconds due to voice arrests. In a 109-word conversational speech sample, 69% of words were disfluent. Some words or syllables were repeated as many as 10 times. Content words were more likely to be disfluent compared to function words. Most disfluencies were at the beginnings of words, but some were also noted in the middle and ends of words.

Little, if any, change in the severity of the disfluency and hyperkinetic motor movements was observed with delayed auditory feedback, metronome pacing, manual pacing with the clinician moving his hand rhythmically, masking noise, and/or electronic pitch-altered feedback. Furthermore, no adaptation effect (e.g., improved fluency) was observed with multiple readings of the same passage.

Of the 60 items on the Perceptions of Stuttering Inventory, WB checked 38 items as being "characteristic of me," including:

- Avoiding talking to people in authority.
- Avoiding asking for information.
- Replying briefly using the fewest words possible.
- Making sudden, jerky, or forceful movements.
- Running out of breath while speaking.
- Avoiding making a purchase.
- Avoiding introducing yourself.
- Giving excuses to avoid talking.
- Straining to talk.
- Avoiding the use of the telephone.
- Perspiring much more than usual while speaking.
- Straining the muscles of your chest or abdomen during speech.
- Having extra and unnecessary eye movements while speaking.
- Breathing forcefully while struggling to speak.

An oral motor examination revealed no facial, tongue, or soft palate asymmetries. Range of motion, speed, and coordination of the tongue during nonspeech tasks were within normal limits. During the oral-facial examination, no hyperkinetic movements of the tongue, lips, or face were observed. Sequential motion rates and alternating motion rates were abnormally slow and irregular, due to the disfluency. WB denied difficulties chewing or swallowing.

Diagnostic therapy was implemented during the assessment. With encouragement, relaxation exercises, and instruction regarding continuous airflow and easy articulatory contacts, WB quickly produced continuous airflow, and smooth, fluent production of continuant sounds and short words was attained. The rapid amelioration of symptoms, normal nonspeech oral motor movements, and the presence of a psychiatric diagnosis (PTSD) led to a diagnosis of psychogenic communication disorder (conversion disorder) (▶ Table 65.1).

Table 65.1 Etiologies of sudden-onset communication disorders. Speech-language pathologists must attempt to differentiate among these etiologies in the case of sudden-onset speech or language disorders that resemble neurogenic disorders: neurologic, psychogenic, and malingering

Etiology	Essential characteristics	Intentionally produced? Secondary gain (external rewards) or primary gain (emotional/psychological reward)?
Neurological Neurogenic communication disorders (e.g., aphasia, dysarthria, neurogenic stuttering) as a result of neurologic insult or disease	Symptoms consistent with known neurological patterns; evidence of neurologic dysfunction. Symptoms not readily reversible.	Not intentionally produced No secondary (external) gain No primary (psychological) gain
Psychogenic (conversion disorder) Patient has no conscious intention to deceive	Symptoms suggest a neurological condition but presentation of symptoms typically do not conform to known neurological patterns. Conflicts or psychological stress may precede symptoms. Symptoms may be bizarre. May be history of psychiatric disorder (e.g., anxiety disorder). Symptomatic therapy may yield fairly rapid reversal of symptoms.	Not intentionally produced Primary (psychological/emotional) gain
Malingering Patient consciously fakes disorder for secondary gain (e.g., to win a legal settlement or obtain insurance benefits)	Patients often uncooperative, give suboptimal effort in testing, and fail to follow through on therapy recommendations. Symptoms or test performance may be inconsistent. May fail very easy assessment tasks (e.g., practice items on a diagnostic test).	Intentionally produced Secondary (e.g., monetary) gain

65.4 Questions and Answers for the Reader

1. Which of the following best describes the role of the speech-language pathologist in the assessment and treatment of individuals with psychogenic communication disorders?
   a) Because there is no organic cause for the problem, the assessment and treatment of psychogenic communication disorders are outside the scope of practice of speech-language pathologists.
   b) If the speech-language pathologist suspects an individual has a psychogenic communication disorder, the patient should be referred to a psychiatrist or psychologist for treatment.
   c) Speech-language pathologists can often effectively treat psychogenic communication disorders.

Answer: c is correct. Speech-language pathologists can be effective in the treatment of these disorders. With symptomatic therapy and encouragement, patients with psychogenic communication disorders often make rapid gains.

a is incorrect. The American Speech Language Hearing Association scope of practice documents indicate that speech-language pathologists may work with individuals whose communication disorder is of psychiatric etiology.

b is incorrect. Because individuals with psychogenic communication disorders believe they have an organic problem, they may not initially follow through on referrals to mental health professionals. The speech-language pathologist can first provide supportive counseling, informing the patient that psychological changes such as stress can interfere with voluntary control of the muscles needed for normal speech. This may serve as a conversational gateway to psychiatric or psychological referral, and at the same time provide the individual with a "face-saving"

explanation for a quick reversal of symptoms following speech therapy.

2. If a patient has evidence of neurologic disease or disorder, then the communication disorder present cannot be psychogenic.
   a) True
   b) False

Answer: b is correct. Psychogenic symptoms can exist in the presence of neurogenic problems such as stroke, traumatic brain injury, or neurologic disease such as multiple sclerosis. Patients can have both neurogenic and psychogenic symptoms. The presence or history of neurologic problems does not preclude a diagnosis of psychogenic communication disorder.

3. A speech-language pathologist must consider many factors when attempting to differentiate neurogenic communication disorder, psychogenic communication disorder, and/or malingering. Which of the following is true regarding this differential diagnosis?
   a) Since WB did not have a history of stuttering in childhood, the adult-onset disfluency must have been psychogenic in origin.
   b) Since WB was taking psychotropic medications that affect the nervous system, his motor speech symptoms were most likely caused by these medications.
   c) WB was most likely malingering, since his brain MRI was normal.
   d) Evidence for the psychogenic nature of WB's speech and motor symptoms came from the case history, the motor speech examination, and the diagnostic therapy.

Answer: d is correct. WB's case history revealed that the speech problem was context specific. His symptoms abated at home (except when he had to speak on the phone), and this is not consistent with a neurological problem. The case history also revealed a history of stressors related to his military service and a history of psychiatric diagnoses (PTSD, anxiety, depression, and sleep disorder). The motor speech examination revealed that the hyperkinetic motor movements of his articulators were not present in nonspeech tasks (e.g., sticking out his tongue, chewing). This would not be the case in hyperkinetic dysarthria where one sees consistent motor patterns in speech and nonspeech tasks. Finally, the "trial" therapy initiated during the assessment revealed that with support from the therapist, WB could reduce the hyperkinetic motor movements, control his airflow, and produce sounds and words fluently. This quick reversibility of symptoms argues for the psychogenic origin of his speech difficulties.

a is incorrect. Adult-onset disfluency may be neurogenic in origin. Neurogenic stuttering has been reported after traumatic brain injury, stroke, and other neurological problems.

b is incorrect. Some medications, and combinations of medications, have been shown to sometimes produce speech disorders; however, since WB's speech problems did not coincide with medication changes, and his disfluencies abated at home, the medications were not a likely cause of his stuttering.

c is incorrect. WB was almost certainly not malingering. There were no external incentives for him to feign the symptoms; he had already been honorably discharged from the military, and he was not involved in any lawsuits. He was not seeking compensation for his difficulties, he was very cooperative in therapy, and he appeared to be truly suffering from his disorder.

65.5 Description of Disorder and Recommended Treatment

WB presented with a psychogenic speech disorder resembling stuttering. In WB's case, a neurologic explanation of the symptoms was inconsistent with the context-dependent nature of the symptoms, normal nonverbal oral movements, normal chewing and swallowing, and reversibility of symptoms. Malingering was not suspected, as there was no obvious external gain and he was cooperative and followed therapy recommendations.

In therapy, he practiced slow, relaxed speech with continuous airflow. He learned to monitor signs of muscular tension to promote smooth, fluent speech. He was quickly able to produce fluent speech in noncommunicative contexts such as reading word lists and sentences.

65.6 Outcome

By the sixth therapy session, WB was able to produce fluent conversational speech with the therapist and the hyperkinetic motor movements were greatly reduced in severity and frequency. The remaining five sessions targeted maintaining fluent speech at the conversational level, improving natural prosody, and generalizing these skills to new conversational partners and places. WB had improved functional outcomes as well; he began making and receiving phone calls at home and began leaving the house more often, although he still generally avoided social situations outside his home.

65.7 Key Points

- Adult sudden-onset communication disorders may be neurologic, psychogenic, or malingered. Psychogenic symptoms are often incompatible with neurologic findings (e.g., normal MRI, normal nonverbal oral movements in the presence of dysarthric-like speech). Patients with psychogenic symptoms frequently have a history of stress, trauma, or psychiatric diagnoses such as anxiety disorder.
- Psychogenic communication disorders are not intentional efforts to deceive. These patients believe they have a disorder with a physical basis.
- One of the hallmarks of psychogenic communication disorders is that the symptoms are often quickly reversed with symptomatic therapy.
- Psychogenic communication disorders can be effectively treated by a speech-language pathologist, and such treatment is in the speech-language pathologist's scope of practice.

Suggested Readings

[1] Baumgartner J, Duffy JR. Psychogenic stuttering in adults with and without neurologic disease. J Med Speech Lang Pathol. 1997; 5(2):75–95

[2] Baizabal-Carvallo JF, Jankovic J. Speech and voice disorders in patients with psychogenic movement disorders [serial online]. J Neurol. 2015; 262(11): 2420–2424

[3] Duffy JR. Acquired psychogenic and related nonorganic speech disorders. In: Duffy JR, Ed. Motor Speech Disorders: Substrates, Differential Diagnosis, and Management. 3rd ed. St. Louis, MO: Mosby; 2013:331–354

[4] Duffy JR. Functional speech disorders: clinical manifestations, diagnosis, and management. Handb Clin Neurol. 2016; 139:379–388

66 Aural Rehabilitation of a Sequential Bilateral Cochlear Implant User

Sara J. Toline

66.1 Introduction

Rehabilitation of a bilateral sequential cochlear implant (CI) user presents many unique challenges. Patients go through an "early acclimation period" with their device as they begin to listen through electrical stimulation presented by the CI. For a bilateral sequential user, the adjustment period will vary based on length of deafness and prior use of amplification. In addition, despite extensive counseling, patients often have preconceived expectations regarding outcomes. A multidisciplinary team is critical to effective management. Furthermore, communication between disciplines ensures patients maximize the use of their devices and support their goals for better listening and spoken communication.

66.2 Clinical History and Description

WM was a 69-year-old woman diagnosed with bilateral progressive sensorineural hearing loss due to otosclerosis as a senior in high school. Subsequent to a stapedectomy, she wore hearing aids bilaterally. Her hearing continued to deteriorate and at the age of 58 years, she was referred for CI evaluation. Testing revealed profound hearing loss in the right ear and a mild-to-severe hearing loss in the left ear. At that time, she received a CI in the right ear. Over the next 10 years, her hearing worsened in her left ear and at the age of 68 years, she received an implant in that ear. Following the second implant, she reported difficulty monitoring speech production, voice quality, and loudness of speech. She reported missing parts of conversations, requested clarification frequently, and was a passive communicator in conversations. She felt isolated from family and friends at gatherings and her self-esteem had declined.

66.3 Clinical Testing

WM was evaluated 1 month postactivation of her second CI. A functional listening assessment was completed utilizing the framework of an auditory developmental hierarchy. All testing was completed in a quiet therapy room by a speech-language pathologist. WM provided information on how her speech was perceived subjectively. She indicated she was still adjusting to the quality of speech. Her volume and pitch fluctuated, indicating little awareness of prosodic features (stress, pitch, rate, and loudness). Speech production was deemed clear and intelligible based on accurate production of sounds in conversation. Some abnormal shifts between nasal versus nonnasal speech sounds were observed.

WM demonstrated awareness of speech sounds across the frequency spectrum utilizing the Ling Six Sound Test. She detected and identified low-frequency vowels /a, u, i/, mid-frequency consonant /ʃ/, and high-frequency consonant /s/. An open-set word list, AB short word list, consisting of basic consonant–vowel–consonant combinations was used to determine her ability to perceive speech sounds at the word level and to identify speech-perception errors. Speech perception was assessed in four conditions: (1) bilaterally in quiet, (2) bilaterally in noise, (3) left side alone, and (4) right side alone. All testing was completed in auditory-only modalities with the use of an acoustic hoop. Her perception of specific linguistic structures was analyzed and she often maintained voice and manner features of sounds. She struggled most in perceiving low-frequency information, including recognition of vowels and discriminating between stop voiced consonants. Her speech perception in noise was only slightly reduced. Functional speech perception testing was in a quiet therapy room by a speech pathologist, as opposed to testing with the audiologist. All words and sentences presented were not calibrated in a soundproof booth. Items were read by the clinician and were repeated by WM. ▶ Table 66.1 depicts the results.

The *Helen sentence test* was developed by Geoff Plant to assess auditory comprehension and identification of questions and/or statements both in quiet and competing background noise. WM had little difficulty identifying sentences in quiet conditions. When simulating noise through a phone application, she omitted words in sentences that were unstressed and less predictable.

Table 66.1 One month postactivation of sequential CI

	Bilateral (quiet)	Bilateral (noise)	Left CI	Right CI
Initial consonants	70%	70%	40%	70%
Vowels	90%	80%	60%	70%
Final consonants	80%	60%	70%	70%
Whole words	60%	50%	30%	40%

CI, cochlear implant.

66.4 Questions and Answers for the Reader

1. **What factors might have influenced how WM performed with her new device?**
   a) Patient expectations.
   b) Length of deafness.
   c) Age.
   d) Need for more auditory training.
   e) All of the above.
   Answer: e is correct. All of the above factors impact performance with a CI.

   a is incorrect. She required ongoing counseling to set realistic expectations, ensure goals were attainable, and make sure her emotions were not hindering the success of using effective communication.

   b is incorrect. The long duration of deafness required a period of adjustment and may have impacted how she performed.

   c is incorrect. Age is a factor that could have impacted on how she performed.

   d is incorrect. Improvements in performance were noted after a course of therapy; therefore, participation in auditory training may have influenced performance.

2. **What change would not alter the course of therapy?**
   a) Brain adaptation.
   b) Rate of progress.
   c) Changes in auditory development.
   d) Device failure.
   e) Use of wireless accessories.
   Answer: e is correct. Auditory therapy sessions provide support with the CI device and any accessory components. Device support would be easily incorporated into a session and would not alter therapy.

   a is incorrect. Brain adaptation is occurring and programming parameters are constantly changing. It is important for the clinician to constantly assess skill level and change targets when appropriate.

   b is incorrect. If the patient makes rapid progress, she would need less frequent training and she may begin a home maintenance sooner. If the patient makes minimal progress, the clinician would need to reevaluate the effectiveness of therapeutic techniques used.

   c is incorrect. Initially, WM had difficulty perceiving low-frequency consonants; she started to have difficulty perceiving high-frequency consonants in the subsequent therapy sessions. She rapidly improved in her ability to identify familiar common phrases and the clinician began to use unfamiliar sentence stimuli.

   d is incorrect. If there is a failure with the device, it is important to make the appropriate referral to her audiologist and surgeon who placed the device. This may cause an abrupt lapse in services.

3. **Based on her performance in the initial evaluation, what would be a typical error observed?**
   a) Detection of final /s/ and /z/ fricatives.
   b) Discrimination of final /b/ and /g/ stops.
   c) Discrimination of final /p/ and /t/ stops.
   d) Detection of vowels in isolation.
   e) Identification of predictable words in quiet.
   Answer: b is correct. It was found that she had difficulty discriminating voiced stop consonants, which include /b/ and /g/ phonemes.

   a is incorrect. In her initial evaluation, WM did not display errors in her ability to detect sounds in words. She had more difficulty with discrimination of sounds in words.

   c is incorrect. She did not display difficulty discriminating high-frequency sounds in her initial evaluation, but this became an issue when retesting after a course of therapy.

   d is incorrect. WM had difficulty discriminating vowels in words, but she detected and accurately identified vowel sounds in isolation.

   e is incorrect. Her performance in quiet was considerably better than her performance in noise. She did have difficulty identifying less predictable words in sentences within the presence of background noise.

66.5 Description of Disorder and Recommended Treatment

WM was diagnosed with a speech and language disorder due to a bilateral, profound, sensorineural hearing loss. Clinical assessments, observations, and subjective reports revealed that her difficulties were affecting her quality of life. It was recommended she receive weekly 45-minute therapy sessions for 3 months. Therapy was conducted through auditory-only modalities and in three conditions: left CI alone, right CI alone, and integration of the two devices. In addition, it was recommended that she spend 30 minutes each night utilizing her newer implant alone. The plans for therapy consisted of the following:

- Device education and support (using devices and wireless accessories and providing support tools specific to the implant company).
  - WM had a CI on the right side for nearly 10 years, so she had knowledge of the parts. She knew how to change and utilize programs and features specific to her device.
- Counseling on the emotional impact hearing loss has as it relates to communication difficulties.
- Training on use of compensatory communication strategies for difficult listening situations.
  - We discussed her level of confidence in her listening abilities. Compensatory strategies offered her support when confronted with poor signal-to-noise ratios, multiple speakers, and speaking from various distances.
  - She began requesting clarification more often and became a more assertive communicator. She was better equipped to advocate for herself in conversations.
  - Anticipation strategies were discussed for specific scenarios.
- Providing direct, functional auditory training.
  - Analytic approach—She identified words in an open-set context and any errors in vowel and consonant sounds were drilled in minimal pair contrasts. Auditory bombardment of high-frequency consonants in syllables and words was used for training.
  - Synthetic approach—Sentence-identification tasks were used for common scenarios, including phrases often heard

at a restaurant, grocery store, and doctor's office. Auditory comprehension was trained through following directions and auditory transfer activities.

- Instructing and providing feedback on the use of prosodic features.
  - She initially demonstrated difficulty with breath support, pitch, resonance, and loudness, but with ongoing treatment and feedback, she began to better monitor these speech skills.
- Training in difficult listening contexts (close vs. distant listening, quiet vs. noisy environment, live vs. recorded speech).
- Encouraging the use of computerized training programs and support applications available.
- Recommending local support groups or online adult CI blogs.
  - WM started her own blog for her emotional support and to assist others with profound hearing loss.

66.6 Outcome

Postimplant audiological testing revealed a marked improvement in speech recognition in the left ear and binaurally at 3 months poststimulation. Results of pre- and postimplant audiological testing are provided in ▶ Fig. 66.1 and ▶ Fig. 66.2.

Her functional speech perception scores on the *AB short word list* improved slightly in all conditions, except performance in

noise, which remained stable. Results of functional speech-perception testing are presented in ▶ Table 66.2.

Subjectively, WM reported increased confidence and comfort with conversations in the context of multiple speakers at gatherings. Noisy restaurants were still difficult for her and she used communication strategies that were discussed and practiced in therapy. She was able to self-monitor her speech and voice quality. When she had difficulty, she effectively used compensatory strategies in addition to taking advantage of her device accessories specifically to support listening in noise. She began employing several strategies to increase perception, including requesting repetition, requesting use of slower speech, requesting the first and/or last word, repeating back what was heard, asking for a paraphrase, asking for a spelling, or requesting key words.

WM continued to utilize an at-home computerized training program, which was created by the CI device manufacturer. She began meeting friends in places she would typically avoid, such as busy restaurants and social gatherings.

66.7 Key Points

- Sequential bilateral implant users present challenges to the user and the clinician.
- Therapeutic techniques will evolve over time dependent on the progress and needs of the patient.

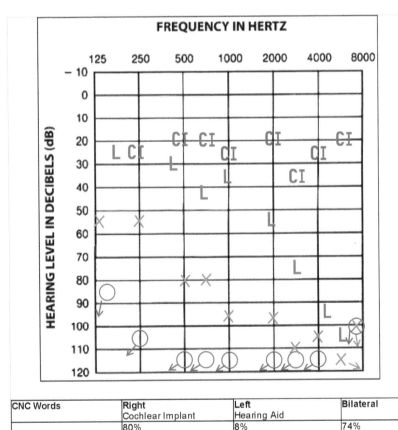

Fig. 66.1 Preimplant audiological testing.

CNC Words	Right Cochlear Implant	Left Hearing Aid	Bilateral
	80%	8%	74%

Az-Bio Sentences (Quiet)	Right Cochlear Implant	Left Hearing Aid	Bilateral
	93%	7%	92%

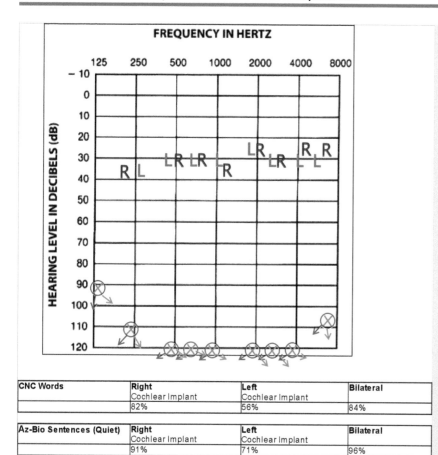

Fig. 66.2 Postimplant audiological testing.

CNC Words	Right Cochlear Implant	Left Cochlear Implant	Bilateral
	82%	56%	84%

Az-Bio Sentences (Quiet)	Right Cochlear Implant	Left Cochlear Implant	Bilateral
	91%	71%	96%

Table 66.2 Results of functional speech perception testing—3 months postactivation of sequential CI

	Bilateral (quiet)	Bilateral (noise)	Left CI	Right CI
Initial consonants	80%	70%	40%	70%
Vowels	100%	80%	100%	100%
Final consonants	90%	60%	70%	70%
Whole words	70%	50%	50%	60%

CI, cochlear implant.

- A multidisciplinary approach to treatment will assure the most optimal performance.
- In addition to direct therapy, a patient can utilize computerized home training to support development of auditory skills.

Suggested Readings

[1] Luterman DM. Counseling Persons with Communication Disorders and Their Families. 5th ed. Austin, TX: Pro-ed; 2008

[2] Tye-Murray N. Foundations of Aural Rehabilitation Children, Adults, and Their Family Members. 3rd ed. Clifton Park, NY: Delmar Cengage Learning; 2009

[3] Adunka OF, Dillon MT, Buchman CA. Auditory outcomes in the adult population. In: Waltzman SB, Roland JT, Eds. Cochlear Implants. 3rd ed. New York, NY: Thieme; 2014:167–181

67 Benign VF Lesions: The Role of Stimulability Testing and Voice Therapy

James Curtis

67.1 Introduction

The impact of inefficient voice use patterns on voice-related symptoms can often be overlooked or underappreciated in the presence of large benign vocal fold lesions. If voice symptoms improve with voice efficiency modifications despite the presence of large benign vocal fold lesions, behavioral therapy may be the only intervention required despite a desire for surgical excision.

67.2 Clinical History

HG was a 56-year-old male businessman with a history of right vocal fold scar and left vocal fold cyst referred for interdisciplinary speech-language pathology (SLP) and laryngology (MD) evaluation. HG reported a 3-year history of voice impairment characterized by increased vocal effort, vocal pain, and vocal fatigue following short periods of continuous voice use (e.g., during business presentations), and a rough, breathy, and inconsistent voice quality. He reported symptom onset may have coincided with a gradual increase in professional voice demands, but denied any specific inciting event. He previously underwent a course of voice therapy in India where he spends 3 to 6 months of every year; this therapy included vocal rest and improved vocal hygiene. HG noted that, at that time, voice rest tended to temporarily relieve his pain, effort, and fatigue symptoms. However, his baseline dysphonia persisted. He was recently seen by an outside physician who recommended surgical intervention for the vocal fold cyst; however, he was not interested in surgery at that time and sought a second opinion regarding intervention.

67.3 Clinical Testing

Clinical assessment of voice included a thorough case history and patient interview, perceptual assessment of voice, rigid laryngostroboscopic evaluation, and stimulability testing.

Perceptual assessment of voice was judged using a 0 (*none*) to 3 (*severe*) GRBAS scale, which revealed moderate overall dysphonia (2/3), moderate roughness (2/3), mild-to-moderate breathiness (1.5/3), and moderate strain (2/3). Perceptual assessment of voice and resonance also revealed a posterior/pharyngeal locus of resonance and reduced phonatory airflow, with intermittent diplophonia during sustained phonation at high pitches. Perceptual assessment of perilaryngeal muscle tension was judged using a subjective 0 (*none*) to 3 (*severe*) scale upon palpation of the perilaryngeal musculature. Findings from palpation revealed moderate bilateral tension in the masseters (2/3), submental region (2/3), suprahyoid/base of tongue region (2/3), thyrohyoid space (2/3; mildly increased with phonation), infrahyoid muscles (2/3), and sternocleidomastoid (2/3). Of note, HG reported moderate tenderness in the thyrohyoid space upon palpation, left greater than right.

Laryngoscopic and stroboscopic findings (▶ Fig. 67.1):
- Supraglottic hyperfunction characterized by lateral compression of the ventricular folds.
- Large, discrete, sessile, broad-based lesion on the left midmembranous vocal fold.
- Mucosal grooving on the medial edge of the right midmembranous vocal fold.
- Vertical phase difference (VPD) and mucosal wave were absent on the right vocal fold at site of grooving, and reduced on the left vocal fold at site of lesion.
- Hourglass phonatory closure pattern at all pitches.

Trial therapy was used to assess HG's awareness of voice use and tension-holding patterns and to assess stimulability for improved reduced perilaryngeal tension and improved voice efficiency. Stimulability was performed indirectly in response to the rigid endoscopic evaluation, and directly during introduction of flow phonation and resonant voice therapy tasks. HG was immediately stimulable for reduced thyrohyoid and suprahyoid tension, reduced vocal strain and roughness, and

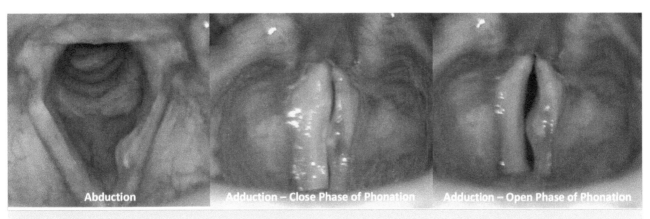

Fig. 67.1 Laryngoscopic and stroboscopic findings on initial evaluation.

improved balance of phonatory airflow and anterior oral resonance. Breathiness was consistent and persisted despite unloading of tension.

67.4 Questions and Answers for the Reader

1. What findings from the patient history and clinical assessment might lead you to believe he may benefit from behavioral intervention?
   a) The presence of abnormal perilaryngeal tension and vocal strain.
   b) The presence of a vocal fold cyst.
   c) The patient report of vocal effort and pain.
   d) a and c.

Answer: d is correct. While voice therapy cannot be guaranteed to improve resolution of benign vocal fold lesions, symptoms related to vocal effort and vocal fatigue can very likely be related to inefficient voice use and tension-holding patterns—both of which are primary targets of behavioral voice therapy. Given that these symptoms are reported by the patient, therapy should be trialed to ameliorate these symptoms, even if surgery is initially or ultimately recommended.

a is partially correct. Perilaryngeal tension and vocal strain are behaviors that can lead to symptoms of vocal effort, pain, and a dysphonic voice quality. Because tension and strain are modifiable behaviors, patients presenting with tension and strain may benefit considerably from voice therapy. Targeting reductions in tension and strain can therefore lessen complaints associated with vocal effort and laryngeal pain and, in some cases, improve smoothness of voice quality in the presence of a lesion (by facilitating consistent phonatory airflow and periodic vibration).

c is partially correct. Vocal effort and pain are likely related to vocal efficiency and laryngeal tension, rather than presence of cyst. As effort and pain are associated with the modifiable behaviors of tension and strain, trial course of behavioral intervention is certainly warranted.

b is incorrect. The presence/absence of a lesion does not dictate whether someone may or may not benefit from therapy. For example, a patient may have a vocal fold cyst and be asymptomatic, and therefore therapy would not be warranted.

2. What findings from the clinical assessment might lead you to believe that the dysphonia is related, at least in part, to voice use patterns, and may benefit from voice therapy?
   a) Audible vocal strain.
   b) Response to stimulability testing.
   c) a and b.

Answer: c is correct. Vocal strain is the result of hyperfunctional glottic valving, which can often result in reduced phonatory airflow and vocal roughness. Responses to stimulability testing revealed that the patient was able to reduce vocal strain and vocal roughness. Therefore, while the dysphonic breathy quality persisted, other parameters of dysphonia were improved with behavioral intervention, further supporting the role for voice therapy for this patient.

a is partially correct. Vocal strain is a function of how someone produces voice, rather than presence of any anatomic abnormalities (e.g., cyst). Vocal strain can reduce the amount and consistency of phonatory airflow, thereby contributing to aperiodicity (roughness) of voice production. Because vocal strain is likely contributing to this patient's dysphonia, and strain is a behavioral target, you may consider that the patient would benefit from voice therapy.

b is partially correct. Given that the patient was stimulable for change, and the change resulted in smoother and more efficient voice quality, he would likely benefit from therapy to target consistent, long-term carryover.

3. What would be your primary goal for voice therapy with this patient?
   a) Improved voice efficiency.
   b) Improved voice quality.
   c) Resolution of vocal fold lesion.

Answer: a is correct. As behavioral therapists, our primary goal should be to improve efficiency of voice production (as able)—ideally to a level that is sustainable for the patient. Typically, in patients with muscle tension dysphonia, this may include reducing perilaryngeal tension at rest and during phonation, and reducing vocal strain to a level that is sustainable for the patient (i.e., where it does not contribute to any perceivable voice changes), while improving balance of easy oral resonance and phonatory airflow.

b is incorrect. Improved voice quality does not always equate to improve voice efficiency and sustainable voice production, and therefore should not be the primary focus of therapy. Individuals with a large vocal fold cyst may achieve "improved voice quality" by straining/pressing over the lesion to achieve a complete phonatory closure pattern to eliminate perceived breathiness. This will likely lead to vocal fatigue, pain, and exacerbation of benign vocal fold lesion.

c is incorrect. If a patient is able to produce an efficient voice in the presence of a lesion, and their symptoms resolve, then the presence/absence of the vocal fold lesion is insignificant.

67.5 Description of Disorder and Recommended Treatment

Impressions from the initial evaluation revealed a diagnosis of left vocal fold cyst, right vocal fold sulcus, and muscle tension dysphonia. Interdisciplinary SLP/MD impressions suggested that the majority of his symptoms were the result of muscle tension dysphonia characterized by reduced phonatory airflow, vocal strain, and perilaryngeal tension. The benign vocal fold lesions likely contributed mainly to the dysphonic breathy quality, the result of incomplete vocal fold closure at site of lesions. Voice therapy was recommended with the goal of improved voice efficiency (i.e., reduced strain, and improved balance of phonatory airflow and easy, anterior oral resonance), and ultimately reduced vocal pain, vocal effort, vocal fatigue, and, to some extent, improved overall voice quality.

Five sessions of voice therapy were completed over the course of 2 months. Specific recommended therapy targets included:

- Education regarding normal laryngeal anatomy and physiology, mechanics of efficient voice production, and current voice use and tension-holding patterns.
- Perilaryngeal massage to reduce, manage, and build awareness of inefficient perilaryngeal tension-holding patterns. Awareness of tension was explored within the context of massage and in conjunction with voicing tasks.
- Voice efficiency tasks as defined by improved balance of airflow, easy oral resonance, and minimal perilaryngeal muscle engagement during phonation. Training involved a brief introduction of stretch-and-flow and semi-occluded vocal tract basic training gestures (e.g., /u/ and /f/-to-/v/ phonation) with near-immediate carryover of concepts and sensations into sentences and conversation.
- Awareness and discrimination tasks aimed to build accuracy in identification between efficient and inefficient voice use by exploring physiologic sensations at the basic training gesture level (e.g., sensation of airflow on fingers during sustained phonation of /f/ and /v/), and by utilizing negative practice to alter between efficient physiologic sensations (e.g., easy, anterior, oral resonance) or inefficient physiologic sensations (e.g., pharyngeal focus resonance).
- Vocal cool downs were recommended to promote tissue remodeling and wound healing. These cool downs were recommended following periods of increased voice use leading to exacerbation of symptoms.

67.6 Outcome

HG completed his scheduled course of voice therapy with near 100% adherence to therapy recommendations, per his report. By the end of therapy, he demonstrated consistent of therapy concepts and efficient voice production during spontaneous conversation with the clinicians, accurately and consistently produced efficient and inefficient voice productions upon cueing, and reported consistent use of efficient voicing at work. He reported awareness that he would intermittently "slip" into inefficient voice use patterns, but was able to quickly modify back into an efficient voice.

Upon his post-therapy follow-up evaluation completed 1 month after the last therapy session and about 3 months after the initial evaluation, HG reported complete resolution of vocal pain, no observable vocal effort, and increased/functional vocal stamina. He also noted that voice quality, while still breathy from time to time, was no longer unstable or unpredictable, and was felt to be consistently smoother and less dysphonic. Perceptual assessment by both the SLP and MD revealed improved voice quality, now with minimal breathiness, intermittent strain and roughness, and minimal thyrohyoid and jaw tension. Laryngoscopic evaluation revealed persistent right vocal fold scar and left vocal fold cyst that was reduced in size compared to initial evaluation (▶ Fig. 67.2). Stroboscopic evaluation revealed improved VPD and mucosal wave and complete closure at all pitches elicited (▶ Fig. 67.2).

The primary goal of voice therapy was intended to entrain efficient voice production to manage patient symptoms, despite the presence of vocal fold lesions. This goal was largely obtained based on patient report and findings at follow-up evaluation. Awareness of voice use patterns allowed empowered HG to identify inefficient patterns, and negative practice throughout the course of therapy provided him with the tools to modify back and forth between efficient and inefficient voice use. Although the primary goal of therapy was not lesion resolution, dramatic reduction in the size of the left vocal fold cyst was observed. HG immediately achieved smooth and efficient voice in the presence of vocal fold scar and large left vocal fold cyst at initial presentation. However, reduction in lesion size allowed for more flexibility with regard to efficient voice production.

67.7 Key Points

- Large benign lesions may not be the primary contributing factor to voice impairment.
- A thorough clinical history, patient interview, and stimulability testing during the initial evaluation are critical to identify the contributions of anatomic and physiologic findings underlying patient symptoms.
- Clinicians should not underestimate the contribution of muscle tension and inefficient voice use patterns in patient symptoms, particularly in the presence of large benign vocal fold lesions. Symptoms may be well managed with voice

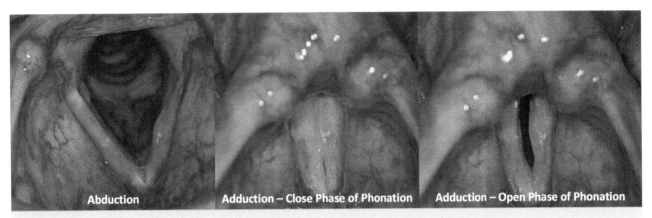

Abduction   **Adduction – Close Phase of Phonation**   **Adduction – Open Phase of Phonation**

Fig. 67.2 Laryngoscopic and stroboscopic findings after completion of voice therapy.

therapy alone if stimulability testing indicates potential for a functionally efficient voice, regardless of lesion management.

Suggested Readings

[1] Verdolini Abbott K, Li NYK, Branski RC, et al. Vocal exercise may attenuate acute vocal fold inflammation. J Voice. 2012; 26(6):814.e1–814.e13

[2] Gartner-Schmidt J, Gherson S, Hapner ER, et al. The development of conversation training therapy: a concept paper. J Voice. 2016; 30(5):563–573

[3] Gillespie AI, Gartner-Schmidt J. Immediate effect of stimulability assessment on acoustic, aerodynamic, and patient-perceptual measures of voice. J Voice. 2016; 30(4):507.e9–507.e14

68 Dystussia and Dysphagia in Parkinson's Disease

Michelle S. Troche, Jordanna M. Sevitz, and Alease M. Holden

68.1 Introduction

Aspiration pneumonia is the leading cause of death in Parkinson's disease (PD) and much of this pulmonary sequelae can likely be attributed to the concomitant presence of swallowing (dysphagia) and cough (dystussia) disturbances, which are often present in PD.[1-4] This case highlights the need to evaluate and manage behaviors across the continuum of airway protection (from cough to swallowing) for improved long-term health outcomes.

68.2 Clinical History and Description

GB was a 69-year-old man who presented with Hoehn and Yahr stage III PD with symptom onset 8 years prior. His medical history was also significant for right unilateral subthalamic nucleus (STN) deep brain stimulation (DBS) surgery followed by left globus pallidus interna (GPi) DBS surgery 3 years later. Of note, DBS has evolved as the management option of choice for persons with PD. The two subcortical structures most commonly targeted during surgery for the treatment of PD are the STN and GPi. Although STN and GPi DBS are generally considered safe and effective for the treatment of people with PD, less is known about the impact of DBS on airway protection. Recent work suggests that STN DBS may result in adverse effects to swallowing function, which are not observed with GPi DBS.[5,6]

GB was referred to our outpatient clinic due to a progressive swallowing disturbance adversely affecting oral intake and quality of life. GB and his wife reported that over the past year, he developed significant coughing with meals, particularly when drinking liquids. He also reported that it was taking him much longer to eat. His wife also noticed that he was drooling more often and coughing throughout the day even in the absence of food or liquid. They also reported marked speech difficulties. GB's wife was particularly worried about his reduced loudness in conversation. GB and his wife reported that his speech function worsened with DBS, but were most concerned about his swallowing dysfunction. Prior to being seen in our clinic, GB had undergone several swallowing evaluations and subsequent treatment at other facilities. He reported that his swallowing therapy consisted of oral motor exercises, the Shaker exercise, and effortful swallow. Additionally, a neurologist recommended he employ a chin tuck when drinking thin liquids. GB had no history of aspiration pneumonia or recent weight loss. He was quite active, participating in weekly exercise classes, cognitive therapy, and a PD support group. He and his wife were very motivated to address these swallowing concerns, but were adamantly opposed to any form of enteral feeding.

68.3 Clinical Testing

Videofluoroscopic evaluation of swallowing (VFES; ▶ Video 68.1) was performed. This examination revealed aspiration of sequential thin liquid boluses and consistent penetration to the level of the vocal folds with sequential presentation of nectar-thick liquids. GB did not cough in response to the aspiration and/or penetration. GB coughed when cued, but the cough was ineffective in clearing the aspirate/penetrant material from the airway. His swallowing was also characterized by reduced extent and duration of pharyngoesophageal segment opening, moderate pharyngeal residue, pooling in the valleculae with pudding and solid boluses, and reduced pharyngeal contraction. Oral transit time was increased, especially for solid and pudding boluses. A chin tuck was trialed with thin liquids, given that it had been recommended by a prior neurologist; however, persistent aspiration was noted even with the chin tuck.

Voluntary and reflex cough testing was conducted to comprehensively assess airway protection in this patient. Voluntary cough airflow dynamics were measured via spirometry during three key phases of the cough: inspiratory phase, compression phase, and expiratory phase (▶ Fig. 68.1). GB was cued to "cough like something went down the wrong pipe" into a facemask to assess the effectiveness of his voluntary cough. Various measures of cough effectiveness were made from the airflow data. Previous data suggested a predictive relationship between voluntary cough airflow and penetration/aspiration in neurodegenerative populations. GB's peak expiratory flow rate (PEFR) was reduced, his compression phase duration was prolonged, and his cough volume acceleration (CVA) was markedly reduced (▶ Fig. 68.2). Reflex cough testing was also conducted. GB was instructed to breathe into a handheld device containing nebulized distilled

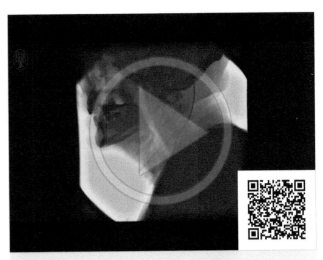

Video 68.1 Videofluoroscopic evaluation of swallowing

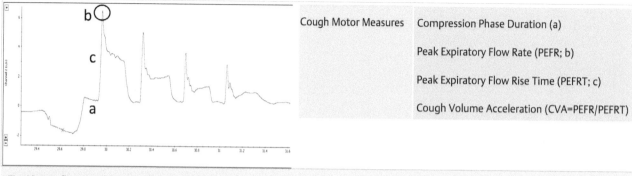

Fig. 68.1 Airflow signal from a normal sequential cough

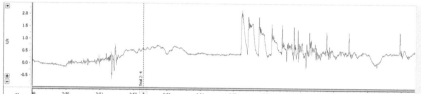

Fig. 68.2 Airflow signal from a sequential cough produced by GB

water (FOG) and cough if necessary.[7] He did not cough in response to the FOG and reported *no urge* to cough (on a modified Borg-scale where 0 indicates no urge and 10 indicates a *very severe urge*). Additionally, maximum expiratory (MEP) and maximum inspiratory (MIP) pressures were evaluated to determine the potential role of decreased respiratory muscle force generation on cough outcomes. GB's average MEP was 77 cm H_2O and his average MIP was 60 cm H_2O.

68.4 Discussion Questions

1. Based on the outcomes of the clinical testing, why is it important to address both the swallowing and cough deficits in this patient?
2. What are two rehabilitation approaches you would try with this patient and why? Have studies identified the efficacy of these approaches?
3. What would you counsel this patient regarding his prognosis, the benefit of rehabilitation, and the importance of home maintenance?

68.5 Questions and Answers for the Reader

1. When analyzing cough airflow in PD, the presence of atussia (i.e., absent cough) and/or dystussia (i.e., disordered cough) may be indicated by (choose all that apply):
   a) Decreased PEFR.
   b) Increased PEFR.
   c) Decreased CVA.
   d) Increased CVA.
   Answer: a is correct. Patients with PD often demonstrate reduced PEFR. When this is the case, it indicates decreased shearing forces that are necessary for forceful ejection of endogenous material from the lower airways. Thus, reduced PEFR is an indication of dystussia in this population.

c is correct. Patients with PD often demonstrate reduced CVA. When this is the case, it indicates decreased shearing forces that are necessary for forceful ejection of endogenous material from the lower airways. Thus, reduced CVA is an indication of dystussia in this population.

b is incorrect. Patients with PD often demonstrate decreased PEFR, indicating the presence of dystussia.

d is incorrect. Patients with PD often demonstrate decreased CVA, indicating the presence of dystussia.

2. Which of the following are swallowing-specific rehabilitation approaches that may be indicated for a patient with pervasive airway-protection deficits (choose all that apply)?
   a) Expiratory muscle strength training (EMST).
   b) The Mendelsohn maneuver.
   c) The Masako maneuver.
   Answer: b is correct. The Mendelsohn maneuver consists of voluntarily manipulating laryngeal elevation during the task of swallowing.

a is incorrect. EMST targets increased force generation of the submental and respiratory muscles, but it does not do this during the task of swallowing.

c is incorrect. The Masako maneuver involves swallowing forcefully while placing one's tongue in between one's teeth. This maneuver targets reduced base of tongue and pharyngeal force generation, which may subsequently reduce residue in the pharyngeal cavity, but does not primarily and specifically target improved airway protection.

3. During a VFES, your patient demonstrates several instances of silent aspiration (aspiration without a cough response). When asked to rate his urge to cough on a scale of 0 to 10, your patient responds "8." When asked to explain his reasoning for not coughing given his heightened perception, your patient states, "I always feel a strong tickle when I drink liquids." Is the patient's high urge to cough when aspirating a positive or negative prognostic indicator?
   a) Positive.
   b) Negative.

Answer: a is correct. This patient demonstrates an awareness of the material in the airway. Therefore, this can be utilized as a therapeutic target wherein the patient is taught to upregulate his reflex cough in the presence of the heightened urge or "tickle."

68.6 Description of Disorder and Recommended Treatment

Swallowing and cough share neural substrates and fall on a continuum of airway protective behaviors.[8] Swallowing serves to prevent material from entering the airway, while cough is essential for efficient ejection of material that has errantly entered the airway. PD is often associated with pervasive and progressive disorders of airway protection, presenting with swallowing, voluntary, and reflex cough deficits, consistent with GB's presentation. GB presented with a moderate-to-severe sensorimotor dysphagia characterized by changes throughout the swallowing mechanism. He also presented with deficits of both reflex and voluntary cough. Most concerning for swallowing safety was his consistent aspiration of thin liquids, reduced sensation of this material (evidenced by no urge to cough and no cough response to aspirate material), and ineffective reflex cough. Cough evaluation revealed decreased PEFR and CVA; both measures indicate decreased shearing forces necessary for clearing the lower airways of endogenous material. Thickening liquids to nectar and chin tuck were only minimally effective in reducing airway compromise and often were associated with increased pharyngeal residue.

A multifaceted treatment approach to management was initiated, addressing both swallowing and cough disorders for maximum benefit to overall airway protection. The management plan included EMST for improved respiratory and submental muscle force generation to support cough and swallowing, swallowing-specific exercises including the effortful swallow, Masako (tongue hold) and Mendelsohn maneuvers, and a home training program.[9],[10] During the initial session, it became clear that GB would not be able to complete the Mendelsohn maneuver, given the high cognitive demand, which is common when treating patients with neurological conditions. Therefore, this treatment approach was eliminated from the treatment plan. The effortful swallow was paired with electromyography to provide biofeedback. Finally, GB's EMST device was set to 58 cm H_2O 75% of his MEP. GB was instructed to complete 25 breaths, 5 days a week.

GB was seen weekly for treatment over 6 weeks. During that time, he also completed a home program consisting of EMST, repetitions of effortful swallowing and Masako maneuvers, and voluntary coughs through a peak-flow meter to target increased cough effectiveness.[11] The peak flow device provided a visual readout of PEFR, allowing GB to monitor his cough airflow and attempt to increase it with practice.

68.7 Outcome

Following the 6 weeks of treatment, GB returned for swallowing evaluation. His VFES revealed improved swallowing safety with no aspiration of nectar thick liquids and reduced aspiration of single sips of thin liquids. However, he still demonstrated aspiration of sequential thin liquid presentations. Cough effectiveness also improved. Overall, GB responded positively to treatment; however, he did not demonstrate complete resolution of airway protective symptoms, which is common in PD and other degenerative conditions. Success in therapy is most often *not* complete resolution of symptoms, but some improvement in symptoms and slowing down of the trajectory of airway protective degeneration. Detraining after the removal of treatment or exercise is seen in all people, but is more rapid in degenerative conditions and in patients with more severe baseline functioning.[12] Maintenance programs are a necessary component of the management plan for persons with degenerative disease.

GB was provided with a rigorous home training program. It was recommended that he return for consistent follow-up and reevaluation. This level of follow-up is especially important when patients like GB are not interested in enteral feeding. In those cases, close follow-up should focus on determining the least restrictive diet, modifying exercise-based training, and providing the most effective compensations with special attention to oral hygiene and physical activity. A multifaceted and holistic approach to management helps prevent pulmonary sequelae while also balancing a positive quality of life.

68.8 Key Points

- Swallowing and cough are on a continuum of airway protective behaviors; swallowing serves to protect the airway from endogenous material and cough serves to eject material that has errantly entered the airway. Both swallowing and cough have been found to be disordered in PD and likely contribute to aspiration pneumonia being a leading cause of death in this population.
- Quantitative measures of cough effectiveness should form a part of our evaluation of airway protection in patients with PD, therefore allowing for the more specific identification of therapeutic targets.
- Management of swallowing dysfunction in PD should be accompanied by the targeting of reflex cough dysfunction as well. This can be achieved through both strength training and skill-based exercises.
- Owing to the degenerative nature of PD, intensive home practice, maintenance programs, and consistent follow-up are essential for long-term airway protective health and quality of life.

Suggested Readings

[1] Troche MS, Brandimore AE, Okun MS, Davenport PW, Hegland KW. Decreased cough sensitivity and aspiration in Parkinson disease. Chest. 2014; 146(5):1294–1299

[2] Troche MS, Brandimore AE, Foote KD, et al. Swallowing outcomes following unilateral STN vs. GPi surgery: a retrospective analysis. Dysphagia. 2014; 29 (4):425–431

[3] Troche MS, Brandimore AE, Godoy J, Hegland KW. A framework for understanding shared substrates of airway protection. J Appl Oral Sci. 2014; 22(4): 251–260

[4] Troche MS, Okun MS, Rosenbek JC, et al. Aspiration and swallowing in Parkinson disease and rehabilitation with EMST: a randomized trial. Neurology. 2010; 75(21):1912–1919

References

[1] Hegland KW, Okun MS, Troche MS. Sequential voluntary cough and aspiration or aspiration risk in Parkinson's disease. Lung. 2014; 192(4):601–608

[2] Troche MS, Brandimore AE, Okun MS, Davenport PW, Hegland KW. Decreased cough sensitivity and aspiration in Parkinson disease. Chest. 2014; 146(5):1294–1299

[3] Pitts T, Bolser D, Rosenbek J, Troche M, Sapienza C. Voluntary cough production and swallow dysfunction in Parkinson's disease. Dysphagia. 2008; 23(3): 297–301

[4] Pitts T, Troche M, Mann G, Rosenbek J, Okun MS, Sapienza C. Using voluntary cough to detect penetration and aspiration during oropharyngeal swallowing in patients with Parkinson disease. Chest. 2010; 138(6):1426–1431

[5] Troche MS, Brandimore AE, Foote KD, et al. Swallowing outcomes following unilateral STN vs. GPi surgery: a retrospective analysis. Dysphagia. 2014; 29 (4):425–431

[6] Troche MS, Brandimore AE, Foote KD, Okun MS. Swallowing and deep brain stimulation in Parkinson's disease: a systematic review. Parkinsonism Relat Disord. 2013; 19(9):783–788

[7] Hegland KW, Troche MS, Brandimore A, Okun MS, Davenport PW. Comparison of two methods for inducing reflex cough in patients with Parkinson's disease, with and without dysphagia. Dysphagia. 2016; 31(1):66–73

[8] Troche MS, Brandimore AE, Godoy J, Hegland KW. A framework for understanding shared substrates of airway protection. J Appl Oral Sci. 2014; 22(4): 251–260

[9] Troche MS, Okun MS, Rosenbek JC, et al. Aspiration and swallowing in Parkinson disease and rehabilitation with EMST: a randomized trial. Neurology. 2010; 75(21):1912–1919

[10] Wheeler KM, Chiara T, Sapienza CM. Surface electromyographic activity of the submental muscles during swallow and expiratory pressure threshold training tasks. Dysphagia. 2007; 22(2):108–116

[11] Silverman EP, Carnaby-Mann G, Pitts T, Davenport P, Okun MS, Sapienza C. Concordance and discriminatory power of cough measurement devices for individuals with Parkinson disease. Chest. 2014; 145(5):1089–1096

[12] Troche MS, Rosenbek JC, Okun MS, Sapienza CM. Detraining outcomes with expiratory muscle strength training in Parkinson disease. J Rehabil Res Dev. 2014; 51(2):305–310

69 Injury Prevention for a Touring Professional Singer with Phonotrauma

Aaron Ziegler

69.1 Introduction

Professional singers who incur vocal injury on tour have a complex set of risk factors and injury mechanisms, making them unique in their voice rehabilitation needs. Guided by an injury-prevention framework, this case describes the role of the speech-language pathologsit (SLP; and laryngology, obliquely) in managing a touring female singer with mild-to-moderate dysphonia secondary to vocal fold nodules.

69.2 Clinical History and Description

JD was a 23-year-old female seen for an 8-week history of worsening hoarseness while performing on tour as a professional second soprano in a 3-hour musical. As lead actress, her performance demands included "belt-style" singing frequently paired with intense choreography and loud, animated character speaking. At initial evaluation, JD reported increased difficulty with singing despite completing daily vocal warm-ups. Specific singing complaints included poor vocal endurance, raspy and strained voice quality, reduced vocal power, pitch breaks, and difficulty with register transitions. She also perceived increased vocal effort in singing certain pitches in her upper range after five weekend performances. These vocal issues improved somewhat with voice rest. She denied a history of voice problems with previous roles or performance opportunities, and had no prior history of voice therapy.

Her vocal hygiene profile was significant for risk factors that could compromise vocal fold tissue health. Regarding superficial dehydration, she reported exposure to desiccated air in hotels, planes, and performance spaces as well as intense choreographic demands that likely require oral, nonhumidified breathing. The performance requirements were intense and perspiration could potentially contribute to systemic dehydration. Nonphonatory inflammation might be an issue, given her history of acid reflux events associated with late night eating and alcohol consumption. She reported modest benefit from prescription medication for her gastroesophageal reflux disease (GERD) with ongoing intermittent heartburn. Finally, JD experienced repeated acute phonotraumatic (RAP) events with substantial social and professional voice use. The term "phonotrauma" is preferred over other expressions such as vocal abuse and misuse related to the negative connotations associated with these terms.[1] Protective factors in her profile included lifetime nonsmoker, limited caffeine intake, graduate of a musical theater training program, and use of amplification and floor monitors in the current production.

69.3 Clinical Testing

JD engaged in a comprehensive voice evaluation[2] with SLP and laryngology. Her speaking voice quality was rated using the Consensus Auditory-Perceptual Evaluation of Voice (CAPE-V)[3,4] and revealed overall mild-to-moderate dysphonia characterized by mild-to-moderate vocal strain, mild roughness, and intermittent glottal fry at phrase boundaries. JD's speaking pitch in conversation was somewhat low for her age and gender; loudness was slightly increased. Her singing voice was characterized by a mild-to-moderate pressed, nasal vocal quality that worsened when belting. Her breathing pattern was predominantly low abdominal in conversation, and in singing she appeared to overdrive her respiratory system. Baseline acoustic data were collected and those data confirmed the auditory-perceptual findings (▶ Table 69.1). Abnormal acoustic findings included reduced maximum phonation time, decreased fundamental frequency and increased vocal intensity in connected speech, and elevated cycle-to-cycle variability in amplitude (i.e., shimmer). Phonatory frequency range was mildly restricted in the high end, and attempts to access her upper range required increased vocal strain. Her voice changes were associated with a moderate handicap of the speaking and singing voice, as determined by the Voice Handicap Index-10 (VHI-10) and Singing VHI-10, respectively.[5,6]

Laryngeal imaging was performed using a flexible distal chip laryngoscope with stroboscopy to evaluate structural and functional deficits of the larynx. Range of motion for vocal fold abduction and adduction was within normal limits bilaterally during inspiration and phonation, respectively. Vocal fold elongation and contraction during ascending and descending pitch glides were normal. Vocal fold appearance suggested recurrent acute injury (i.e., phonotrauma) as evidenced by mild-to-moderate erythema (redness) and small, bilateral, pliable mid-membranous vocal fold swellings that were coated with mucous. With both speaking and singing voice, phonatory physiology was characterized by increased supraglottic activity with mild-to-moderate lateral squeezing of the false vocal folds that was reduced with trial therapy of flow phonation and oral–nasal resonance balancing. During stroboscopy, glottic closure was complete with sustained phonation; however, hourglass deformity was present when unloading laryngeal muscle tension during trial voice therapy. The propagating mucosal wave was minimally reduced bilaterally over the lesions, and symmetry in vibratory phase and amplitude was observed.

Table 69.1 Clinical findings from JD's baseline comprehensive voice evaluation and her 1-year follow-up

Measure	Baseline	1-year follow-up	Pre–Post Δ	Normative data[33] mean (range)
Maximum phonation time (MPT)[a]	12 s	13 s	8.3%	20.9 (11.8–32.0 s)
Fundamental frequency (F_0) [a]				
• Vowel /a/ (pitch)	225 Hz (A_3)	222 Hz (A_3)	−1.3%	
• Reading (*Rainbow Passage*)[34]	230 ± 50.4 Hz	238 ± 47.8 Hz	3.5%	224.3 Hz (192–275 Hz)
• Monologue (pitch)	208 ± 40.3 Hz (G_3)	222 ± 38.6 Hz (A_3)	6.7%	210.3 Hz (179–256 Hz)
Phonatory frequency range[a]				
• Minimum F_0 (pitch)	145 Hz (D_3)	156 Hz (D_3)	6.2%	140.2 Hz (98–196 Hz)
• Maximum F_0 (pitch)	960 Hz (B_5)	1,071 Hz (C_6)	11.6%	1,121.5 Hz (587–2,093 Hz)
• Total F_0 range (pitch range) semitones (ST)	815 Hz (D_3–B_5) 32.7 ST	915 Hz (D_3–C_6) 33.4 ST	12.2% 2.1%	981.3 Hz 37.0 ST
Vocal intensity (SPL)[a]				
• Vowel (/a/)	78 dB	81 dB	3.8%	75.0 ± 4.5 dB SPL
• Reading (*Rainbow Passage*[34])	80 ± 4.4 dB	79 ± 4.7 dB	−1.25%	68.2 ± 2.51 dB SPL
• Monologue	78 ± 4.2 dB	79 ± 4.7 dB	1.3%	
Perturbation (/a/; type 1 signal)[b]				
• Jitter	0.578%	0.313%	(−45.8%)	0.633 ± 0.351%
• Shimmer	0.316 dB	0.282 dB	(-10.7%)	0.176 ± 0.220 dB
• Noise-to-harmonic ratio	0.108	0.098	(−9.2%)	0.112 ± 0.009
CAPE-V[3,4]	24 (out of 100)	6	(−75.0%)	Abnormal > 10
VHI-10[5]	22 (out of 40)	3	(−86.4%)	2.83 ± 3.9; abnormal > 11
SVHI-10[6]	21 (out of 40)	7	(−66.7%)	8.4 ± 0.5; abnormal > 9
Vocal fold appearance				

CAPE-V, Consensus Auditory-Perceptual Evaluation of Voice; VHI-10, Voice Handicap Index-10; SVHI-10, Singing Voice Handicap Index-10.

[a]Normative data for MPT, F_0, total F_0 range, and vocal intensity data only.

[b]Multidimensional Voice Profile (MDVP), Computerized Speech Lab (CSL) Normative Database (Pentax Medical, Montvale, NJ).

Note: To collect a monologue, the patient spoke for 1 minute about where she grew up.

A significant challenge in the management of hoarseness/dysphonia in touring singers is identifying the causes (i.e., risk factors and injury mechanisms) for the onset and maintenance of the current voice problem. Both performer-related and environmental factors have been shown to increase the risk of injury in Broadway and West End musical theater performers.[7,8] A commonly employed injury-prevention framework known as the Haddon matrix is a useful tool to delineate pertinent risk factors and causal mechanisms that contribute to injury.[9,10] The Haddon matrix assumes that injury is due to an interaction among three factors: host, agent of injury, and environment. In this view of injury, the host is an individual who sustains injury and the agent of injury is some form of energy transfer (i.e., mechanical, thermal, electrical, ionizing radiation, or chemical). Mechanisms responsible for energy transfer include inanimate objects such as guns, knives (i.e., vehicle), or humans (i.e., vector). The environment is the context that leads to injury, which consists of the physical surroundings and the sociocultural environment. The Haddon matrix also distinguishes among temporal phases of the injury event to appreciate the time sequence of an injury (i.e., pre-event, event, and post-event). To illustrate the range of risk factors and injury mechanisms involved in JD's vocal injury genesis, her historical information and clinical testing results are summarized in ► Table 69.2.

Table 69.2 Haddon matrix[9,10] applied to the vocal injury of a touring singer

	Host (performer at risk of injury)	Agent of vocal injury (bio-mechanical and chemical energy transfer)	Physical environment (setting characteristics)	Sociocultural environment (norms/practices)
Pre-vocal injury (period just before tour)	(-) Lacked vocal cool down routine	(-) Large nonessential voice use (-) High professional voice use demands with rehearsal	(-) Resided in loud urban environment	(-) Felt social and economic pressures to get hired as singer
Vocal injury (period on tour before evaluation)	(-) Surface dehydration from oral inhalation of dry air with dancing and exposure to dry air in planes and hotels (-) Systemic dehydration from sweating and exhaling water vapor with dancing, and insufficient water intake given physical demands (-) Acid reflux from agitation of stomach with singing and dancing, late night eating, and nightly alcohol consumption (- - -) Lacked vocal cool down routine	(-) Chemical energy transfer from acid reflux exposure (- -) Large nonessential voice use (- - -) Large performing voice use (- -) Biomechanical energy transfer with inefficient vocal technique in loud voice and belt voice (-) Biomechanical energy transfer with use of high modal register with character voice production	(- -) Performed in large spaces with poor acoustics (-) Exposure to stage fog chemicals (-) Wore costuming that restricted breathing for speaking and singing	(- -) Production contract issues included high number of weekly performances, two performances on same day, same-day practice and performance (- -) Inadequate rest time with performances and social activities
Post–vocal injury (period after evaluation)	(-) Anxiety and stress over vocal condition, increasing laryngeal muscle tension	(-) High, but reduced, vocal demands with the implementation of vocal dose reduction strategies (-) Ongoing complaints of excess throat mucous and heartburn	(- -) Upcoming performances in less than ideal venues	(- -) Bound by contract terms (- -) Desire to be resilient singer (-) Hired as cruise ship singer after tour and did not complete full course of voice therapy

Notes: The Haddon Matrix can be used to define risk factors as in this case report, but it also can be used to help identify intervention strategies. Ratings to indicate the relative contribution of risk factors and injury mechanisms to her vocal injury: -, low; - -, moderate; - - -, high.

Analysis using the Haddon matrix indicated a new onset of speaking and singing voice problems in the setting of (1) vocally unhealthy lifestyle choices (i.e., host factor), (2) large amounts of biomechanical energy transfer with high vocal demands and possible chemical energy transfer with a diagnosis of GERD (i.e., agents of injury), and (3) expansive performance spaces with poor acoustics, exposure to desiccated air in performance venues, lodging, and airplanes (i.e., physical environmental factors), and increased performance pressures associated with the rules, policies, and norms around the performance schedule, contract, and production (i.e., sociocultural environmental factors). Focusing on the agent of injury, clinical testing identified inefficiency of the speaking and singing voice that most likely increased vocal fold impact stress and resulted in large biomechanical energy transfer to the vocal fold mucosa as the vocal folds collide during voicing. Specifically, JD underutilized abdominal breathing at spoken phrase boundaries, demonstrated compensatory laryngeal muscle tension with speaking, and exhibited intermittent laryngeal–pharyngeal vocal focus during conversation. Inefficiencies in the belt singing voice were unnecessarily high exhalatory drive, increased laryngeal and lingual muscle tension, and overly nasal resonance. In terms of the timing of JD's current vocal injury, the onset most likely occurred during a timeframe characterized by increased biomechanical energy transfer given the phonotraumatic nature of her lesions. Thus, temporal analysis using the Haddon matrix suggests the vocal injury was sustained over a 2-month period of touring at which time she experienced an accumulation of phonotraumatic and acid reflux events that reached a critical threshold, produced negative vocal fold tissue changes, and compromised vocal function. As demonstrated, the Haddon matrix is a useful approach for evaluating the relative contribution to vocal injury of different host, agent of injury, and environmental attributes, as well as temporal factors.

69.4 Questions and Answers for the Reader

1. A 23-year-old singer presents with a gradual onset of an 8-week history of hoarseness (dysphonia) that has worsened in severity while on tour in a musical. Given JD's history and clinical testing results, what are possible contributing factors to the onset and maintenance of her voice problem?

   a) JD's voice problem is likely due to increased muscle tension from psychological stress associated with production and tour demands. Given her formal singing voice training, it is unlikely her speaking and singing voice technique is a factor in the development of her vocal injury.

   b) She did not have risk factors in her profile that would impact vocal fold tissue health by causing dehydration or nonphonatory inflammation. Her voice problem can be attributed to inefficient speaking and singing voice technique alone.

c) Her voice problem is likely due to her diagnosis of GERD that compromises vocal fold tissue health with exposure to acidic gastric contents.

d) Her voice problem appears related to vocal fold dehydration, nonphonatory inflammation from acid reflux, and phonotrauma related to large nonessential voice use and high-impact stress with belting and loud, animated character voice use.

Answer: d is correct. JD's vocal injury appears related to multiple risk factors and injury mechanisms. Poor vocal fold tissue health increases a person's susceptibility to vocal injury and high vocal fold impact stress in speaking and singing is the presumed cause of phonotraumatic lesions such as vocal fold nodules.

a is incorrect. Although psychological stress may increase laryngeal, pharyngeal, and lingual muscle tension with speaking and singing, JD's profile indicates that other factors were most likely at play in the genesis of her vocal injury. Furthermore, singers can exhibit inefficient voice technique despite formal voice training. Speaking voice technique is sometimes a major factor in voice problems arising in singers.

b is incorrect. Although the cause of vocal fold nodules is phonotrauma associated with high vocal fold impact stress, JD's voice care prior to her evaluation also involved several risk factors known to impact vocal fold tissue health. Vocal fold dehydration and nonphonatory inflammation from acid reflux exposure increase the risk of vocal injury.

c is incorrect. Despite possible vocal fold inflammation with acid reflux exposure, high vocal fold impact stress is the cause of phonotraumatic lesions. Furthermore, GERD is a diagnosis that is often overdiagnosed because of overlapping symptoms between acid reflux and voice problems. The feeling of excess throat mucous could be caused, in part, by phonotrauma.

2. JD reports that she had no prior voice problems before the onset of her current hoarseness (dysphonia). She describes vocal symptoms such as poor vocal endurance, raspy and strained vocal quality, pitch breaks, difficulty with register transitions, and an inability to produce certain pitches in her upper range. Considering JD's history and symptoms, the most likely finding on laryngeal imaging would be:

a) No structural or physiological changes of the larynx. JD is malingering in hopes of ending her tour contract and leaving the production before the tour ends.

b) A structural change of her vocal fold mucosa consistent with RAP events caused by high vocal fold impact stress with belt singing and loud, animated character voice demands.

c) A physiologic change in which she demonstrates primary muscle tension dysphonia in the absence of any structural deficits of the vocal folds. Essentially, she exhibits poor phonatory "form" with voice production as her only issue.

d) A vocal fold motion impairment in which one of the vocal folds is fixed in a far lateral abducted position, creating a large phonatory gap between the vocal folds.

Answer: b is correct. High-impact stress in the context of loud, animated character voices combined with belt singing is the assumed cause of her vocal fold nodules. With RAP

events, the vocal folds demonstrate structural changes that interfere with the vibratory properties of the vocal folds and lead to abnormal voice production. Increased mass of the vocal folds, impaired phonatory closure, and elevated cycle-to-cycle variability in vocal fold vibration from the presence of phonotraumatic lesions can lead to the symptoms described by JD.

a is incorrect. JD did not appear to have a reason to lie about her vocal issues nor did she indicate secondary gain. Furthermore, JD expressed motivation to address her vocal injury and hopes of a Broadway career.

c is incorrect. Although JD demonstrated increased supraglottic activity with speaking and singing, she also demonstrated structural changes of the vocal folds. In fact, her laryngeal hyperfunction is likely to compensate for impaired vocal fold closure with bilateral vocal fold nodules. As a result of glottal incompetence, minimum and average phonatory airflow increases and the voice sounds breathy.

d is incorrect. The onset of vocal fold motion impairment is typically sudden, which does not correspond to JD's description of a gradual onset. Furthermore, the glottal incompetence that results from this motion impairment is usually characterized by an extremely breathy voice quality and reduced loudness, neither of which was described by JD or observed by the SLP.

3. The laryngologist and SLP who evaluated JD recommended a course of voice therapy to rehabilitate JD's vocal injury. However, JD is unable to attend more than one voice therapy session during the current production stopover because of the short timeframe she is in town for the tour. Considering an injury-prevention framework, what are appropriate recommendations/countermeasures that are reasonable to consider for stabilizing the vocal injury of a patient who is on tour?

a) JD should abstain from performing for the remainder of the tour to eliminate the potential hazard associated with the production's vocal demands.

b) JD should develop and implement a personalized voice-care program to optimize vocal fold tissue health and improve vocal fold vibratory behavior. It is not necessary for JD to enroll in voice therapy to change her vocal technique.

c) The SLP should counsel JD to consider a different career given that her vocal fold tissue does not appear to tolerate high vocal demands.

d) The SLP and JD should collaborate to create a realistic treatment plan that includes a personalized voice-care program to implement during the remainder of the tour as well as a course of voice therapy to be completed at the end of the tour.

Answer: d is correct. For patients with phonotraumatic lesions, vocal fold tissue health is important to address to promote healthy vocal fold tissue that vibrates more easily. Furthermore, vocal fold wound healing is accelerated by the use of a semioccluded vocal tract with Lessac-Madsen resonant voice therapy (LMRVT) humming due to vocal fold tissue mobilization that is characterized by large amplitude oscillations.[11]

a is incorrect. Voice rest will only temporarily eliminate the hazard of voice production. However, the vocal fold pathology will likely return or worsen once JD begins to vocalize again if she has not modified her vocal technique.

b is incorrect. Although vocal fold tissue health is critical for optimal vocal function, addressing lifestyle factors alone has not been shown to completely resolve dysphonia in most cases. Because some vocal behaviors are phonotraumatic, JD must also change her vocal technique to manage lesions that manifest from high vocal fold impact stress.

c is incorrect. Genetics may be a factor in the development of vocal fold nodules in some individuals, suggesting that certain singers may be more susceptible to vocal fold injury than others. However, JD denied a history of voice problems with other vocally demanding roles, indicating that the patient's biological makeup was not likely a factor.

69.5 Description of Disorder and Recommended Treatment

The laryngologist diagnosed JD with mild-to-moderate dysphonia secondary to bilateral mid-membranous thickening, suggestive of vocal fold nodules and mild-to-moderate compensatory laryngeal hyperfunction. The vocal fold nodules most likely represent a new vocal fold pathology given her lack of voice problems prior to the tour, and the softness and pliability of the lesions suggest a nascent pathological process. Vocal fold nodules are symmetric phonotraumatic lesions that form from deposition of fibronectin into the mucosa of the vocal folds. With such lesions, the agent of vocal injury is presumed to be biomechanical energy transfer to the vocal fold tissue at intolerable levels during vibration. Specifically, tissue damage occurs from high levels of impact stress as the vocal folds collide repeatedly at midline during voicing.[12] Traditionally, certain vocal behaviors such as a loud, pressed voice at high pitch have been thought to cause benign phonotraumatic lesions like vocal fold nodules.[13,14]

JD appeared stimulable for improved phonatory efficiency with voice therapy techniques that focused on coordination of breathing and voicing in speaking and singing and improved balance of oral–nasal resonance in singing.[15] Thus, she was deemed a good candidate for improvement with voice therapy and referred to an SLP who has a singing voice background. Behavioral voice therapy is an efficacious treatment for vocal fold nodules, and generally involves the acquisition of new voice use patterns.[16] Importantly, managing touring performers requires a treatment plan that takes into account both the production goals and the performer's career aspirations. In this case, the director of the tour was fully supportive of JD's need to undergo voice rehabilitation during the vocal injury phase. Furthermore, JD was highly motivated to address her vocal injury because the dysphonia caused her anxiety and she had aspirations for a Broadway career. Management of JD's dysphonia involved a multiphase treatment plan to address key risk factors and injury mechanisms contributing to the onset of her vocal injury and the maintenance of her dysphonia that were identified in the Haddon matrix.

Treatment recommendations were based on a set of 10 injury-prevention strategies known as Haddon's countermeasures (► Table 69.3).[17,18] Haddon's countermeasures focus on controlling, modifying, and interrupting the amount and rates

of harmful energy transfer likely causing injury to a host. Although Haddon's countermeasures include 10 injury-prevention strategies, their order does not suggest the importance of risk factors or causes contributing to the injury. As such, strategies placed lower on the list of Haddon's countermeasures can be applied before considering those listed higher. This principle is especially important once appreciable injury has occurred, in which case application of injury-prevention strategies 9 and 10 might be applied as immediate measures to stabilize the injury (countermeasure 9: begin to counter damage done by the hazard; countermeasure 10: stabilize, repair, and rehabilitate the object of damage). To that end, JD immediately stopped most voice use as she observed a 1-day absence from the production to allow for a temporary cessation of biomechanical energy transfer with vocal fold impact stress, and to support vocal fold wound healing.[19] She also attended a session of voice therapy to receive counseling on a personalized voice care program developed with her input and to acquire voice therapy techniques that could prevent further vocal fold tissue damage from biomechanical (voice production) and chemical (i.e., GERD) energy transfer.[20]

Another key principle is that larger amounts of energy transfer relative to the structure's ability to withstand damage will necessitate a strategy placed higher in the list of Haddon's countermeasures. Along those lines, healthy vocal fold tissue is more resistant to biomechanical energy transfer and less susceptible to vocal fold injury. Thus, addressing vocal fold tissue health in addition to modifying the amount and rate of phonotrauma is critical to positive and long-term treatment outcomes. Accordingly, her voice-care program involved strategies for optimal vocal fold tissue health, which included the use of a humidifier in her hotel and dressing rooms to improve vocal fold superficial hydration and greater fluid consumption to increase systemic hydration.[21] The program also included a reduction in nightly alcohol consumption to minimize acid reflux exposure. To limit phonotrauma, she agreed to decrease social voice use during times of high professional voice demands and utilize alternative forms of communication.[22,23]

In the case of JD, the contractual requirement to remain on tour meant that JD would continue to be exposed to high amounts and rates of biomechanical energy transfer. Injury-prevention strategies focused on controlling the release of biomechanical energy to assure that harmful damage to the vocal folds did not occur. Accordingly, JD engaged in negative practice by alternating between extreme nasal and oral-only resonance on isolated phonemes /i/ and /o/, and then varied the degree of oral–nasal resonance until balanced. She reported a decrease in laryngeal–pharyngeal tension with resonance balancing. Continuing to maintain balanced resonance, JD phonated through a straw while performing vocal function exercises (VFEs).[24,25] The VFE program includes a set of four phonatory tasks with the aim to rebalance respiratory, laryngeal, and resonatory subsystems during voice production. JD completed the VFE with a straw to promote a reduction in vocal fold impact stress by encouraging barely adducted vocal folds and lower subglottal pressures.[26] As expected, JD observed greater vocal ease with straw phonation. She also placed her hand on her abdomen to monitor abdominal breathing on productions of /hu/ and as a tactile cue for better coordination of exhalation and voicing on functional words and phrases. These respiratory and resonatory voice techniques were applied to her current show material, first singing vowels only and then singing the lyrics, to initiate generalization—the most challenging component of voice therapy.[27] She noted less vocal effort and greater strength of overtones in singing her show repertoire with greater vocal economy.[28] These functional vocal tasks promoted transfer of techniques to real-world vocal situations that, together with immediate improvements in vocal function, provided motivation to

adhere to treatment recommendations. A vocal cool down using resonant voice humming was taught and recommended to accelerate postperformance vocal fold tissue recovery.[29] In addition, a soft singing task was taught as a simple way to monitor for vocal fold inflammation.[30] Finally, the SLP observed JD in performance and offered additional clinical advice to reduce her vocal intensity with group singing and consider alternative, less phonotraumatic options for animated voice use.

Table 69.3 Haddon's countermeasures[17,18] applied to the vocal injury of a touring singer

Countermeasure 1: Prevent the creation of the hazard (voice production, acid reflux)

Take a hiatus from performances by occasionally requesting an understudy to perform one show on days with two performances
To prevent acid reflux, have the largest meal for lunch and eat a small, low fat, low acid dinner

Countermeasure 2: Reduce the amount of hazard (voice production, acid reflux) brought into being

Limit nonessential voice use when rehearsal and performance or two performances occur in 1 day
Teach a healthy whisper, and encourage nonverbal communication when possible (text, email)
Reduce nightly alcohol consumption to limit the number of acid reflux events that occur

Countermeasure 3: Prevent the release of the hazard (voice production, acid reflux)

Mark the voice in rehearsals by not speaking and singing full out to limit vocal dose
Adopt lifestyle behaviors (i.e., chew gum and walk around after meals) to promote gastric emptying and prevent acid reflux events

Countermeasure 4: Modify the rate of release of the hazard (voice production) from its source

Work with the sound engineer on optimizing amplification and feedback in each new space to reduce vocal dose
Adjust speaking and singing vocal technique to be less phonotraumatic by addressing respiratory–phonatory coordination and balance of oral–nasal resonance

Countermeasure 5: Separate the hazard (voice production) from that which is to be protected by time and space

Observe vocal naps during production times when the singer is not performing on stage to reduce vocal dose
Test the acoustics of each new performance space and determine any necessary adjustments in vocal technique
Teach vocally healthy character voices that minimize vocal fold impact stress

Countermeasure 6: Separate the hazard (voice production) from that which is to be protected by a physical barrier (surface hydration)

Utilize nebulized hydration treatments after musical numbers that induce heavy oral breathing from execution of intense choreography, and as needed (e.g., dry planes)

Countermeasure 7: Modify relevant basic qualities of the hazard (voice production, acid reflux)

Restart private singing instruction with a voice teacher who has expertise in musical theater vocal styles to learn to produce a healthy belt voice
Take acid reflux medication as prescribed to reduce acidity of refluxed contents and minimize nonphonatory vocal fold inflammation

Countermeasure 8: Make what is to be protected (vocal folds) more resistant to damage (phonotrauma) from the hazard (voice production)

Optimize vocal fold tissue health by improving surface (i.e., use humidifier at hotel and theater to breathe moist air) and systemic hydration (consume more water/fluids). Get adequate sleep, maintain a healthy diet, and practice hand hygiene precautions to lower your risk of respiratory or gastrointestinal infections.

Countermeasure 9: Begin to counter damage (phonotrauma) done by the hazard (voice production)

Take 1 day off from the current production to observe a full day of complete voice rest
Attend one session of voice therapy during current production stopover to stabilize the vocal injury. Complete vocal warm-ups of VFEs with straw phonation as a rehabilitation program until able to attend a full course of voice therapy in New York City
Incorporate a vocal cool down routine of RV humming taught to reduce postperformance vocal fold inflammation
Use soft singing as a screening tool to detect vocal fold swelling; seek medical care early

Countermeasure 10: Stabilize, repair, and rehabilitate the object of damage (vocal folds)

Follow up with laryngology as needed during tour for ongoing medical support
Complete four to six sessions of voice therapy with an SLP at the end of the tour to fully restore vocal function
Undergo laryngologic evaluation upon discharge from voice therapy to confirm vocal fold status

SLP, speech-language pathologist; VFEs, vocal function exercises; RV, resonant voice.

69.6 Outcome

The main goal of management for JD's acute vocal injury was stabilization of her vocal deterioration and the underlying pathophysiologic process by applying a set of injury-reduction strategies (i.e., Haddon's countermeasures). As for treatment outcomes, JD returned for follow-up 1 year later after just ending a contract with a cruise ship and expressed satisfaction with her current vocal situation. She adopted a number of countermeasures from her voice-care program, which was in line with the SLP's instructions that she implement the most feasible and effective strategies. Accordingly, JD eliminated alcohol consumption for the remaining 2 months of the tour, and now drinks only occasionally. She increased her water intake to counteract systemic dehydration with intense choreography and reported daily use of a humidifier to promote vocal fold superficial hydration. She incorporated a more extensive vocal warm-up routine that included VFEs with straw phonation and regularly completed postperformance vocal cool downs with resonant voice humming. She marked her voice at rehearsals and decreased her vocal intensity during group singing. With these countermeasures, she perceived an initial improvement in voice over the remainder of the tour, and a nearly full return of vocal function after the tour ended. Specifically, she described better vocal clarity and ease, improved vocal power, better access to pitches in her upper range, and greater consistency in her singing voice. She demonstrated a noticeable improvement in the overall severity of dysphonia with corresponding changes in acoustic measures (▶ Table 69.1). Vocal fold appearance and vibratory behavior improved; the vocal folds were white, laryngeal hyperfunction was substantially reduced, and the vocal fold nodules had nearly resolved. Only a minimal amount of thickening was visible with soft phonation at high pitches. These clinically meaningful improvements were paralleled by decreased vocal handicap in both speaking and singing.

With improved vocal function, she reported increased confidence in her singing voice that motivated her to participate in auditions for new roles. However, she continued to experience decreased vocal endurance with prolonged singing, although only mildly and after much longer periods of singing. She was encouraged to continue voice rehabilitation with an SLP in her city of residence, but was unable to coordinate SLP services because of a new production contract she took shortly after her tour ended. Accordingly, JD was advised at her follow-up visit to enroll in two to three sessions of voice therapy when she returned home to address laryngeal hyperfunction with the production of character voices and loud voice.

Postevent management of a touring singer with a vocal injury is critical for successful clinical outcomes and to prevent a future voice problem, which is more likely in patients who have a history of dysphonia.[31,32] As a component of her long-term post–vocal injury management, singing instruction from a voice teacher who works with injured singers was recommended to deal with the patient's ongoing complaint of mild vocal fatigue with singing. Guidance by a voice teacher allows singers to navigate difficult song repertoire with improved vocal efficiency (i.e., minimal phonotrauma). Finally, continuous medical care is crucial for singers who use the voice professionally and are at risk for vocal injury. Once voice rehabilitation concludes, whether discharge occurs because the patient successfully meets treatment goals or if vocal function is not fully restored, JD was counseled to follow up with a laryngologist and as needed thereafter. The inclusion of these final two components in her long-term management plan (i.e., singing instruction and ongoing laryngologic medical care) highlights the circular nature of caring for a touring singer. Incorporating countermeasures at the preinjury event phase are critical to avoid a recurrence or the onset of a new vocal injury.

69.7 Key Points

- Voice problems in touring singers typically result from multiple risk factors for suboptimal vocal fold tissue health together with high vocal fold impact stress associated with inefficient vocal technique in speaking and singing as an agent of vocal injury.
- The major challenge of diagnosing and managing touring singers is distinguishing between preexisting and new laryngeal pathology, which can be facilitated by an analysis of risk factors and vocal injury mechanisms according to a vocal injury event stage using the Haddon matrix.
- SLPs managing touring singers should consider the patient's career aspirations as well as contractual agreements that dictate production demands and performance schedules when developing a treatment plan.
- Voice rehabilitation, which can be guided by Haddon's countermeasures, involves personalized voice care to optimize vocal fold tissue health, voice therapy strategies that facilitate wound healing and counter existing vocal fold tissue damage, and functional voice tasks that promote generalization of voice therapy techniques to performances and daily communication.
- Successful treatment outcomes for touring singers require stabilization of vocal injury during the acute injury stage and long-term clinical care post–vocal injury to fully rehabilitate vocal function.

69.8 Acknowledgments

The author thanks Dr. Carol W. Runyan, Professor of Epidemiology and Director of the Program for Injury Prevention, Education and Research (PIPER) at the Colorado School of Public Health, for providing a critical review of the injury epidemiology concepts explained in this case report and for offering her technical assistance with the application to this case of the Haddon matrix and Haddon's countermeasures.

Suggested Readings

[1] Leborgne WD, Rosenberg M. The Vocal Athlete. San Diego, CA: Plural Publishing; 2014
[2] Titze IR. Principles of Voice Production. Iowa City, IA: National Center for Voice and Speech; 2004
[3] Titze IR, Verdolini Abbott K. Vocology: The Science and Practice of Voice Habilitation. Salt Lake City, UT: National Center for Voice and Speech; 2012

[4] Ziegler A, Johns MM. Health promotion and injury prevention education for student singers. J Sing. 2012; 68(5):531–541

References

[1] Verdolini K. Critical analysis of common terminology in voice therapy: a position paper. Phonoscope. 1999; 2(1):1–8

[2] Mehta DD, Hillman RE. Voice assessment: updates on perceptual, acoustic, aerodynamic, and endoscopic imaging methods. Curr Opin Otolaryngol Head Neck Surg. 2008; 16(3):211–215

[3] Kempster GB, Gerratt BR, Verdolini Abbott K, Barkmeier-Kraemer J, Hillman RE. Consensus auditory-perceptual evaluation of voice: development of a standardized clinical protocol. Am J Speech Lang Pathol. 2009; 18(2):124–132

[4] Zraick RI, Kempster GB, Connor NP, et al. Establishing validity of the Consensus Auditory-Perceptual Evaluation of Voice (CAPE-V). Am J Speech Lang Pathol. 2011; 20(1):14–22

[5] Rosen CA, Lee AS, Osborne J, Zullo T, Murry T. Development and validation of the voice handicap index-10. Laryngoscope. 2004; 114(9):1549–1556

[6] Cohen SM, Statham M, Rosen CA, Zullo T. Development and validation of the singing voice handicap-10. Laryngoscope. 2009; 119(9):1864–1869

[7] Evans RW, Evans RI, Carvajal S, Perry S. A survey of injuries among Broadway performers. Am J Public Health. 1996; 86(1):77–80

[8] Evans RW, Evans RI, Carvajal S. Survey of injuries among West End performers. Occup Environ Med. 1998; 55(9):585–593

[9] Haddon W, Jr. A logical framework for categorizing highway safety phenomena and activity. J Trauma. 1972; 12(3):193–207

[10] Runyan CW. Introduction: back to the future–revisiting Haddon's conceptualization of injury epidemiology and prevention. Epidemiol Rev. 2003; 25(1):60–64

[11] Titze IR, Abbott KV. Vocology: The Science and Practice of Voice Habilitation. Salt Lake City, UT: National Center for Voice and Speech; 2012

[12] Verdolini K, Rosen CA, Branski RC, Eds. Classification Manual for Voice Disorders-I. Mahwah, NJ: Lawrence Erlbaum Associates; 2006

[13] Titze IR. Mechanical stress in phonation. J Voice. 1994; 8(2):99–105

[14] Jiang JJ, Titze IR. Measurement of vocal fold intraglottal pressure and impact stress. J Voice. 1994; 8(2):132–144

[15] Van Stan JH, Roy N, Awan S, Stemple J, Hillman RE. A taxonomy of voice therapy. Am J Speech Lang Pathol. 2015; 24(2):101–125

[16] Ziegler A, Gillespie AI, Abbott KV. Behavioral treatment of voice disorders in teachers. Folia Phoniatr Logop. 2010; 62(1–2):9–23

[17] Haddon W, Jr. Energy damage and the ten countermeasure strategies. Hum Factors. 1973; 15(4):355–366

[18] Haddon W, Jr. Advances in the epidemiology of injuries as a basis for public policy. Public Health Rep. 1980; 95(5):411–421

[19] Branski RC, Verdolini K, Sandulache V, Rosen CA, Hebda PA. Vocal fold wound healing: a review for clinicians. J Voice. 2006; 20(3):432–442

[20] Nanjundeswaran C, Li NY, Chan KM, Wong RK, Yiu EM, Verdolini-Abbott K. Preliminary data on prevention and treatment of voice problems in student teachers. J Voice. 2012; 26(6):816.e1–816.e12

[21] Sivasankar M, Leydon C. The role of hydration in vocal fold physiology. Curr Opin Otolaryngol Head Neck Surg. 2010; 18(3):171–175

[22] Titze IR, Hunter EJ. Comparison of vocal vibration-dose measures for potential-damage risk criteria. J Speech Lang Hear Res. 2015; 58(5):1425–1439

[23] Titze IR, Svec JG, Popolo PS. Vocal dose measures: quantifying accumulated vibration exposure in vocal fold tissues. J Speech Lang Hear Res. 2003; 46(4):919–932

[24] Stemple JC, Lee L, D'Amico B, Pickup B. Efficacy of vocal function exercises as a method of improving voice production. J Voice. 1994; 8(3):271–278

[25] Sabol JW, Lee L, Stemple JC. The value of vocal function exercises in the practice regimen of singers. J Voice. 1995; 9(1):27–36

[26] Titze IR. Voice training and therapy with a semi-occluded vocal tract: rationale and scientific underpinnings. J Speech Lang Hear Res. 2006; 49(2):448–459

[27] Ziegler A, Dastolfo C, Hersan R, Rosen CA, Gartner-Schmidt J. Perceptions of voice therapy from patients diagnosed with primary muscle tension dysphonia and benign mid-membranous vocal fold lesions. J Voice. 2014; 28(6):742–752

[28] Berry DA, Verdolini K, Montequin DW, Hess MM, Chan RW, Titze IR. A quantitative output-cost ratio in voice production. J Speech Lang Hear Res. 2001; 44(1):29–37

[29] Verdolini Abbott K, Li NY, Branski RC, et al. Vocal exercise may attenuate acute vocal fold inflammation. J Voice. 2012; 26(6):814.e1–814.e13

[30] Bastian RW, Keidar A, Verdolini-Marston K. Simple vocal tasks for detecting vocal fold swelling. J Voice. 1990; 4(2):172–183

[31] Miller MK, Verdolini K. Frequency and risk factors for voice problems in teachers of singing and control subjects. J Voice. 1995; 9(4):348–362

[32] Verdolini K, Ramig LO. Review: occupational risks for voice problems. Logoped Phoniatr Vocol. 2001; 26(1):37–46

[33] Baken RJ, Orlikoff RF. Clinical Measurement of Speech and Voice. 2nd ed. San Diego, CA: Cengage Learning; 2000

[34] Fairbanks G. Voice and Articulation Drillbook. New York City, NY: Harper & Row; 1960

70 Dysphagia in Generalized Dystonia following Deep Brain Stimulation

Erin Yeates

70.1 Introduction

Dystonia is a movement disorder characterized by involuntary and often sustained muscle contractions, causing twisting, repetitive movements, and abnormal postures.[1] Dystonia can be part of another disorder (i.e., a symptom of Parkinson's disease) or a primary condition. Generalized dystonia is differentiated from focal dystonias; generalized dystonia affects multiple areas of the body, while a focal dystonia impacts a certain area (i.e., cervical dystonia affecting the neck muscles or spasmodic dysphonia affecting the laryngeal musculature only during speaking).[2] This case describes the signs and symptoms of dysphagia and dysarthria in an individual with progressive generalized dystonia, a hyperkinetic movement disorder.

70.2 Clinical History and Description

FT was a 42-year-old man referred to an outpatient swallowing clinic for instrumental assessment of dysphagia. He was diagnosed with early-onset generalized dystonia, with typical development up until age 5 years, at which time he developed dysarthria. His symptoms progressed to include dystonic posturing including right hand clenching and toe walking by 8 years old. By age 13, he required a wheelchair for mobility. His dystonia was progressive and impacted all four limbs, trunk, cervical, and oromandibular regions. He had bilateral globus pallidus interna deep brain stimulators (GPi DBS) implanted 2 years ago with the aim of reducing dystonia; mild improvements in truncal and limb dystonia were offset by worsened speech, swallowing, and drooling. Previous medical imaging (MRI brain) showed bilateral encephalomalacia to the basal ganglia. In addition to the DBS, his dystonia was treated with baclofen (antispasmodic medication). He had no other medical conditions.

70.3 Clinical Testing

FT reported that his main issue was difficulty chewing. This issue was present prior to DBS insertion, but was now worse. Chewing was fatiguing and prolonging meal time. He lost some weight, with pre-DBS weight at 180 lb, and within a year post-surgery, he was down to 170 lb. He admitted he was having so much trouble self-feeding and chewing that he avoided eating all day long while at work and during his commute. He was fasting continuously upward of 10 hours per day. He reported he was able to eat lunch at his office before DBS. FT's oral dystonia worsened with stimulation on; he only got relief if he turned stimulation off. His speech intelligibility decreased. He denied any episodes of pneumonia or lung infection pre- or post-DBS.

Oral mechanism exam revealed mildly reduced right lip retraction. There was evidence of bilateral restricted tongue range of motion and strength. The soft palate appeared retracted at baseline on mouth opening, without phonation. Dentition was normal. FT reported pain and tightness secondary to dystonia in the bilateral neck and cheeks; palpation revealed hard, tight muscle tone. Dysarthria assessment revealed strained-strangled voice quality. He had difficulty initiating speech at times, and intermittent vocal tremor was noted. Resonance was hypernasal. Intelligibility was variable. Dysarthria was consistent with a mixed dysarthria with hyperkinetic and spastic features.

Clinical swallowing examination revealed grossly timely and adequate hyolaryngeal excursion on palpation. One episode of strong coughing after swallowing liquids (out of five trials) was observed. He was unable to coordinate drinking from a cup without spilling, and habitually drank from a water bottle with an attached straw. Self-feeding was challenging and laborious. Chewing was incomplete with a loss of adequate rotary jaw motion, but no obvious signs or symptoms of aspiration with pureed or soft solids were observed. Multiple swallows per bolus, concerning for pharyngeal residue, were noted across textures.

Videofluoroscopy assessed swallowing physiology and evaluated the risk for silent aspiration. Swallow onset delay was observed with thin liquids, with the bolus head reaching just beyond the vallecular space prior to swallow initiation. Anterior hyoid excursion was mildly reduced. Arytenoid to epiglottic contact was complete, but delayed with thin liquids, leading to one episode of trace aspiration followed by immediate coughing. FT's cough was effective in clearing the barium from the airway (Penetration-Aspiration Scale score of 4). Nectar-thickened liquids created more pharyngeal residue, primarily in the valleculae. The upper esophageal sphincter opened adequately. The most significant issue was with chewing. Mastication was prolonged and disorganized, resulting in aggregation of solid, unchewed soft solid bolus in the pyriforms prior to swallow initiation.

70.4 Questions and Answers for the Reader

1. Based on the clinical and instrumental exams, what phase of swallowing was the most significant concern for FT?
   a) The oral phase.
   b) The pharyngeal phase.
   c) The esophageal phase.

Answer: a is correct. FT's report that he had difficulty self-feeding and chewing to the extent that he regularly avoided eating in public (i.e., at work) was concerning for oral phase dysphagia. His oromandibular and cervical dystonias led to twisting, uncontrolled movements of the neck and articulators even during patterned motions such as chewing. He also denied episodes of pneumonia, suggesting that he is thus far avoiding respiratory compromise despite his difficulties. Mastication was deemed impaired on the videofluoroscopy, with solid unchewed pieces of the bolus spilling into the pharynx in an uncontrolled manner during chewing.

b is incorrect. While there were pharyngeal phase concerns related to delay swallow onset, vallecular residue, and an isolated incident of penetration–aspiration, his primary deficits originated in the oral phase.

c is incorrect. There was nothing in FT's history or presentation that suggested esophageal phase dysphagia.

2. What would be the suggested diet based on the videofluoroscopy and clinical history?
   a) Pureed solids and nectar-thickened liquids.
   b) Minced/soft solids as tolerated and regular thin liquids.
   c) Regular diet and regular thin liquids.
   d) NPO (nil per os) with enteral nutrition.

Answer: b is correct. Minced/soft solids and regular thin liquids; given that mastication is such a challenge, FT was advised to minimize hard, difficult-to-chew foods to minimize his risk of airway obstruction. This, however, did need to be balanced with his desire to minimize the restrictions on his diet, as well as his self-feeding challenges, which made finger foods easier to manage than using utensils. Thin liquids appear appropriate at this time.

a is incorrect. While this may well be the safest and most conservative diet for FT, it places significant restrictions on his quality of life. The single episode of trace aspiration effectively ejected from the airway in an individual without any history of respiratory compromise does not suggest a pattern of consistent aspiration or poor airway clearance. Given that FT wishes to minimize dietary restrictions, thickened liquids are unlikely to be adhered to in the community.

c is incorrect. Regular solids place too many demands on his oral phase, specifically with respect to mastication.

d is incorrect. This approach is too conservative and would drastically impair FT's quality of life.

3. What factor(s) impact FT's nutrition status?
   a) Weight loss in the context of worsened dysphagia.
   b) Avoidance of eating in social settings due to worsened dysphagia and difficulty self-feeding.
   c) Inefficiency of chewing.
   d) All of the above.

Answer: d is correct. All of these factors suggest that FT may have suboptimal nutrition, and a registered dietician consult would be beneficial. Since his DBS, FT has had more difficulty chewing and swallowing. His more laborious self-feeding in the context of uncontrollable dystonic movements is leading to longer, less efficient meals. It takes him longer to chew and swallow a single bite and to complete a meal. When a person must work so hard for every bite, nutrition strategies provided by our dietician colleagues can help an individual get the most protein

and energy out of every bite so they can maintain their weight and remain healthy.

a is partially correct, see d above.

b is partially correct, see d above.

c is partially correct, see d above.

70.5 Description of Disorder and Recommended Treatment

The primary therapy for dystonia is botulinum toxin injections, which tend to have a limited effect on generalized dystonia. FT tried Botox in the past with limited therapeutic success; he was not currently receiving injections. Surgical management of medically refractory dystonia has become more common in recent years, with the target generally being the globus pallidus interna (GPi)[1] as performed in FT. It is not uncommon, anecdotally, for patients post-DBS to report improvement in some symptoms (i.e., mobility), but seemingly worse speech and swallowing. Review of the literature by Troche and colleagues[3] found no clinically significant improvement or decline in dysphagia after DBS. However, longer-term follow-up of these patients shows significant improvement in mobility and overall disability, but the most commonly reported stimulation-related side effects are on speech and swallowing.[4] Stimulation adjustment can be a long process measured in months and even years in the generalized dystonia population. FT was advised to review his concerns regarding worsened speech and swallowing with his movement disorders neurologist, and to determine whether further adjustments to his stimulation parameters might make a difference in his symptoms.

70.6 Outcome

Based on the exam, FT was advised to continue with thin liquids and soft, well-moistened or minced solids. For solids, he avoided many harder, drier, chewier solids, and it was reinforced that these types of items were best avoided given his inefficient and disorganized chewing, as well as uncontrolled posterior spillage with chewable solids. He refused a pureed diet. For liquids, the single episode of trace aspiration was met with effective coughing. Given that he had no history of respiratory compromise, it was felt that he was able to tolerate occasional small amounts of aspiration. Head positioning strategies such as chin down were impossible given his cervical dystonia.

The registered dietician was consulted in conjunction with the SLP and given that FT was able to continue with thin liquids and was able to self-feed relatively easily from a straw, suggestions were provided for smoothies and nutritional supplements. He agreed to a meal replacement from the straw; although he may cough occasionally, he would feel more socially acceptable than trying to eat a solid meal when in public. The dietician also suggested high-calorie, high-protein meal ideas (i.e., adding more nutrient dense oils and sauces to foods).

FT was seen at 1 year later for repeat swallowing assessment. He reported that his dysarthria and dysphagia were slightly better, but still problematic. He continued quarterly follow-up for device programming with his neurologist and had found a DBS program that better balanced the improvements in limb dystonia with the worsening of the cervical and oromandibular dystonias. Repeat videofluoroscopy showed mild improvements, mostly in terms of swallowing delay. The delay with thin liquids was less prominent, and no episodes of airway invasion were observed. However, mastication did not seem significantly improved and continued to be laborious. FT reported he had essentially continued his usual diet since the previous visit, but he consumed a smoothie mixed with a nutritional supplement at lunch by straw. His weight was stable (although he did not return back to his baseline weight) and he felt like he could sit in the lunch room with his coworkers again and be part of the meal.

70.7 Key Points

- Patients with dystonia have unique, individual presentations of dysphagia and dysarthria, but impaired mastication efficiency and bolus control can lead to significant oropharyngeal dysphagia.

- DBS treatment may impact some symptoms (i.e., mobility) more effectively than others (i.e., speech and swallowing).
- Community-dwelling patients require a nuanced, realistic approach to develop strategies and recommendations for swallowing that promote safety and efficiency of swallowing, as well as the patient's personal goals.

References

[1] Hu W, Stead M. Deep brain stimulation for dystonia. Transl Neurodegener. 2014; 3(1):2
[2] Barkmeier-Kraemer JM, Clark HM. Speech-language pathology evaluation and management of hyperkinetic disorders affecting speech and swallowing function. Tremor Other Hyperkinet Mov. 2017; 7:489
[3] Troche MS, Brandimore AE, Foote KD, Okun MS. Swallowing and deep brain stimulation in Parkinson's disease: a systematic review. Parkinsonism Relat Disord. 2013; 19(9):783–788
[4] Isaias IU, Alterman RL, Tagliati M. Deep brain stimulation for primary generalized dystonia: long-term outcomes. Arch Neurol. 2009; 66(4):465–470

71 Speech Therapy Telepractice Program for a Client with Aphasia

Judy P. Walker

71.1 Introduction

Telepractice is the service delivery method of using technology to provide rehabilitation services at a distance. The purpose of this case study is to demonstrate a successful speech therapy telepractice program for a client with aphasia.

71.2 Clinical History and Description

CP was a 68-year-old, right-handed female who was referred for speech therapy telepractice services 6 months following a left hemisphere stroke. At the time of her stroke, a computed tomography (CT) scan revealed a left middle cerebral artery (MCA) cerebrovascular accident (CVA) in the parietal and temporal lobe regions, which was accompanied by severe fluent aphasia and mild oral dysphagia. CP was seen for inpatient speech therapy, followed by outpatient services for 5 months and reportedly made improvements in receptive and expressive language and functional communication using an iPad. Past medical history was significant for diabetes, hypertension, and bilateral carpal tunnel syndrome. CP was a high school graduate and retired bookkeeper. She lived at home with her 92-year-old mother and had two supportive daughters: one lived close by and the other in a nearby state.

71.3 Clinical Testing

CP was evaluated in person in her home to determine her current level of functioning and to assess her computer skills as well as her equipment and Internet access to ensure that she was appropriate for telepractice services. One daughter and CP's mother were present during the evaluation. CP was alert and ambulatory with no evidence of motor difficulties. Although she appeared to understand questions, CP had difficulty verbally conveying thoughts and frequently requested that her daughter or mother provide responses to questions.

Pure tone hearing screening presented at 250, 500, 1000, 2000, and 4000 Hz was within normal limits (WNL) bilaterally. CP wore glasses for corrected visual acuity. An oral peripheral examination was WNL. No evidence of motor speech difficulties was observed. Speech intelligibility was 100%. CP was currently eating a regular oral diet and her daughter confirmed that CP swallowed without difficulty. Attention and executive functioning were observed to be WNL. Language was assessed using the Western Aphasia Battery-Revised (WAB-R),[1] and results indicated an aphasia quotient of 48 (scale of 0–100), indicating severe aphasia (▶ Table 71.1). Auditory comprehension was

moderately impaired for sentences of increased length and complexity beyond simple subject + verb + direct object grammatical constructions. Verbal expression was fluent and severely impaired at word/sentence level. Spontaneous speech consisted primarily of jargon, containing numerous semantic paraphasias and neologisms with periodic recognizable automatic expressions (e.g., I don't know, don't worry). CP benefited from a combination of phonemic cueing and writing the first letters of words to assist with word finding. Repetition was moderate/severely impaired for sentences of increased length and complexity. Reading comprehension was moderately impaired beyond simple sentence constructions. Writing was moderate/severely impaired at word/sentence level. CP frequently used a writing compensatory strategy to assist with lexical access when speaking.

Table 71.1 Comparisons of CP's pre- and posttherapy raw scores and aphasia quotients from the Western Aphasia Battery-R

Subtest	Pretherapy results	Posttherapy results
Spontaneous speech		
• Information content	4/10	6/10
• Fluency	7/10	7/10
Auditory comprehension		
• Yes/no questions	53/60	57/60
• Word recognition	43/60	48/60
• Sequential commands	34/80	41/80
Repetition	34/100	40/100
Naming		
• Object naming	17/60	26/60
• Word fluency	2/20	3/20
• Sentence completion	6/10	6/10
• Responsive speech	6/10	8/10
Aphasia quotient	48	57.2
Reading		
• Comprehension of sentences	10/40	12/40
• Reading commands	7/20	9/20
• Word–object matching	6/6	6/6
Writing		
• Writing on request	4/6	5/6
• Written output	6/34	15/34
• Writing to dictation	0/10	0/10

Source: Kertesz.[1]

Note: Interpretation of the WAB-R aphasia quotient is as follows: 0 to 25 = very severe; 26 to 50 = severe; 51 to 75 = moderate; 76 and above = mild.

The ASHA Functional Communication Skills for Adults (ASHA FACS)[2] was completed with the assistance of CP's daughter as a standardized measure of functional communication (▶ Table 71.2). Additionally, the Walker Functional Checklist[3] was completed to quantify functional communication abilities in activities of daily living (ADLs) unique to CP (▶ Table 71.3). Cumulatively, CP was able to communicate basic needs and communicate with some help in social situations and in daily planning. She had greater difficulty in reading and writing required for functional tasks. CP's daughter reported that CP periodically used nonverbal cues such as gestures, facial expression, and tone of voice to assist with conveying thoughts. CP also reportedly retrieved objects or attempted to write words related to the topic of discussion to assist in conveying the message, which was very time-consuming.

Table 71.2 Comparison of CP's pre- and posttherapy total and mean scores from the ASHA Functional Communication Skills for Adults (ASHA FACS)

Domain	Total score		Mean score	
	Pretherapy	Posttherapy	Pretherapy	Posttherapy
Social communication	127/147	127/147	6.04	6.04
Communication basic needs	48/49	49/49	6.8	7
Reading/writing	50/70	54.5/70	5	5.5
Daily planning	27/35	33/35	5.4	6.6
Overall communication index mean score			5.81	6.2

Source: Frattali et al.[2]

Note: Interpretation of the ASHA FACS mean score range is as follows: 7 = does independently; 1 = does not do at all.

Table 71.3 Comparisons of pretherapy and posttherapy ratings of CP's ability to complete activities of daily living (ADLs) that were unique to her using an adapted version of the Walker Functional Checklist for people with aphasia

Walker functional checklist										
ADL tasks	Accuracy		Impaired cognitive and linguistic processes							
	Pretherapy	Posttherapy	Sensory	Motor	Attention	Ex. fun.	Aud. comp.	Verb. exp.	Read	Write	Comp. strategy
Easy										
• Housework	+	+						X			Gesture
• Cooking	+	+						X			Gesture
• Yardwork	+	+						X			Gesture
• Self-care	+	+						X			Gesture
Moderate										
• Home repair requests	–	±						X			Gesture/ writing
• Bank	–	+					X	X	X	X	Gesture
• Walmart	–	+					X	X	X	X	Gesture
• Shaw's	–	+					X	X	X	X	Gesture
• Hannaford	–	+					X	X	X	X	Gesture
• Wendy's	–	+					X	X	X	X	Gesture/iPad
• Driving/ directions	–	±					X	X	X	X	Gesture/ writing
Difficult										
• Talking on phone	–	±					X	X			iPad
• Explaining day	–	±					X	X			Gesture/ writing/iPad

Source: Walker.[3]

Note: Interpretation of the accuracy ratings are as follows: (+) independent, (±) somewhat independent, (–) dependent.

Aud. comp., auditory comprehension; Comp. strategy, compensatory strategy; Ex. fun., executive functioning; Verb. exp., verbal expression;

71.4 Questions and Answers for the Reader

1. Based on CP's history, select one area that you would *not* assess in your evaluation.
   a) Language.
   b) Functional communication.
   c) Dysphagia.
   d) Hearing and vision.
   e) Verbal reasoning and problem-solving.

Answer: e is correct. Since this patient has language deficits, the validity of results for assessing verbal reasoning and problem-solving would be in question. This patient may not fully understand questions due to auditory comprehension deficits and may not be able to answer questions due to verbal expression deficits.

a is incorrect. The primary complaint for this patient is language difficulties associated with a left hemisphere stroke. Therefore, you want to evaluate all language modalities to determine her level of functioning in each modality.

b is incorrect. The patient reportedly was able to use strategies to assist with functional communication. You want to determine what strategies the patient uses and how successful she is at using these strategies to communicate.

c is incorrect. Any patient with neurological damage may have difficulty with swallowing. Therefore, it is essential to determine whether a patient has a safe swallow as part of any routine assessment of patients who have had strokes. This patient reportedly had an oral dysphagia upon admission to the hospital, which should be addressed in your evaluation.

d is incorrect. Hearing and visual acuity are the first stages in auditory and reading comprehension. Unless hearing and visual acuity are addressed, a clinician will not be able to ascertain whether deficits in auditory and reading comprehension may be attributed to an acuity rather than a language problem.

2. Considering CP's site of lesion as indicated in the CT findings, the results of the evaluation, and behavioral observations, what type of aphasia does CP exhibit?
   a) Broca's.
   b) Anomic.
   c) Global.
   d) Wernicke's.
   e) Transcortical motor.

Answer: d is correct. CP's presentation is consistent with this type of aphasia. Wernicke's aphasia is typically associated with a lesion to the posterior superior temporal gyrus and can be described as a fluent aphasia. Although auditory comprehension is often impaired for words and sentences, verbal expression is the hallmark characteristically described as utterances with relatively intact syntax but containing numerous semantic paraphasias and neologisms, which are devoid of meaning. Repetition tends to mimic verbal expression.

a is incorrect. CP's presentation is not consistent with this type of aphasia. Broca's aphasia is associated with lesions to the frontal lobe and can be described as a nonfluent aphasia. Auditory comprehension for simple sentences is relatively good, but verbal expression and repetition consists of halting, telegraphic utterances containing a preponderance of nouns, and verbs, but missing function words.

b is incorrect. CP's presentation is not consistent with this type of aphasia. Although anomic aphasia is often associated with lesions to the temporal and parietal lobes, this mild fluent aphasia is described primarily as difficulty with word finding with relatively preserved auditory comprehension and repetition.

c is incorrect. CP's presentation is not consistent with this type of aphasia. Global aphasia is associated with large perisylvian lesions with very severe deficits in all modalities. These patients have difficulty understanding simple words, and verbal expression is often limited to repetitive automatic utterances.

e is incorrect. CP's presentation is not consistent with this type of aphasia. Transcortical motor aphasia is associated with a frontal lobe lesion and has similar language characteristics as a Broca's aphasia, except repetition is relatively good compared to verbal expression.

3. Speech therapy telepractice is recommended for CP. What would be considered a negative prognostic indicator for improvement in language functioning from speech therapy telepractice services in this case?
   a) Patient motivation.
   b) Time post onset.
   c) Severity of stroke.
   d) Family support.
   e) Medical history.

Answer: c is correct. The strongest predictor of short- and long-term outcome is severity of stroke. CP had a relatively large MCA stroke in the temporal and parietal lobes and continued to demonstrate persistent moderate to severe language deficits 6 months after the stroke.

a is incorrect. Motivation is a key factor in making progress during recovery. CP was very motivated to engage in speech therapy telepractice sessions. She completed all homework assignments, which facilitated carryover of skill development between sessions.

b is incorrect. Most improvement of language occurs within the first few months and patients tend to plateau after 1 year where only smaller gains can be seen. CP is 6 months post onset, which is still within the spontaneous recovery time frame.

d is incorrect. The patient had a strong multigenerational support system living in her home or close by who assisted her within and between sessions. One of CP's daughters, who lived further away, remotely joined sessions from her home computer assisted with homework assignments from a distance.

e is incorrect. Diabetes and hypertension are controllable risk factors for stroke.

4. You will see this patient for two 1-hour speech therapy telepractice sessions per week. What is the best treatment approach to use with this patient given her deficits and current living situation?
   a) Functionally oriented treatment approach that will focus only on improving compensatory strategies for communication.
   b) Impairment-based treatment approach that will only target therapy goals for improving linguistic processes.

c) Combined impairment-based and functionally oriented approaches that will target improving linguistic processes while simultaneously teaching the patient compensatory strategies for communication.

Answer: c is correct. A combined approach that will help the patient recover language while simultaneously providing her with a means to communicate in everyday life is the most comprehensive type of treatment program for this patient.

a is incorrect. Although the brain is the most plastic during the first month following a stroke, spontaneous recovery can still occur up to a year, at which time patients tend to plateau. Therefore, it is essential to assist the brain in recovering neural networks that are associated with linguistic processes during this crucial time through language therapy.

b is incorrect. While it is crucial to treat linguistic processes to assist in language recovery, this patient is living at home and in her community. For reasons involving safety and quality of life issues, this patient needs to have ways to communicate when language is not available. For instance, CP had difficulty talking on the phone. So, her house telephone was equipped with a direct dial to the police station and automatic address message to alert authorities in case of an emergency.

71.5 Description of Disorder and Recommended Treatment

At 6 months following left MCA CVA, CP presented with moderate Wernicke's aphasia. Auditory comprehension was moderately impaired at word/sentence level. Verbal expression was fluent and moderate/severely impaired at word level. Spontaneous speech was characterized primarily by neologistic jargon embedded in sentences, which appeared to have some semblance of grammar and also contained the periodic presence of automatic utterances. Repetition was moderate/severely impaired at sentence level. Reading was moderately impaired at sentence level. Writing was severely impaired at word level. Hearing and visual acuity were WNL. Motor speech, swallowing, attention, and executive functioning were WNL. Functionally, CP's communication deficits interfered with her ability to perform ADLs independently within and outside of the home environment. Within the home, CP had established compensatory strategies of using writing, inconsistent gesturing, and limited use of her iPad to assist her in conveying her wants/needs/ideas to her daughter and mother. They reported that CP was successful in communicating her thoughts less than 50% of the time.

Speech therapy telepractice was recommended two times a week for 6 months. The therapy focused on using an impairment-based approach[4] to directly target the improvement of linguistic processes combined with a functionally oriented approach[4] to improve CP's ability to communicate using any means possible in ADLs that were unique to her. Prognosis for improvement of linguistic abilities was guarded based on the severity of the CVA and severity of residual deficits. Prognosis for improvement of functional communication was good based on CP's intact cognitive abilities, motivation, and family support. She was an excellent candidate for telepractice speech therapy given her advanced computer skills.

71.6 Outcome

The impairment-based treatment goals targeted (1) auditory comprehension at a sentence and conversational level, (2) verbal expression at word and sentence levels using a combined grapheme–phoneme cueing strategy to aid in the lexical access of nouns and verbs related to functional contexts, (3) reading and writing at word or sentence level as related to functional contexts. The functionally oriented treatment goals targeted strategies to compensate for language deficits, such as gestures, writing words, and using smart technology, which assisted CP in conveying her thoughts within functionally based ADLs.

Speech therapy telepractice sessions were provided from the speech therapy telepractice lab on the University of Maine campus using a secure interactive video conferencing system that connected CP from her home computer to a computer in the campus lab through high-speed Internet access. Each computer was equipped with high-definition audio and video to ensure the highest quality connection and service delivery. The system allowed for adaptation of the impairment-based treatment approach through desktop presentations of custom-made materials/activities, which were developed from photos and videos taken at CP's home and within her community. An example can be seen in Video 71.1, where the student clinician worked with CP on a verbal expression, sentence-building activity related to driving using a combined grapheme–phoneme cueing strategy to aid in word retrieval. Since CP drove independently, CP's daughters were concerned that she would not have the language skills to verbally convey information about her location should she become lost. The telepractice platform allowed for the desktop presentation of photos related to driving and the use of eTools to enable both the clinician and CP to simultaneously write on the desktop while using the combined phoneme–grapheme cueing strategies to assist with lexical access. Each singular photo slide was followed by a slide containing an audio file of the first sound accompanied by the first letter of the target word, then another slide containing an audio file of the spoken word associated with the written word. Although they were not used in the activity, these additional slides were embedded in the activity for CP to practice at home when the clinician was not present to provide her with the grapheme–phoneme cues and confirmation of the correct words. The telepractice platform also supported a functionally oriented treatment approach through sharing websites and browsers to create highly enriched activities that targeted CP's ADLs within virtual environments in her home and community. As shown in Video 71.2, the aforementioned sentence-building activity was expanded into a supported conversation activity[5] using Google Earth[6] to create a virtual environment of CP's neighborhood and community. CP was asked to give directions for driving her typical route to a local restaurant while being supported by the clinician and her daughter to provide clarifying information. These types of therapy activities were used to improve CP's language and communication abilities so she could successfully converse about ideas, places, and things in her world. When CP had achieved criteria for language and functional communication goals within each activity of daily living, the clinician addressed the functional checklist to identify another activity of daily living. New sets of therapy materials were

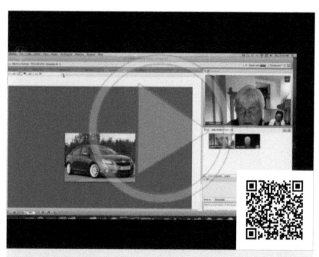

Video 71.1 Example of sentence-building activity related to driving.

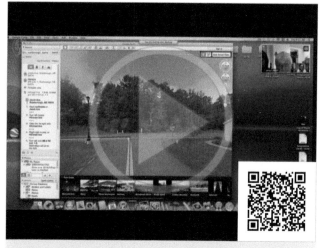

Video 71.2 Example of a supported conversation activity related to driving using Google Earth.

developed with the aid of CP and her family members who took photos and videos of CP within that specific activity of daily living.

At the end of 6 months of therapy, CP was reevaluated using the WAB-R and the ASHA FACS. As shown in ▶ Table 71.1 and ▶ Table 71.2, CP made improvements in linguistic and functional communication abilities. Her WAB-R aphasia quotient increased from a 48 to 57.2 with specific areas of improvement especially noted in auditory comprehension, verbal expression in producing words that contained greater meaning, along with written output. Functional communication also improved especially in areas related to reading/writing and daily planning. Additionally, CP made significant progress in achieving therapy goals as they related to ADLs that were unique to her. As shown in ▶ Table 71.3, CP gained greater independence in communicating wants and needs using combined language and functional communication strategies in several easy and moderate ADLs that were previously problematic. She continued to require assistance with communication in difficult ADLs. CP and her family reported great satisfaction with the successful outcome of the speech therapy telepractice program and stated that they would strongly recommend this program to other individuals with aphasia.

71.7 Key Points

- Classification of aphasia is determined through consideration of neuroimaging findings, diagnostic results, and behavioral observations.
- Several important factors regarding language, functional abilities, and patient environment must be taken into consideration when designing a comprehensive evaluation for aphasia.
- Several prognostic indicators must be taken into consideration when determining a prognosis for a person with aphasia.
- Telepractice technology is a viable and highly creative service delivery model for providing successful treatment programs for people with aphasia.

Suggested Readings

[1] Towey MP. Speech telepractice: installing a speech therapy upgrade for the 21st century. Int J Telerehabil. 2012; 4(2):73–78

[2] Walker JP. University of Maine, Speech Therapy Telepractice and Technology Program Manual. University of Maine Faculty Monographs. Book 220. 2015. http://digitalcommons.library.umaine.edu/fac_monographs/220

References

[1] Kertesz A. Western Aphasia Battery-Revised. San Antonio, TX: Pearson; 2006

[2] Frattali C, Thompson C, Holland A, Wohl C, Ferketic M. Functional Assessment of Communication Skills for Adults. Rockville, MD: American Speech-Language-Hearing Association; 1995

[3] Walker JP. Functional outcome: a case for mild traumatic brain injury. Brain Inj. 2002; 16(7):611–625

[4] Galletta EE, Barrett AM. Impairment and functional interventions for aphasia: having it all. Curr Phys Med Rehabil Rep. 2014; 2(2):114–120

[5] Kagan A. Supported conversation for adults with aphasia: methods and resources for training conversation partners. Aphasiology. 1998; 12(9):851–864

[6] Google Earth [computer program]. Version 7.1.2.2041. Mountain View, CA: Google; 2013

72 Linguistic and Cognitive Deficits in Autoimmune Encephalopathy

Alejandro E. Brice and Jamie Swartz

72.1 Introduction

Autoimmune encephalopathies (AEs) occur when antibodies attack cell surfaces or synaptic proteins[1] and can be associated with widespread and/or focal nervous system involvement. AE can affect patients of all ages with some preference for young children, women, and young adults, and they can develop with or without concurrent tumors. With AE, all areas of cognition can be impaired with the most common clinical symptom consisting of a rapid and progressive dementia that can be mistaken for Creutzfeldt–Jakob disease.[2]

72.2 Clinical History

SJ was a 32-year-old woman admitted to the emergency room with bilateral arm and leg numbness, heaviness, and tingling sensations in addition to confusion. She reported a bandlike sensation around her upper arm (like a tight strap) and her leg numbness was more pronounced on the left side. Blood tests revealed antinuclear antibody, a test for autoimmune disorders, of 1:40, which was not significant. SJ also presented with decreased protein S, which is associated with a blood disorder and increased risk of thrombosis (e.g., formation of a clot in a blood vessel). At that time, SJ was diagnosed with an undifferentiated connective tissue disorder (i.e., where the body attacks its own tissues) and was treated with steroids. Four years later, SJ returned to the emergency room after suffering altered mental state (e.g., three episodes of lost consciousness causing motor vehicle accidents). She was disoriented and presented with short-term memory loss, inability to express herself, and slowed processing.

72.3 Clinical Testing

SJ reported that she experienced disorientation, memory loss, word-retrieval difficulties, and problems with pragmatic context as well as difficulties with focus and concentration. The Rey Auditory Verbal Learning Test (RAVLT),[3] Boston Naming Test (BNT),[4] and an examination of verbal fluency (semantic and letters) were administered by a licensed psychologist. SJ was not seen by a speech-language pathologist at that time as she was functional in activities of daily living including her work. The psychologist reported that verbal, immediate memory from the RAVLT scores were low average to average; verbal delayed memory from the RAVLT scores were low average to average and recognition cues did not substantially improve recall. Confrontation naming from the BNT was within normal limits (BNT = 54/60). Letter and semantic fluency scores were reported to be borderline to low average. No alexia or agraphia was reported.

SJ was also assessed by a neurologist using the Mini-Mental State Examination (MMSE)[5] and oriented to person, place, and time, but not context; difficulty with serial sevens (counting down from 100 using 7, i.e., 100–93–86–79–72–65,...); and

inability to spell the word "world" backward. SJ scored 25/30 on the MMSE. In addition, the Montreal Cognitive Assessment (MoCA),[6] an assessment similar to the MMSE, was administered. The MoCA consists of a 30-point scale and measures the following: (1) memory recall; (1) visuospatial abilities; (3) phonemic fluency; (4) executive function; (5) verbal abstraction; (6) attention, concentration, and working memory; (7) serial subtraction; (8) confrontation naming; (9) sentence repetition; and (10) orientation to time and place. A score of 26 or greater is considered normal.[5] SJ scored 25/30, suggestive of altered cognitive abilities. She had difficulty with drawing a clock with the numbers outside of the circle and with attention and repetition issues (i.e., reading list of digits and letters and repeating them forward and backward). SJ could not remember items even with a multiple choice format. She was eventually diagnosed with encephalopathy of unknown origin.

SJ underwent a comprehensive medical workup. The magnetic resonance imaging (MRI) indicated ovoid (egg-shaped) T2 (imaging indicating abnormally high water content) hyperintensity (patches of damaged cell tissue that shows up as white spots on the MRI, sometimes indicative of multiple sclerosis, dementia, or diabetes) in the frontal lobe. Also, a punctuate lesion in the parietal lobe was found. These lesions were not identified during her prior workup. Due to her autoimmune hypercoagulable state, SJ had a series of subsequent pulmonary emboli. After treatment with high-dose steroids, the immediate pulmonary symptoms began to dissipate; however, it took several months for full recovery.

72.4 Questions and Answers for the Reader

1. AEs are part of a spectrum of inflammatory central nervous system disorders. Three types of AEs exist, which are:
   a) Encephalopathies without cancer, encephalopathies with cancer, and Hashimoto's encephalopathies.
   b) Encephalopathies without cancer, paraneoplastic encephalopathies, and peripheral nervous system vasculitis.
   c) Encephalopathies without cancer, paraneoplastic encephalopathies, and central nervous system vasculitis.
   d) Paraneoplastic encephalopathies, Hashimoto's encephalopathies, and central nervous system vasculitis.

Answer: c is correct. The three types of encephalopathies consist of those without cancer, those pertaining to metabolic effects of cancer and changes produced in tissues remote from a tumor or its metastases, and inflammation of central nervous system blood vessels.

a is incorrect. Hashimoto's encephalopathy is one type under those with cancer. Encephalopathies with cancer are paraneoplastic encephalopathies, where the body's immune system is fighting cancer; it is a systemic disturbance associated but not directly related to the cancer.

b is incorrect. The third type of encephalopathy involves the central nervous system and not the peripheral nervous system.

d is incorrect. Hashimoto's encephalopathy is one type under those with cancer.

2. SJ scored poor to low average on tests. These tests included:
   a) Focus and divided attention, short-term memory, visual memory, and delayed memory.
   b) Focus and divided attention, sustained attention, short-term memory, verbal short-term memory, delayed memory, letter and semantic memory, visuoconstruction skills, and nonverbal reasoning.
   c) Focus and divided attention, sustained attention, short-term memory, verbal short-term memory, delayed memory, letter and semantic memory, and visual short-term memory.
   d) Focus and divided attention, sustained attention, short-term memory, verbal short-term memory, delayed memory, letter and semantic memory, visual short-term memory, and time- and set-sequencing tasks.

Answer: b is correct. SJ scored low on items concerning attention, memory, nonverbal reasoning, and visuoconstruction skills. These deficits are typical of AE and associated dementias.

a is incorrect. SJ also scored low on sustained attention; verbal short-term memory, letter, and semantic memory were also affected; she also scored impaired on time- and set-sequencing tasks.

c is incorrect. Visual short-term memory was average. In addition, verbal short-term memory, delayed memory, letter and semantic memory, visuoconstruction skills, time sequencing, set sequencing, and nonverbal reasoning were also affected.

d is incorrect. Time- and set-sequencing tasks were borderline.

3. Encephalopathies affect _____ areas of cognition and memory loss is present in about _____ of patients with AEs.
   a) Some; one-third.
   b) Some; one-half.
   c) All; one-third.
   d) All; one-half.

Answer: d is correct. Memory is affected in one-half of all AEs and nearly all aspects of cognition are affected.

a is incorrect. AEs affect all areas of cognition and about one half of patients exhibit memory loss.

b is incorrect. AEs affect all areas of cognition.

c is incorrect. About one-half of patients exhibit memory loss.

4. AEs can affect:
   a) Patients of all ages.
   b) Preference for children, young women, and young adults.
   c) Preference for young men.
   d) a and b.
   e) a and c.

Answer: d is correct. AEs can affect anybody; however, there is a preference for children, young adults, adults, and women.

a is incorrect. AEs also show preference for children, young women, and young adults.

b is incorrect. AEs can affect patients of all ages.

c is incorrect. AEs show preference for children, young women, and young adults.

e is incorrect. AEs show preference for children, young women, and young adults.

72.5 Description of Disorder and Recommended Treatment

AEs are part of a spectrum of inflammatory central nervous system disorders that may include limbic encephalitis, which is noted by subacute onset, memory loss, altered senses, seizures, possible personality changes, and/or personality or mood changes.[7] Encephalopathies affect all areas of cognition,[2] with memory loss present in about half the patients with AEs. Cognitive communication disorders in AEs may include difficulties with memory, attention, organization, problem-solving, and executive functioning.[8] All areas of language may be affected (i.e., phonologic, morphologic, syntactic, semantic, pragmatic).[8]

Three types of AEs exist: (1) encephalopathies without cancer, but with serologic evidence of autoimmunity including Hashimoto's encephalopathy; (2) paraneoplastic encephalopathies including syndromes caused by the body's immune system fighting cancer; and (c) central nervous system vasculitis.[7] Hashimoto's encephalopathy along with other encephalopathy etiologies are often misunderstood.[9] Caselli et al.[10] stated that "diagnosis of an autoimmune encephalopathy is difficult and often inferred from serologic, electroencephalopathy, and spinal fluid findings" (p. 879).

However, AEs display common symptoms consisting of rapid onset, headaches, mild hyperthermia, and frequent cerebrospinal fluid (CSF) pleocytosis (an elevated number of lymphocytes or white blood cells in the CSF). Electroencephalograms are more than likely to be abnormal showing focal slow activity often associated with epileptic activity.[1]

SJ was subsequently evaluated by a speech-language pathologist and presented with flaccid dysarthria (low muscle tone) and generalized weakness on the left side of her face and body. Flaccid dysarthria is a lower motor neuron disorder, or a disorder causing disruption in the communication between neurons in the spinal cord and skeletal muscles in the arms, legs, chest, face, throat, and tongue. SJ was clinically diagnosed with myasthenia gravis, an autoimmune disease that leads to fluctuating muscle weakness and fatigue. Voluntary muscle weakness is the main symptom; muscles become weaker with continued physical activity. Dysphagia (difficulty swallowing), dysarthria (slurred speech), and breathing difficulties can also be outcomes.

Results of naming and memory tests, that is, the BNT, the MMSE, and the MoCA, indicated low-to-average performance (BNT = 54/60; MMSE 25/30; MoCA = 25/30). In addition, the neurologist and psychologist both reported that SJ scored poor-to-low average on tests regarding attention. This was true in tests of focused and/or divided attention. SJ answered quickly and inaccurately in the poor to borderline range on tasks of sustained attention. Short-term memory scores were low average to average, with difficulty in verbal short-term memory tasks opposed to visual short-term memory, which was average. Delayed memory scores were also low average to average and cues did not significantly enhance results. Letter and semantic verbal fluency scores were also low average to average. Visuo-constructional skills were borderline due to poor planning. SJ scored impaired to borderline on a time-sequencing and set-shifting task. Borderline scores were also present on complex reasoning tasks. Nonverbal reasoning was low average to average. Verbal fluency was borderline. According to the neurologist, SJ presented with "mild subcortical dysfunction" with frontoparietal location consistent with lesions found in the front and left parietal areas as revealed by repeated MRI studies.

Cognitive-language therapy was not formally provided as SJ was functional in both activities of daily living and work activities. SJ did not receive conventional speech-language therapy. However, SJ's sister was a speech-language pathologist and offered strategies, including word naming tasks, reading, writing, word memory tasks, auditory attention tasks, divided attention tasks, working memory tasks, and cognitive speed tasks.[11-14]

72.6 Outcome

Four months after the onset of symptoms, SJ reported that her episodes of confusion and cognitive issues ceased. After a 3-day course of high-dose Solu-Medrol (a corticosteroid), symptoms dramatically improved, that is, sustained attention and recall and retrieval of information. SJ reported near immediate improvement of memory and attention-related skills. SJ continued treatment (methotrexate and intravenous immunoglobulin) for myasthenia gravis and undifferentiated connective tissue disorder, both autoimmune disorders. In addition, SJ received anticoagulation therapy for autoimmune blood coagulation dysfunction. SJ reported that tasks of attention when presented sequentially and slowly have the highest degree of success. Short-term and delayed memory tasks continue to be facilitated by the use of calendars, note-taking applications and programs, and recording of sequentially based tasks. Activities undertaken systematically and slowly have a higher rate of completion and success. SJ's cognitive function improved; her pre- and postintervention performances, as measured by the BNT and the MMSE, were as follows: (1) BNT preintervention = 54/60 and postintervention = 60/60, and (2) MMSE preintervention = 25/30 and postintervention = 30/30.

72.7 Key Points

- AEs can affect patients of all ages.
- Treatment may consist of corticosteroid drug intervention along with cognitive-language therapy.
- Compensatory strategies may include note-taking applications, recording events on a sequential basis, systematically

slowing down tasks for higher completion rates, and/or use of calendars.

Suggested Readings

[1] Ancelin ML, Carrière I, Helmer C, et al. Steroid and nonsteroidal anti-inflammatory drugs, cognitive decline, and dementia. Neurobiol Aging. 2012; 33(9): 2082–2090

[2] Wolkowitz OM, Lupien SJ, Bigler ED. The "steroid dementia syndrome": a possible model of human glucocorticoid neurotoxicity. Neurocase. 2007; 13 (3):189–200

References

[1] Leypoldt F, Armangue T, Dalmau J. Autoimmune encephalopathies. Ann NY Acad Sci. 2015; 1338:94–114

[2] Flanagan EP, Caselli RJ. Autoimmune encephalopathy. Semin Neurol. 2011; 31 (2):144–157

[3] Rey A. L'examen psychologique dans les cas d'encéphalopathie traumatique. Arch Psychol. 1941; 28:21

[4] Kaplan EF, Goodglass H, Weintraub S. The Boston Naming Test. 2nd ed. Philadelphia, PA: Lea & Febiger; 1983

[5] Folstein MF, Folstein SE, McHugh PR. "Mini-mental state." A practical method for grading the cognitive state of patients for the clinician. J Psychiatr Res. 1975; 12(3):189–198

[6] Nasreddine ZS, Phillips NA, Bédirian V, et al. The Montreal Cognitive Assessment, MoCA: a brief screening tool for mild cognitive impairment. J Am Geriatr Soc. 2005; 53(4):695–699

[7] McKeon A. Immunotherapeutics for autoimmune encephalopathies and dementias. Curr Treat Options Neurol. 2013; 15(6):723–737

[8] American Speech-Language-Hearing Association. Knowledge and skills needed by speech-language pathologists providing services to individuals with cognitive-communication disorders [knowledge and skills]. 2005. Available at: http://www.asha.org/policy/KS2005-00078/. Last accessed October 30, 2016. doi:10.1044/policy.KS2005-00078

[9] Mijajlovic M, Mirkovic M, Dackovic J, Zidverc-Trajkovic J, Sternic N. Clinical manifestations, diagnostic criteria and therapy of Hashimoto's encephalopathy: report of two cases. J Neurol Sci. 2010; 288(1–2):194–196

[10] Caselli RJ, Drazkowski JF, Wingerchuk DM. Autoimmune encephalopathy. Mayo Clin Proc. 2010; 85(10):878–880

[11] Acerson A. Cognitive therapy for mild traumatic brain injury. 2013. Available at: https://thespeechclinic.wordpress.com/2013/02/28/cognitive-therapy-for-mild-traumatic-brain-injury/. Last accessed January 28, 2015

[12] Ylvisaker M, Szekeres S, Feeney T. Communication disorders associated with traumatic brain injury. In: Chapey R, Ed. Language Intervention Strategies in Aphasia and Related Neurogenic Communication Disorders. Philadelphia, PA: Lippincott Williams & Wilkins; 2001:745–208

[13] Hopper T, Bayles K. Management of neurogenic communication disorders associated with dementia. In: Chapey R, Ed. Language Intervention Strategies in Aphasia and Related Neurogenic Communication Disorders. Philadelphia, PA: Lippincott Williams & Wilkins; 2001:829–846

[14] Murray L, Chapey R. Assessment of language disorders in adults. In: Chapey R, Ed. Language Intervention Strategies in Aphasia and Related Neurogenic Communication Disorders. Philadelphia, PA: Lippincott Williams & Wilkins; 2001:55–126

73 Stroke-Induced Aphasia and Dysphagia: Acute and Long-Term Implications

Kerry Lenius

73.1 Introduction

Dysphagia and aphasia following stroke can yield complex challenges to the speech-language pathologists (SLPs), both acutely and more long term. In particular, challenges with health care communication within and across the continuum of care can pose significant obstacles to the implementation of effective rehabilitation strategies.

73.2 Clinical History and Description

SB was a 64-year-old male with a history of hypertension, prior stroke, atrial fibrillation, hepatitis C, and cirrhosis. He was admitted to the university medical center after an anterior division left middle cerebral artery stroke, resulting in damage to the left frontal lobe (▶ Fig. 73.1). He was followed by an SLP in the acute care setting for both speech/language and swallowing deficits. At that time, SB presented with global aphasia, apraxia, and oropharyngeal dysphagia. A nasogastric tube was acutely employed for nutrition and a gastrostomy tube (G-tube) was eventually placed prior to discharge. He returned to an outpatient clinic 6 months after

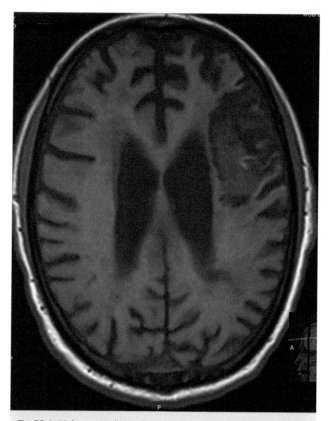

Fig. 73.1 SB brain MR demonstrating left anterior middle cerebral artery stroke with frontal lobe damage.

his stroke. He was wheelchair bound with global aphasia and remained dependent on G-tube feedings.

73.3 Clinical Testing

Upon admission immediately following the stroke, the Nurse Swallow Screen was completed,[1] which SB failed due to somnolence and dysarthria. On the second day of hospitalization, the SLP assessed SB using the Mann Assessment of Swallowing Ability (MASA)[2] and the bedside version of the Western Aphasia Battery Revised.[3] Results are presented in ▶ Table 73.1 and ▶ Table 73.2. Verbal output was limited and unintelligible. SB

Table 73.1 MASA assessment results. Higher scores reflect less impairment

Scored item	Score/possible	Description
Alertness	10/10	Awake/alert
Cooperation	10/10	Willing to participate/cooperative
Auditory comprehension	2/10	No response to speech
Respiration	10/10	Clear chest on chest X-ray
Respiratory rate for swallow	3/5	Uncoordinated
Dysphasia	2/5	No functional speech
Dyspraxia	2/5	Groping
Dysarthria	2/5	Speech attempts are unintelligible
Saliva	3/5	Drooling at times
Lip seal	3/5	Unilaterally weak
Tongue movement	4/10	Minimal movement
Tongue strength	2/10	Gross weakness on assessment
Tongue coordination	5/10	Gross incoordination
Oral prep	8/10	Oral bolus escape
Gag	1/5	No gag detected
Palate	2/10	No volitional movement due to apraxia
Bolus clearance	5/10	Some clearance
Oral transit	4/10	>10-s delay
Cough reflex	3/5	Weak reflexive cough
Voluntary cough	2/10	Unable to produce volitional cough; apraxia
Voice	10/10	Good quality with minimal voicing attempts
Trache	10/10	No tracheostomy
Pharyngeal phase	8/10	Slow initiation subjective judgment as not visualized with imaging
Pharyngeal response	5/10	Throat clearing after PO trials
Total score	**116/300**	**Severe dysphagia**

Table 73.2 WAB-R bedside assessment results (higher scores reflect less impairment)

Scored item	Score/possible	Description
Spontaneous speech: content	0/10	No meaningful responses
Spontaneous speech: fluency	0/10	Nonfluent
Auditory verbal comprehension (yes/no)	0/10	No response
Sequential commands	0/10	Unable
Repetition	0/10	Unable
Object naming	0/10	None
Bedside aphasia score	**0/100**	**Severe global**

was unable to follow verbal directions and displayed signs of oral and limb apraxia. Recommendations were made for continued aphasia therapy and for SB to remain NPO (nil per os) with the goal of instrumental evaluation of swallow function once oral acceptance improved at the bedside.

One week after the stroke, SB participated in a modified barium swallow (MBS) study for further assessment of dysphagia. The study revealed severe oral and mild pharyngeal dysphagia. Oral and pharyngeal swallow initiation was delayed with severe postswallow oral residue. However, only minimal pharyngeal residue with one instance of supraglottic penetration was observed with thin liquids during a secondary swallow, which cleared with completion of the swallow. Given his oral deficits and inconsistent ability to take trials by mouth (PO) at bedside, continued nothing by mouth (NPO) status was recommended; however, he had a good prognosis for return to PO diet with rehabilitation. On day 8 post stroke, a G-tube was placed to support ongoing nutritional needs in preparation of discharge to a subacute facility. At day 11, SB's ability to accept and clear PO trials from the oral cavity with the SLP improved. A puree solid/thin liquid diet, with supplemental G-tube feedings, was recommended. SB was discharged on day 12, a Saturday, with continued global aphasia and NPO status. It is possible that, in the haste of discharge, the SLP oral diet recommendation was overlooked as nutritional needs were already addressed via G-tube.

73.4 Questions and Answers for the Reader

1. Did the clinical findings in this case match anticipated findings given the stroke location?
   a) No, I would have anticipated Wernicke's aphasia.
   b) No, I would have anticipated severe pharyngeal dysphagia.
   c) Yes, global aphasia, apraxia, and dysphagia are typical of SB's infarct location.
   d) It is not possible to predict clinical impairments based on stroke location.

Answer: c is correct. Left frontal lobe damage often results in nonfluent aphasia and apraxia, and can result in dysphagia.

a is incorrect as temporal lobe damage is the area associated with Wernicke's aphasia and SB had frontal lobe involvement.

b is incorrect. Severe pharyngeal dysphagia is more common with brainstem strokes.

d is incorrect. Predictions can be made based on neurological findings, although a clinical assessment is still required.

2. Which suggestion would be the most helpful to SB's caregiver?
   a) Tell SB exactly what you want him to do and expect him to follow your instructions. If he does not, then he is being manipulative.
   b) Teach SB American sign language (ASL) to communicate.
   c) Stay home and keep SB away from family and friends. They are not able to communicate with him, so it would just be frustrating for them.
   d) Allow behaviors (eating and conversation attempts) to be as stress-free and natural as possible. Provide simple picture and gesture supports to get your message across.

Answer: d is correct. Automatic tasks are easier to perform for individuals with apraxia and use of pictures and gestures can support comprehension.

a is incorrect. SB has impaired language comprehension and is not likely to understand verbal instructions.

b is incorrect. ASL is a language and therefore difficult for someone with aphasia and apraxia to utilize effectively. However, training simple gestures may be beneficial.

c is incorrect. Individuals with aphasia are often excluded from conversations and social interactions. This exclusion negatively impacts people with aphasia on a psychosocial level.

3. Which is *not* a key factor that often delays discharge to a subacute facility?
   a) Establishing a method for nutrition and hydration.
   b) Ability to communicate wants and needs.
   c) Insurance coverage.
   d) Bed availability.

Answer: b is correct. The inability to communicate does *not* delay subacute placement. This is one reason why many physicians may believe it is only important for the SLP to address swallowing in acute care.

a is incorrect. Establishing a nutrition route is crucial prior to acute care discharge. In our region of the country (Florida), most skilled nursing facilities will not accept a patient for placement with a nasogastric tube.

c is incorrect. Insurance is a key factor in determining whether a patient will be accepted into a facility. Some facilities do hold charity beds for those without insurance.

d is incorrect. Bed availability, especially if long-term care is anticipated, is often problematic as space is limited.

4. SB resided at the skilled nursing facility (SNF) for 4 months before returning home. He was not initiated on an oral diet at the SNF. What could the SNF speech pathologist have done to facilitate returning this patient to oral intake?
   a) Review acute care records, contact the hospital SLP if records are not available, assess SB's current ability, and, if still indicated, request SB to be started on oral intake supplemented by tube feeding as needed.

b) Continue NPO and repeat the MBS 1 month after he arrived to the skilled facility.

c) Tell the physician at the skilled facility that because SB did not aspirate on his swallow study, he should immediately be placed on a regular diet and tube feedings should be terminated.

d) Initiate electrical stimulation to target pharyngeal contraction and laryngeal closure.

Answer: a is correct. The oral apraxia and difficulty initiating a swallow were main contributors to the dysphagia. Reinstating at least some oral intake as soon as possible would have been beneficial to reestablish motor patterns for oral swallow, prevent disuse atrophy, and improve quality of life and functional ability.

b is incorrect. This would prolong SB's NPO status and, while an MBS could be repeated, that study is done in a stressful, structured environment, which is often less successful for individuals with impaired motor planning.

c is incorrect. Though SB did not have aspiration on his MBS, his oral phase of swallow was not efficient and he may not have been able to meet nutritional needs on an oral diet alone. A dietitian can assist with transitioning from PO with tube feeding supplements to PO alone once adequate oral intake was established.

d is incorrect. Pharyngeal contraction and laryngeal closure were not impaired.

73.5 Description of Disorder and Recommended Treatment

73.5.1 Communication

During his acute care hospital stay, SB was unable to reliably communicate information effectively due to global aphasia and apraxia. Due to these deficits, a yes/no board with hand-over-hand rehearsal to initially assist motor planning (due to an associated limb apraxia) was employed to answer simple questions. Even after the motor planning rehearsal, answers were only 40% reliable, but this method provided an outlet and starting point for communication. Acute care therapy focused on establishing the most reliable communication methods and educating nursing and family members on aphasia and communication strategies to use with SB. His nurse, while with good intention, placed a 20-item picture board at his bedside and expected him to independently respond to her questions. Additionally, during one visit, SB's wife was present and the SLP used that opportunity to educate her on aphasia, the impact on communication, and communication strategies.

73.5.2 Swallowing

SB also presented with a significant oropharyngeal dysphagia characterized primarily by delayed swallow initiation and oral residue. In a hospital acute care setting, swallowing is frequently seen as a priority for rehabilitation.[4] Oral dysphagia

and difficulty with motor planning were the predominant factors characterizing SB's dysphagia, which presented a challenge for direct intervention as he was largely unable to follow commands. As is often the case with apraxia of swallow, SB was more successful with oral consumption when he was allowed to independently hold a cup and spontaneously feed himself. During SLP sessions in acute care, therapeutic PO trials of various consistencies were offered. However, his swallowing success was inconsistent. His performance ranged from successfully and efficiently consuming 8 ounces of liquid to being unable to adequately transfer material from the cup into his mouth to simply holding the bolus in his oral cavity without initiating a swallow.

73.6 Outcome

Records of his care at the subacute facility were unavailable; however, SB returned to our hospital clinic 6 months later for an outpatient MBS. During that period, he remained NPO, continued to present with severe communication impairment, and had a significant right hemiplegia. At the time of the outpatient evaluation, SB lived at home without continued therapy services. His spouse accompanied him to the appointment; he remained wheelchair bound and G-tube-dependent.

SB's wife reported difficulty managing tube feedings at home and requested reevaluation for SB to possibly return to an oral diet. MBS revealed delayed swallow, resulting in spillage to the vallecular space before the swallow. However, he spontaneously compensated with early laryngeal vestibule closure without aspiration (▶ Fig. 73.2). Oral initiation and oral clearance had improved in comparison to his past assessment and he was able to masticate solids. Based on these results, an oral diet was recommended (regular solids and liquids) and that the G-tube be

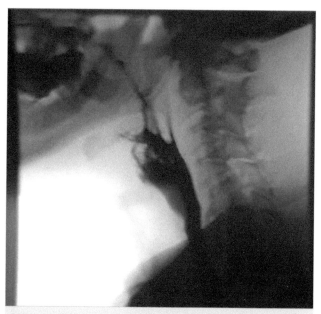

Fig. 73.2 Image from SB's first rehab swallow study in lateral view during thin liquid swallows.

removed once SB demonstrated that he was able to consume a total oral diet without the need for supplemental nutrition. Occupational therapy was also consulted to evaluate the potential for adaptive feeding utensils to improve self-feeding.

When SB's wife was asked about her husband's aphasia at the outpatient visit, her response was, "Aphasia? What's that?" She did not recall hearing the term, despite the extensive education provided during his acute care and likely during his subacute hospitalization. This situation highlights how caregivers are often overwhelmed by terms and information during the acute phases of stroke and additional reinforcement throughout the rehabilitation continuum is required.[5] Informal language testing revealed persistent global aphasia, but he did respond to yes/no questions provided in an aphasia-friendly format (picture supports) with 70% accuracy. SB's wife expressed concern regarding a lack of community resources and support. She reported that they did not have access to personal transportation and were dependent on the city bus to get to the hospital and appointments. Transferring SB into the bus was particularly challenging, and therefore they rarely left the house. Due to transportation concerns, follow-up aphasia services were recommended with home health care. Finally, the team provided SB and his wife with information regarding free community resources such as a local aphasia support group.

73.7 Key Points

- It is imperative that SLPs assess patients to determine the most appropriate augmentative communication options including access methods and device complexity.
- Following verbal instructions is *not* a requirement for swallowing. Many individuals with aphasia and/or dementia do retain the ability to swallow even when unable to comprehend verbal instructions.
- Do not assume people know and understand the word "aphasia" even if they are the primary caregiver for someone with aphasia. Reeducate at every opportunity.
- Aspiration and aspiration risk are not the only reasons someone may be NPO following acute stroke.
- People with aphasia are often impacted at all levels of the International Classification of Functioning, including personal and environmental factors.

Suggested Readings

[1] Simmons-Mackie N, Kagan A. Application of the ICF in aphasia. Semin Speech Lang. 2007; 28(4):244–253

[2] Wilmskoetter J, Herbert TL, Bonilha HS. Factors associated with gastrostomy tube removal in patients with dysphagia after stroke. Nutr Clin Pract. 2017; 32(2):166–174

References

[1] Titsworth WL, Abram J, Fullerton A, et al. Prospective quality initiative to maximize dysphagia screening reduces hospital-acquired pneumonia prevalence in patients with stroke. Stroke. 2013; 44(11):3154–3160

[2] Mann G. MASA: The Mann Assessment of Swallowing Ability. Albany, NY: Singular Thomson Learning; 2002

[3] Kertesz A. The Western Aphasia Battery. New York, NY: Grune & Stratton; 1982

[4] Foster A, O'Halloran R, Rose M, Worrall L. "Communication is taking a back seat": speech pathologists' perceptions of aphasia management in acute hospital settings. Aphasiology. 2016; 30(5):585–608

[5] Danzl MM, Harrison A, Hunter EG, et al. "A lot of things passed me by": rural stroke survivors' and caregivers' experience of receiving education from health care providers. J Rural Health. 2016; 32(1):13–24

74 Cognitive Rehabilitation for a Combat-Injured Veteran with Mild TBI and Comorbid Conditions

Donald L. MacLennan and Leslie Nitta

74.1 Introduction

Mild traumatic brain injury (TBI), also called concussion, is the signature injury of the wars in Iraq and Afghanistan, although there is nothing "mild" about these injuries. Mild TBI in combat-injured veterans is typically complicated by comorbid conditions, such as posttraumatic stress disorder (PTSD), depression, anxiety, chronic pain, and sleep disturbance, all of which contribute to cognitive symptoms that impact the integration of combat veterans into home and community.

74.2 Clinical History and Description

RJ, a 23-year-old male Army veteran, presented 2 years after sustaining a mild TBI related to an armored vehicle accident while under fire in Afghanistan. He experienced no loss of consciousness, but reported feeling dazed. He experienced headache and trouble concentrating, symptoms that resolved within 2 days allowing him to return to duty without further complaint. Approximately 6 months after his return to the United States, he began experiencing problems with concentration and memory that coincided with the diagnosis of PTSD, anxiety, depression, sleep disturbance, and chronic pain (headache, low back pain). At the time of evaluation by the VA Polytrauma Team, RJ was a full-time student in a bachelor's degree program in psychology and has the long-term goal of completing a master's degree in industrial and organizational psychology. He expressed concern that cognitive challenges were undermining his academic performance. Specifically, he reported significant distractibility when listening to lectures, taking notes, and struggling to recall information during examinations.

74.3 Clinical Testing

Interview: The clinician and veteran engaged in an interview/ conversation in which the veteran endorsed cognitive concerns described above. He described how these difficulties impacted daily functioning at home and school, and his expectations for therapy. He also described treatment he was receiving for comorbid conditions.

Table 74.1 Repeatable Battery for the Assessment of Neuropsychological Status (RBANS)

Index	Score	Percentile
Immediate memory	125	96
Visuospatial/con-structional	100	50
Language	113	81
Attention	113	81
Delayed memory	81	10

Testing included a combination of objective testing and self-report measures including the *Repeatable Battery for Assessment of Neuropsychological Status*[1] (RBANS). The RBANS is a cognitive screening tool with excellent reliability and validity. Performance on measures of attention, immediate memory, visual/constructional skills, and language were within the normal range. Mild impairment in delayed verbal memory was observed (▶ Table 74.1).

Repeatable Battery for the Assessment of Neuropsychological Status Self-report measures, the *Behavioral Rating Inventory of Executive Functions-Adult*[2] (BRIEF-A), and the *Return to School Needs Assessment*[3] were completed. RJ reported the perception of impaired metacognitive aspects of executive functions, including severe challenges in working memory and milder challenges in task monitoring, planning and organization, and initiation (▶ Table 74.2). He was particularly concerned about academic readiness, and specifically (1) focusing on lectures, (2) taking good notes in class, and (3) remembering what he had learned when taking tests (▶ Table 74.3). He confirmed significant difficulty in these areas. He was receiving mostly Cs in his classes and expressed concern that he would not have a sufficient GPA for graduate school.

Behavioral Rating Inventory of Executive Functions-Adult
Return to School Needs Assessment[3]:
Responses on a 5-point scale (*not at all difficult* to *extremely difficult*).

Interpretation: RJ presented with normal performance on objective cognitive measures with the exception of mild impairment in delayed verbal memory. However, self-Report Measures identified significant challenges in a variety of cognitive areas. This disparity between objective and self-report instruments is frequently seen and does not necessarily suggest that RJ did not put forth adequate effort on the objective measures. In this case, the veteran had shown excellent effort during testing. His symptoms were validated and discussed in terms of potential response to cognitive rehabilitation strategies.

Table 74.2 Behavioral Rating Inventory of Executive Functions-Adult (BRIEF-A)

Index	T-score	Comment
Behavioral index	64, just below cut-off for impairment	Reflects a perception of mild challenges in the areas of inhibition of behavior and the ability to shift behavioral set
Metacognitive index	72, above cut-off for impairment	Reflects a perception of significant challenges in the areas of working memory, task monitoring, and planning and organization; and mild challenges in the area of initiation
Global executive component	72	Reflects a perception of significant challenges in executive functions

Table 74.3 Return to School Needs Assessment

Moderately degree of difficulty	Staying awake in class; listening to instructor and taking notes at the same time; and keeping emotions under control toward instructors and classmates
Quite a bit of difficulty	Maintaining attention in class, when reading, when at work or school; organizing notes from lecture; remembering to bring completed assignments to class; working with others on group assignments; writing in a clear manner; keeping a balance between school and other life activities
Extreme degree of difficulty	Selecting a topic for a paper, recalling learned information when taking a test, and focusing while reading a home

74.4 Questions and Answers for the Reader

1. What is the typical recovery trajectory of neurocognitive symptoms for the vast majority of individuals who have sustained a concussion/mild TBI without abnormal findings on traditional neuroimaging (i.e., MRI, CT)?
   a) Possible significant cognitive symptoms during the first 72 hours following the inciting event, with resolution of significant symptoms within 1 to 3 weeks for athletes and up to 3 months for most individuals.
   b) Some individuals may experience neurocognitive symptoms beyond 3 months; however, cognitive difficulties would be expected to be subtle.
   c) Some individuals may experience severe neurocognitive symptoms beyond 3 months that require up to 3 years of cognitive rehabilitation to achieve grossly functional status.
   d) Persistent severe symptoms beyond 3 months postinjury can result in lifelong disability.
   e) a and b.

Answer: e is correct. See explanations below.

a is partially correct. The majority of people with uncomplicated mild TBI show recovery in days to weeks after the injury.

b is partially correct. A small proportion of people show mild persisting symptoms beyond 3 months postinjury.

c is incorrect. Individuals who report severe cognitive problems after sustaining a single uncomplicated concussion/mild TBI are believed to experience symptoms that are multifactorial in nature and unlikely to be a result of a discrete uncomplicated concussion/mild TBI.

d is incorrect. Clinicians should be aware that extended treatment of reported cognitive problems related to an uncomplicated concussion/mild TBI is highly likely to create an impression of disability that may have lifelong negative consequences to the client.

2. What factors could contribute to the self-perception of "severe" executive function impairment revealed through responses on the BRIEF-A?
   a) A remote concussion/mild TBI.
   b) A mental health condition.
   c) Perfectionism.
   d) Malingering.
   e) b and c.

Answer: e is correct. See explanations below.

b is partially correct. Concentration and memory problems are so common among those who experience depression and anxiety disorders that they are included among the diagnostic criteria.

a is incorrect. Individuals who experience persistent cognitive complaints after mild TBI 3 months or greater after sustaining a concussion are atypical and would be expected to, at most, have subtle cognitive problems for which they would likely be able to compensate through use of strategies; a persistent "severe" cognitive impairment is more likely to be seen in those who have experienced a more severe head injury or dementia.

c is partially correct. Biopsychosocial conceptualization of poor outcome from mild TBI cites many factors that contribute to postconcussion symptoms. People characterized as perfectionistic are likely to perceive normal lapses of concentration or memory as symptoms of impairment.

d is incorrect. While malingering may occur, it is far from typical. This veteran showed excellent effort on objective testing and performed well on formal effort measures in neuropsychological testing.

3. What are some of the reasons for everyday memory lapses? For example, have you ever personally experienced any of these memory "failures"? If so, what are the factors that may have contributed to your own memory "failures"?
   a) Poor organizational skills or a time management lapse.
   b) Decreased motivation.
   c) Inattention.
   d) All or any combination of the above.

Answer: d is correct. Everyone forgets something from time to time. It is probably no accident that virtually every mobile phone has native reminder apps that help us remember future appointments, deadlines, phone numbers, addresses, etc.

4. Cognitive symptoms occur after mild TBI and are associated with comorbid conditions such as PTSD, anxiety, depression, chronic pain, and sleep disturbance. What is true about the appropriate time to initiate cognitive rehabilitation after mild TBI with comorbid conditions?
   a) Cognitive rehabilitation should begin when comorbid conditions have resolved.
   b) Treatment should begin with promoting positive expectation for recovery while simultaneously addressing psychiatric symptoms, somatic complaints, and self-care routines.

c) Low-dose cognitive rehabilitation may be used as an adjunct treatment for comorbid conditions.

d) Provide cognitive rehabilitation when cognitive symptoms persist beyond 3 months postinjury.

e) b and c.

Answer: e is correct. See explanations below.

b is partially correct. As comorbid conditions may resolve quickly with treatment and are likely the primary cause of cognitive complaints, early treatment may eliminate the need for formal cognitive rehabilitation.

a is incorrect. Comorbid conditions may persist over time and the cognitive symptoms associated with those conditions may negatively impact function at home, school, or work.

c is partially correct. Cognitive symptoms and associated maladaptive responses may interfere with treatments for comorbid conditions. For example, problems with memory and distractibility may affect a person's ability to follow through with treatment recommendations. When this occurs, cognitive rehabilitation delivered concurrently with other behavioral therapies may help with adherence and implementation of therapeutic activities such as taking medications and completing therapy-related assignments.

d is incorrect. Comorbid conditions may persist over time and the cognitive symptoms associated with those conditions may negatively impact function at home, school, or work. This may further increase stress and anxiety and amplify the comorbid conditions. Cognitive strategies that facilitate success in resuming everyday activities diminish stress and anxiety and provide a better foundation for recovery of comorbid conditions.

74.5 Description of Problem and Recommended Treatment

RJ identified challenges with working memory and distractibility in particular. He identified distractibility as the underlying cognitive challenge impacting his ability to focus on lectures and take complete notes in class. His method of study, reading and rereading notes without self-testing, raised questions as to whether he had sufficient judgment of learning to discriminate learned from unlearned material in his notes.

Initial treatment focused on education regarding the nature of his injury so as to foster positive expectations for recovery and to promote more accurate attribution of symptoms to mental health conditions rather than to a mild brain injury. Misattribution of symptoms as a result of brain injury can maintain the perception of cognitive disability. Cognitive rehabilitation was provided in the context of a dynamic coaching approach in which RJ had the autonomy to select goals and strategies of treatment. The clinician served as a coach to model and explicitly teach self-regulatory skills critical to problem-solving as he implemented strategies at school. RJ selected self-talk, silently telling himself to "focus" at intervals during lectures, as a metacognitive strategy to enhance attention to lectures. He selected the use of a smartpen, an assistive technology strategy that audio records lectures in such a way that the recording is anchored to specific locations on his notes, as a strategy to efficiently retrieve missed notes after the lecture. He took notes using the Cornell Note Taking method and used key words on the left side of his notes to self-test learning after a delay, enabling him to more accurately identify learned from unlearned information.

74.6 Outcome

Testing: Performance on objective testing using the RBANS at the end of treatment did not significantly differ from initial evaluation. However, RJ's self-report measures showed significant symptom reduction. Although he continued to report challenges with working memory on self-report measures, the magnitude of those challenges was greatly reduced and the metacognitive strategy portion of the BRIEF-A was below the threshold for impaired performance. His perceived academic difficulty also decreased on the Return to School Needs Inventory. He reported mild difficulty focusing on lectures, mild difficulty remembering what he had learned when taking tests, and no difficulty taking good notes in class.

Academic performance: RJ's grades improved from mostly Cs to mostly As with some Bs. His professors commented on the improvements in the quality of his work and he felt confident in his ability to achieve his academic goals. The effectiveness of his strategies remained stable during times of increased stress, as when buying a house, and he reported continued success in school at 3- and 6-month follow-up appointments.

74.7 Key Points

- For many combat-injured veterans with mild TBI, persisting cognitive symptoms may be associated with comorbid conditions (PTSD, anxiety, depression, chronic pain, sleep disturbance) rather than the mild TBI. Such cases show a symptom trajectory of immediate presentation of cognitive symptoms at the time of injury with rapid resolution followed by delayed onset of cognitive symptoms coinciding with the diagnosis of comorbid conditions.

- Combat veterans with mild TBI often perform normally or near normally on objective measures of cognitive performance. However, they often report significant cognitive symptoms on self-report. This disparity does not mean that such symptoms are not "real." Clinicians are advised to validate these symptoms and treat cognitive deficits regardless of etiology.

- Cognitive symptoms respond well to strategy-based approaches to cognitive rehabilitation that employ a combination of metacognitive strategies and assistive technology for cognition. Awareness training is typically not required as combat-injured veterans show excellent awareness of their strengths and challenges, and may hyperfocus on those symptoms.

- The effectiveness of cognitive rehabilitation is enhanced by a collaborative approach that emphasizes patient autonomy and positive expectation for recovery. Active ingredients for this approach include education regarding the nature and recovery trajectories of mild TBI and comorbid conditions, use of motivational interviewing techniques, and a dynamic coaching approach to cognitive rehabilitation that empowers the veteran to select his/her own goals and strategies and to self-evaluate the effectiveness of the strategies.

Suggested Readings

[1] Working Group to Develop a Clinician's Guide to Cognitive Rehabilitation in mTBI for Military Service Members and Veterans. Clinician's Guide to Cognitive Rehabilitation in Mild Traumatic Brain Injury: Application for Military Service Members and Veterans. Rockville, MD: American Speech-Language-Hearing Association; 2016. Available at: http://www.asha.org/uploadedFiles/ASHA/Practice_Portal/Clinical_Topics/Traumatic_Brain_Injury_in_Adults/Clinicians-Guide-to-Cognitive-Rehabilitation-in-Mild-Traumatic-Brain-Injury.pdf. Last accessed December 12, 2017

[2] Cooper DB, Bowles AO, Vanderploeg R, et al. Study of Cognitive Rehabilitation Effectiveness (SCORE) Study Manuals. 2016. Available at: http://dvbic.dcoe.mil/study-manuals. Last accessed December 12, 2017

[3] Iverson GL, Silverberg N, Lange RT, Zasler ND. Conceptualizing outcome from mild traumatic brain injury. In: Arciniegas DB, Bullock MR, Kreutzer JS, Eds. Brain Injury Medicine. Principles and Practice. 2nd ed. New York, NY: Demos Medical Publishing; 2013:470–497

References

[1] Randolph, C. Repeatable Battery for the Assessment of Neuropsychological Status (RBANS): Test Manual. San Antonio, TX: Harcourt; 1998

[2] Roth RM, Isquith PK, Gioia GA. Behavior Rating Inventory of Executive Function–Adult Version: Test Manual. Lutz, FL: Psychological Assessment Resources; 2005

[3] Zarzecki MA, Crawford E, Smith-Hammond C. Return to School Needs Assessment. Unpublished; 2009

75 Interdisciplinary Collaboration for a Client with Alzheimer's Disease

Robert Maxwell

75.1 Introduction

It is estimated that by the year 2050 approximately 16 million Americans alone will suffer from Alzheimer's disease.[1] Speech-language pathologists play a crucial and evolving role in the interdisciplinary management of the cognitive-linguistic and physical complications associated with this progressive neurological condition.

75.2 Clinical History and Description

JK was an 81-year-old male who transitioned to an assisted living environment after a brief acute care hospitalization following a fall at home. His spouse reported JK had become agitated during an attempt to assist him with dressing, causing him to lose his balance and fall. During his acute care admission, JK was dehydrated and experiencing unintentional weight loss warranting treatment with intravenous fluids and observation. Despite guided orientation to the assisted living community and attempts by facility nursing staff to develop rapport, JK remained resistant to assisted care and documentation reported multiple incident reports of aggression and verbal abuse directed toward staff. JK's spouse reported a gradual change in personality and cognitive function, with increasing falls over the last several years with no clear etiology despite multiple consultations with his general practitioner. Hospital discharge paperwork and neurology consult indicated no evidence of acute injury related to the recent fall or evidence of vascular insult in the available imaging studies. Discharge planning recommended ongoing involvement by an area geriatric psychologist for assistance with suspected Alzheimer's disease and medical management of existing medications to assist with mood regulation and cognitive functioning.

75.3 Clinical Testing

JK was referred to speech-language pathology by nursing for comprehensive individualized assessment of functional communication secondary to frequent communication breakdowns and noncompliance with verbal directives related to assisted care. The referral form noted deficits in short-term memory and frequent frustration when communicating with facility staff. JK was evaluated in his apartment; his spouse, who continued to reside outside of the facility, was not available at the time of assessment. The clinician contacted JK's spouse via telephone to conduct a clinical interview and to review the initial evaluation findings. JK's spouse was invited to join treatment sessions to allow for direct caregiver education and to promote carryover of functional communication strategies designed and implemented throughout the course of treatment.

Table 75.1 Subtest calculated scores and overall cognitive domain scores from the Cognitive Linguistic Quick Test (CLQT) at initial testing

Cognitive domain score table	
Cognitive domain: attention	**Overall score: 86**
Subtest	Calculated score
• Symbol cancellation	63
• Story retelling	8
• Symbol trails	0
• Design memory	6
• Mazes	8
• Design generation	1
Cognitive domain: memory	**Overall score: 85**
Subtest	Calculated score
• Personal facts	28
• Story retelling	24
• Generative naming	3
• Design memory	30
Cognitive domain: executive functions	**Overall score: 6**
Subtest	Calculated score
• Symbol trails	0
• Generative naming	3
• Mazes	2
• Design generation	1
Cognitive domain: language	**Overall score: 19**
Subtest	Calculated score
• Personal facts	4
• Confrontation naming	8
• Story retelling	4
• Generative naming	3
Cognitive domain: visuospatial skills	**Overall score: 33**
Subtest	Calculated score
• Symbol cancellation	14
• Symbol trail	0
• Design memory	12
• Mazes	6
• Design generation	1
Composite severity rating: 1.8	

Interpretation of the CLQT composite severity rating is as follows: 4.0–3.5 = within normal limits; 3.4–2.5 = mild; 2.4–1.5 = moderate; 1.4–1.0 = severe.

JK's cognitive-linguistic evaluation consisted of both informal and formal assessment. During conversation, the clinician noted intermittent episodes of anomia resulting in communication abandonment and frustration. JK's retention of verbally presented directives embedded in conversation was also limited, consistent with spouse and nursing reports. Reading comprehension was screened informally to ensure appropriateness of potential written prompts to be used during intervention, and revealed functional comprehension with sentence-length written material. A review of JK's available medical record indicated no relevant comorbidities, citing only his progressive cognitive-linguistic decline and newly noted probable Alzheimer's disease notation from the supervising neurologist. No significant history of visual or hearing loss was noted.

Through the use of high-interest topics, as noted by JK's initial admission paperwork completed by his spouse, the clinician was able to maintain engagement and progress the initial encounter to include completion of standardized assessments. Feasible assessment tools were selected based on JK's case history and clinical presentation, including the Brief Cognitive Assessment Tool (BCAT)[2] and the Cognitive Linguistic Quick Test (CLQT)[3] to gather additional information to assist in plan of care development. The BCAT was designed as a multidomain cognitive screening tool to assess contextual memory, executive functions, and attentional capacity. JK achieved a total BCAT score of 23, indicating the upper range of moderate cognitive impairment consistent with formal dementia. Question analysis revealed significant impairments in both verbal memory skills and executive functioning related to problem-solving and safety awareness (▶ Table 75.1). The CLQT was also administered to further assess the cognitive domains of attention, memory, language, executive functions, and visuospatial skills. JK achieved a composite severity rating of 1.8, also indicating a moderate cognitive linguistic decline (▶ Table 75.2).

75.4 Questions and Answers for the Reader

1. Based on the available information describing JK's history and current clinical presentation, would the speech-language pathologist include an assessment of swallowing functioning in the initial evaluation?
   a) Yes.
   b) No.

Answer: a is correct. Although the direct nursing referral only cited deficits in functional communication, a review of the medical record indicates recent episodes of both dehydration and unintentional weight loss. Although these conditions may be complications of behaviors associated with JK's progressive cognitive decline, such as lack of initiation or memory impairment, they are also possible complications of difficulty with swallowing warranting a dysphagia screen.

b is incorrect. Although initial referrals serve as a starting point for clinical interview and potential assessment tool selection, speech-language pathologists must remain sensitive to all available information and client reports to allow for adaptation of planned assessments and treatment approaches based on functional presentation and performance.

2. As a member of an interdisciplinary team within the assisted living community, which of the following disciplines should be considered for referral to further assess JK's functional ability?
   a) Physical therapy.
   b) Occupational therapy.
   c) Dietician.
   d) All of the above.

Table 75.2 Subtest and overall scores from the Brief Cognitive Assessment Tool (BCAT) at initial testing

BCAT score table	
Orientation	4
Immediate verbal recall	3
Visual recognition/naming	3
Attention	
• Letter list	0
• Mental control: count backward 20–1	1
• Mental control: recite days of the week backward from Sunday	0
• Digits: forward	1
• Digits: backward	0
Abstraction	3
Language	
• Repeat	1
• Fluency	0
Executive	
• Cognitive shifting	0
• Arithmetic reasoning	1
• Judgment	0
Visuospatial	
• Design	2
• Clock	1
Delayed verbal recall	0
Immediate story recall	1
Delayed visual memory	0
Delayed story recall	0
Story recognition	2
BCAT total score	23

Interpretation of the BCAT total score is as follows: 46–50 = normal; 34–46 = mild cognitive impairment; 26–34 = mild dementia; 0–25 = moderate–to–severe dementia.

Answer: d is correct. As part of an interdisciplinary team, the speech-language pathologist must not only assess and treat the areas associated with their own scope of practice, but also advocate for their clients by connecting them to additional community resources and professionals as determined by functional presentation.

a is incorrect. Although the speech-language pathologist should consider a referral to physical therapy to assess recent loss of balance and noted fall history, a is not the best possible answer.

b is incorrect. Although the speech-language pathologist should consider a referral to occupational therapy to assess noted reports of JK requiring assistance from his spouse to complete dressing tasks and other activities of daily living, b is not the best possible answer.

c is incorrect. Although the speech-language pathologist should consider a referral to the dietician secondary to recent episodes of dehydration and unintentional weight loss, c is not the best possible answer.

3. Medical testing was previously completed to rule out both acute and chronic medical conditions potentially associated

with cognitive-linguistic decline. Which of the following conditions or scenarios may have been medically relevant, if present, in cases involving reports of cognitive-linguistic decline?

a) Initiation of new medication to assist with musculoskeletal pain management.
b) Exacerbation of congestive heart failure.
c) Identification of a new onset urinary tract infection.
d) History of major depressive disorder.
e) All of the above.

Answer: e is correct. See explanations below.

a is partially correct. A wide variety of medications result in changes in cognitive functioning as a potential side effect. Pain medications, including opioids, are known to potentially impact cognitive performance.

b is partially correct. Congestive heart failure negatively impacts the heart's ability to pump the necessary blood throughout the body, including to the brain. Any disruption to the necessary supply of nutrients and oxygen in the brain can negatively impact cognition.

c is partially correct. Any identified systemic infection in the body may negatively impact cognition. Urinary tract infections, especially in elderly populations, are often associated with rapid changes in cognition, also known as delirium.

d is partially correct. Many seemingly unrelated medical conditions, such as depression, can negatively impact cognitive functioning. Speech-language pathologists should complete a thorough review of the client's medical history and consider any such conditions that may be contributing to or serving as the underlying catalyst of cognitive decline.

75.5 Description of Problem and Recommended Treatment

Upon admission to the assisted living facility, JK presented with a recent acute care hospitalization secondary to fall behavior, dehydration, unintentional weight loss, and caregiver reports of exacerbation of progressive cognitive-linguistic decline. Clinical observation noted frequent communication breakdowns and episodes of frustration when assisted care was attempted. Clinical interview of his primary caregiver and review of medical record indicated no known comorbidities impacting cognitive-linguistic abilities and diagnosis of Alzheimer's disease was assigned along with referrals to skilled rehabilitation for further assessment. Formalized assessment of functional communication indicated both expressive and receptive deficits characterized by intermittent episodes of anomia, with no self-directed attempts to repair, and difficulty processing multistep verbal directives embedded in typical conversation. Deficits in attention, executive function, and problem-solving interfered with JK's ability to manage activities of daily living and required caregiver cueing and assistance to sequence activities. A screen of oral mechanisms was within normal limits and no overt signs and symptoms of aspiration were noted with oral intake, indicating recent issues involving dehydration and uninten-

tional weight loss were likely attributed to complications associated with noted cognitive-linguistic deficits versus a true dysphagia. Facility interdisciplinary team monitored oral intake and relevant clinical data to ensure proper nutrition.

Speech-language pathology intervention was recommended five times per week for 1 month. Therapy focused on the development and implementation of a caregiver-driven functional maintenance program to promote the use of compensatory strategies to assist with functional communication when word-finding deficits occurred. Furthermore, sessions focused on strategies to repair communication breakdowns via caregiver use of verbal segmentation and implementation of a cueing hierarchy when presenting verbal directives. All interventions were developed and implemented with a person-centered approach consistent with the International Classification of Functioning, Disability, and Health (ICF) model.[4]

Functional treatment goals targeted the following:

- Auditory comprehension of verbally presented stimuli at the sentence level.
- Use of communication repair strategies during episodes of anomia with only minimal communication partner multimodal cueing.
- Reading comprehension at the phrase and sentence level to allow the introduction of environmental signage in JK's immediate environment to assist with memory and sequencing of daily routines.

Treatment sessions were held in JK's assisted living apartment and common areas to maximize environmental context for desired activities. JK's spouse and immediate facility caregivers were incorporated into treatment sessions to allow for education and modeling related to assisted word retrieval and communication repair strategies in daily care. Semantic-based word retrieval strategies[5] were demonstrated and modeled for both JK and caregivers to improve his functional ability to not only express his basic wants and needs, but also more effectively participate in clinical care plan meetings and desired social activities. The clinician provided direct instruction regarding the listing of semantic features when desired target words could not be retrieved and caregivers were provided instruction on a cueing hierarchy to promote this strategy when JK did not self-initiate. In addition, the clinician participated in assisted care tasks provided by facility nursing staff and modeled verbal segmentation of directives to decrease auditory processing demands and JK's frustrations. By embedding goals directly in functional daily activities, similar to inclusion techniques in a classroom setting, the clinician also demonstrated linguistic mapping of task components to assist in sequencing and overall task completion.

75.6 Outcome

As successful communication strategies were identified, the treating clinician educated JK's spouse and potential communication partners within JK's community setting to improve functional communication with key support personnel, including physical therapy staff, occupational therapy staff, activities staff, nursing, dietary aides, and housekeeping. To maximize functional carryover of communication strategies, the clinician facilitated creation of reminiscing books[6] based on photos and personal memorabilia items provided by JK's spouse. Additional high-interest items for discussion were introduced via the use of technology items, such as the It's Never 2 Late (iN2L)[7] and Google Earth.[8]

Signage was also created and placed at key touch points within JK's room to help prompt the completion of desired tasks and to assist with memory of necessary appointments, relevant safety precautions, etc. As accommodations were implemented to address JK's cognitive-linguistic deficits, his spouse and caregivers reported improved engagement and acceptance of care. Functional communication strategies allowed for increased socialization and participation in facility activities designed to offer both cognitive stimulation and physical exercise. Prior to completion of skilled speech-language pathology services, the clinician provided final recommendations and strategies to maximize functional ability in the form of a functional maintenance plan for JK's caregivers and provided education on monitoring for future changes in functional communication and other speech-language pathology–related areas as JK's medical condition progressed.

75.7 Key Points

- Effective care plan development for individuals with Alzheimer's disease and other forms of dementia requires both informal and formal assessment of functional abilities to ensure interventions will be meaningful to the individual and translate into daily living.
- Speech-language pathologists working with clients with dementia must operate as part of a larger interdisciplinary team that addresses functional concerns in a holistic manner to maximize functional outcomes and carryover.

- Technology and environmental modification can assist clinicians in creating environments that offer context and direction in the absence of direct communication partner cueing.
- When addressing current functional deficits in the context of progressive neurological disorders, the speech-language pathologist must also provide extensive education to caregivers and offer insight regarding the future speech-language-swallowing needs as the underlying illness progresses.

Suggested Readings

[1] Brookshire RH, ed. Introduction to Neurogenic Communication Disorders. 8th Ed. St. Louis, MO: CV Mosby; 2015
[2] Giebel C, Challis D. Translating cognitive and everyday activity deficits into cognitive interventions in mild dementia and mild cognitive impairment. Int J Geriatr Psychiatry. 2015; 30(1):21–31

References

[1] Alzheimer's Association. 2017 Alzheimer's Disease: Facts and Figures 2017. Available at: https://www.alz.org/documents_custom/2017-facts-and-figures.pdf. Last accessed January 14, 2018
[2] Mansbach WE, MacDougall EE, Rosenzweig AS. The Brief Cognitive Assessment Tool (BCAT): a new test emphasizing contextual memory, executive functions, attentional capacity, and the prediction of instrumental activities of daily living. J Clin Exp Neuropsychol. 2012; 34(2):183–194
[3] Helm-Estabrooks N. Cognitive Linguistic Quick Test. San Antonio, TX: PsychCorp; 2001
[4] World Health Organization. International Classification of Functioning, Disability and Health (ICF). Geneva: World Health Organization; 2001
[5] Murry L, Paek E. Behavioral/nonpharmacological approaches to addressing cognitive-linguistic symptoms in individuals with dementia. Perspect ASHA Spec Interest Groups. 2016; 1(15):12–25
[6] O'Shea E, Devane D, Cooney A, et al. The impact of reminiscence on the quality of life of residents with dementia in long-stay care. Int J Geriatr Psychiatry. 2014; 29(10):1062–1070
[7] It's Never 2 Late (iN2L) [Adaptive engagement/rehab technology] 2017. Centennial, CO, www.iN2L.com
[8] Google Earth [Computer program] Version 7.1.5.1557. Mountain View, CA: Google; 2013

76 Efficacy of Transcranial Direct Current Stimulation in Posttraumatic Stress Disorder

Jyutika Mehta

76.1 Introduction

Posttraumatic stress disorder (PTSD) is a psychiatric disorder that can develop after exposure to a traumatic event and affects approximately 3.5% of the adult population in the United States, and is recognized as global mental health concern.[1] Deficits in working memory are observed in PTSD.[2] Memory problems reduce the neurological resources available to PTSD patients and can impact their ability to engage in and respond to treatment with associated negative occupational and social outcomes.[3,4]

76.2 Clinical History and Description

ZM, a 40-year-old male, is a military veteran and diagnosed[2] with combat-associated PTSD presented with memory-related deficits. His presenting concern was difficulty with word recall, which often led to anxiety in social and professional situations. A history of combat-related psychological counseling was reported. There was no history of head injury with loss of consciousness, no neurological or psychiatric condition other than PTSD, no presence of deep brain stimulator, no history of alcohol/drug dependence, or seizures. ZM was prescribed Zoloft (50 mg/day) for anxiety and for mild-to-moderate depression. He was married and his wife reported episodes of difficulty recalling names of familiar friends and family members as well as appropriate words in conversations, which led to frequent frustration and social disengagement.

76.3 Clinical Testing

The primary outcome measure was Wechsler Adult Intelligence Scale (WAIS; Fourth Edition).[5] The test scores provide four indices: Verbal Comprehension Index (VCI), Perceptual Reasoning Index (PRI), Working Memory Index (WMI), and Processing Speed Index (PSI). The VCI is designed to measure verbal reasoning and concept formation. The PRI is designed to measure fluid reasoning in the perceptual domain with tasks that assess nonverbal concept formation, visual perception and organization, visual-motor coordination, learning, and the ability to separate figure and ground in visual stimuli. The WMI measures sustained attention, concentration, and executive functions, while the PSI is an indication of the rapidity with which simple or routine information is processed. All the indices were calculated as standard scores with a mean of 100 and standard deviation of 15. The secondary outcome measures were changes on (1) Beck Depression Inventory-II (BDI-II)[6] and World Health Organization's Quality of Life Questionnaire-Brief Version (WHOQOL-BREF).[7] BDI-II is a screening instrument to quantify

depression symptoms. It is a self-administered, 21-item survey that is scored on a scale of 0 to 3 in a list of four statements arranged in increasing severity about a particular symptom of depression. Quality of life measurement extends beyond measures of disease and pathology and captures important aspects of survey participants' daily social contexts. Primary and secondary outcome measures were administered 1 week prior to transcranial direct current stimulation (tDCS) sessions and 1 week after the 12th treatment.

76.4 Questions and Answers for the Reader

1. What is tDCS?
   a) Transcranial direct current stimulation.
   b) Transcranial direct cranium stimulation.
   c) Transdermal direct current stimulation.
   d) Transformational direct current solution.

Answer: a is correct. Transcranial direct current stimulation (tDCS) is a noninvasive brain stimulation treatment that uses direct electrical currents to stimulate specific parts of the brain.

b is incorrect. "c" in tDCS is current.

c is incorrect. "t" in tDCS is transcranial.

d is incorrect. "t" in tDCS is transcranial and "s" is stimulation.

2. How does tDCS work?
   a) By getting the neurons to fire.
   b) By altering neuron polarity.
   c) By changes in action potential.

Answer: b is correct. tDCS causes polarity-dependent alterations in cortical excitability and activity.

a is incorrect. tDCS does not get neurons to fire but may possibly increase their likelihood of firing.

c is incorrect. tDCS does not influence action potential, but may bring about subthreshold modulation of resting membrane potential.

3. What is working memory?
   a) A type of memory used in procedural tasks.
   b) A type of short-term memory.
   c) A type of long-term memory.

Answer: b is correct. A part of short-term memory that is concerned with perceptual and linguistic processing.

a is incorrect. Working memory is primarily used in linguistic tasks.

c is incorrect. Working memory is part of short-term memory.

4. What is 10–20 International EEG placement?
   a) Recognized method to apply scalp electrodes.

b) Recognized method to study EEG.

c) Recognized method to study neuronal topography.

Answer: a is correct. The International 10–20 system is a recognized method to describe and apply the location of scalp electrodes. This method was developed to ensure standardized reproducibility so that studies could be compared over time and subjects.

b is incorrect. Although used to collect EEG, it is not necessarily a method to study EEG.

c is incorrect. This method can be used to locate appropriate underlying neuronal tissue based on scalp topography, but its primary purpose is to determine electrode placement.

76.5 Description of Problem and Recommended Treatment

A substantial proportion of individuals with PTSD show limited benefit from pharmacological and/or behavioral therapy, and this seems especially true for PTSD-related memory dysfunction. Moreover, pharmacological management often has serious side effects and may lead to poor compliance. Studies have evaluated the efficacy of existing approaches in management of PTSD, and these treatments may have better acceptability in PTSD patients if fewer side effects were noted. In the present case, no serious adverse effect was noted during or after application of tDCS and the patient exhibited improvement in memory measures and overall PTSD symptoms.

Clinical use of tDCS has been reported in the treatment of psychiatric and neurological conditions and has demonstrated

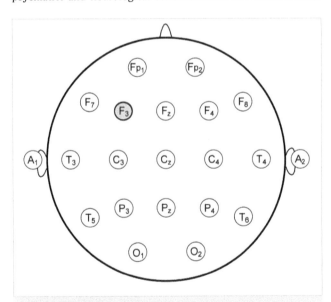

Fig. 76.1 dLPFC corresponds to electrode F3 position on the 10–20 International system of electrode placement.

facilitation of improvements in cognition and working memory.[8] tDCS involves application of weak direct electrical currents to the scalp via sponge electrodes to polarize underlying neurons, which leads to changes in cortical excitability. It is theorized that this excitability extends beyond the period of stimulation. Through this polarity-dependent shift, low-intensity dc current influences neuronal function by inducing neurochemical changes and influences nonneuronal cellular components of the central nervous system.

For ZM, tDCS was applied thrice a week (MWF) for 4 weeks for a total of 12 sessions. Anodal electrode was placed over the left dorsolateral prefrontal cortex (dLPFC) and cathodal electrode was placed on contralateral (right) shoulder according to the 10–20 EEG placement system (▶ Fig. 76.1). This electrode montage was adopted because anodal tDCS of the dLPFC is known to enhance working memory.[8] Precise positioning of electrodes ensures that current is directed to appropriate neuronal tissue. Intensity of current was maintained at 2 mA for 30 minutes during each visit. ZM was monitored throughout the session and asked to report any adverse effect like scalp pain, tingling, itching, or any other discomfort. He did not report any adverse event during the treatment. ZM continued with counseling and medication regimen during the treatment sessions.

76.6 Outcome

ZM showed remarkable response to tDCS treatment sessions. Improvement in working memory as well as marked reduction

Table 76.1 Results of tDCS treatment sessions

Scale	Preintervention score	Postintervention score	Interpretation
Verbal Comprehension Index	101[a]	105[a]	Overall verbal comprehension scores remain unchanged
Perceptual Reasoning Index	92[a]	95[a]	Overall nonverbal reasoning scores remain unchanged
Working Memory Index	75[a]	98[a]	Improved significantly
Processing Speed Index	82[a]	95[a]	Improved significantly
BDI-II	19 (borderline clinical depression)	12 (mild mood disturbance)	Improved significantly

BDI-II, Beck Depression Inventory-II.
[a]Scores are standard scores with mean = 100 and SD = 15. Verbal Comprehension Index and Perceptual Reasoning Index did not change significantly, while Working Memory Index and Processing Speed Index showed significant improvement. BDI scores improved depression classification from borderline clinical depression to mild mood disturbance.

in anxiety and depression symptoms appears to have made significant positive impact on the patient's quality of life. Results were qualitatively analyzed and summarized in ▶ Table 76.1. Overall, verbal comprehension and nonverbal processing did not change as a result of tDCS. However, working memory and processing speed showed significant improvement as a result of tDCS intervention. Specifically, the WMI index improved by over 20 points (over 1 SD), which can be considered a meaningful clinical gain. BDI-II scores were also lowered considerably, resulting in a change of category from "borderline clinically depressed" to "mild mood disturbance." Further, ZM reported increased interest in daily family and social routines, as well as noticeably less difficulty with word recall. His wife reported similar outcomes and stated that ZM appears to be happier and "not as frustrated" leading to a "more harmonious" social interactions and relationships. WHOQOL-BREF responses showed improvement across all domains and a marked reduction in avoidance of social interaction.

76.7 Key Points

- tDCS appears to have improved ZM's ability to recall and resulted in an increase in the rate and in the total amount of recovery of memory functions.
- Although the results in this case are based on single participant and should be interpreted with appropriate caution, such findings can provide empirical evidence upon which a larger clinical trial can be developed.
- Novel approaches are needed to address concerns in the neurorehabilitation field. If noninvasive brain stimulation such as tDCS, either singly or in combination with other therapeutics,

is found to accelerate rate and/or extent of neurocognitive recovery, it will have wide-reaching application in both cost of rehabilitation and quality of life.

Suggested Readings

[1] Baddeley A. Working memory: looking back and looking forward. Nat Rev Neurosci. 2003; 4(10):829–839

[2] Jasper HH. Report of the committee on methods of clinical examination in electroencephalography. Electroencephalogr Clin Neurophysiol. 1958; 10(2): 370–375

References

[1] Friedman MJ, Keane TM, Resick PA, Eds. Handbook of PTSD: Science and Practice. New York, NY: Guilford Press; 2015

[2] American Psychiatric Association. Diagnostic and Statistical Manual of Mental Disorders. 5th ed. Arlington, VA: American Psychiatric Publishing; 2013

[3] Wrocklage KM, Schweinsburg BC, Krystal JH, et al. Neuropsychological functioning in veterans with posttraumatic stress disorder: Associations with performance validity, comorbidities, and functional outcomes. J Int Neuropsychol Soc. 2016; 22(4):399–411

[4] Geuze E, Vermetten E, de Kloet CS, Hijman R, Westenberg HG. Neuropsychological performance is related to current social and occupational functioning in veterans with posttraumatic stress disorder. Depress Anxiety. 2009; 26(1):7–15

[5] Wechsler D. Wechsler Adult Intelligence Scale. 4th ed. San Antonio, TX: Pearson; 2008

[6] Beck AT, Steer RA, Brown GK. Manual for the Beck Depression Inventory-II. San Antonio, TX: Psychological Corporation; 1996

[7] The WHOQOL Group. Development of the World Health Organization WHOQOL-BREF quality of life assessment. Psychol Med. 1998; 28(3):551–558

[8] Fregni F, Boggio PS, Nitsche M, et al. Anodal transcranial direct current stimulation of prefrontal cortex enhances working memory. Exp Brain Res. 2005; 166(1):23–30

77 Management of Patients at End of Life

Joseph Murray

77.1 Introduction

The frail elder experiences physical decline and reduced capacity to adapt to stressors. Those stressors may include multiple disease processes, iatrogenic effects of pharmaceutical treatments for the medical problems as well as the intangible effects of isolation, loss of a spouse, exhaustion of caregivers, and difficulty in organizing and completing health care directives. In the elder with failure to thrive (FTT), the decline is frequently more dramatic than a single diagnosis and the synergy of stressors may lead to unexplained weight loss, malnutrition, and functional deficits.

77.2 Clinical History and Description

FH was a 90-year-old man with a history of heart disease, mild signs of Parkinson's disease (PD), hypothyroidism, gastroesophageal reflux disease, severe esophageal dysmotility, cervical spondylosis, and kyphosis. FH was in a normal state of health and living alone until 1 year ago when he was seen at the emergency department on several occasions related to falls at home resulting in chronic paraspinal and cervical muscular pain. Shortly thereafter, FH was admitted following a fall at his home. He was unable to right himself and was stationary for 2 days until a neighbor found him. He was admitted to a local hospital and underwent a short period of inpatient rehabilitation. Following discharge, FH moved in with his 88-year-old ex-wife who served as his primary caregiver. She had her own health concerns, including heart disease, chronic obstructive pulmonary disorder (COPD), and progressive dementia.

FH's pharmacological management included medications for heart disease and Sinemet for PD. Notably, he was prescribed opioids for chronic pain for the cervical spondylitis and new muscular and orthopedic pain from the recent fall. Several months following discharge, he was readmitted for dyspnea and suspected aspiration pneumonitis versus pneumonia following witnessed aspiration during an emesis event and subsequent difficulty handling oral secretions. He complained of increased pain and increasing dysphagia. He underwent an extensive evaluation including computed tomography of the neck, laryngoscopy, barium esophagram, esophagogastroduodenoscopy, and modified barium swallow (MBS). He was made NPO (nil per os, "nothing by mouth") and percutaneous endoscopic gastrostomy (PEG) feedings were initiated. He was discharged home after declining placement in a rehabilitation facility.

Two months later, he was readmitted following a fall. He was in severe pain related to the fall and pain management was challenging (▶ Fig. 77.1). Although he received enteral feeding at the designated rate and volume, he had lost weight (▶ Fig. 77.2). His symptoms related to PD had progressed with increased cogwheeling and rigidity. His Sinemet dose was increased, and he again declined rehabilitation placement and was discharged home. Several weeks later, his PEG tube became dislodged. He was admitted for replacement of the PEG and was severely dehydrated with moderate nutritional compromise thought to be related to chronic diarrhea. His tube feeding was adjusted and he was rehydrated following a short stay and was discharged home. A synopsis of the course of his workup is provided in ▶ Table 77.1.

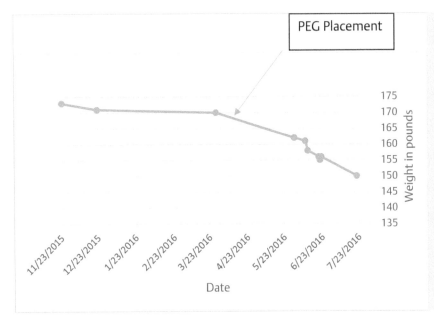

Fig. 77.1 Weight during period of decline.

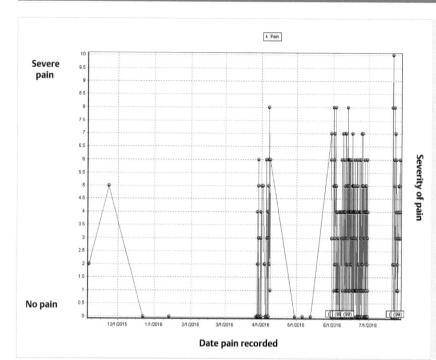

Fig. 77.2 Pain ratings recorded during period of decline.

Table 77.1 Testing and results

Testing	Result
Neck CT (3/28)	No evidence of acute fracture or cortical disruption Anterior osteophyte complex at C5–C6 Thickening of piriformis Recommend ENT evaluation
Laryngoscopy (3/28)	Visible stream of secretions being aspirated Does not cough or respond to the secretions in any way Distal pharyngeal soft-tissue fullness Placed gastroenterology consult
Gastroenterology EGD (3/29)	Grade B esophagitis Dilation with food in the entire esophagus No apparent structural outlet obstruction, lesions, or strictures Recommended barium esophagram
Barium esophagram (3/30)	Severely limited examination secondary to patient condition and kyphosis Severe aspiration of contrast Tertiary contractions and stasis of contrast with severe dysmotility Recommendation for dedicated speech pathology oropharyngeal exam
Clinical swallowing evaluation (3/31)	Speech/voice • Hypophonia with wet dysphonic quality • No festination of speech • No dysarthria Sensorimotor exam • Unable to produce volitional cough • Generalized weakness of oromotor systems • Sensory system normal • Increase in adventitious airway signs with ice chips/water sips • Recommend modified barium swallow to confirm findings
Modified barium swallow (3/31)	Confirmation of anterior cervical osteophytes at C5–C6 Generalized weakness of propulsive components of swallow Moderate/severe postswallow retention • All bolus textures midpharynx

Table 77.1 continued

Testing	Result
	• Without subsequent spontaneous clearing swallows Silent gross aspiration of all boluses greater than 2–3 mL in volume • Cued coughing ineffective in clearing aspirant Recommendation for short-term NPO status with enteral feeding until patient becomes more robust with reassessment for readiness to initiate safe oral feedings
Clinical swallowing evaluation (4/3)	Largely unchanged from previous assessment Patient lethargic and not requesting oral intake Recommend palliative care consult to evaluate goals of care Failing to thrive and in a state of terminal frailty Family meeting is called Patient is unable to participate in meeting due to somnolence Goals of care reviewed with family who decide that full code and all life-sustaining efforts be enacted in continued care for patient
EGD (4/4)	Externally removable PEG placement successfully completed
Clinical bedside exam (7–21)	Somnolent but awake and interactive Paucity of speech but requesting food and liquid Speech/voice • Grossly hypophonic with severe wet dysphonic quality • No festination of speech • No dysarthria Sensorimotor exam • Unable to produce volitional cough • Generalized weakness of oromotor systems • Sensory system normal Increase in adventitious airway signs with ice chips/water sips

CT, computed tomography; EGD, esophagogastroduodenoscopy; ENT, ear, nose, and tongue; NPO, nil per os, "nothing by mouth"; PEG, percutaneous endoscopic gastrostomy.

77.3 Questions and Answers for the Reader

1. PEG tube feeding in an adult with FTT is guaranteed to result in the following:
   a) Improved nutrition and hydration.
   b) Direct delivery of nutrients into the enteral system bypassing the oral route.
   c) Increase in weight.
   d) Pain and suffering on the part of the patient.

Answer: b is correct. Food and liquid are delivered via a tube into the stomach bypassing the oral cavity. Although aspiration of food and liquid may not occur, patients with enteral feeding tubes can still aspirate oropharyngeal secretions and/or aspirate refluxed materials. In some patients, including elders with dementia, enteral feeding is not protective for aspiration pneumonia, reduced length of hospital stay, or mortality.

a is incorrect. This response is sometimes true, but not guaranteed. Enteral feeding formulas may offer enough calories and nutrients, but may not be processed in the same way food is. Further, the anabolic systems that combine to convert nutrients into glucose may become aberrant in patients with certain diseases leading to catabolic processes where the body preferentially converts stored fats and muscle into glucose instead of nutrients that enter the alimentary system through the mouth or even a feeding tube.

c is incorrect. Some patients may gain weight. Some patients may lose weight as a result of diarrhea, which is a common side effect of nonoral feeding.

d is incorrect. Although some patients find nasogastric tube feeding and PEG placement unpleasant, others find that it is tolerable and preferred to the chronic discomfort associated with aspiration events and/or fatigue that may occur during meals in particularly weak patients.

2. In an adult patient, FTT is defined as:
   a) An expected functional outcome from a primary disease diagnosis such as lung cancer or diabetes.
   b) Progressive debility after common and reversible causes of frailty are detected and seemingly managed.
   c) A state of socioeconomic poverty with an inability to pay for expensive health care.
   d) A state of diminished health resulting from noncompliance with medical regimens.

Answer: b is correct. Frail elders frequently present with symptoms that are more severe than expected given existing, known disease and/or other health conditions. Typically, their symptoms are outsized and not fully explained following seemingly effective treatments.

a is incorrect. Typically, the decline of the patient and inability to recover from a reversible condition is out of line with the presentation of a single disease.

c is incorrect. Socioeconomic stressors can contribute to and amplify functional disability in a frail elder. It is not typically a singular cause of FTT.

d is incorrect. Even patients who are closely managed and monitored in modern health care systems can become frail and suffer from intractable decline in physical function.

3. Short-term tube feeding may result in improved outcomes for elderly subjects with acute but reversible health deficits.
   a) True
   b) False

Answer: a is correct. Some frail patients may "bounce back" after a short period of improved nutrition and rehabilitation. All efforts should be made to help the patient regain enough functional reserve to return to baseline. It is important to communicate that enteral feedings are reversible and to be sure that the patient and family are well informed regarding the intent of short-term enteral nutrition.

b is incorrect. Although some patient populations (i.e., demented elders) have been shown to have worse outcomes with enteral feeding, considerable evidence suggests that many patients do well with the associated improved nutrition.

4. Decision making at the end of life …:
   a) Can be guided by a well-constructed decision-making chart.
   b) Is based on the number of disease processes present and the degree of debility of the patient.
   c) Should be individually constructed and determined by the patient and family after an informed discussion.
   d) Should be left to the professional medical team.

Answer: c is correct. Sustaining autonomy and dignity at the end of life are essential.

a is incorrect. Each patient should be treated as an individual with unique value systems and requirements for sustaining dignity at the end of life. Some patients require complete autonomy and direction to sustain dignity at the end of life. Others may require the consensus of a family group. Principals in making decisions may demonstrate resolve to engage in complete life-sustaining treatment only to change their mind as they reflect further and integrate information and witness the burden of life-sustaining treatments.

b is incorrect. Projections of the timing and nature of death are difficult to predict.

d is incorrect. Medical professionals should guide an informed patient through treatment options and to deliver those treatments and procedures in a way that sustains dignity.

77.4 Description of Disorder and Recommended Treatment

MBS revealed generalized weakness of the propulsive components of the swallow resulting in retention of the bolus in the pharynx (i.e., postswallow residue). An anterior cervical osteophyte complex obstructed bolus transit with reduced pharyngeal clearance. FH's generally inefficient pharyngeal stage, likely secondary to PD and the presence of cervical osteophytes, synergistically resulted in bolus retention. Both components were evident and perceived by FH, but were not clinically significant when he was stronger and possessed adequate functional muscle reserve. In that context, he maintained his weight and overall health. The immobility resulting from his recent fall, pain, and iatrogenic effect of reduced sensorium related to the opioid pain management likely contributed to reduced functional reserve and debility. Intervention in the form of enteral feeding was appropriate initially. Some patients regain the functional reserve necessary to sustain safe oral intake after a short bout of enteral feeding during acute illness. Other patients may continue to have trouble managing pain and/or may not be capable of undergoing aggressive rehabilitation. These patients may spiral into further loss of function and debility related to the acute stressor (i.e., the fall), the baseline effect of multiple comorbidities (i.e., a mild form of PD, cervical osteophytes, and COPD), and iatrogenic effects of pharmaceutical management for pain (i.e., reduction in sensorium and somnolence with immobility).

77.5 Outcome

FH was readmitted shortly thereafter with a urinary tract infection, dyspnea, and suspected pneumonia. Although previously ambulating with a walker, he was now nonambulatory at home. His caregiver reported that she was unable to assist in his activities of daily living. He was identified as failing to thrive. FH was somnolent, but when awake and interactive, he requested oral intake at times and the family wished to comply with this request. A clinical bedside examination of swallowing was performed with identical findings from previous visits. The issue of pleasure feeds was initiated by the speech pathologist, which led to further discussion with the palliative care team regarding goals of care. A family meeting ensued and FH was subsequently admitted to a hospice care center where he expired surrounded by family shortly after admission.

77.6 Key Points

- Multiple, mild comorbidities and polypharmacy following an unrelated acute event, such as a fall, may result in a functional profile that is marked by greater impairment than would be expected.
- Patients and families may not agree when to initiate end-of-life care. The care team should be sensitive to these unique perspectives and allow patients and families to make informed choices.
- Enteral feeding may have a favorable short-term effect in some patients and allow for recovery of strength to allow for rehabilitation.
- Some patients may acquire aspiration pneumonia even when NPO and receiving enteral feeding secondary to aspiration of oropharyngeal secretions or aspiration of tube feeding secondary to dysmotility or reflux.

Suggested Readings

[1] Abraham RR, Girotra M, Wei JY, Azhar G. Is short-term percutaneous endoscopic gastrostomy tube placement beneficial in acutely ill cognitively intact elderly patients? A proposed decision-making algorithm. Geriatr Gerontol Int. 2015; 15(5):572–578

[2] Hwang TL, Lue MC, Nee YJ, Jan YY, Chen MF. The incidence of diarrhea in patients with hypoalbuminemia due to acute or chronic malnutrition during enteral feeding. Am J Gastroenterol. 1994; 89(3):376–378

[3] Periyakoil VS. Frailty as a terminal illness. Am Fam Physician. 2013; 88(6): 363–368

78 Augmentative and Alternative Communication for a Client with Broca's Aphasia

Amber Thiessen

78.1 Introduction

This case history focuses on the process of implementing augmentative and alternative communication (AAC) intervention for improved functional communication and life participation for EB, a woman with aphasia. Many people with aphasia experience chronic language deficits that affect their life participation. Often, these individuals benefit from the use of AAC supports, including speech-generating devices, low-technology communication books and boards, and various techniques and strategies to maximize their communication.

78.2 Clinical History and Description

EB was a 68-year-old woman who suffered left hemisphere cerebrovascular accident resulting in Broca's aphasia. Approximately 10 months ago, EB was admitted to a local hospital presenting with right-sided weakness and difficulty speaking. Computed tomography scan revealed an ischemic stroke in the left middle cerebral artery. EB received appropriate medical treatment and was later evaluated to determine the extent of her deficits. Assessment revealed symptoms consistent with Broca's aphasia, including the production of short, agrammatic utterances and difficulty with written expression. Her expressive language was significantly more affected than her receptive language. In addition, EB presented with right-sided hemiplegia resulting in an inability to use her right arm and difficulty ambulating.

EB received inpatient therapy for 8 weeks focused on improved language expression and physical functioning. During this time, she regained function in her right leg; however, her language deficits and hemiparesis of her right arm persisted. She then transitioned back to her home with her husband, a retired teacher. Prior to her stroke, EB was an active member of her community. She regularly attended social outings with her friends and enjoyed spending time with her two adult children and her grandchildren. Since returning home, EB had become increasingly isolated. She spent most of her time at home, but expressed a desire to return to her previous hobbies and social schedule. As such, EB began receiving outpatient speech therapy to address her ongoing communication deficits and participation limitations.

78.3 Clinical Testing

EB underwent a comprehensive assessment including the Aphasia Quotient portion of the Western Aphasia Battery-Revised[1] to determine the severity and type of aphasia. EB achieved a 48.2 with characteristics consistent with her diagnosis of Broca's aphasia. In addition to formal testing, informal assessment was performed to determine which modes of communication EB spontaneously utilized to communicate. EB relied most on verbal production; however, facial expressions and gestures including referential pointing were also observed. EB did not spontaneously attempt to draw to express herself, and when prompted to do so, she was reluctant. Additional informal assessments were completed to examine EB's literacy skills and ability to recognize objects depicted in images. EB recognized sight words with 85% accuracy during a picture–word matching test; however, she demonstrated more difficulty when attempting to write common words (e.g., lamp, table).

EB and her husband were also interviewed to better understand her communication needs and the support network currently in place. Specific information gathered included important topics of conversation, hobbies and interests, and social roles (e.g., parent, spouse, friend). In addition, EB and her husband were questioned about the people with which she communicated and the environments in which she frequented before and after her stroke as well as communication situations that were most challenging since the stroke.

78.4 Questions and Answers for the Reader

1. What type of AAC intervention would be most appropriate for EB?
   a) Unaided AAC strategies only.
   b) Low-technology AAC supports only.
   c) High-technology AAC supports only.
   d) A combination of unaided and high- and low-technology AAC supports.
   e) EB is not an appropriate candidate for AAC intervention.

Answer: d is correct. Like most people, EB communicates in a variety of settings about a range of topics with communication partners ranging from strangers to family members. Creating an intervention plan that incorporates various aided and unaided AAC techniques and supports will allow her to meet her diverse communication needs more effectively. For example, for individuals who are more familiar with EB's communication style, unaided strategies paired with existing speech may be effective; however, for people who are less familiar with EB, aided forms of AAC including high- and low-technology supports may be necessary. Having several options available will allow EB to choose the most effective strategy to express herself in a variety of situations.

a is incorrect. Unaided AAC strategies include gestures, facial expressions, and other methods of communication that do not require external supports. Although unaided AAC methods would benefit EB, this technique alone will be insufficient to meet her needs.

b is incorrect. Low-technology AAC supports include communication books and boards and other nonelectronic communication aids. Although low-technology supports would be beneficial for EB, solely using these supports would not be sufficient to meet EB's diverse communication needs.

c is incorrect. High-technology AAC supports, also referred to as speech-generating devices, are electronic devices that produce synthesized speech output. The benefits of using high-technology supports are numerous; however, there are times when they may not be the most efficient or effective choice. For example, EB may be able to produce a gesture or use a low-technology communication book more effectively in certain instances than finding that information in a high-technology AAC system. Having several options available will allow EB to use the most effective communication strategy for each situation.

e is incorrect. EB still has some preserved natural speech; however, she frequently experiences communication breakdowns that limit her ability to participate in everyday activities. Because she cannot meet her functional communication needs through natural speech alone, EB is a candidate for AAC intervention to augment her existing communication capabilities.

2. When is it appropriate to implement AAC strategies for someone with aphasia?
   a) Early in the recovery process.
   b) Six months after stroke.
   c) One year after stroke.
   d) When the client asks for it.
   e) It is never appropriate.

Answer: a is correct. AAC intervention is designed to support the immediate and future needs of individuals with complex communication disorders such as aphasia. As such, AAC should not be considered a treatment of last resort. Instead, supports should be identified early in the treatment process and should be modified as the individual makes gains in therapy.

b and c are incorrect. Speech therapy for aphasia can be broadly divided into restorative and compensatory treatment approaches. The goal of restorative intervention is to reduce the language impairment experienced by a person with aphasia by restoring their level of functioning as closely to their prestroke state as possible. The goal of compensatory intervention is to compensate for the language deficits experienced by people with aphasia. AAC is a compensatory treatment designed to allow people to participate functionally in situations and environments that require communication. It is essential that clinicians focus both on restoring lost function and compensating for current and future deficits to improve their clients' function and to give them a way to communicate with their language deficits.

d is incorrect. Clinicians should consider their client's wishes; however, many clients are not aware that AAC is an option. Hence, it is essential that clinicians provide their clients with any and all appropriate treatment options to maximize recovery and well-being.

e is incorrect. AAC intervention is appropriate for any client who cannot meet his/her functional communication needs through natural speech. For those with residual capabilities, AAC can be used to augment current communication, and for those with very little speech communication, AAC can be used as an alternative communication method.

3. Why is it beneficial to have a family member or close friend involved in the assessment and treatment process for someone with aphasia?
   a) So they can be provided information about the vocabulary and communication needs of the person with aphasia.
   b) So they can learn how to modify their own communication style to more effectively communicate with the person with aphasia.
   c) So they can learn how to maintain the AAC supports used by the person with aphasia.
   d) All of the above.
   e) They should not be part of the assessment and treatment process.

Answer: d is correct. Family members and close friends play a critical and often multifaceted role in supporting the communication of people with aphasia. They have intimate knowledge of vocabulary needs and can serve as informants regarding communication needs. Family members and friends also provide the day-to-day support necessary for AAC system maintenance. In addition to these roles, family members and close friends need to learn how to modify their own communication style to ensure that the person with aphasia comprehends their messages.

a is partially correct. The family members and friends of people with aphasia can act as communication informants by describing potential topics and environments/situations in which the person with aphasia needs to be able to communicate. However, their role is not limited to providing this type of information, so this answer is only partially correct.

b is partially correct. Many people with aphasia experience deficits in receptive language. As such, communication partners often must modify their own communication style to ensure that the person with aphasia can comprehend their messages. This requires training. Clinicians must provide family and friends with training on ways to augment their communication (e.g., writing key words, lowering speaking rate). Providing augmented input is only one reason why family and friends should participate in the assessment and treatment process; therefore, this answer is only partially correct.

c is partially correct. Formal therapy time is limited for most people with aphasia. Hence, family members and friends often are called upon to provide the support necessary to maintain AAC systems (e.g., adding/removing photos and content, technical maintenance). Clinicians must train family members and friends to assume this role, and being active participants in the therapy process can be beneficial. Although AAC system maintenance is an important function served by family and friends, it is not their only role, so this answer is only partially correct.

e is incorrect. The input of family members and friends is important for assessment and treatment planning. Their input can be beneficial when designing AAC support, and they might be needed to assist in system maintenance once formal therapy has ended.

78.5 Description of Problem and Recommended Treatment

EB presented with characteristics consistent with Broca's aphasia. She had received prior therapy focused on restoring language expression abilities; however, little improvement was observed from this intervention. Given her desire to return to social routines, the decision was made to implement AAC supports to compensate for her language deficits. Recognizing the benefits of a multimodal communication approach, an appropriate high-technology AAC device was identified and EB was also trained on other communication strategies including communicative drawing and the use of gestures and facial expressions to increase communicative effectiveness.

EB trialed three high-technology devices during communication activities in therapy sessions to determine the most effective device to address her communication needs. The clinician observed EB using these devices. After using each device, EB and her husband provided input on their strengths and weaknesses. This information was taken into consideration, and a final device was ordered for EB. The selected device was a lightweight tablet that EB found easy to carry given her continued issues with hemiparesis. In addition, the device allowed EB to take photos and import them as communication supports.

78.6 Outcome

Upon receiving her AAC device, EB and her husband attended 12 therapy sessions over the course of 6 weeks focused on programming and functional use of the device. As recommended by the clinician, EB and her husband identified two key times of the day during which they felt that communication was an obstacle and that they had time to devote to incorporating AAC. It was during these specific times that they were instructed to practice using AAC and to document any challenges that arose from those interactions. They then met with the clinician to discuss the documented challenges and to develop appropriate strategies to improve their interactions. After approximately 3 weeks of gradual implementation of the AAC system and receiving feedback from the clinician, EB and her husband began to report increased communication success. Further treatment was provided to increase the time they spent focused on AAC implementation. Recognizing that EB would need consistent ongoing support with her AAC system, the clinician also provided EB's husband and adult daughter with training on programming the device and assisting her with communication breakdowns.

After discharging from therapy, EB began attending individual and group therapy at a local university clinic focused on the use of the camera in device to document her day for future communication interactions and on improved verbal and written expression abilities. Although retesting using the WAB-R indicated minimal improvement, EB and her husband reported that she had returned to some of her former social routines. She began to attend a weekly lunch with old friends and started to go to church again. EB's children reported that she is more engaged and appears happier than she was before she began outpatient therapy. She particularly enjoys attending group therapy, and although she still gets frustrated with communication challenges, she remained hopeful of continued improvement and increased independence.

78.7 Key Points

- Although restorative therapy is essential for individuals with aphasia, it is imperative that clinicians also identify effective compensatory communication methods. EB's initial therapy focused solely on improved expression, but she was unable to meet her communication needs. Effective AAC supports should be a focus of treatment early in recovery along with restorative interventions.
- It is essential to assess the unique needs of each client with aphasia to design the most effective AAC systems possible. A needs assessment must address communication partners, frequent environments, important topics, and hobbies.
- People who rely on AAC often benefit from the support of a facilitator for programming and maintenance of AAC systems and for assistance when interacting with less familiar communication partners. As such, clinicians should consider identifying a facilitator for clients who rely on AAC.

Suggested Reading

[1] Simmons-Mackie N, King JM, Beukelman DR, Eds. Supporting Communication for Adults with Acute and Chronic Aphasia. Baltimore, MD: Brookes; 2013

Reference

[1] Kertesz A. Western Aphasia Battery-Revised (WAB-R). San Antonio, TX: Pearson; 2006

79 Utilization of Self-Help Activities for an Adult Who Stutters

Mitchell Trichon, Annie Bradberry, and Shane Wilmoth

79.1 Introduction

Stuttering has often been defined by the overt features that can be heard or seen when speaking. To many people who stutter (PWS), such definitions ignore some aspects that affect quality of life, such as negative thoughts and feelings associated with speech or the decision not to speak to avoid stuttering. Such negative feelings can include helplessness, shame, fear, embarrassment, frustration, and loneliness.[1,2] The impact of stuttering is far-reaching and can impact a person's personality, education, relationships, and career.[2,3] Connecting PWS through self-help activities can lessen the negative impact stuttering can have by providing positive experiences, which can be beneficial in improving quality of life. Self-help activities are an underutilized resource for many people with communication disorders. However, more PWS are seeking these activities as they are increasingly accessible through self-help organizations (e.g., National Stuttering Association and Friends – The National Association of Young People Who Stutter) and Internet-based options such as Facebook groups and video-conferencing communities (e.g., Stutter Social). In addition, evidence now suggests that participation in such activities is helpful to PWS.[4,5,6,7]

79.2 Clinical History and Description

DR was a 41-year-old male who stuttered; he self-referred for therapy following an increase in stuttering. He attributed the increase in disfluency to increased stress at work as a result of a job change requiring more verbal communication with teenagers. DR reported that he had stuttered since age 5 and had a grandfather who reportedly outgrew his stuttering as a child. DR received therapy from elementary school through high school. He reported that, during early elementary school, he and his clinician worked on using a metronome and tapping his

hand to his leg to control his speech rate. He found both to be ineffective at improving fluency and attributes them as contributing factors to his secondary behaviors. He also reported using filler words to avoid or delay stuttering. In his early 20 s, he attended a university clinic where he learned fluency-shaping skills, including easy onsets and pausing/phrasing to improve his fluency. He found that the easy onsets helped him to communicate more easily until he returned home from college when he discontinued regular use of these skills.

79.3 Clinical Testing

The initial evaluation took place at a university clinic. Oral peripheral examination was within normal limits and hearing screening revealed normal responses to pure tone screening at 20 dB at 500 Hz, 1,000 Hz, 2,000 Hz, and 4,000 Hz in both ears. DR reported increased difficulty talking under time pressure, with smaller groups, and on the telephone. He reported that stuttering interfered with work and social relationships, but had little impact on family relationships. DR also reported that he lacked self-confidence, and often felt lonely, anxious, and frustrated. He described positive experiences with previous therapy and was interested in participating in a support group.

The Stuttering Severity Instrument-Fourth Edition (SSI-4)[8] was administered to assess the severity of overt features of stuttering (i.e., frequency, duration, physical concomitants). DR's overall score was a 42, which corresponded to a "very severe" fluency disorder, as shown in ▶ Table 79.1, based on a reading and speaking task, both with over 300 syllables.

The Overall Assessment of the Speaker's Experience of Stuttering-Adult Version (OASES-A)[9] was also administered to evaluate four different aspects of DR's perception of observable stuttering behaviors, his reactions to stuttering, challenges with communication in daily situations, and how stuttering interfered with quality of life. The 100-item questionnaire includes questions on a 5-point scale, with 5 meaning the most severe negative impact of stuttering. DR's scores of each section and the total are presented in ▶ Table 79.2.

Table 79.1 Stuttering Severity Instrument-Fourth Edition (SSI-4) results

SSI-4 categories	Data	Task score
Frequency	Percentage of stuttered syllables—reading 10%; speaking 17%	15
Duration	5.7 seconds average of longest three	12
Physical concomitants	High pitch during prolongation, throat clearing, open mouth articulatory posture, eye twitching, reduced eye contact, head turning, laryngeal tension, limb movements	15
Total		42

Table 79.2 Overall Assessment of the Speaker's Experience of Stuttering (Adults) (OASES-A) results

Section	Impact score	Impact rating
I—General information	3.33	Moderate/severe
II—Your reaction to stuttering	3.31	Moderate/severe
III—Communication in daily situations	3.22	Moderate/severe
IV—Quality of life	2.90	Moderate
Total	3.19	Moderate/severe

An informal fluency probe was also conducted to determine which fluency-enhancing behaviors were optimal for fluency-focused therapy. DR successfully implemented easy-onset phonation 10/10 times (100%) at both word and sentence levels with clinician modeling. DR was also able to use light articulatory contacts 10/12 times (83%) at both word and sentence levels with clinician modeling. DR had difficulty with pausing and phrasing during a reading task but successfully implemented reduced speech rate to increase his fluency.

DR was cooperative throughout the assessment. He expressed motivation to gain more control of his stuttering and expressed an interest in revisiting strategies he previously had success with, including easy onsets and light articulatory contacts. He was also open to other recommendations.

79.4 Questions and Answers for the Reader

1. Why is it important to assess the client's perceptions and attitudes about their stuttering and communication, in addition to the severity of the observable features of stuttering?
   a) Severity of observable features of stuttering are not a good indicator of how stuttering impacts a client's daily life.
   b) Client perceptions and attitudes of their stuttering and communication may provide valuable information that can guide therapy and help address specific challenging situations.
   c) Client perceptions and attitudes help the clinician to understand how the client experiences their stutter, instead of how others experience the client's stuttering.
   d) All of the above.

Answer: d is correct. The observable severity of a person's stutter often does not correlate with how stuttering impacts their life. For example, someone who may be good at avoiding stuttering may be severely impacted by their stuttering. As stated in b, assessing the client's perceptions and attitude about their stuttering can give the clinician valuable information about what to do in therapy. As stated in c, it provides insight into the client's thoughts and feelings about their stuttering and provides a potential way to discuss feelings and attitudes with clients when reviewing the assessment with them.

a, b, and c by themselves are incorrect. They leave out the other correct answers.

2. Which of the following benefits is least likely to occur by participating in a self-help activity for PWS (with verbal communication)?
   a) Receive training in the mechanics of particular speech skills.
   b) Learn about others' experiences of using various speech skills.
   c) Have a supportive forum to potentially practice speech skills that they learned in therapy.
   d) Receive exposure to various views and ideas about stuttering and being a person who stutters.

Answer: a is correct. A person who participates in a self-help activity is not likely to receive training in the mechanics of speech skills. This may be a topic of discussion but speech training is usually discouraged by self-help activity leaders. If speech training is involved in such a forum by a licensed professional, then it should be labeled as a therapy group.

b is incorrect. PWS often discuss their experiences of current or past therapies or speech skills that were used. This is especially true when someone is asking questions about using a particular approach or speech skill.

c is incorrect. Many PWS use verbal self-help activities as a supportive environment in which they can practice or use speech skills or a therapy approach that they have previously learned.

d is incorrect. One of the benefits of participating in self-help activities for PWS is learning about how PWS have different attitudes and ideas about stuttering and being a PWS. This often results in giving clients more options related to their stuttering and related feedback about how others manage challenging situations.

3. A client presents with severe stuttering (observable features). The client also reports that he avoids verbal communication because of the shame and embarrassment associated with stuttering. Which of the following statements is least likely to be a possible successful therapy outcome for this client?
   a) Reduced number of moments of stuttering (frequency) inside and outside of the clinic.
   b) Reduced amount of physical struggle when stuttering (duration of moments of stuttering/secondary characteristics), but has not necessarily reduced frequency of stuttering outside of the clinic.
   c) Increased everyday conversation initiation with less fear of speaking, with no or minimal change in observable stuttering severity.
   d) Increased fluent speech in the clinic by using speech skills, but chooses not to use speech skills outside of the clinic because of self-reported unnatural sounding speech.
   e) Increased fluent speech in the clinic by using speech skills, but chooses not to use speech skills outside of the clinic because his new sense of self-acceptance and reduced stigma associated with stuttering.

Answer: d is correct. A client who has learned skills to speak more fluently but chooses not to use these skills due to his/her belief about the social acceptability of the technique (social validity) should not be considered as having achieved a successful therapy outcome since the learned speech skills will not result in improved verbal communication or reduction of stigma.

a is incorrect. A reduction of stuttering frequency that can be generalized to everyday communication and should be considered a successful therapy outcome.

b is incorrect. A reduction of the physical struggle, which includes shorter durations of moments of stuttering and reduction of secondary characteristics or physical concomitants of stuttering, should be considered a successful therapy outcome, even without a reduction of frequency of stuttering since it would result in improved verbal communication.

c is incorrect. An increase in everyday conversation initiation by someone who avoided conversation due to embarrassment should be considered a successful therapy outcome since it would result in increased verbal communication with less fear of stigmatization of stuttering.

e is incorrect. A client who has learned speech skills to speak more fluently who chooses not to use speech skills in everyday conversation because he feels more empowered and less stigmatized by his stuttering should be considered as having achieved a successful therapy outcome.

79.5 Description of Problem and Recommended Treatment

DR was a good candidate for therapy and was recommended to work with a speech-language pathologist once per week for 6 months before reevaluation. Since DR was motivated to gain more control of his stuttering and was stimulable for easy-onset and light articulatory contacts, it was important to include working on these skills as a component of treatment. DR also reported that he was fearful of speaking situations and often tried to avoid stuttering, which had negatively impacted aspects of his life.

DR expressed a willingness to meet with other PWS. He was given information about the National Stuttering Association (NSA) and their local chapter(s) and it was recommended that he look into connecting with the local chapter for support.

79.6 Outcome

DR attended therapy and reported that he did not benefit much because he was increasingly focused on becoming fluent instead of improving communication, including reduced struggle when stuttering, reduced fear, increased initiation of conversation, and increased fluency. Despite the original recommendation, DR did not pursue a self-help group, but after a year of treatment, DR found a website/organization called Stutter Social. The organization is an Internet-based community of PWS with voluntary hosts who guide supportive discussions through scheduled video conferences. DR became a regular weekly participant and integrated his experiences in the group and the topics they discussed into discussions within his on-campus therapy sessions.

In communicating with other PWS, DR learned about various self-help organizations, including the NSA and their supportive activities. After a year of learning about people's experiences with the NSA through Stutter Social, DR traveled to and participated in an annual NSA conference and reported it to be "life-changing." He attributed his self-acceptance of stuttering to his experiences of participating in these various self-help activities. During the next half year of treatment, DR became open to the idea of using the strategy "voluntary stuttering" in his speech as a way to stutter more easily. He had reported some success in using this technique as one of his strategic options. A year and a half after becoming involved with the self-help stuttering community, DR decided to terminate speech therapy services. Although DR's observable stuttering behavior remained severe, he reported a reduction of stigmatization of stuttering, which he attributed to the supportive relationships built through self-help organizations for PWS. DR also reported that he took com-

fort in knowing that he could go back to using his speech skills such as easy onsets and voluntary stuttering if he wished.

DR continued his regular attendance in Stutter Social's scheduled video-conference meetings. He also became more involved in the NSA by regularly attending regional and annual conferences and taking on leadership roles to help other PWS.

79.7 Key Points

- Participation in self-help activities for PWS has the potential to reduce stigma and improve quality of life, empowerment, and self-acceptance. Self-help activities are also a supportive forum to practice therapy techniques and conversational speech outside of the clinic and can assist with maintenance and transfer of therapy techniques to real-life situations.
- Depending on the therapy approach, some speech skills may require cognitive or attitudinal changes for the client to begin to use the new speech skill outside of the clinic and be generalized to everyday use. For example, empowerment and self-acceptance may be necessary to implement voluntary stuttering as a viable speech skill in everyday communication.
- Success in stuttering treatment can be defined in various ways, including reduced struggle of stuttering, increased fluency, reduced fear of speaking, and increased enjoyment of speaking.
- Self-acceptance of stuttering often reduces the negative feelings associated with stuttering and can support a drive to manage one's stuttering.

Suggested Reading

[1] Trichon M, Tetnowski J. Self-help conferences and change in the experience of stuttering: preliminary findings and implications for self-help activities. Paper presented at: Proceedings of the Tenth World Congress of the International Fluency Association, July 6–8, 2015; Lisbon, Portugal

References

[1] Corcoran JA, Stewart M. Stories of stuttering: A qualitative analysis of interview narratives. J Fluency Disord. 1998; 23(4):247–264

[2] Trichon M. Self-help Conferences for People Who Stutter: An Interpretive Phenomenological Analysis [dissertation]. Lafayette, LA: University of Louisiana at Lafayette; 2010

[3] Klompas M, Ross E. Life experiences of people who stutter, and the perceived impact of stuttering on quality of life: personal accounts of South African individuals. J Fluency Disord. 2004; 29(4):275–305

[4] Boyle MP. Psychological characteristics and perceptions of stuttering of adults who stutter with and without support group experience. J Fluency Disord. 2013; 38(4):368–381

[5] Raj EX, Daniels DE. Psychosocial support for adults who stutter: Exploring the role of online communities. Speech Lang Hear. 2017; 20(3):144–153

[6] Trichon M, Raj EX. Peer-support for people who stutter: history, benefits, and accessibility. In: Amster BJ, Klein E, Eds. More than Fluency: The Social, Emotional, and Cognitive Dimensions of Stuttering. San Diego, CA: Plural Publishing; 2018:187–214

[7] Trichon M, Tetnowski J. Self-help conferences for people who stutter: a qualitative investigation. J Fluency Disord. 2011; 36(4):290–295

[8] Riley GD. Stuttering Severity Instrument. 4th ed. Austin, TX: Pro-Ed; 2009

[9] Yaruss JS, Quesal RW. OASES-A: Overall Assessment of the Speaker's Experience of Stuttering (Adults). McKinney, TX: Stuttering Therapy Resources 2016

80 Targeting Social Communication Skills for an Adult Client with Autism Spectrum Disorder

Jarrod B. Zinser

80.1 Introduction

Deficits in social communication skills are a hallmark of autism spectrum disorders (ASDs) (DSM-5, 2013). This case provides a framework to address social communication deficits in a young adult with ASD.

80.2 Clinical History and Description

TB was a 25-year-old male college student diagnosed with ASD in 2012 at a local behavioral health clinic after being admitted for attempted suicide. He cited a "difficult home life" as well as an inability to establish lasting connections with his peers (specifically females) as catalysts to this attempt. TB initially sought improved understanding of his diagnosis and skills to better interact with others, both socially and professionally. He reported difficulties maintaining various jobs, as well as dating. TB reported no previous speech-language treatment; he denied speech, language, or hearing difficulties in his family. TB lived at home with both parents, hoping to move out postgraduation. At the time of his initial evaluation, he was a junior at Florida State University, majoring in criminology. He was a member of the university's marching band and was also a client of Vocational Rehabilitation Services.

80.3 Clinical Testing

TB was evaluated at a university speech and hearing clinic to assess his pragmatic language skills, formally and informally. TB was compliant throughout testing, completing each task without complaint. He produced minimal to no emotion during formal and informal measures and his eye gaze rarely deviated from the treatment room table.

Both hearing screening and oral mechanism exams were unremarkable. TB then participated in a conversational exchange/sample. He avoided eye contact upon greeting, lacked a greeting upon arrival, and often responded with brief or limited information. Because TB produced brief responses, conversational probes were utilized (see ▶ Table 80.1). The Comprehensive Assessment of Spoken Language (CASL; Carrow-Woolfolk, 1999)-Book Three was administered to assess TB's supralinguistic and pragmatic language skills. He completed the following four subtests: Nonliteral Language, Meaning from Context, Ambiguous Sentences, and Pragmatic Judgment. TB's standard score for each subtest fell two standard deviations below the mean (100), indicating below-average performance. Nonverbal intelligence was also assessed to rule out cognitive deficits that impact his ability to interact with others. Using the Test of Nonverbal Intelligence, Fourth Edition (TONI-4; Brown, Sherbenou, Johnsen, 2010),

Table 80.1 Probes for eliciting conversational behavior in adults

"Tell me about the type of job you want."
"Where do you see yourself in five years?"
"What types of music do you listen to? Why is that your favorite?"
"What genres of movies do you like? Tell me about it."
"Tell me about your hobbies. How do you spend your down time?"
"Are you currently dating? Is that one of your personal goals?"
"Tell me about your friends. What do you do together? How often did you see each other?"

TB achieved a standard of 90, a low-average score. The Making Inferences subtest of the Social Language Development Test - Adolescent (SLDT-A; Bowers, Huisingh, LoGiudice, 2010) was also administered informally to assess TB's ability to detect nonverbal and context clues in a picture of a person or people, assume the perspective of a specific person in the picture, infer what the person is thinking, express the person's thought as a relevant, direct quotation, and state the visual clue that suggests what the person is thinking using an "I" statement. TB received a score of 0 out of 10 possible points, indicating a weakness in this area. Speech, voice, and fluency were all subjectively judged to be within normal limits.

80.4 Questions and Answers for the Reader

1. Why is assessing narrative skills imperative for those diagnosed with ASD?
   a) The ability to understand and produce a narrative monologue is an important aspect of typical pragmatic development.
   b) To obtain a mean length of utterance (MLU).
   c) To assess literacy skills.

Answer: a is correct. A cohesive narrative is required for effective conversational exchanges.

b is incorrect. Collecting MLU is inappropriate. It is typically used with children to measure language proficiency.

c is incorrect. Assessing TB's reading and writing skills will not provide information regarding his communicative interactions with others.

2. Based on the information reported earlier, what is the best treatment approach to use with this TB?
   a) Improve narrative skills.
   b) Improve discourse management skills.
   c) Improve communicative intent.
   d) a and b.
   e) All of the above.

Answer: d is correct. See explanations in a and b below.

a is partially correct. Testing revealed deficits in narrative production. Much of communication requires being able to tell a story.

b is partially correct. Informal measures revealed weak conversation skills. Thus, discourse management must be targeted for this client to meet his goals of forming relationships and improved job retention.

c is incorrect. Communicative intent is typically targeted in young children with ASD.

e is incorrect. a and b are the most appropriate skills to target.

3. Why would an observational rating scale be useful in this type of case?
   a) It is a norm-referenced method.
   b) Observational rating scales can be used to evaluate conversational or narrative skills.
   c) It is a way to measure your own interactions with the client.

Answer: b is correct. Observational rating scales can help identify areas of disordered behavior.

a is incorrect. Typically, norms for these instruments are not provided. Their purpose is not to compare to typical development.

c is incorrect. Observational rating scales are typically client-centered.

4. What would be considered a negative prognostic indicator in TB's case?
   a) Client motivation.
   b) Current level of cognitive functioning.
   c) Severity of disorder.

Answer: c is correct. Autism is defined as an impairment in social communication and interaction.

a is incorrect. TB was highly motivated to improve his communication skills.

b is incorrect. TB did not display any cognitive deficits that may contribute to his communication difficulties. His nonverbal intelligence score was considered average.

80.5 Description of Problem and Recommended Treatment

TB presented with a severe impairment in pragmatic language skills characterized by deficits in making inferences, understanding nonliteral language, gathering meaning from context, responding appropriately to various social scenarios, and understanding ambiguous statements. Treatment was recommended twice a week for 1-hour sessions. TB's program specifically targeted his ability to produce a cohesive narrative (see ▶ Table 80.2 for suggested scoring rubric) as well as the social use of language in conversation, including correctly interpreting supralinguistic aspects of communication. Improved job interview skills and the use of appropriate language in the workplace were also recommended. Participation in an adult social skills group was also discussed. Prognosis for improvement of these skills was judged to be guarded; however, positive prognostic indicators included TB's willingness to participate in treatment, as well as his motivation to improve these skills.

Table 80.2 Scoring rubrics for narratives

Weak: Narrative consists of descriptions and poorly organized, uninteresting stories.
Adequate: Stories take one of four forms:
a) An account of events without a high point or climax.
b) A minimal narrative without elaboration.
c) A story without a resolution.
d) A confusing narrative with some strong descriptive elements.
Good: Narratives are captivating stories that contain problems and resolutions, but they may contain organizational weaknesses.
Strong: Narratives are easily understood and contain clear, integrated story lines; elaboration; interesting word choices; and some captivating features, such as a climax or plot twist or compelling personal voice.

Adapted from Paul R, Norbury C. Language Disorders from Infancy to Adolescence. 4th ed. St. Louis, MO: Elsevier Mosby; 2012:444.

80.6 Outcome

TB spent a total of four consecutive semesters in treatment. He made progress across goals targeting facial expression identification and rationale, identifying appropriate interview behaviors, and improved awareness of nonverbal communication behaviors in multiple partners. However, TB continued to demonstrate difficulties managing his role throughout conversational exchanges. He was often rated as overly talkative, producing out-of-sync content, confusing accounts, topic perseveration, providing insufficient background information, inadequate clarification, and scripted/stereotyped sentences/discourse. TB's intonation was judged to be unusual and his eye gaze rarely assisted his communicative attempts.

Across the targeted goals, TB displayed weaknesses demonstrating reciprocity in conversational exchanges, generalizing nonliteral concepts, and initiating greetings with familiar and unfamiliar partners. Cueing was often required to assist with goal completion. Repetitions, providing binary choices, and modeling proved to be the most effective.

Throughout treatment, TB required operational definitions regarding friendship (e.g., acquaintance vs. best friend) and dating. The PEERS (Program for the Education and Enrichment of Relational Skills) curriculum was then introduced to assist TB in making and maintaining relationships. He did not readily accept these skills based on previous failed relationships and, thus, cognitive behavior therapy was recommended to identify and address dysfunctional thoughts about interacting with others that may be inhibiting progress. TB had weekly appointments at the university counseling center. Treatment was discontinued at the request of the client once he obtained a full-time job.

80.7 Key Points

- New diagnostic criteria for ASD were provided by the Diagnostic and Statistical Manual of Mental Health Disorders-Fifth Edition (DSM-5).
- Know the difference between the diagnostic criteria for autism and social (pragmatic) communication disorder.
- For treatment, rating forms must be developed to track and measure progress regarding conversation skills. Landa et al.'s pragmatic rating scale is incredibly useful.[1]

- Homework should include real-world applications. Clients should rate their use of pragmatic skills targeted in treatment.

Suggested Readings

[1] McPartland JC, Klin A, Volkmar FR. Asperger Syndrome. 2nd ed. New York, NY: Guilford Press; 2014

References

[1] Landa R, Piven J, Wzorek MM, Gayle JO, Chase GA, Folstein SE. Social language use in parents of autistic individuals. Psychol Med. 1992; 22(1):245–254

[2] Gantman A, Kapp SK, Orenski K, Laugeson EA. Social skills training for young adults with high-functioning autism spectrum disorders: a randomized controlled pilot study. J Autism Dev Disord. 2012; 42(6):1094–1103

Index

Note: Page numbers set **bold** or *italic* indicate headings or figures, respectively.